T0210916

Lecture Notes in Computer Science 9003

Commenced Publication in 1973
Founding and Former Series Editors:
Gerhard Goos, Juris Hartmanis, and Jan van Leeuwen

Editorial Board

David Hutchison
  Lancaster University, Lancaster, UK
Takeo Kanade
  Carnegie Mellon University, Pittsburgh, PA, USA
Josef Kittler
  University of Surrey, Guildford, UK
Jon M. Kleinberg
  Cornell University, Ithaca, NY, USA
Friedemann Mattern
  ETH Zurich, Zürich, Switzerland
John C. Mitchell
  Stanford University, Stanford, CA, USA
Moni Naor
  Weizmann Institute of Science, Rehovot, Israel
C. Pandu Rangan
  Indian Institute of Technology, Madras, India
Bernhard Steffen
  TU Dortmund University, Dortmund, Germany
Demetri Terzopoulos
  University of California, Los Angeles, CA, USA
Doug Tygar
  University of California, Berkeley, CA, USA
Gerhard Weikum
  Max Planck Institute for Informatics, Saarbrücken, Germany

More information about this series at http://www.springer.com/series/7412

Daniel Cremers · Ian Reid
Hideo Saito · Ming-Hsuan Yang (Eds.)

Computer Vision – ACCV 2014

12th Asian Conference on Computer Vision
Singapore, Singapore, November 1–5, 2014
Revised Selected Papers, Part I

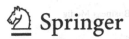 Springer

Editors
Daniel Cremers
Technische Universität München
Garching
Germany

Ian Reid
University of Adelaide
Adelaide, SA
Australia

Hideo Saito
Keio University
Yokohama, Kanagawa
Japan

Ming-Hsuan Yang
University of California at Merced
Merced, CA
USA

Videos to this book can be accessed at
http://www.springerimages.com/videos/978-3-319-16864-7

ISSN 0302-9743   ISSN 1611-3349   (electronic)
Lecture Notes in Computer Science
ISBN 978-3-319-16864-7   ISBN 978-3-319-16865-4   (eBook)
DOI 10.1007/978-3-319-16865-4

Library of Congress Control Number: 2015934895

LNCS Sublibrary: SL6 – Image Processing, Computer Vision, Pattern Recognition, and Graphics

Springer Cham Heidelberg New York Dordrecht London
© Springer International Publishing Switzerland 2015
This work is subject to copyright. All rights are reserved by the Publisher, whether the whole or part of the material is concerned, specifically the rights of translation, reprinting, reuse of illustrations, recitation, broadcasting, reproduction on microfilms or in any other physical way, and transmission or information storage and retrieval, electronic adaptation, computer software, or by similar or dissimilar methodology now known or hereafter developed.
The use of general descriptive names, registered names, trademarks, service marks, etc. in this publication does not imply, even in the absence of a specific statement, that such names are exempt from the relevant protective laws and regulations and therefore free for general use.
The publisher, the authors and the editors are safe to assume that the advice and information in this book are believed to be true and accurate at the date of publication. Neither the publisher nor the authors or the editors give a warranty, express or implied, with respect to the material contained herein or for any errors or omissions that may have been made.

Printed on acid-free paper

Springer International Publishing AG Switzerland is part of Springer Science+Business Media
(www.springer.com)

Preface

ACCV 2014 received a total of 814 submissions, a reflection of the growing strength of Computer Vision in Asia. We note, particularly, that a number of Area Chairs commented very positively on the overall quality of the submissions. The conference had submissions from all continents (except Antarctica, a challenge for the 2016 organizers perhaps) with 64 % Asia, 20 % from Europe, and 10 % from North America.

The Program Chairs assembled a geographically diverse team of 36 Area Chairs who handled between 20 and 30 papers each. Area Chairs recommended reviewers for papers, and each paper received at least three reviews from the 638 reviewers who participated in the process. Paper decisions were finalized at an Area Chair meeting held in Singapore in September 2014. At this meeting, Area Chairs worked in triples to reach collective decisions about acceptance, and in panels of 12 to decide on the oral/poster distinction. The total number of papers accepted was 227, an overall acceptance rate of 28 %. Of these, 32 were selected for oral presentation.

We extend our immense gratitude to the Area Chairs and Reviewers for their generous participation in the process – the conference would not be possible if it were not for this huge voluntary investment of time and effort. We acknowledge particularly the contribution of 35 reviewers designated as "Outstanding Reviewers" (see page 14 in this booklet for a full list) who were nominated by Area Chairs and Program Chairs for having provided a large number of helpful, high quality reviews.

The Program Chairs are also extremely grateful for the support, sage advice, and occasional good-natured prompting provided by the General Chairs. Each of them helped with matters that in other circumstances might have been left to the Program Chairs, so that it regularly felt as if we had a team of seven, not four Program Chairs. The PCs are very grateful for this.

Finally, we wish to thank the authors and delegates. Without their participation there would be no conference. The conference was graced with a uniformly high quality of presentations and posters, and we offer particular thanks to the three eminent keynote speakers, Stephane Mallat, Minoru Etoh, and Dieter Fox, who delivered outstanding talks.

Computer Vision in Asia is growing, and the quality of ACCV steadily climbing so that it is now, rightly, considered as one of the top conferences in the field. We look forward to future editions.

November 2014

Daniel Cremers
Ian Reid
Hideo Saito
Ming-Hsuan Yang

Organization

Organizing Committee

General Chairs

Michael S. Brown	National University of Singapore, Singapore
Tat-Jen Cham	Nanyang Technological University, Singapore
Yasuyuki Matsushita	Microsoft Research Asia, China

Program Chairs

Daniel Cremers	Technische Universität München, Germany
Ian Reid	University of Adelaide, Australia
Hideo Saito	Keio University, Japan
Ming-Hsuan Yang	University of California at Merced, USA

Organizing Chair

Teck Khim Ng	National University of Singapore, Singapore
Junsong Yuan	Nanyang Technological University, Singapore

Workshop Chairs

C.V. Jawahar	IIIT Hyderabad, India
Shiguang Shan	Institute of Computing Technology, Chinese Academy of Sciences, China

Demo Chairs

Bohyung Han	POSTECH, Korea
Koichi Kise	Osaka Prefecture University, Japan

Tutorial Chairs

Chu-Song Chen	Academia Sinica, Tawain
Brendan McCane	University of Otago, New Zealand

Publication Chairs

Terence Sim	National University of Singapore, Singapore
Jianxin Wu	Nanjing University, China

Industry Chairs

Hongcheng Wang	United Technologies Corporation, USA
Brian Price	Adobe, USA
Antonio Robles-Kelly	NITCA, Australia

Steering Committee

In-So Kweon	KAIST, Korea
Yasushi Yagi	Osaka University, Japan
Hongbin Zha	Peking University, China

Honorary Chair

Katsushi Ikeuchi	University of Tokyo, Japan

Area Chairs

Lourdes Agapito	Queen Mary University of London/University College London, UK
Thomas Brox	University of Freiburg, Germany
Tat-Jun Chin	University of Adelaide, Australia
Yung-Yu Chuang	National Taiwan University, Taiwan
Larry Davis	University of Maryland, USA
Yasutaka Furukawa	Washington University in St. Louis, USA
Bastian Goldluecke	University of Konstanz, Germany
Bohyung Han	POSTECH, Korea
Hiroshi Ishikawa	Waseda University, Japan
C.V. Jawahar	IIIT Hyderabad, India
Jana Kosecka	George Mason University, USA
David Kriegman	University of California, San Diego, USA
Shang-Hong Lai	National Tsing-Hua University, Taiwan
Ivan Laptev	Inria Rocquencourt, France
Kyoung Mu Lee	Seoul National University, Korea
Vincent Lepetit	École Polytechnique Fédérale de Lausanne, Switzerland
Jongwoo Lim	Hanyang University, Korea
Simon Lucey	CSIRO/University of Queensland, Australia
Ajmal Mian	University of Western Australia, Australia
Hajime Nagahara	Kyushu University, Japan
Ko Nishino	Drexel University, USA
Shmuel Peleg	The Hebrew University of Jerusalem, Israel
Imari Sato	National Institute of Informatics, Japan
Shin'ichi Satoh	National Institute of Informatics, Japan
Stefano Soatto	University of California, Los Angeles, USA
Jamie Shotton	Microsoft Research, UK
Ping Tan	Simon Fraser University, Canada
Lorenzo Torresani	Dartmouth College, USA
Manik Varma	Microsoft Research, India
Xiaogang Wang	Chinese University of Hong Kong, China
Shuicheng Yan	National University of Singapore, Singapore
Qing-Xiong Yang	City University of Hong Kong, Hong Kong
Jingyi Yu	University of Delaware, USA

Junsong Yuan   Nanyang Technological University, Singapore
Hongbin Zha   Peking University, China
Lei Zhang   Hong Kong Polytechnic University, Hong Kong,
                    China

Program Committee Members

Catherine Achard	Xun Cao	Jen-Hui Cheng
Hanno Ackermann	Gustavo Carneiro	Liang-Tien Chia
Haizhou Ai	Joao Carreira	Chen-Kuo Chiang
Emre Akbas	Umberto Castellani	Shao-Yi Chien
Naveed Akhtar	Carlos Castillo	Minsu Cho
Karteek Alahari	Turgay Celik	Nam Ik Cho
Mitsuru Ambai	Antoni Chan	Jonghyun Choi
Dragomir Anguelov	Kap Luk Chan	Wongun Choi
Yasuo Ariki	Kwok-Ping Chan	Mario Christoudias
Chetan Arora	Bhabatosh Chanda	Wen-Sheng Chu
Shai Avidan	Manmohan Chandraker	Albert C.S. Chung
Alper Ayvaci	Sharat Chandran	Pan Chunhong
Venkatesh Babu	Hong Chang	Arridhana Ciptadi
Xiang Bai	Kuang-Yu Chang	Javier Civera
Vinceth Balasubramanian	Che-Han Chang	Carlo Colombo
Jonathan Balzer	Vincent Charvillat	Yang Cong
Atsuhiko Banno	Santanu Chaudhury	Sanderson Conrad
Yufang Dao	Yi-Ling Chen	Olliver Cossairt
Adrian Barbu	Yi-Lei Chen	Marco Cristani
Nick Barnes	Jieying Chen	Beleznai Csaba
John Bastian	Yen-Lin Chen	Jinshi Cui
Abdessamad Ben Hamza	Kuan-Wen Chen	Fabio Cuzzolin
Chiraz BenAbdelkader	Chia-Ping Chen	Jeremiah D. Deng
Moshe Ben-Ezra	Yi-Ting Chen	Alessio Del Bue
AndrewTeoh Beng-Jin	Tsuhan Chen	Fatih Demirci
Benjamin Berkels	Xiangyu Chen	Xiaoming Deng
Jinbo Bi	Xiaowu Chen	Joachim Denzler
Alberto Del Bimbo	Haifeng Chen	Anthony Dick
Horst Bischof	Hwann-Tzong Chen	Julia Diebold
Konstantinos Blekas	Bing-Yu Chen	Thomas Diego
Adrian Bors	Chu-Song Chen	Csaba Domokos
Nizar Bouguila	Qiang Chen	Qiulei Dong
Edmond Boyer	Jie Chen	Gianfranco Doretto
Steve Branson	Jiun-Hung Chen	Ralf Dragon
Hilton Bristow	MingMing Cheng	Bruce Draper
Asad Butt	Hong Cheng	Tran Du
Ricardo Cabral	Shyi-Chyi Cheng	Lixin Duan
Cesar Cadena	Yuan Cheng	Kun Duan
Francesco Camastra	Wen-Huang Cheng	Fuqing Duan

Zoran Duric
Michael Eckmann
Hazim Ekenel
Naoko Enami
Jakob Engel
Anders Eriksson
Francisco Escolano
Virginia Estellers
Wen-Pinn Fang
Micha Feigin
Jiashi Feng
Francesc Ferri
Katerina Fragkiadaki
Chi-Wing Fu
Yun Fu
Chiou-Shann Fuh
Hironobu Fujiyoshi
Giorgio Fumera
Takuya Funatomi
Juergen Gall
Yongsheng Gao
Ravi Garg
Arkadiusz Gertych
Bernard Ghanem
Guy Godin
Roland Goecke
Vladimir Golkov
Yunchao Gong
Stephen Gould
Josechu Guerrero
Richard Guest
Yanwen Guo
Dong Guo
Huimin Guo
Vu Hai
Lin Hai-Ting
Peter Hall
Onur Hamsici
Tony Han
Hu Han
Zhou Hao
Kenji Hara
Tatsuya Harada
Mehrtash Harandi
Jean-Bernard Hayet
Ran He

Shengfeng He
Shinsaku Hiura
Jeffrey Ho
Christopher Hollitt
Hyunki Hong
Ki Sang Hong
Seunghoon Hong
Takahiro Horiuchi
Timothy Hospedales
Kazuhiro Hotta
Chiou-Ting Candy Hsu
Min-Chun Hu
Zhe Hu
Kai-Lung Hua
Gang Hua
Chunsheng Hua
Chun-Rong Huang
Fay Huang
Kaiqi Huang
Peter Huang
Jia-Bin Huang
Xinyu Huang
Yi-Ping Hung
Mohamed Hussein
Cong Phuoc Huynh
Du Huynh
Sung Ju Hwang
Naoyuki Ichimura
Ichiro Ide
Yoshihisa Ijiri
Sei Ikeda
Nazli Ikizler-Cinbis
Atsushi Imiya
Kohei Inoue
Yani Ioannou
Catalin Ionescu
Go Irie
Rui Ishiyama
Yoshio Iwai
Yumi Iwashita
Arpit Jain
Hueihan Jhuang
Yangqing Jia
Yunde Jia
Kui Jia
Yu-Gang Jiang

Shuqiang Jiang
Xiaoyi Jiang
Jun Jiang
Kang-Hyun Jo
Matjaz Jogan
Manjunath Joshi
Frederic Jurie
Ioannis Kakadiaris
Amit Kale
Prem Kalra
George Kamberov
Kenichi Kanatani
Atul Kanaujla
Mohan Kankanhalli
Abou-Moustafa Karim
Zoltan Kato
Harish Katti
Hiroshi Kawasaki
Christian Kerl
Sang Keun Lee
Aditya Khosla
Hansung Kim
Kyungnam Kim
Seon Joo Kim
Byungsoo Kim
Akisato Kimura
Koichi Kise
Yasuyo Kita
Itaru Kitahara
Reinhard Klette
Georges Koepfler
Iasonas Kokkinos
Kazuaki Kondo
Xiangfei Kong
Sotiris Kotsiantis
Junghyun Kown
Arjan Kuijper
Shiro Kumano
Kashino Kunio
Yoshinori Kuno
Cheng-hao Kuo
Suha Kwak
Iljung Kwak
Junseok Kwon
Alexander Ladikos
Hamid Laga

Antony Lam
Francois Lauze
Duy-Dinh Le
Guee Sang Lee
Jae-Ho Lee
Chan-Su Lee
Yong Jae Lee
Bocchi Leonardo
Marius Leordeanu
Matt Leotta
Wee-Kheng Leow
Bruno Lepri
Frederic Lerasle
Fuxin Li
Hongdong Li
Rui Li
Jia Li
Yufeng Li
Yongmin Li
Yung-Hui Li
Cheng Li
Xin Li
Peihua Li
Xirong Li
Annan Li
Xi Li
Chia-Kai Liang
Shu Liao
T. Warren Liao
Jenn-Jier Lien
Joseph Lim
Ser-Nam Lim
Huei-Yung Lin
Haiting Lin
Weiyao Lin
Wen-Chieh (Steve) Lin
Yen-Yu Lin
RueiSung Lin
Yuanqing Lin
Yen-Liang Lin
Haibin Ling
Hairong Liu
Cheng-Lin Liu
Qingzhong Liu
Miaomiao Liu
Jingchen Liu
Ligang Liu

Haowei Liu
Guangcan Liu
Feng Liu
Shuang Liu
Shuaicheng Liu
Xiaobai Liu
Si Liu
Lingqiao Liu
Chen Change Loy
Feng Lu
Tong Lu
Zhaojin Lu
Le Lu
Huchuan Lu
Ping Luo
Lui Luoqi
Ludovic Macaire
Arif Mahmood
Robert Maier
Yasushi Makihara
Koji Makita
Yoshitsugu Manabe
Rok Mandeljc
Al Mansur
Gian-Luca Marcialis
Stephen Marsland
Takeshi Masuda
Thomas Mauthner
Stephen Maybank
Chris McCool
Xing Mei
Jason Meltzer
David Michael
Anton Milan
Gregor Miller
Dongbo Min
Ikuhisa Mitsugami
Anurag Mittal
Daisuke Miyazaki
Henning Müller
Thomas Moellenhoff
Pascal Monasse
Greg Mori
Bryan Morse
Yadong Mu
Yasuhiro Mukaigawa
Jayanta Mukhopadhyay

Vittorio Murino
Atsushi Nakazawa
Myra Nam
Anoop Namboodiri
Liangliang Nan
Loris Nanni
P.J. Narayanan
Shawn Newsam
Thanh Ngo
Bingbing Ni
Jifeng Ning
Masashi Nishiyama
Mark Nixon
Shohei Nobuhara
Vincent Nozick
Tom O'Donnell
Takeshi Oishi
Takahiro Okabe
Ryuzo Okada
Takayuki Okatani
Gustavo Olague
Martin Oswald
Wanli Ouyang
Yuji Oyamada
Paul Sakrapee
  Paisitkriangkrai
Kalman Palagyi
Hailang Pan
Gang Pan
Sharath Pankanti
Hsing-Kuo Pao
Hyun Soo Park
Jong-Il Park
Ioannis Patras
Nick Pears
Helio Pedrini
Pieter Peers
Yigang Peng
Bo Peng
David Penman
Janez Pers
Wong Ya Ping
Hamed Pirsiavash
Robert Pless
Dilip Prasad
Dipti Prasad Mukherjee
Andrea Prati

Vittal Premachandran
Brian Price
Oriol Pujol Pujol
Pulak Purkait
Zhen Qian
Xueyin Qin
Bogdan Raducanu
Luis Rafael Canali
Visvanathan Ramesh
Ananth Ranganathan
Nalini Ratha
Edel Garcia Reyes
Hamid Rezatofighi
Christian Riess
Antonio Robles-Kelly
Mikel Rodriguez
Olaf Ronneberger
Guy Rosman
Arun Ross
Amit Roy Chowdhury
Xiang Ruan
Raif Rustamov
Fereshteh Sadeghi
Satoshi Saga
Ryusuke Sagawa
Fumihiko Sakaue
Mathieu Salzmann
Jorge Sanchez
Nong Sang
Pramod Sankar
Angel Sappa
Michel Sarkis
Tomokazu Sato
Yoichi Sato
Jun Sato
Harpreet Sawhney
Walter Scheirer
Bernt Schiele
Frank Schmidt
Dirk Schnieders
William Schwartz
McCloskey Scott
Faisal Shafait
Shishir Shah
Shiguang Shan
Li Shen

Chunhua Shen
Xiaohui Shen
Shuhan Shen
Sanketh Shetty
Boxin Shi
YiChang Shih
Huang-Chia Shih
Atsushi Shimada
Nobutaka Shimada
Ilan Shimshoni
Koichi Shinoda
Abhinav Shrivastava
Xianbiao Shu
Gautam Singh
Sudipta Sinha
Eric Sommerlade
Andy Song
Li Song
Yibing Song
Mohamed Souiai
Richard Souvenir
Frank Steinbruecker
Ramanathan Subramanian
Yusuke Sugano
Akihiro Sugimoto
Yasushi Sumi
Yajie Sun
Weidong Sun
Xiaolu Sun
Deqing Sun
Min Sun
Ju Sun
Jian Sun
Ganesh Sundaramoorthi
Jinli Suo
Rahul Swaminathan
Yuichi Taguchi
Yu-Wing Tai
Taketomi Takafumi
Jun Takamatsu
Hugues Talbot
Toru Tamaki
Xiaoyang Tan
Robby Tan
Masayuki Tanaka
Jinhui Tang

Ming Tang
Kevin Tang
João Manuel R.S. Tavares
Mutsuhiro Terauchi
Ali Thabet
Eno Toeppe
Matt Toews
Yan Tong
Akihiko Torii
Yu-Po Tsai
Yi-Hsuan Tsai
Matt Turek
Seiichi Uchida
Hideaki Uchiyama
Toshio Ueshiba
Norimichi Ukita
Julien Valentin
Pascal Vasseur
Ashok Veeraraphavan
Matthias Vestner
Xiaoyu Wang
Dong Wang
Ruiping Wang
Sheng-Jyh Wang
Shenlong Wang
Lei Wang
Song Wang
Xianwang Wang
Yang Wang
Yunhong Wang
Yu-Chiang Frank Wang
Hanzi Wang
Hongcheng Wang
Chaohui Wang
Chen Wang
Cheng Wang
Changhu Wang
Li-Yi Wei
Longyin Wen
Gordon Wetzstein
Paul Wohlhart
Chee Sun Won
Kwan-Yee
  Kenneth Wong
John Wright
Jianxin Wu

Xiao Wu	Jimei Yang	Cha Zhang
Yi Wu	Chih-Yuan Yang	Hong Hui Zhang
Xiaomeng Wu	Bangpeng Yao	Hui Zhang
Rolf Wurtz	Jong Chul Ye	Guofeng Zhang
Tao Xiang	Mao Ye	Xiao-Wei Zhao
Yu Xiang	Sai Kit Yeung	Rui Zhao
Yang Xiao	Kwang Moo Yi	Gangqiang Zhao
Ning Xu	Alper Yilmaz	Shuai Zheng
Li Xu	Zhaozheng Yin	Yinqiang Zheng
Changsheng Xu	Xianghua Ying	Zhonglong Zheng
Jianru Xue	Ryo Yonetani	Weishi Zheng
Mei Xue	Ju Hong Yoon	Wenming Zheng
Yasushi Yagi	Kuk-Jin Yoon	Lu Zheng
Koichiro Yamaguchi	Lap Fai Yu	Baojiang Zhong
Kota Yamaguchi	Gang Yu	Lin Zhong
Osamu Yamaguchi	Xenophon Zabulis	Bolei Zhou
Toshihiko Yamasaki	John Zelek	Jun Zhou
Takayoshi Yamashita	Zheng-Jun Zha	Feng Zhou
Pingkun Yan	De-Chuan Zhan	Feng Zhu
Keiji Yanai	Kaihua Zhang	Ning Zhu
Jie Yang	Tianzhu Zhang	Pengfei Zhu
Ruigang Yang	Yu Zhang	Cai-Zhi Zhu
Ming Yang	Zhong Zhang	Zhigang Zhu
Hao Yang	Yinda Zhang	Andrew Ziegler
Meng Yang	Xiaoqin Zhang	Danping Zou
Xiaokang Yang	Liqing Zhang	Wangmeng Zuo
Yi Yang	Xiaobo Zhang	
Yongliang Yang	Changshui Zhang	

Best Paper Award Committee

James Rehg	Georgia Institute of Technology, USA
Horst Bischof	Graz University of Technology, Austria
Kyoung Mu Lee	Seoul National University, South Korea

Best Paper Awards

1. Saburo Tsuji Best Paper Award

A Message Passing Algorithm for MRF inference with Unknown Graphs and Its Applications
Zhenhua Wang (University of Adelaide), Zhiyi Zhang (Northwest A&F University), Geng Nan (Northwest A&F University)

2. Sang Uk Lee Best Student Paper Award [Sponsored by Nvidia]

Separation of Reflection Components by Sparse Non-negative Matrix Factorization
Yasuhiro Akashi (Tohoku University), Takayuki Okatani (Tohoku University)

3. Songde Ma Best Application Paper Award [Sponsored by NICTA]

Stereo Fusion using a Refractive Medium on a Binocular Base
Seung-Hwan Baek (KAIST), Min H. Kim (KAIST)

4. Best Paper Honorable Mention

Singly-Bordered Block-Diagonal Form for Minimal Problem Solvers
Zuzana Kukelova (Czech Technical University, Microsoft Research Cambridge),
Martin Bujnak (Capturing Reality), Jan Heller (Czech Technical University),
Tomas Pajdla (Czech Technical University)

5. Best Student Paper Honorable Mention [Sponsored by Nvidia]

On Multiple Image Group Cosegmentation
Fanman Meng (University of Electronic Science and Technology of China),
Jianfei Cai (Nanyang Technological University), Hongliang Li
(University of Electronic Science and Technology of China)

6. Best Application Paper Honorable Mention [Sponsored by NICTA]

Massive City-scale Surface Condition Analysis using Ground and Aerial Imagery
Ken Sakurada (Tohoku University), Takayuki Okatani (Tohoku Univervisty),
Kris Kitani (Carnegie Mellon University)

ACCV 2014 – Outstanding Reviewers

Emre Akbas	Catalin Ionescu	Bernt Schiele
Jonathan Balzer	Suha Kwak	Chunhua Shen
Steve Branson	Junseok Kwon	Sudipta Sinha
Sanderson Conrad	Fuxin Li	Deqing Sun
Marco Cristani	Chen-Change Loy	Yuichi Taguchi
Alessio Del Bue	Scott McCloskey	Toru Tamaki
Anthony Dick	Xing Mei	Dong Wang
Bruce Draper	Yasushi Makihara	Yu-Chiang Frank Wang
Katerina Fragkiadaki	Guy Rosman	Paul Wohlhart
Tatsuya Harada	Mathieu Salzmann	John Wright
Mehrtash Harandi	Pramod Sankar	Bangpeng Yao
Nazli Ikizler-Cinbis	Walter Scheirer	

ACCV 2014 Sponsors

Platnium   Singapore Tourism Board

Gold   Omron
            Nvidia
            Garena
            Samsung

Silver   Adobe
            ViSenze

Bronze   Lee Foundation
            Morpx
            Microsoft Research
            NICTA

Contents – Part I

Recognition

Deep Representations to Model User 'Likes'

Sharath Chandra Guntuku[1]([✉]), Joey Tianyi Zhou[1],
Sujoy Roy[2], Lin Weisi[1], and Ivor W. Tsang[3]

[1] School of Computer Engineering, Nanyang Technological University,
Singapore, Singapore
sharathc001@e.ntu.edu.sg, wslin@ntu.edu.sg
[2] Institute for Infocomm Research, Singapore, Singapore
sujoy@i2r.a-star.edu.sg
[3] QCIS, University of Technology, Sydney, Australia
ivor.tsang@uts.edu.au

Abstract. Automatically understanding and modeling a user's liking for an image is a challenging problem. This is because the relationship between the images features (even semantic ones extracted by existing tools, viz. faces, objects etc.) and users' 'likes' is non-linear, influenced by several subtle factors. This work presents a deep bi-modal knowledge representation of images based on their visual content and associated tags (text). A mapping step between the different levels of visual and textual representations allows for the transfer of semantic knowledge between the two modalities. It also includes feature selection before learning deep representation to identify the important features for a user to like an image. Then the proposed representation is shown to be effective in learning a model of users image 'likes' based on a collection of images 'liked' by him. On a collection of images 'liked' by users (from Flickr) the proposed deep representation is shown to better state-of-art low-level features used for modeling user 'likes' by around 15–20 %.

1 Introduction

This work investigates the answer to the question - "Why did a user like an image?". If there was only one image and we had no clue about the user, it would be a very hard question to answer. But, given a collection of images that the user has 'liked', it should be possible to model the user's taste and infer more on - "What 'kind' of images the user 'likes'?". Based on this knowledge, images that the user has not seen and may probably 'like' can be recommended. Conversely, given an image and a set of users, we should be able to predict the user(s) who will 'like' the image.

The notion of 'like' is very subjective and subtle, and hence hard to describe by methods or processes. This makes the process of modeling user's taste hard. If we know a set of pictures that a user has 'liked', then computationally we can consider several factors that can contribute towards the user liking the images, namely, the affective factors,the objects in the image and their perspectives/poses, the setting of the image, colors or no colors, the context of the

---

These authors 'S.C. Guntuku and J.T. Zhou' contributed equally.

© Springer International Publishing Switzerland 2015
D. Cremers et al. (Eds.): ACCV 2014, Part I, LNCS 9003, pp. 3–18, 2015.
DOI: 10.1007/978-3-319-16865-4_1

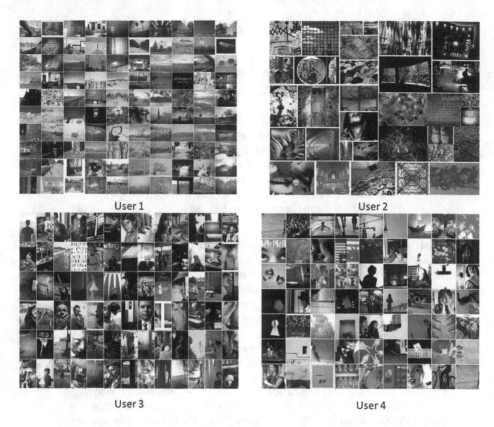

User 1   User 2

User 3   User 4

Fig. 1. Users have innate preferences which draw them to different 'kinds' of images.

image, etc., all of which induce the user to have some emotional connection with the image. The question this work investigates is "How do these factors influence the user's liking for an image?" For example, Fig. 1 shows the set of images liked by four different users. The difference between Users 1, 2 and 3, 4 is that while one group (Users 3 & 4) tends to like images with a lot of people and faces, the other group (Users 1 & 2) likes images without people. Even within Users 3 & 4 we can see that User 3 tends to like black and white images whereas User 4 tends to like color images. Similarly User 1 tends to like images which are spread out and natural whereas User 2 tends to like images with high clutter and which have some tinge of graphics in them.

While visual content does play a significant role in capturing the users' preferences, we note that tags associated with images often enhance the information conveyed by visual features or sometimes compliment them by conveying information about the image which visual features fail to convey [1]. Users tend to like an image because it is a place that they have visited before or because they relate to the person in the image or the scene in the image triggers a memory from their past and so on. This 'contextual' value associated with images is often captured by the tags associated with an image [2]. While tags primarily

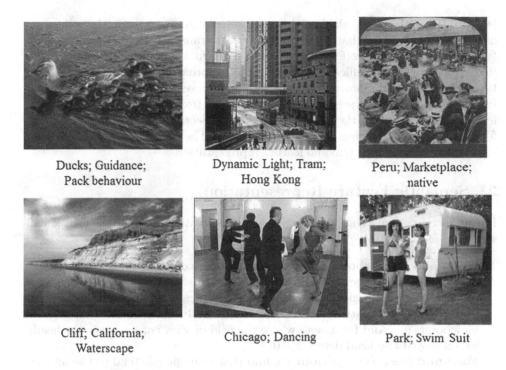

Ducks; Guidance; Pack behaviour	Dynamic Light; Tram; Hong Kong	Peru; Marketplace; native
Cliff; California; Waterscape	Chicago; Dancing	Park; Swim Suit

Fig. 2. Tags can show perspectives which Visual features can fail to convey.

convey the concepts in an image which visual detectors can be trained to detect (for example the objects in the image etc.), they many a time convey semantic concepts that go beyond what traditional visual detectors can be trained to detect. We can also attribute the varieties in 'likes' to the users psychophysical nature or personality. The role of personality in influencing preferences has been studied in several domains (viz. music [3,4], images [5,6]). However, in this work we are not trying to learn the users' personality. Rather we aim to learn deep representations for the image based on all the factors we can think of and how they combine to induce a user to 'like' the image (Fig. 2).

Difference from Deep Learning for Concepts Detection: The images we consider are accompanied with associated textual information (tags). Visual and textual information have been used in the computer vision literature to model contents for tasks like categorization, image search and so on. We wish to highlight that predicting 'likes' is different from visual concept detection as the supervisory information for modeling 'likes' is subtle and cannot be visually verified. Modeling such subtle response would intuitively involve a combination of several higher level semantic factors viz. context, affective and aesthetic. The goal is to look for mid-level representation that can help model user 'likes'.

Contributions: (1) Unlike [7], this work investigates the user 'like' modeling problem based on a larger collection of semantic, syntactic, aesthetic and contextual features. (2) A deep bimodal knowledge representation from the initial collection of features is proposed that allows for knowledge transfer between the modalities (visual and text). These features are used to learn a model for predicting user 'likes' for images. The efficacy of the proposed approach (usage of high-level features and the learning process of deep bimodal representations) is evaluated in an image recommendation scenario. Throughout the text, we use the phrase 'high-level features' to denote the features mentioned in Sect. 2 and the phrase 'low-level features' to denote the features mentioned in [7]. The proposed deep representation is denoted as 'deep bimodal feature representation'.

2   Semantic Feature Representation

In this section we give a short description and motivation for using the mentioned semantic features (Table 1).

1. **Head and Upperbody recognition:** Presence of people plays a significant role in the way images are perceived [8]. And most images have persons who are only partially visible. The field of view typically shows only their upper body. For this situation, we used an upper-body detector for near frontal viewpoints [9]. And for images where the field of view consists only the head, we employed the head detector [10].
2. **Face and Pose recognition:** We find that some people tend to like images where people are looking away from the camera, and others tend to like images where people are looking at the camera. We extracted the relative area of the bounding boxes returned by the algorithm [11], along with the pose angle to categorise a face as a profile/frontal face.
3. **Gender identification:** Images with people are found to be liked and commented upon heavily by members of the opposite gender [12]. Output from the face detection was used as input for the IntraFace [13] to enable it to detect distribution of gender in the images users liked.
4. **Scene Features:** What is in an image can be 'summarised' by its scene. We selected the PRICoLBP feature [14] which was shown to be effective for scene classification task.
5. **Computer Graphics image:** With the advancement of computer graphics, very attractive images can be rendered, which capture the attention of people. Flickr even has groups [15] where computer graphics images are exclusively posted and discussed about. At the same time there are users who like natural images. They can be distinguished using geometry features [16].
6. **Saliency: threshold count:** Saliency gives a possible point of attention of a viewer. We find that saliency also gives an idea of the scale of the image. Zoomed-in images usually have spread out saliency, which tells that there is nothing explicit in the image grabbing the attention of the user. This is also the case with images which have a scenic backdrop. But iconic images or images with clear objects show sharp saliency spikes. To capture if users like iconic images or otherwise, we used saliency [17] to compute the average number of maximal intensity points in an image relative to a threshold.

7. **Black and white vs. color image:** People who like black & white images are believed to be attracted by the focus, subtlety of tones and versatility in those images [18–20].
8. **Visual Clutter:** People characterized by anxious and tense behavior tend to have different tastes when compared with people with peaceful and easygoing outlook. To capture this cue, we use visual clutter which can be a good descriptor to measure the busy-ness of an image.
   It can also be used as an alternative to the number of objects in the scene as the latter is difficult to measure for natural scenes. We used the feature congestion measure [21] for measuring clutter.
9. **Tags:** We construct a dictionary of tags (with an average of 9.1 tags per image). We removed some stop words like camera names ('kodak', 'fujifilm', 'canon' etc.), lens characteristics ('70 mm', 'eos' etc.), and 'generic' words like 'image' and 'photo', just having a single letter ('a–Z') or number ('0–9'). The tag feature matrix is binary and sparse unlike the visual feature matrix. We then apply sparse SVD to convert the sparse tags feature matrix into a compressed representation (refer [2]).

Table 1. List of features (with newly added features on the right-hand column)

List of features used	
Color: avg. intensity of RGB	**Head and upperbody recognition**
#Edges: Canny edge detection	**Face and pose recognition**
Texture index	**Gender identification**
Regions: using mean shift segmentation algorithm	**Scene classification**
#Objects: using deformable parts models	**Computer graphics vs. Natural image**
#Number of faces: using Voila Jones detector	**Saliency**
GIST descriptors	**Black & White vs. Color image**
	Visual clutter
Entropy	**Tags**

3   Proposed Approach

The framework for modeling user 'likes' is depicted in Fig. 3. This includes the design steps for bimodal deep knowledge representation and the process of training a model for predicting user 'likes'. There are two separate parts in this framework. (a) Identifying the features in the initial feature collection which influence a user the most in liking the image (Sect. 3.1). This gives us an idea of the features among the initial collection of features that would be considered relevant if we did not have mid-level representations. (b) Learning the deep bimodal representation of images (described in Sect. 3.2).

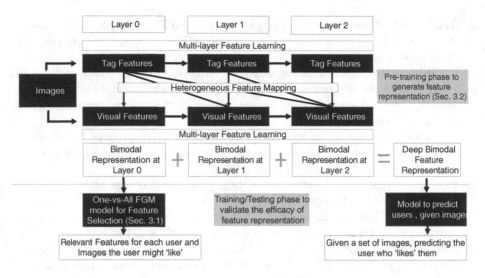

Fig. 3. Framework for modeling user 'likes'.

3.1 User-Specific Feature Selection

The features described in Sect. 2 are semantic concepts to represent an image. However it is not clear what influences a user to 'like' an image as intuitively, only a specific set of features might contribute for each user to like an image. Formally, the selection of most informative features for users can be expressed as solving a sparse SVM formulation as follows (similar to [22]):

$$\min_{\mathbf{d}} \min_{\mathbf{w}, \epsilon, \rho} \frac{1}{2}\|\mathbf{w}\|_2^2 + \frac{C}{2}\sum_{i=1}^n \epsilon_i^2 - \rho \tag{1}$$

$$s.t. \quad y_i \mathbf{w}^\top (\mathbf{x}_i \odot \mathbf{d}) \geq \rho - \epsilon_i, \tag{2}$$

where $\mathbf{d} \in \mathcal{D} = \{\|\mathbf{d}\|_0 \leq B, \mathbf{d}_j \in \{0,1\}\}$ and 1, 0 indicate that the feature is selected or not respectively. $\mathbf{x}$ denotes the feature vector, $\mathbf{w}$ denotes the weight vector, ρ is the bias, ϵ_i is the ith instances loss incurred by classifiers, B is the number of features to be selected and C is the trade-off parameter. Solving the above optimization is a NP-hard problem with lots of possible combinations of features. To reduce the computation cost, we adopt the Feature Generation Machine (FGM) [22] method to learn $\mathbf{d}$ and $\mathbf{w}$ simultaneously, which represent the index of selected features and their corresponding weight. For more details of solving this problem, please refer to [22].

3.2 Learning Deep Bimodal Feature Representation

Multi-view fusion has been widely studied in machine learning to improve performance of various tasks. [23–25]. Especially, several methods for fusing visual and textual information related to images have been proposed (e.g.: CCA [2]). These methods essentially find linear projections of two random vectors that are maximally correlated. While these approaches have been very successful in applications like image search and so on, it must be noted that mapping features to user 'likes' is by nature non-linear and hence such linear approaches could fail. Although kernel versions of such linear projection based methods exist (KCCA [26]), the time required to train (i.e., to compute the joint representations of two domains) scales poorly with training data size. We also note that while kernel methods are aimed at finding higher dimensional space where data can be linearly separable, the motivation of this problem necessitates finding better feature representations (which are not necessarily separable in higher dimensions).

Recently, there have also been works [27] which learn multimodal representations of images using deep learning methods. However, we use deep networks to learn multi-layer nonlinear representations of both tag and visual features individually. At every layer, we "translate" the features from tag domain into visual domain. We concatenate the visual features and the "translated" tag features at every layer and use this as the representation for every image. The entire process is described formally in Algorithm 1. The initial idea of feature translation is inspired from [28] where heterogenous feature mapping was done on text domain of different languages. However, our proposed method is different from [28] in two aspects:

- The algorithm in [28] is for heterogeneous transfer learning [29], while we focus on learning multimodal representations by augmenting features for classification.
- The deep structure in [28] learns feature representation in the same layer across domains, however we propose a new architecture for multi-modal representations shown in Fig. 4 based on the intuitions presented in Sect. 3.2. The translators learnt across layers are expected to aid in capturing more information about user likes, thereby increasing the model performance.

Multi-layer Homogeneous Feature Learning. Marginalized Stacked Denoising Autoencoders (mSDA) [30] are used to form a deep network wherein layerwise nonlinear transformations of the Visual and Textual features of an image are learned. We choose mSDA because of its advantages like faster training time and implementation simplicity, when compared to other forms of Autoencoders. The mid-level representations thus learned by the deep network are found to be very effective features for classification with SVMs [27,28].

In presenting the formulation, we follow the notations used in [30] for simplicity. We absorb a constant feature into the selected feature vector as $\mathbf{x}_V = [\mathbf{x}_V^\top \ 1]^\top$ or $\mathbf{x}_T = [\mathbf{x}_T^\top \ 1]^\top$, and incorporate a bias term $\mathbf{b}$ within the weight matrix as $\mathbf{W}_V = [\mathbf{W}_V \ \mathbf{b}_V]$. We further denote $\mathbf{X}_V$ as Visual Domain data, and $\mathbf{X}_V$ the union tag domain data.

Firstly, for the Visual Domain data, we apply mSDA on $\mathbf{X}_V$ to learn a weight matrix $\mathbf{W}_V \in \mathbb{R}^{(d_V+1) \times (d_V+1)}$ by minimizing the squared reconstruction loss as

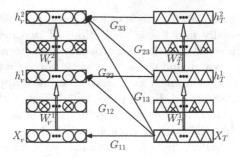

Fig. 4. Learning deep feature representation.

follows,

$$\sum_{i=1}^{m}\left\|\mathbf{X}_V - \mathbf{W}_V\mathbf{X}_V^{(i)}\right\|_F^2,\tag{3}$$

where $\mathbf{X}_V^{(i)}$ denotes the i-th corrupted version of $\mathbf{X}_V$. The solution to (3) depends on how the original features are corrupted which can be explicitly expressed as follows,

$$\mathbf{W}_V = \mathbf{P}\mathbf{Q}^{-1} \quad \text{with} \quad \mathbf{Q} = \widetilde{\mathbf{X}}_V\widetilde{\mathbf{X}}_V^\top \quad \text{and} \quad \mathbf{P} = \widehat{\mathbf{X}}_V\widetilde{\mathbf{X}}_V^\top,\tag{4}$$

where $\widehat{\mathbf{X}}_V = [\mathbf{X}_V\ \mathbf{X}_V\ \cdots\ \mathbf{X}_V]$ denotes the m-times repeated version of $\mathbf{X}_V$, and $\widetilde{\mathbf{X}}_V$ is the corrupted version of $\widehat{\mathbf{X}}_V$. In general, to alleviate bias in estimation, a large number of m over the training data with random corruptions are required, which is computationally expensive. To address this issue, mSDA introduces a corruption probability p to model infinite corruptions, i.e., $m \longrightarrow \infty$. Then a feature vector $\mathbf{q} = [1-p,\cdots,1-p,1]^\top \in \mathbb{R}^{d_V+1}$ is defined, where $\mathbf{q}_i$ represents the probability of a feature indexed by i "surviving" after the corruption. Thus, we can obtain the expectation of (3), and its solution can be written analytically as

$$\mathbf{W}_V = \mathbb{E}[\mathbf{P}]\mathbb{E}[\mathbf{Q}]^{-1},\tag{5}$$

where $\mathbb{E}[\mathbf{P}]_{ij} = \mathbf{S}_{ij}\mathbf{q}_j$, $\mathbf{S} = \mathbf{X}_V\mathbf{X}_V^\top$, and

$$\mathbb{E}[\mathbf{P}]_{ij} = \begin{cases} \mathbf{S}_{ij}\mathbf{q}_i\mathbf{q}_j, & \text{if } i \neq j, \\ \mathbf{S}_{ij}\mathbf{q}_i, & \text{otherwise.} \end{cases}\tag{6}$$

After $\mathbf{W}_V$ is learned, the nonlinearity of features is injected through the nonlinear encoder function $h(\cdot)$ that is learned together with the reconstruction weights $\mathbf{W}_V$, mSDA applies a nonlinear squashing-function, e.g., the hyperbolic tangent function $\tanh(\cdot)$, on the outputs of mSDA, $\mathbf{h}_V = \tanh(\mathbf{W}_V\mathbf{X}_V)$, to generate nonlinear features.

Cross-Layer Heterogeneous Feature Mapping. So far, in a specific layer k of feature learning, we have learned a pair of reconstruction weights $\mathbf{W}_V^k$ and $\mathbf{W}_T^k$, and higher-level feature representations $\mathbf{h}_V^k$ and $\mathbf{h}_T^k$ for the visual and tags domain data respectively (architecture shown in Fig. 4). By denoting $\mathbf{h}_V^k$ and $\mathbf{h}_T^j$ the layer k and layer j feature representations of the cross-domain corresponding instances in the visual and tag domains respectively, we now introduce how to learn a feature mapping across heterogeneous features $\mathbf{h}_V^k$ and $\mathbf{h}_T^j$.

Algorithm 1. Deep Heterogenous Feature Mapping.

Input: tag domain data $\mathbf{D}_T = \{\mathbf{x}_{T_i}\}_{i=1}^{n_1}$, visual domain data $\mathbf{D}_V = \{(\mathbf{x}_{V_i}, y_{V_i})\}_{i=1}^{n_2}$, a feature corruption probability p in mSDA, a trade-off parameter λ, and the number of layers K.

Initializations: $\mathbf{X}_V$, $\mathbf{X}_T$, $\mathbf{h}_V^1 = \mathbf{X}_V$, $\mathbf{h}_T^1 = \mathbf{X}_T$, and learn $\mathbf{G}_1$ by solving

$$\min_{\mathbf{G}_{1,1}} \|\mathbf{h}_V^1 - \mathbf{G}_{1,1}\mathbf{h}_{T,1}\|_F^2 + \lambda\|\mathbf{G}_{1,1}\|_F^2.$$

Run FGM to select relevant features
for $i = 2, ..., K$ **do**
    1: Apply mSDA on $\mathbf{h}_V^{i-1}$ and $\mathbf{h}_T^{i-1}$:

$$\{\mathbf{W}_V^i, \mathbf{h}_V^i\} = \text{mSDA}(\mathbf{h}_V^{i-1}, p),$$
$$\{\mathbf{W}_T^i, \mathbf{h}_T^i\} = \text{mSDA}(\mathbf{h}_T^{i-1}, p).$$

end for
for $j = 1, ..., K$ **do**
    for $k = j + 1, ..., K$ **do**
        2: Learn heterogeneous feature mapping $\mathbf{G}_{k,j}$:

$$\min_{\mathbf{G}_{k,j}} \|\mathbf{h}_V^k - \mathbf{G}_{k,j}\mathbf{h}_T^j\|_F^2 + \lambda\|\mathbf{G}_{k,j}\|_F^2.$$

    end for
end for
Do feature augmentation on visual domain data and mapped tag domain data

$$\mathbf{Z}_V = [\mathbf{h}_V^{k^\top} \cdots \mathbf{G}_{k,j}\mathbf{h}_T^{K^\top}]^\top,$$

and train a classifier f with $\{\mathbf{Z}_V, \mathbf{Y}_V\}$.
Output: f, $\{\mathbf{G}_{k,j}\}_{k,j=1}^K$, $\{\mathbf{W}_V^k\}_{k=2}^K$, and $\{\mathbf{W}_T^k\}_{k=2}^K$.

Specifically, from layer j of text domain to layer k of visual, we aim to learn a feature transformation $\mathbf{G}_{k,j} \in \mathbb{R}^{(d_V+1)\times(d_T+1)}$, where a bias term is incorporated by minimizing the following objective,

$$\|\mathbf{h}_V^k - \mathbf{G}_{k,j}\mathbf{h}_T^j\|_F^2 + \lambda\|\mathbf{G}_{k,j}\|_F^2, \tag{7}$$

where $\lambda > 0$ is a parameter of the regularization term on $\mathbf{G}_{k,j}$, which controls the tradeoff between the alignment of heterogeneous features and the complexity of $\mathbf{G}_{k,j}$. It can be shown that the optimization problem (7) has a closed form solution which can be written as follows,

$$\mathbf{G}_{k,j} = (\mathbf{h}_V^k {\mathbf{h}_T^j}^\top)({\mathbf{h}_T^j}{\mathbf{h}_T^j}^\top + \lambda\mathbf{I})^{-1}, \qquad (8)$$

where $\mathbf{I}$ is the identity matrix of the dimensionality $d_T + 1$.

We note that learning the feature mapping between a layer of tags and all the corresponding higher layers of visual features might probably capture the semantics of the image better than mapping between the same layers. For example, given a picture of sunset - tag associated with it might be 'sunset', whereas the visual features will depict the colors in the image like 'red', 'yellow' and low clutter in the image and so on. We can see that the tag features are in this case are at a higher level of semantics when compared to visual features, therefore making the mapping between this layer of tags and higher layers of visual features more meaningful.

4   Experiments

4.1   Dataset

For the experiments, from Flickr we crawled 200 images (and tags associated with each image) each marked as favorite by 20 random users (i.e., a total of 4000 images). For every image, we extract the features mentioned in Sect. 2 using default-parameters of the of the softwares provided by the cited works along with low-level features mentioned in [7].

4.2   Results and Analysis

We attempt to investigate the following questions in this section:

1. How do high-level features compare with low-level features in representing user 'likes'? Can we represent a user's 'likes' more efficiently with high-level visual features?
2. What features influence a user the most in 'liking' an image?
3. How well do the bimodal deep representations perform in modeling users' preferences when compared to individual modalities?

While the first two questions deal with the efficacy of using the proposed high-level features (without any deep learning involved) in representing user 'likes', the third question deals with the efficacy of using the learned bimodal deep representations in representing user 'likes'.

Comparing high-level features with low-level features: For answering the first question, we compare the performance of high-level features and low-level features in discriminating users' 'likes'. For each user, we divide the data (images) into training and test sets (with three splits (a) 25 %/75 % (b) 50 %/50 % and (c) 75 %/25 %) and build a one-vs-all user classification module using FGM

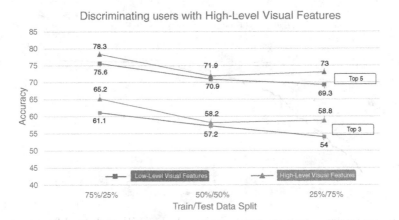

Fig. 5. High-level features require lesser amount of training data to capture users' preferences when compared to low-level features.

(described in Sect. 3.1). For each split we note the accuracy of user being correctly predicted for the test images (shown in Fig. 5). When low-level features are used, the model's performance varies based on the amount of training data, but when high-level features are used, the model performs well with less amount of training data. The reason for this can be ascertained to the amount of information the model is able to gather with each image based on the features. While low-level features would need a lot of examples to identify the patterns in users' preferences, this would not be required in case of high-level features.

Using the above one-vs-all models, we ranked the test images for each user based on the score given by the classifiers and we obtained the mean recall curves with high-level features and low-level features (shown in Fig. 6). For many users, the model also retrieves images in top-k which were not actually tagged as favorite by the user, but upon visual inspection we found that they had very similar characteristics to that of the images that the user tagged as favorite. These so-called 'false-positives' are expected because the user is not expected to have seen all the images that other users have tagged as favorite and therefore we cannot rule out the possibility that the user would like the image, provided the user sees it. As we know only the relevant images (user 'likes'), we use recall as the metric to measure the model's performance. For every user a total of 3800 images are provided as test images and within the images ranked as top 100, high-level features can retrieve about 30 % of the images 'liked' by the user while low-level features can retrieve only 15 %. Also high-level features are able to retrieve all the images 'liked' by the user around 15 % faster than low-level features. This again confirms the results shown in the previous experiment (in Fig. 5).

Features Relevant to each User: While conducting the above experiment, we also note the features selected by FGM to answer the second question. As mentioned in Sect. 1, we find that most users have preferences which can be

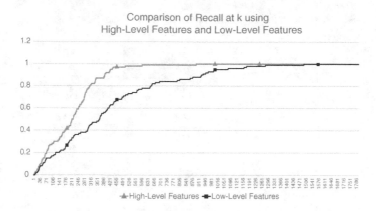

Fig. 6. Image retrieval performance to users is higher with high-level features than by using low-level features.

captured by high-level semantic features. The weights learnt, along with random images liked by three users, are depicted in Fig. 7.

We observe that User C likes images which have pictures with people (predominantly women), User B likes colorful images and User A likes cluttered images which have a tinge of graphics in them. Also we note that there are users who have certain common preferences - for example both Users A and B prefer high clutter in images. Similarly there were other instances in the data set where more than one users had similar preferences for the presence of people in the image (for example User's 3 and 4 in Fig. 1). This observation can be used to build many interesting applications of which one is providing recommendations to a group a people (by clustering them according to personality, culture etc.).

Comparing bimodal deep representation with individual modalities: We then train multiple layers of features for each modality using the model and use heterogenous feature mapping described in Sect. 3.2 to learn mapping from the tag features to visual features. The intuition behind using stacked auto-encoder is that pre-training multiple layers of features can help in capturing the characteristics of an image better (due to the non-linearities). Then, we concatenate features in all the layers to form the 'deep-feature' vector. To verify the intuition behind multi-layer pre-training and also to examine the efficacy of the trained bimodal (visual + tag) representation, we compare the performance of every layer of individual modalities in discriminating the users' 'likes' with that of the combined bimodal representation. This is shown in Fig. 8.

We train a SVM model (using a 5-fold cross validation setting) on the combined (visual + tag) features. We randomly divide the data set into 25 %/75 % training and test sets. To see if the features are able to distinguish between users' preferences, we test the accuracy of predicting the right user, given an image. Modeling user likes is a personalization problem which is user centric where the number of images liked by each user might play a more important role than the number of users themselves. Keeping this issue in mind, we considered 200

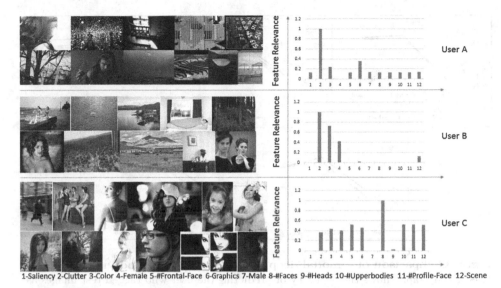

1-Saliency 2-Clutter 3-Color 4-Female 5-#Frontal-Face 6-Graphics 7-Male 8-#Faces 9-#Heads 10-#Upperbodies 11-#Profile-Face 12-Scene

Fig. 7. Features weighted for three users and a sample of images they tagged as favorite. Users' preferences can be represented using high-level visual features.

images for each user, which is similar to that used by [5,7]. And we test the method used in [7] on our dataset and use that as the baseline for comparing the performance of our method.

The results (in Fig. 8) show a comparison of the performance of the above model under different settings (i.e., using visual features alone, using tag features alone, using bimodal features). The following observations can be made based on the Fig. 8:

- 15 %–20 % increase in performance is achieved at each top-k setting by using the deep bimodal representation when compared to baseline performance.
- Hierarchical representations give to 5–10 % increase in performance when compared to shallow models trained on corresponding individual modalities.
- From top-1 to top-5 there is an improvement of over 35–40 % using bimodal deep representation.
- Visual features model user 'likes' better than tag features (by 20–30 %) which is different from the applications like image search etc. where tag features are more important.
- When compared with individual modalities, the combined representation improves the performance by 10–30 % which shows that a combination of multiple modalities can model user 'likes' better than individual modalities.

We also found in our experiments that simple concatenation of visual and tag features give inferior performance (5 %–10 % at each the layer) when compared with learning a bimodal representation using feature mapping from tag

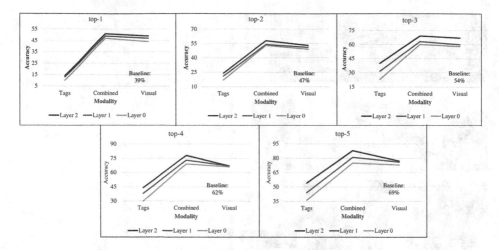

Fig. 8. Comparison of bimodal deep representation with individual modalities. Each graph shows the accuracy of predicting the user who tagged test images as favorite in top-k attempts. The baseline performance (with features used in [7]) is mentioned for each top-k setting. Learning multi-layer bimodal representation gives better performance than using shallow individual modalities. Layer 0 indicates the original features and Layers 1&2 the deep features for each modalities. 'Combined' indicates the performance of the bimodal representation at each layer.

domain to visual domain. This confirms that simple concatenation of features from different domains does not lead to a good representation [2] and feature mapping is necessary to learn effective bimodal representations to model user 'likes'.

5   Conclusion

In this paper, we attempted to model users 'likes' using bimodal deep representation of images on a Flickr data set. Several syntactic, semantic, aesthetic and contextual features were used to build a deep knowledge representation for images (using visual and textual information). A feature selection strategy was applied to learn the most influential features for a user to like an image. Deep bimodal representation was learnt using novel approach for knowledge transfer between tag domain and visual domain of images to model user 'likes'. A 15 %–20 % increase in performance was achieved when compared to shallow models trained on low-level features (and a 5 %–10 % increase when compared to shallow models trained on high-level features). Further work on understanding what the mid-level representations mean and testing our method on large scale dataset is under progress.

References

1. Kennedy, L., Naaman, M., Ahern, S., Nair, R., Rattenbury, T.: How flickr helps us make sense of the world: context and content in community-contributed media collections. In: Proceedings of the 15th International Conference on Multimedia. MULTIMEDIA 2007, pp. 631–640. ACM, New York (2007)
2. Gong, Y., Ke, Q., Isard, M., Lazebnik, S.: A multi-view embedding space for modeling internet images, tags, and their semantics. Int. J. Comput. Vis. **106**, 210–233 (2014)
3. Lampropoulos, A.S., Lampropoulou, P.S., Tsihrintzis, G.A.: A cascade-hybrid music recommender system for mobile services based on musical genre classification and personality diagnosis. Multimedia Tools Appl. **59**, 241–258 (2012)
4. Mairesse, F., Walker, M.A., Mehl, M.R., Moore, R.K.: Using linguistic cues for the automatic recognition of personality in conversation and text. J. Artif. Intell. Res. (JAIR) **30**, 457–500 (2007)
5. Cristani, M., Vinciarelli, A., Segalin, C., Perina, A.: Unveiling the multimedia unconscious: implicit cognitive processes and multimedia content analysis. In: Proceedings of the 21st ACM International Conference on Multimedia. MM 2013, pp. 213–222. ACM, New York (2013)
6. Guntuku, S.C., Roy, S., Weisi, L.: Personality modeling based image recommendation. In: He, X., Luo, S., Tao, D., Xu, C., Yang, J., Hasan, M.A. (eds.) MMM 2015, Part II. LNCS, vol. 8936, pp. 171–182. Springer, Heidelberg (2015)
7. Lovato, P., Perina, A., Sebe, N., Zandonà, O., Montagnini, A., Bicego, M., Cristani, M.: Tell me what you like and i'll tell you what you are: discriminating visual preferences on flickr data. In: Lee, K.M., Matsushita, Y., Rehg, J.M., Hu, Z. (eds.) ACCV 2012, Part I. LNCS, vol. 7724, pp. 45–56. Springer, Heidelberg (2013)
8. Judd, T., Ehinger, K., Durand, F., Torralba, A.: Learning to predict where humans look. In: 2009 IEEE 12th International Conference on Computer Vision, pp. 2106–2113. IEEE (2009)
9. Eichner, M., Marin-Jimenez, M., Zisserman, A., Ferrari, V.: 2d articulated human pose estimation and retrieval in (almost) unconstrained still images. Int. J. Comput. Vis. **99**, 190–214 (2012)
10. Marin-Jimenez, M., Zisserman, A., Eichner, M., Ferrari, V.: Detecting people looking at each other in videos. Int. J. Comput. Vis. **106**, 282–296 (2014)
11. Zhu, X., Ramanan, D.: Face detection, pose estimation, and landmark localization in the wild. In: 2012 IEEE Conference on Computer Vision and Pattern Recognition (CVPR), pp. 2879–2886 (2012)
12. Ploderer, B., Howard, S., Thomas, P., Reitberger, W.: "Hey world, take a look at me!": appreciating the human body on social network sites. In: Oinas-Kukkonen, H., Hasle, P., Harjumaa, M., Segerståhl, K., Øhrstrøm, P. (eds.) PERSUASIVE 2008. LNCS, vol. 5033, pp. 245–248. Springer, Heidelberg (2008)
13. Xiong, X., De la Torre, F.: Supervised descent method and its applications to face alignment. In: IEEE Conference on Computer Vision and Pattern Recognition (CVPR) (2013)
14. Qi, X., Xiao, R., Guo, J., Zhang, L.: Pairwise rotation invariant co-occurrence local binary pattern. In: Fitzgibbon, A., Lazebnik, S., Perona, P., Sato, Y., Schmid, C. (eds.) ECCV 2012, Part VI. LNCS, vol. 7577, pp. 158–171. Springer, Heidelberg (2012)
15. Flickr, H.: Freecg (2014)

16. Ng, T.T., Chang, S.F.: Classifying Photographic and Photorealistic Computer Graphic Images using Natural Image Statistics. ADVENT Technical report, No. 220-2006-6, Columbia University (2004)
17. Judd, T., Ehinger, K., Durand, F., Torralba, A.: Learning to predict where humans look. In: IEEE International Conference on Computer Vision (ICCV) (2009)
18. Rowse, D.: Why black and white photography (2014). http://digital-photography-school.com/why-black-and-white-photography/(Retrived)
19. Machajdik, J., Hanbury, A.: Affective image classification using features inspired by psychology and art theory. In: Proceedings of the International Conference on Multimedia, MM 2010, pp. 83-92. ACM, New York (2010)
20. Datta, R., Joshi, D., Li, J., Wang, J.Z.: Studying aesthetics in photographic images using a computational approach. In: Leonardis, A., Bischof, H., Pinz, A. (eds.) ECCV 2006. LNCS, vol. 3953, pp. 288-301. Springer, Heidelberg (2006)
21. Rosenholtz, R., Li, Y., Mansfield, J., Jin, Z.: Feature congestion: a measure of display clutter. In: Proceedings of the SIGCHI Conference on Human Factors in Computing Systems, pp. 761-770. ACM (2005)
22. Tan, M., Wang, L., Tsang, I.W.: Learning sparse SVM for feature selection on very high dimensional datasets. In: ICML, pp. 1047-1054 (2010)
23. Blum, A., Mitchell, T.: Combining labeled and unlabeled data with co-training. In: Proceedings of the 11th Annual Conference on Computational Learning Theory, pp. 92-100 (1998)
24. Sindhwani, V., Niyogi, P.: A co-regularized approach to semi-supervised learning with multiple views. In: Proceedings of the ICML Workshop on Learning with Multiple Views (2005)
25. Zhou, J.T., Pan, S.J., Qi, M., W Tsang, I.: Multi-view positive and unlabeled learning. In: Proceedings of the 4th Asian Conference on Machine Learning, ACML 2012, Singapore, 4-6 November 2012, pp. 555-570 (2012)
26. Zheng, W., Zhou, X., Zou, C., Zhao, L.: Facial expression recognition using kernel canonical correlation analysis (KCCA). IEEE Trans. Neural Netw. **17**, 233-238 (2006)
27. Srivastava, N., Salakhutdinov, R.: Multimodal learning with deep Boltzmann machines. In: Advances in Neural Information Processing Systems, pp. 2222-2230 (2012)
28. Zhou, J.T., Pan, S.J., Tsang, I.W., Yan, Y.: Hybrid heterogeneous transfer learning through deep learning. In: Twenty-Eighth AAAI Conference on Artificial Intelligence (2014)
29. Zhou, J.T., W Tsang, I., Pan, S.J., Tan, M.: Heterogeneous domain adaptation for multiple classes. In: Proceedings of the Seventeenth International Conference on Artificial Intelligence and Statistics, pp. 1095-1103 (2014)
30. Chen, M., Xu, Z.E., Weinberger, K.Q., Sha, F.: Marginalized denoising autoencoders for domain adaptation. In: ICML (2012)

Submodular Reranking with Multiple Feature Modalities for Image Retrieval

Fan Yang[1]([✉]), Zhuolin Jiang[2], and Larry S. Davis[1]

[1] University of Maryland College Park, College Park, MD, USA
{fyang,lsd}@umiacs.umd.edu
[2] Noah's Ark Lab, Huawei Technologies, Hong Kong, China
zhuolin.jiang@huawei.com

Abstract. We propose a submodular reranking algorithm to boost image retrieval performance based on multiple ranked lists obtained from multiple modalities in an unsupervised manner. We formulate the reranking problem as maximizing a submodular and non-decreasing objective function that consists of an information gain term and a relative ranking consistency term. The information gain term exploits relationships of initially retrieved images based on a random walk model on a graph, then images similar to the query can be found through their neighboring images. The relative ranking consistency term takes relative relationships of initial ranks between retrieved images into account. It captures both images with similar ranks in the initial ranked lists, and images that are similar to the query but highly ranked by only a small number of modalities. Due to its diminishing returns property, the objective function can be efficiently optimized by a greedy algorithm. Experiments show that our submodular reranking algorithm is effective and efficient in reranking images initially retrieved by multiple modalities. Our submodular reranking framework can be easily generalized to any generic reranking problems for real-time search engines.

1 Introduction

Numerous approaches have been proposed to improve the performance of content-based image retrieval (CBIR) systems. Most of them adopt a single feature modality such as bag-of-words (BoW) [1], Fisher vectors [2,3] or vector locally aggregated descriptors (VLAD) [4]. Various extensions based on a single feature modality have been proposed, such as query expansion [5,6], spatial verification [7] and Hamming embedding [8]. However, a single feature modality only captures one "view" of an image. Often, a lower-ranked but relevant retrieved image from one feature modality may be highly ranked by another modality. By fusing retrieval results from multiple feature modalities, we may discover both agreement and inconsistency among them to improve retrieval quality. Recent work combines multiple feature modalities for reranking by multi-modal graph-based learning [9],

---

Electronic supplementary material The online version of this chapter (doi:10.1007/978-3-319-16865-4_2) contains supplementary material, which is available to authorized users.

© Springer International Publishing Switzerland 2015
D. Cremers et al. (Eds.): ACCV 2014, Part I, LNCS 9003, pp. 19–34, 2015.
DOI: 10.1007/978-3-319-16865-4_2

query-specific graph fusion [10] or Co-Regularized Multi-Graph Learning [11]. In [9] requires a large number of queries to compute relevance scores for initially retrieved images, which is only suitable for large sets of queries. In [10], initial ranked lists were converted to undirected graphs, which were linearly combined without considering the inter-relationships between modalities. In [11] is a supervised learning based on image attributes, so it is not suitable for unsupervised reranking tasks.

We present a submodular objective function for reranking images retrieved by multiple feature modalities, which is very efficient and fully unsupervised. Submodularity [12] has been applied to various optimization problems in vision due to the availability of efficient approximate optimization methods based on its diminishing returns property - which means that as the incremental optimization algorithm proceeds, each item added to the evolving solution has less and less marginal value as the solution set grows. Our submodular objective function consists of two terms: an information gain term and a relative ranking consistency term. To compute the information gain, we first represent each initial ranked list as an undirected graph, where nodes are retrieved dataset images and edges represent similarities between images. The graph structure is then modeled as a transition matrix under the assumption of a random walk on a graph. Edge weights between nodes are converted to the probability of walking from a node to its neighbors. We select a subset of retrieved images by maximizing the information gain over the graph, which maximizes the mutual information between the selected subset and unselected nodes in the graph. The information gain takes pairwise relationships of retrieved images into consideration, and favors compact clusters of retrieved images which are similar to the query.

The relative ranking consistency term exploits the inter-relationships among multiple ranked lists obtained by different feature modalities. Specifically, if relative ranks between two images are consistent across multiple ranked lists, the ranking relationship between them is considered reliable and captured by our relative ranking consistency term. Additionally, our relative ranking consistency term encourages selecting images that are similar to the query but only found and highly ranked by a small number of modalities.

The final submodular objective function combines both the relationships among retrieved images from a single modality and the relative ranks of image pairs across different modalities, thereby improving initial retrieval results obtained by multiple independent modalities. Our approach only utilizes pairwise similarities between images in terms of appearance information without using any prior knowledge, hence it is fully unsupervised. Moreover, although we evaluate our submodular reranking algorithm on natural image retrieval, it only involves similarity graphs and initial ranked lists. Therefore, it can be easily extended to other generic retrieval tasks with multiple independent ranked lists returned by heterogeneous and non-visual features, such as audio and text. The main contributions of our work are summarized as follows:

- We address the problem of reranking natural images with multiple feature modalities by maximizing a submodular objective function, which is done by an efficient greedy algorithm.

- We model the image-level relationships for each modality as a graph and apply information gain theory to find the most similar images to the query. Only pairwise similarities between images are used to construct the graph. Our approach is unsupervised without using any label information.
- We propose a relative ranking consistency term to exploit the inter-relationships of multiple ranked lists across different modalities. The relative ranking consistency term effectively selects images that have consistent relative ranks across multiple modalities. It also discovers images that are similar to the query but only found by one or a few modalities.

2 Related Works

The majority of image retrieval approaches are based on a single feature modality. They usually adopt the bag-of-words (BoW) feature as an image representation, and then compute the similarities between a query image and dataset images for retrieval [1]. Many works focus on learning good feature representations for retrieval problems. Jégou et al. [4] proposed the vector locally aggregated descriptor as a compact representation. It achieved good results while requiring less storage compared to the BoW feature. Multi-VLAD [13] was later proposed to construct and match VLAD features of multiple levels from an image to improve localization accuracy. RootSIFT [14] was proposed to address the burstiness problem with standard BoW features. To compensate for the spatial information loss in the standard BoW-based approach, spatial verification [7] was proposed to match SIFT descriptors between images at the cost of extra storage space. Vocabulary trees [15] were proposed to improve efficiency in codebook construction and descriptor quantization by using hierarchical clustering. Contextual weighting [16] was further applied to vocabulary trees to increase the discriminative ability of visual words. Instead of quantizing a descriptor to a single visual word, assigning it to multiple words results in more discriminative BoW vectors and thus achieves better performance [17,18]. Query expansion [5,6,14] has been widely applied to rerank initially retrieved images, where a small portion of top ranked images serve as additional queries and are fed into the retrieval system again to further explore similar images. Some improvements such as Hamming embedding with geometric constraints [8], dataset-side feature augmentation [14] and co-occurrences of visual words [19] have achieved state-of-the-art results.

Although a single feature modality can achieve good retrieval results, better performance is anticipated if retrieved results from multiple feature modalities are properly fused. This is because they usually describe images from complementary perspectives. Recent work on fusing multiple feature modalities for image retrieval has been proposed, such as multi-modal graph learning [9], query-specific graph fusion [10] and Co-Regularized Multi-Graph Learning [11]. In [9] proposed a graph-based learning algorithm to infer weights of modalities. However, it requires a large number of queries beforehand to estimate relevance scores of initially retrieved images, which is not feasible if only a small number of queries are available.

In [10] constructed a graph for each initial ranked list based on a single feature modality using k-reciprocal nearest neighbors. In [11] imposed intra-graph and inter-graph constraints in a supervised learning framework which requires image attribute information. However, image attributes are not always available and the training process may be time-consuming for larger graphs. In contrast, our reranking approach considers both image-level and modality-level relationships, and does not require any attribute information or label information.

Submodularity, as a discrete analog of convexity, is widely studied in combinatorial optimization [12] due to its diminishing returns property: adding an element to a smaller set contributes more than adding it to a larger set. Various submodular functions have been proposed and successfully applied to many vision applications, such as image segmentation [20,21], dictionary selection/learning [22,23], saliency detection [24], object recognition [25] and video hashing [26]. A few works applied submodular functions to diversified ranking [27–29], where elements in the reranked list are similar to the query but also diversified. For diversified ranking, submodular functions are designed to seek a trade-off between similarity and diversity. It should be noted that [27–29] are not similar to our submodular reranking, since we encourage elements in the reranked list to be similar to the query and homogenous rather than diversified.

3   Submodular Reranking

We formulate the reranking problem as selecting and rearranging a subset of retrieved images from initial ranked lists obtained from multiple modalities. Our submodular objective function utilizes similarities of pairs of images to exploit relationships between retrieved images within each modality. It also considers the relative ranking between retrieved images across multiple ranked lists.

3.1   Preliminaries

Submodularity. Let $\mathcal{V}$ be a finite set. A set function $f : 2^{\mathcal{V}} \to \mathbb{R}$ is submodular if it satisfies $f(\mathcal{S} \cup a) - f(\mathcal{S}) \geq f(\mathcal{T} \cup a) - f(\mathcal{T})$ for all $\mathcal{S} \subset \mathcal{T} \subseteq \mathcal{V}, a \in \mathcal{V} \backslash \mathcal{T}$. This is called the *diminishing returns property*: adding a to a small set has a bigger impact than adding it to a larger set. The gain of the function value $f(\mathcal{S} \cup a) - f(\mathcal{S})$ is called the *marginal gain* of f when adding a to $\mathcal{S}$.

Monotonicity. A set function $f : 2^{\mathcal{V}} \to \mathbb{R}$ is monotone (or non-decreasing) if for every $\mathcal{S} \subseteq \mathcal{T} \subseteq \mathcal{V}, f(\mathcal{S}) \leq f(\mathcal{T})$ and $f(\emptyset) = 0$.

3.2   Information Gain with Graphical Models

Graph Construction. Given M feature modalities, we obtain M initial ranked lists of retrieved images for each query image. For efficient reranking, we select only the top K retrieved images from each ranked list. Note that the top K images are generally not the same across different modalities. Given an initial ranked list consisting of K retrieved images from modality m, we represent it as an undirected graph $\mathcal{G}_m = (\mathcal{V}_m, \mathcal{E}_m)$ where nodes $v_m \in \mathcal{V}_m$ are images and $e_m(i,j) \in \mathcal{E}_m$ denotes the edge that connects $v_m(i)$ and $v_m(j)$. An affinity matrix $\mathbf{A}_m \in \mathbb{R}^{K \times K}$ is used to represent the graph with the element $a_m(i,j)$ corresponding to the edge weight of $e_m(i,j)$, which is the pairwise similarity between images $v_m(i)$ and $v_m(j)$[1]. To facilitate the objective function construction (see Sect. 3.2), we do not include self-loops $e_m(i,i)$ of nodes $v_m(i)$ in the graph. Therefore, $a_m(i,i)$ is set to 0. For notational convenience, we denote $\mathcal{V}$ as the union of all nodes from the M undirected graphs, so that $\mathcal{V} = \mathcal{V}_1 \cup \mathcal{V}_2 \cup \cdots \cup \mathcal{V}_M$. We aim to select a subset of nodes $\mathcal{S}$ from $\mathcal{V}$ which are the most similar to the query image and arrange them in order to obtain the reranked result. Furthermore, $\mathcal{U}$ denotes the set of images which are not selected, so that $\mathcal{U} \cap \mathcal{S} = \emptyset$ and $\mathcal{V} = \mathcal{S} \cup \mathcal{U}$.

Information Gain. Given M graphs, we seek a method to combine them so that complementary modalities may help discover images similar to the query in a joint manner. Although the same graph construction is used for all ranked lists, pairwise similarities from different modalities are usually of incomparable scales, making a direct graph combination infeasible. To address this problem, we resort to information gain theory with graphical models [30], which is based on a simple probabilistic model.

We start from the random walk model on a graph $\mathcal{G}_m$. The random walk model can be interpreted as a Markov process: a walker stays at a node in the graph at time t and randomly walks to one of its neighboring nodes under some probability at time $t+1$. The probability of "walking" between nodes is called the transition probability and is defined as $\mathbf{P}_m = \mathbf{D}_m^{-1}\mathbf{A}_m$, where $\mathbf{D}_m \in \mathbb{R}^{K \times K}$ is a diagonal matrix with the diagonal element $d_m(i,i) = \sum_j a_m(i,j)$. The transition matrix $\mathbf{P}_m$ is a row-stochastic matrix indicating the transition probabilities of a random walk on the graph. $p_m(i,j)$ represents the conditional probability of walking from node $v_m(i)$ to node $v_m(j)$, which indicates the similarity between $v_m(i)$ and $v_m(j)$ based on the observation of $v_m(i)$. With the transition matrix $\mathbf{P}_m$, edge weights are converted to probabilities. Then we adopt information gain as a direct measure of the value of information of our graphical models. We start from a single graph $\mathcal{G}_m$, and define the information gain as

$$F_m(\mathcal{S}) = H(\mathcal{V}_m \backslash \mathcal{S}) - H(\mathcal{V}_m \backslash \mathcal{S} | \mathcal{S}) \tag{1}$$

where $\mathcal{S}$ is the subset we select from $\mathcal{V}$, and $\mathcal{V}_m \backslash \mathcal{S}$ is the set $\mathcal{V}_m$ with $\mathcal{S}$ removed. $H(\mathcal{V}_m \backslash \mathcal{S})$ is the entropy of unselected nodes in graph $\mathcal{G}_m$. $H(\mathcal{V}_m \backslash \mathcal{S} | \mathcal{S})$ is the conditional entropy of remaining nodes on graph $\mathcal{G}_m$ after we have observed $\mathcal{S}$. Specifically, $H(\mathcal{V}_m \backslash \mathcal{S} | \mathcal{S})$ and $H(\mathcal{V}_m \backslash \mathcal{S})$ are defined as

$$H(\mathcal{V}_m \backslash \mathcal{S} | \mathcal{S}) = - \sum_{v \in \mathcal{V}_m \backslash \mathcal{S}, s \in \mathcal{S}} p_m(v,s) \log p_m(v|s)$$

$$H(\mathcal{V}_m \backslash \mathcal{S}) = - \sum_{v \in \mathcal{V}_m \backslash \mathcal{S}} p_m(v) \log p_m(v) \tag{2}$$

---

[1] Please see experiment section about how to compute pairwise similarities.

where $p_m(v, s) = p_m(v|s)p_m(s)$. $p_m(v|s)$ is the transition probability of walking to a node v in graph $\mathcal{G}_m$ when the walker is at node s. $p_m(s)$ and $p_m(v)$ are the marginal probabilities of nodes s and v being similar to the query from modality m. $p_m(v|s)$ can be directly obtained from $\mathbf{P}_m$. To calculate the marginal probability $p_m(v)$, we use the normalized similarities between the query and retrieved images. We denote the similarities between the top K retrieved images and the query image from modality m as $\mathbf{c}_m = (c_{m,1}, c_{m,2}, ..., c_{m,K})^\top$. ℓ_1 normalization is then applied to $\mathbf{c}_m$ to obtain $p_m(v) = c_{m,v}/|\mathbf{c}_m|_1$.

We have the following proposition stating that the information gain with our graphical model is submodular.

Proposition 1. $F_m : 2^{\mathcal{V}_m} \to \mathbb{R}$ *is a submodular and monotone function.*

The proof is presented in the supplementary material. F_m is essentially the mutual information $I(\mathcal{V}_m\backslash\mathcal{S}; \mathcal{S})$ capturing the mutual dependence between subset $\mathcal{S}$ and unselected nodes $\mathcal{V}_m\backslash\mathcal{S}$, which measures how much $\mathcal{S}$ is representative of the graph with respect to the query. That F_m is non-decreasing is obvious, because the addition of any node to $\mathcal{S}$ always provides information or does not provide information at all, since "information never hurts". Submodularity comes from the observation that the information gain of adding a node to $\mathcal{S}$ becomes less in a later stage because it is more likely similar to elements in $\mathcal{S}$ as $\mathcal{S}$ grows.

To combine graphs, we need to determine the importance of each graph. Here we adopt the heuristic of simply summing up the information gains of the individual graphs to obtain the total information gain:

$$R(\mathcal{S}) = -\sum_m \left(\sum_{v\in\mathcal{V}\backslash\mathcal{S}} p_m(v) \log p_m(v) - \sum_{v\in\mathcal{V}\backslash\mathcal{S}, s\in\mathcal{S}} p_m(v, s) \log p_m(v|s) \right) \quad (3)$$

The information gain on a graph takes relationships between dataset images into account, so it propagates information about a dataset image to its neighbors, and better exploits dataset images that are similar to the query than simple pairwise comparisons. The combination seeks an agreement with respect to pairwise similarities derived from multiple modalities, so explores relationships of modalities to some extent. Note that since the top K images retrieved from different modalities may not be the same, $p_m(v)$ and $p_m(v|s)$ are set to 0 if an image is not included in graph $\mathcal{G}_m$, so it does not contribute to the objective function. An image discovered by most modalities contributes more to the information gain, therefore is selected to be in $\mathcal{S}$ with greater chance.

Since $F_m(\mathcal{S})$ is submodular and monotonically increasing, the linear combination of submodular functions, $R(\mathcal{S})$, is also submodular and non-decreasing. Since the information gain exploits the pairwise relationships between retrieved images, maximizing $R(\mathcal{S})$ is equivalent to selecting a group of images that are similar to the query and closely related to each other. Intuitive examples are shown in Fig. 1.

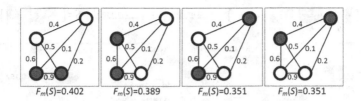

Fig. 1. The importance of information gain for selecting nodes into subset S. The number next to the edges is weight (similarity) between nodes. Red dots represent the selected subset S while white dots are remaining nodes $V_m \setminus S$. The marginal probability of all nodes is set to $1/4$. Four cases of selection are presented, where the corresponding value of $F_m(S)$ is shown under each sub figure. By computing the information gain, we observe that it prefers images that are closely related to each other to be selected into S, resulting in a compact cluster. Therefore, relationships of dataset images are exploited to facilitate reranking (Color figure online).

3.3 Relative Ranking Consistency

Simply summing up initial ranks obtained from different modalities for an image is not suitable, as a higher rank may be overly diluted by other lower ranks. Although complementary information from multiple modalities is used by integrating the $F_m(S)$, information gain does not completely utilize the inter-relationships between modalities. Additionally, it only considers pairwise similarities between images. However, the initial ranks of retrieved images from different modalities provide additional information that can further improve performance. For example, an image that is similar to the query and ranked lower by one modality may be ranked higher when it is perceived from a different perspective (*i.e.*, different modality). We propose a simple yet effective relative ranking consistency measure to model inter-relationships of multiple ranked lists.

Our measure is based on two criterion. First, relationships of relative ranks between retrieved images should be maintained. Images with similar ranks in the initial ranked lists from different modalities should also be ranked closely after reranking. Second, images with consistent ranks across multiple modalities should have their ranks preserved after reranking. An image that is similar to the query but highly ranked by only a smaller number of modalities should also be captured. In contrast to the information gain term, this relative ranking consistency measure models inter-relationships of modalities at a higher level: using ranks themselves rather than pairwise similarities between images.

Again, as in Sect. 3.2, we only consider the top K images from each ranked list and denote V as the union of all retrieved images. Our goal is to select a subset of retrieved images $S \subseteq V$. We first define the *relative ranking* between a pair of images and then use it to measure the "inter-rank" consensus amongst multiple ranked lists.

Let $\mathbf{r}_m \in \mathbb{R}^K$ denote the positions of the top K images in the initial ranked list by modality m, $\mathbf{r}_m = (r_{m,1}, r_{m,2}, ..., r_{m,K})^\top$, where $r_{m,i}$ is the position of image I_i in the m-th ranked list. Smaller value means higher rank. The relative

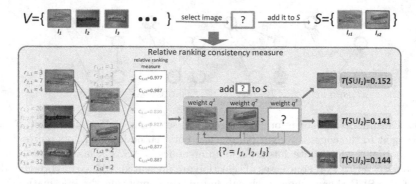

Fig. 2. The effectiveness of the relative ranking consistency measure. The set $\mathcal{V}$ contains $K = 100$ images, from which we need to select an image into $\mathcal{S}$, which currently contains two images. Starting from initial ranks from the 3 modalities, we compute the relative ranking consistency measure between images in $\mathcal{V}$ and $\mathcal{S}$. For illustration purposes, we only show the values of the relative ranking consistency measure for 3 images (I_1, I_2 and I_3) in the set $\mathcal{V}$. I_1 in $\mathcal{V}$, which is initially ranked close to images in $\mathcal{S}$ across all modalities, has the largest relative ranking consistency $\mathcal{C}$. The relative ranking consistency of I_3, which is highly ranked by only a single modality, is larger than that of I_2 in $\mathcal{V}$, which is lower ranked by all modalities. Therefore, the relative ranking consistency term favors adding I_1 to $\mathcal{S}$ as it produces the largest function value for $T(\mathcal{S})$. Then it favors adding I_3 over I_2, which has the smallest function value. Our relative ranking consistency successfully captures inter-relationships amongst multiple ranked lists and uses them to select images.

ranking between two images is defined as

$$rr_m(v_i, v_j) = |r_{m,v_i} - r_{m,v_j}|, \quad v_i, v_j \in \mathcal{V} \qquad (4)$$

where v_i and v_j correspond to images I_i and I_j in the graph representations. If either v_i or v_j is not included in the top K images by modality m, $rr_m(v_i, v_j)$ is set to K. The relative ranking considers the difference between ranks of retrieved images. Similarly, for modality m', we also have the relative ranking, $rr_{m'}(v_i, v_j)$, of the same image pair in a different modality. On the one hand, the consensus between $rr_m(v_i, v_j)$ and $rr_{m'}(v_i, v_j)$ indicates that the rank relationship between v_i and v_j is reliable and should be maintained after reranking, which is related to the "consistency" between ranked lists. On the other hand, we also aim to discover images which are similar to the query but highly ranked by only a small number of modalities, thereby capturing the "distinctiveness" of specific modalities. To enforce both consistency and distinctiveness constraints, we define a relative ranking consistency measure across multiple ranked lists as

$$\mathcal{C}(v_i, v_j) = \frac{1}{Z} \sum_{m, m' \in M, m \neq m'} 1 - \frac{\min(rr_m, rr_{m'})}{K} \qquad (5)$$

where $Z = \frac{M(M-1)}{2}$ is a normalization factor corresponding to the number of all possible modality pairs. With this measure, if images I_i and I_j are ranked similarly across multiple modalities, they will also have similar ranks in the reranked list, *i.e.*, they both will be selected and highly ranked in $\mathcal{S}$ or both will be excluded from $\mathcal{S}$. This results from the constraint on relative ranking consistency. Now consider the situation in which an image I_i is ranked closely to a visually similar image I_j only in a small number of modalities. In this case, we still discover such similarity due to the use of the min function, and rank these images appropriately. If either v_i or v_j is not included in the top K images by modalities m and m', $1 - \frac{\min(rr_m, rr_{m'})}{K} = 0$, which indicates that these two images have disparate ranks and should contribute nothing to the objective function. Therefore, we take the inter-relationships amongst multiple ranked lists into account with respect to the relative ranking between two images. Several examples are shown in Fig. 2 with more explanations.

Finally, we define a set function based on the rank biased overlap (RBO) similarity [31], incorporating the aforementioned relative ranking consistency measure. RBO similarity was proposed in [31] but they did not observe or take advantage of its submodularity property. We extend the basic idea from [31] that highly ranked images should be more important than lower ranked images in our objective function. Suppose the images in $\mathcal{S}$ are ordered and that the position of image I_i in the new ranked list is r_{v_i}. The relative ranking consistency term is defined as

$$T(\mathcal{S}) = (1 - q) \sum_{s=1}^{|\mathcal{S}|} q^s \cdot \frac{1}{s} \sum_{v_i, v_j \in \mathcal{S}, r_{v_i} < r_{v_j} = s} \mathcal{C}(v_i, v_j) \tag{6}$$

where the term $\frac{1}{s} \sum_{v_i, v_j \in \mathcal{S}, r_{v_i} < r_{v_j} = s} \mathcal{C}(v_i, v_j)$ allows us to select the image v_j with new rank s and compute the average relative ranking measure between v_j and all other s images with higher new ranks than v_j (see Fig. 2). $|\mathcal{S}|$ is the cardinality of $\mathcal{S}$. With the requirement that highly ranked images should have more weight in the objective function than lower ranked images, we introduce a weight parameter q for each image according to its new rank in $\mathcal{S}$. q controls the steepness of weight decay, so that a higher ranked image contributes more to the function value. Starting from the top ranked image with $s = 1$, the function assigns weight q^s to this image v_j and iteratively computes the average relative ranking between v_j and other higher ranked images v_i ($r_{v_i} < r_{v_j}$). Maximizing this function leads to a subset of images $\mathcal{S}$, where images are highly ranked and similarly ranked with each other in the initial ranked list. Since at least two images are needed to compute the relative ranking consistency measure, a phantom item v_p is included into $\mathcal{S}$ to select the first image. In practice, we use the query itself as the phantom with rank $r_{v_p} = 0$. Then we have the following proposition with the proof in the supplementary material.

Proposition 2. $T : 2^{\mathcal{V}} \to \mathbb{R}$ *is a submodular and monotone function if elements in $\mathcal{S}$ are ordered with respect to a phantom item $v_p \in \mathcal{S}$ and $r_{v_p} = 0$.*

3.4   Optimization

Combining the information gain and relative ranking consistency terms, we obtain the final objective function $Q(\mathcal{S}) = R(\mathcal{S}) + \lambda T(\mathcal{S})$ for the reranking problem. The solution is obtained by maximizing the objective function:

$$\max_{\mathcal{S}} \quad R(\mathcal{S}) + \lambda T(\mathcal{S})$$
$$s.t. \quad \mathcal{S} \subseteq \mathcal{V}, |\mathcal{S}| \leq K_s \tag{7}$$

where λ is a pre-defined weighting factor balancing the two terms. K_s is the largest number of selected images, which means we only select and rerank at most K_s images. Equation 7 is submodular and non-decreasing since it is a linear combination of submodular and non-decreasing functions. Direct optimization of Eq. 7 is a NP-hard problem, but it can be approximately optimized by a greedy algorithm. Starting from an empty set $\mathcal{S} = \emptyset$, the greedy algorithm iteratively adds a new element to $\mathcal{S}$ which provides the largest marginal gain at each iteration, until K_s elements have been selected. Specifically, during each iteration, we search for an image $a^* \in \mathcal{V} \backslash \mathcal{S}$, which gives the largest combined marginal gain from the information gain and relative ranking consistency terms, add it to $\mathcal{S}$ and set its rank to $r_{a^*} = \rho^{cur}$, where ρ^{cur} indicates the iteration step. The iteration terminates when $|\mathcal{S}| = K_s$. The reranked images are those from $\mathcal{S}$, and ranks are also obtained. We can tune K_s to control the efficiency and accuracy of the algorithm. The entire process is presented in Algorithm 1. The constraint on the number of reranked images leads to a uniform matriod $\mathcal{M} = (\mathcal{V}, \mathcal{I})$, where $\mathcal{I}$ is the collection of subsets $\mathcal{S} \subseteq \mathcal{V}$ satisfying the constraint that the number of reranked images is less than K_s. Maximizing a submodular function with a uniform matriod constraint yields a $(1 - 1/e)$ approximation to the optimal solution [12].

To further accelerate the optimization, we adopt lazy evaluation [23] to avoid recomputing the function value for each node $a^* \in \mathcal{V} \backslash \mathcal{S}$ during each iteration. The basic idea is maintaining a list of images with corresponding marginal gains in descending order. Only the top image is re-evaluated during each iteration. Other images are evaluated only if the top image does not remain at the top after re-evaluation. Lazy evaluation is based on the diminishing returns property: the function value of an element cannot increase during iterations. The lazy greedy algorithm leads to a speed-up of more than 40, as we will show in the experiments.

Algorithm 1. Submodular Reranking

Input: Graphs $\{\mathcal{G}_1, ..., \mathcal{G}_M\}$, initial ranked lists $\{\mathbf{r}_1, ..., \mathbf{r}_M\}$, K_s and λ

Output: Reranked list $\mathbf{r}$ and final retrieved images $\mathcal{S}$

Initialization: $\mathcal{S} \leftarrow \emptyset$, $\rho^{cur} \leftarrow 0$, $\mathbf{r} \leftarrow 0$

while $|\mathcal{S}| < K_s$ **do**
    $a^* = \underset{\mathcal{S} \cup \{a\} \in \mathcal{V}}{\arg\max} \; Q(\mathcal{S} \cup \{a\}) - Q(\mathcal{S})$
    if $Q(\mathcal{S} \cup \{a^*\}) \leq Q(\mathcal{S})$ **then**
        break;
    end if
    $\rho^{cur} \leftarrow \rho^{cur} + 1 \quad \mathcal{S} \leftarrow \mathcal{S} \cup \{a^*\}; r_{a^*} \leftarrow \rho^{cur}$
end

---

4 Experiments

4.1 Experimental Setting

Datasets. We evaluate our submodular reranking algorithm on 4 public datasets: *Holidays* [8], *UKbench* [15], *Oxford* [7] and *Paris* [17]. The *Holidays* dataset includes 1491 image from 500 categories, where the first image in each category is used as a query. The *UKbench* dataset contains 10200 images from 2550 objects or scenes. The *Oxford* and *Paris* datasets consist of 5062 and 6412 photos of famous landmarks in Oxford and Paris, respectively. Both datasets have 55 queries, where multiple queries are from the same landmark.

Table 1. Comparisons with state-of-the-art approaches. We use N-S score on *UKbench*, and mAP (in %) on other datasets. "-" means the results are not reported. Results using individual terms of our objective function are shown in the right-most columns.

Datasets	BoW [32]	GIST [33]	Color	Ours [10]		[7]	[8]	[18]	[32]	[16]	[34]	[35]	[19]	IG	RRC
Holidays	77.2	35.0	55.8	**84.9**	84.6	-	75.1	83.9	-	78.0	82.1	76.2	61.4	83.9	73.1
UKbench	3.50	1.96	3.09	**3.78**	3.77	3.45	-	3.64	3.67	3.56	-	3.52	3.36	3.75	3.54
Oxford	67.4	24.2	8.5	**74.3**	-	66.4	54.7	68.5	81.4	-	78.0	75.2	41.3	68.5	33.0
Paris	69.3	19.2	8.4	**74.8**	-	-	-	-	80.3	-	73.6	74.1	-	64.6	39.2

Evaluation Criteria. Following [7,8,17], we use mean average precision (mAP) to evaluate retrieval performance on *Holidays*, *Oxford* and *Paris* datasets. For the *UKbench* dataset, we use N-S score [15] which is the average correct number of top 4 retrieved images.

Features. We use the visual words from [32] to construct BoW vectors except on *Holidays* dataset where we adopt Hessian affine + SIFT descriptor to construct 1M-dimension BoW vectors using single assignment and approximate k-means (AKM) [7]. Standard tf-idf weighting is used. For global representations, we use a 1192-dimension GIST feature [33] and a 4000-dimension HSV color feature with 40 bins for H and 10 bins for S and V components.

Parameters. The similarity between two BoW vectors is computed by cosine similarity. We use a Gaussian kernel to convert Euclidean distance d to a similarity by $\exp(-d/\sigma)$ for GIST and color features. σ are empirically set to 0.34 and 0.14 respectively, and fixed in all experiments. q in Eq. 6 is set to 0.9 and λ in Eq. 7 is set to 0.01, both fixed in all experiments. K equals the number of dataset images in each dataset; while smaller value can be used for very large datasets. $K_s = 1000$ for all datasets.

4.2 Results Comparisons

Comparisons with State-of-the-art Approaches. Our primary focus is a reranking algorithm that improves retrieval performance of multiple ranked lists obtained by multiple independent feature modalities. Although our implementation depends only on pairwise similarities without spatial verification and query expansion, the performance by our submodular reranking is comparable to other state-of-the-art approaches using a single modality, as shown in Table 1.

Since there are limited methods for reranking by fusion for natural image retrieval, we only compare our algorithm to [10], which is also an unsupervised reranking method using multiple feature modalities, as shown in Table 1. Note that [11] is not directly comparable as it requires image attributes for learning. It is clear that our reranking algorithm outperforms [10], although we combine inferior individual modalities compared to [10]^2. Results by our reranking are also comparable to other state-of-the-art approaches, even we only use pairwise similarities without any learning and post-processing techniques, such as query expansion and spatial verification. We improve the best single modality (BoW) by 10.0%, 8.0%, 10.2% and 7.9% on the four datasets, respectively. Additionally, without specifically inferring weight for each modality, our reranking algorithm is very robust against inferior modalities, such as the color feature on *Oxford* and *Paris*, which only achieves less than 9% mAP. Although results on *Oxford* dataset by several approaches using a single modality [32,34,35] are better than those by our reranking algorithm, note that our reranking algorithm does not require SIFT descriptors or BoW vectors as [32,34,35] did, as long as we have pairwise similarities of pairs of images. Therefore, for the scenarios where original features cannot be stored and loaded efficiently due to limited resources, *i.e.*, mobile computing, our algorithm is more suitable than [32,34,35] for improving initial retrieval results. It is reasonable to expect that a higher accuracy might be obtained if we apply our reranking algorithm to fuse features which achieve better individual performance.

Table 2. Comparison of results by our reranking algorithm and other rank aggregation approaches. Runtime (in second) of reranking 1000 images for a single query using direct greedy optimization and lazy evaluation is shown in the right-most columns.

Datasets	Mean [36]	Median [37]	Geo-mean [37]	Robust [38]	Borda [37]	Ours	direct	lazy	speed-up
Holidays	59.2	71.7	76.4	71.5	59.2	**84.9**	16.5	0.40	41x
UKbench	2.89	3.47	3.50	3.33	2.89	**3.78**	55.7	1.34	42x
Oxford	18.6	34.7	40.5	35.6	18.6	**74.3**	38.3	0.74	52x
Paris	24.4	38.5	46.6	39.8	24.4	**74.8**	43.1	0.78	55x

Comparisons of Individual Terms. Our objective function consists of two terms: information gain and relative ranking consistency. These are complementary: the information gain term explores relationships between images and modalities at a fine level by using pairwise similarities, while the relative ranking consistency term exploits the inter-relationships between initial ranked lists in a coarser level as it only uses the ranks themselves. As shown in Table 1, by combining the two terms, our algorithm outperforms each individual term and achieves the best accuracy.

Comparisons with Baselines. We also compare the reranking accuracy of our reranking algorithm with other rank aggregation baseline approaches that combine multiple ranked lists. We use 5 rank aggregation approaches for comparison: mean rank aggregation [36], median rank aggregation [37], geometric mean

---

^{2} In [10], BoW achieved 77.5% mAP on *Holidays* and 3.54 N-S on *UKbench*, while color achieved 62.6% and 3.17, respectively. N-S score by GIST is 2.21 on *UKbench*.

rank aggregation [37], robust rank aggregation [38] and Borda count [36,37]. The results are shown in Table 2.

Our reranking algorithm outperforms all other rank aggregation approaches that do not as effectively use the inter-relationships amongst multiple ranked lists. The results by mean rank aggregation and Borda count are even much worse than those by a single modality (BoW), showing that a higher rank is overly diluted by other lower ranks. Incorporating the information gain and relative ranking consistency, our algorithm effectively exploits relationships of image pairs and multiple ranked lists at both a fine and a coarse level, leading to a higher retrieval accuracy.

4.3 Parameter Analysis

Impact of K_s. The parameter K_s controls the number of images to be reranked, which affects efficiency and reranking accuracy. Smaller K_s leads to fast convergence but may not discover images similar to queries but lower ranked since it discards a large number of initially retrieved images. We investigate the accuracy and execution time of our reranking with respect to K_s.

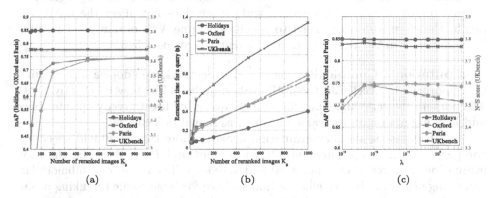

(a)   (b)   (c)

Fig. 3. (a) Change of mAP with respect to K_s. (b) Average reranking time for a single query with respect to K_s. (c) Change of mAP with respect to λ. Best view in color (Color figure online).

The retrieval accuracy in terms of mAP and average reranking time for a single query as K_s is varied are shown in Fig. 3(a), where K_s ranges from 10 to 1000. As we perform reranking on more images, the chance of discovering a similar but lower ranked image increases. Therefore, the mAP gradually improves. More specifically, the mAP rapidly increases as K_s increases from 10 to 500 for *Oxford* and *Paris* datasets. When more images are included in reranking after this point, the improvement of mAP is only incremental, showing that reranking images that are significantly lower ranked does not much benefit retrieval performance. In comparison, the mAP for *Holidays* and *UKbench* datasets reaches its highest value when $K_s < 100$ and remains almost constant thereafter. Images in the *Oxford* and *Paris* datasets have significant variance and each query has a large number of similar dataset images that can be retrieved. Images similar to the query can only be better discovered by a deeper inspection of initial ranked lists. In contrast, similar images in the *Holidays* and *UKbench* datasets are near-duplicates, and most queries have fewer than 10 similar images that are already highly ranked in the initial ranked lists. Therefore, only a smaller number of initially retrieved images need to be reranked.

To evaluate execution time, we calculate the average time spent to rerank K_s retrieved images for a single query in each dataset. From Fig. 3(b), it is not surprising that reranking a larger number of images takes more time. Nevertheless, our algorithm achieves sublinear time to rerank retrieved images for a single query with respect to K_s, showing the efficiency of the greedy algorithm with lazy evaluation. Furthermore, it takes the lazy evaluation less than 1.5 s on a desktop with 3.4 GHz CPU to rerank as many as 1000 images without any code optimization. Therefore, our reranking algorithm is scalable for large-scale image reranking tasks.

Impact of λ. In Eq. 7, we balance the information gain and relative ranking consistency by parameter λ. Since λ controls the importance of individual terms, it also affects the reranking accuracy. We investigate the change of reranking performance with respect to λ, as shown in Fig. 3(c). Our reranking algorithm is very robust: changing λ within a wide range does not affect the mAP too much, therefore we do not need to specifically tune λ to obtain good results. The change of mAP with respect to different λ is at most 5–6 %.

Computational Complexity. As stated in Sect. 3.4, we adopt a lazy evaluation approach to accelerate the optimization process. To show its effectiveness, we compare the reranking time for a single query by direct greedy optimization and lazy evaluation on the same machine, as shown in Table 2.

On all datasets, the lazy evaluation achieves more than a 40-fold speed-up compared to direct optimization. On the *Oxford* and *Paris* datasets, the lazy evaluation achieves more than a 50-fold speed-up. Therefore, our submodular reranking algorithm is very efficient and scalable for larger-scale reranking problems. With proper code optimization and parallel computing, our algorithm can be easily applied to reranking multiple ranked lists for real-time search engines.

5   Conclusions

We address the problem of reranking images that are initially ranked by multiple feature modalities by maximizing a submodular and monotone objective function. Our objective function is composed of an information gain term and a relative ranking consistency term. The information gain term utilizes relationships of initially retrieved images based on a random walk model on a graph. Based on this term, an image initially lower ranked but resembling other retrieved images that are similar to the query will have higher rank after reranking. The relative ranking consistency term measures the relative ranking between two initially retrieved images across multiple ranked lists. It maintains the consistency of relative ranks between two images during reranking, and also captures a high rank of an image that is similar to the query but only discovered by one or a few modalities. The objective function can be efficiently maximized by a lazy greedy algorithm, leading to an ordered subset of initially retrieved images. Experiments show that our reranking algorithm improves overall retrieval accuracy and is computationally efficient.

Acknowledgement. This work was supported by the NSF EAGER grant: IIS1359900, Scalable Video Retrieval.

References

1. Sivic, J., Zisserman, A.: Video google: a text retrieval approach to object matching in videos. In: ICCV, pp. 1470–1477 (2003)
2. Perronnin, F., Liu, Y., Sánchez, J., Poirier, H.: Large-scale image retrieval with compressed Fisher vectors. In: CVPR, pp. 3384–3391 (2010)
3. Douze, M., Ramisa, A., Schmid, C.: Combining attributes and fisher vectors for efficient image retrieval. In: CVPR, pp. 745–752 (2011)
4. Jégou, H., Douze, M., Schmid, C., Pérez, P.: Aggregating local descriptors into a compact image representation. In: CVPR, pp. 3304–3311 (2010)
5. Chum, O., Philbin, J., Sivic, J., Isard, M., Zisserman, A.: Total recall: automatic query expansion with a generative feature model for object retrieval. In: ICCV, pp. 1–8 (2007)
6. Chum, O., Mikulík, A., Perdoch, M., Matas, J.: Total recall II: query expansion revisited. In: CVPR, pp. 889–896 (2011)
7. Philbin, J., Chum, O., Isard, M., Sivic, J., Zisserman, A.: Object retrieval with large vocabularies and fast spatial matching. In: CVPR, pp. 1–8 (2007)
8. Jegou, H., Douze, M., Schmid, C.: Hamming embedding and weak geometric consistency for large scale image search. In: Forsyth, D., Torr, P., Zisserman, A. (eds.) ECCV 2008, Part I. LNCS, vol. 5302, pp. 304–317. Springer, Heidelberg (2008)
9. Wang, M., Li, H., Tao, D., Lu, K., Wu, X.: Multimodal graph-based reranking for web image search. IEEE Trans. Image Process. **21**, 4649–4661 (2012)
10. Zhang, S., Yang, M., Cour, T., Yu, K., Metaxas, D.N.: Query specific fusion for image retrieval. In: Fitzgibbon, A., Lazebnik, S., Perona, P., Sato, Y., Schmid, C. (eds.) ECCV 2012, Part II. LNCS, vol. 7573, pp. 660–673. Springer, Heidelberg (2012)
11. Deng, C., Ji, R., Liu, W., Tao, D., Gao, X.: Visual reranking through weakly supervised multi-graph learning. In: ICCV, pp. 2600–2607 (2013)
12. Nemhauser, G.L., Wolsey, L.A., Fisher, M.L.: An analysis of approximations for maximizing submodular set functions. Math. Program. **14**, 265–294 (1978)
13. Arandjelović, R., Zisserman, A.: All about VLAD. In: CVPR, pp. 1578–1585 (2013)
14. Arandjelović, R., Zisserman, A.: Three things everyone should know to improve object retrieval. In: CVPR, pp. 2911–2918 (2012)
15. Nistér, D., Stewénius, H.: Scalable recognition with a vocabulary tree. In: CVPR, pp. 2161–2168 (2006)
16. Wang, X., Yang, M., Cour, T., Zhu, S., Yu, K., Han, T.X.: Contextual weighting for vocabulary tree based image retrieval. In: ICCV, pp. 209–216 (2011)
17. Philbin, J., Chum, O., Isard, M., Sivic, J., Zisserman, A.: Lost in quantization: improving particular object retrieval in large scale image databases. In: CVPR, pp. 1–8 (2008)

18. Jégou, H., Douze, M., Schmid, C.: On the burstiness of visual elements. In: CVPR, pp. 1169–1176 (2009)
19. Jégou, H., Chum, O.: Negative evidences and co-occurences in image retrieval: the benefit of PCA and whitening. In: Fitzgibbon, A., Lazebnik, S., Perona, P., Sato, Y., Schmid, C. (eds.) ECCV 2012, Part II. LNCS, vol. 7573, pp. 774–787. Springer, Heidelberg (2012)
20. Jegelka, S., Bilmes, J.: Submodularity beyond submodular energies: coupling edges in graph cuts. In: CVPR, pp. 1897–1904 (2011)
21. Kim, G., Xing, E.P., Li, F.F., Kanade, T.: Distributed cosegmentation via submodular optimization on anisotropic diffusion. In: ICCV, pp. 169–176 (2011)
22. Krause, A., Cevher, V.: Submodular dictionary selection for sparse representation. In: ICML, pp. 567–574 (2010)
23. Jiang, Z., Zhang, G., Davis, L.S.: Submodular dictionary learning for sparse coding. In: CVPR, pp. 3418–3425 (2012)
24. Jiang, Z., Davis, L.S.: Submodular salient region detection. In: CVPR, pp. 2043–2050 (2013)
25. Zhu, F., Jiang, Z., Shao, L.: Submodular object recognition. In: CVPR (2014)
26. Cao, L., Li, Z., Mu, Y., Chang, S.F.: Submodular video hashing: a unified framework towards video pooling and indexing. In: ACM Multimedia, pp. 299–308 (2012)
27. Tong, H., He, J., Wen, Z., Konuru, R., Lin, C.Y.: Diversified ranking on large graphs: an optimization viewpoint. In: KDD, pp. 1028–1036 (2011)
28. Zhu, X., Goldberg, A.B., Gael, J.V., Andrzejewski, D.: Improving diversity in ranking using absorbing random walks. In: HLT-NAACL, pp. 97–104 (2007)
29. He, J., Tong, H., Mei, Q., Szymanski, B.K.: GenDeR: a generic diversified ranking algorithm. In: NIPS, pp. 1151–1159 (2012)
30. Krause, A., Guestrin, C.: Near-optimal nonmyopic value of information in graphical models. In: UAI, pp. 324–331 (2005)
31. Webber, W., Moffat, A., Zobel, J.: A similarity measure for indefinite rankings. ACM Trans. Inf. Syst. **28**, 1–38 (2010)
32. Qin, D., Gammeter, S., Bossard, L., Quack, T., Gool, L.J.V.: Hello neighbor: accurate object retrieval with k-reciprocal nearest neighbors. In: CVPR, pp. 777–784 (2011)
33. Oliva, A., Torralba, A.: Modeling the shape of the scene: a holistic representation of the spatial envelope. Int. J. Comput. Vis. **42**, 145–175 (2001)
34. Qin, D., Wengert, C., Gool, L.V.: Query adaptive similarity for large scale object retrieval. In: CVPR (2013)
35. Shen, X., Lin, Z., Brandt, J., Avidan, S., Wu, Y.: Object retrieval and localization with spatially-constrained similarity measure and k-nn re-ranking. In: CVPR, pp. 3013–3020 (2012)
36. Aslam, J.A., Montague, M.H.: Models for metasearch. In: SIGIR, pp. 275–284 (2001)
37. Dwork, C., Kumar, R., Naor, M., Sivakumar, D.: Rank aggregation methods for the web. In: WWW, pp. 613–622 (2001)
38. Kolde, R., Laur, S., Adler, P., Vilo, J.: Robust rank aggregation for gene list integration and meta-analysis. Bioinformatics **28**, 573–580 (2012)

Accurate Scene Text Recognition Based on Recurrent Neural Network

Bolan Su$^{(\boxtimes)}$ and Shijian Lu

Institute for Infocomm Research, 1 Fusionopolis Way,
21-01 Connexis, Singapore, Singapore
{subl,slu}@i2r.a-star.edu.sg

Abstract. Scene text recognition is a useful but very challenging task due to uncontrolled condition of text in natural scenes. This paper presents a novel approach to recognize text in scene images. In the proposed technique, a word image is first converted into a sequential column vectors based on Histogram of Oriented Gradient (HOG). The Recurrent Neural Network (RNN) is then adapted to classify the sequential feature vectors into the corresponding word. Compared with most of the existing methods that follow a bottom-up approach to form words by grouping the recognized characters, our proposed method is able to recognize the whole word images without character-level segmentation and recognition. Experiments on a number of publicly available datasets show that the proposed method outperforms the state-of-the-art techniques significantly. In addition, the recognition results on publicly available datasets provide a good benchmark for the future research in this area.

1 Introduction

Reading text in scenes is a very challenging task in Computer Vision, which has been drawing increasing research interest in recent years. This is partially due to the rapid development of wearable and mobile devices such as smart phones, digital cameras, and the latest google glass, where scene text recognition is a key module to a wide range of practical and useful applications.

Traditional Optical Character Recognition (OCR) systems usually assume that the document text has well defined text fonts, size, layout, etc. and scanned under well-controlled lighting. They often fail to recognize camera-captured texts in scenes, which could have little constraints in terms of text fonts, environmental lighting, image background, etc., as illustrated in Fig. 1.

Intensive research efforts have been observed in this area in recent years and a number of good scene text recognition systems have been proposed. One approach is to combine text segmentation with existing OCR engines, where text pixels are first segmented from the image background and then fed to OCR engines for recognition. Several systems have been reported that exploit Markov Random Field [5], Nonlinear color enhancement [6] and Inverse Rendering [7] to extract the character regions. However, the text segmentation process by itself is a very challenging task that is prone to different types of segmentation errors.

© Springer International Publishing Switzerland 2015
D. Cremers et al. (Eds.): ACCV 2014, Part I, LNCS 9003, pp. 35–48, 2015.
DOI: 10.1007/978-3-319-16865-4_3

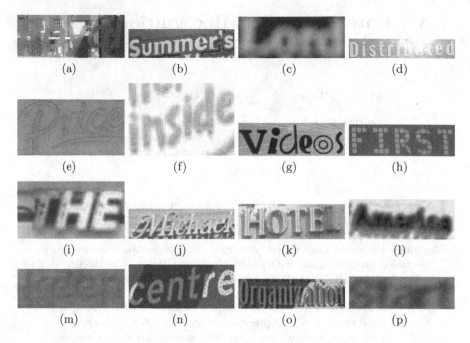

Fig. 1. Word image examples taken from the recent Public Datasets [1–4]. All the words in the images are correctly recognized by our proposed method.

Furthermore, the OCR engines may fail to recognize the segmented texts due to special text fonts and perspective distortion, as the OCR engines are usually trained on characters with fronto-parallel view and normal fonts.

A number of scene text recognition techniques [4, 8–11] have been reported in recent years that tend to train their own scene character classifiers. Most of these methods follow a bottom-up approach to group the recognized characters into a word based on the context information. The grouping process to form a word is usually defined as finding the best word alignment that fits the set of detected characters. Lexicon and n-gram language model are also incorporated as a top-down clue to recover some common errors, such as spelling and ambiguities [6, 7, 10]. On the other hand, these new techniques also require robust and accurate character-level detection and recognition, otherwise the word alignment will lead to incorrect result due to the error accumulation from lower levels to higher levels.

In this paper, we propose a novel scene text recognition technique that treats a word image as an unsegmented sequence and does not require character-level detection, segmentation, and recognition. Figure 2 shows the overall flowchart of our proposed word recognition system. First, a word image is converted into a sequence of column feature, where each column feature is generated by concatenating the HOG features extracted from the corresponding image patches in the same column of the input image. A multi layer recurrent neural network (RNN) with bidirectional Long Short-Term Memory (LSTM) [12] is then trained for

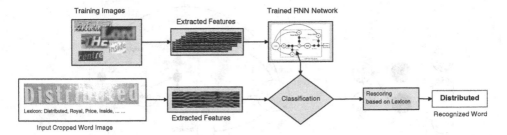

Fig. 2. The overall flowchart of our proposed scene word recognition system.

labelling the sequential data. Finally, the connectionist temporal classification (CTC) [13] technique is exploited to find out the best match of a list of lexicon words based on the RNN output of the sequential feature using.

We apply our proposed technique on cropped word image recognition with a lexicon. The cropped word denotes a word image that is cropped along the word bounding box within the original image as illustrated in Fig. 1. Such word regions can be located by a text detector or with user assistance in different real-world scenarios. The lexicon refers to a list of possible words associated with the word image, which can be viewed as a form of contextual information. It is obvious that the search space can be significantly narrowed down in real world applications. For example, the lexicon can be nearby signboard names collected using Google when recognizing signboards at one location [4]. In other cases, the lexicon can be food names, sporter names, product lists, etc., depending on different scenarios.

The proposed scene text recognition technique has a number of novel contributions. First, we describe an effective way of converting a word image into a sequential signal where techniques used in relevant areas, such as speech processing and handwriting recognition, can be introduced and applied. Second, we adapt RNN and CTC techniques for recognition of texts in scenes, and designed a segmentation-free scene word recognition system that obtains superior word recognition accuracy. Third, unlike some systems that rely heavily on certain local dataset (which are not available to the public) [8,14], our system makes use of several publicly available datasets, hence providing a baseline for easier benchmarking of the ensuing scene text recognition techniques.

2 Related Work

2.1 Scene Text Recognition

In general, the word recognition in natural scene consists of two main steps, text detection and text recognition. The first step usually detects possible regions as character candidates, the second step recognizes the detected regions and groups them into word.

Different visual feature detectors and descriptors have been exploited for the detection and recognition of texts in scenes. The Histogram of Oriented Gradient (HOG) feature [15] is widely used in different methods [4,10,16]. Recently,

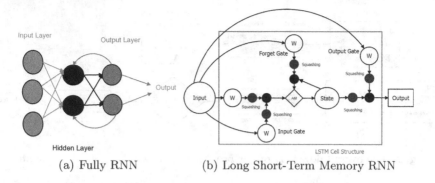

(a) Fully RNN   (b) Long Short-Term Memory RNN

Fig. 3. Illustration of Recurrent Neural Network.

the part-based tree structure [9] is also proposed along with the HOG descriptor to capture the structure information of different characters. In addition, the Co-occurrence HOG feature [17] is developed to represent the spatial relationship of neighbouring pixels. Other features including stroke widths (SW) [18,19], maximally stable extremal regions (MSER) [20,21] and weighted direction code histogram (WDCH) [8] have also been applied for character detection and classification. The HOG feature is also exploited in our proposed system for construction of sequential features of word images.

With large amount training data, the systems reported in [8,14,22] obtain high recognition accuracy with unsupervised feature learning techniques. Moreover, different approaches are proposed to group the detected characters into word using contextual information, including Weighted Finite-State Transducers [11], Pictorial Structure [4,16], and Conditional Random Field Model [9,10]. We propose a novel scene text recognition technique that treat each word image as a whole without requiring character-level segmentation and recognition. The CTC technique [13] is exploited to find the best word alignment for each unsegmented column feature vector and so character-level segmentation and recognition is not needed.

2.2   Recurrent Neural Network

Recurrent Neural Network (RNN) is a special neural network that has been used for handling sequential data, as illustrated in Fig. 3(a). The RNN aims to predict the label of current time stamp with the contextual information of past time stamps. It is a powerful classification model but not widely used in the literature. The major reason is that it often requires a long training process as the error path integral decays exponentially along the sequence [23].

The long short-term memory (LSTM) model [23] was proposed to solve this problem as illustrated in Fig. 3(b). In LSTM, an internal memory structure is used to replace the nodes in the traditional RNN, where the output activation of the network at time t is determined by the input data of the network at time t and the internal memory stored in the network at time $t-1$. The learning procedure under LSTM therefore becomes local and constant. Furthermore, a forget gate is added to determine whether to reset the stored memory [24]. This strategy helps the RNN to remember contextual information and withdraw errors during learning. The memory update and output activation procedure of RNN can be formulated in Eq. 1 as follows:

$$S^t = S^{t-1} \cdot f(W_{forget}X^t) + f(W_{in}X^t) \cdot f(W_c X^t) \tag{1a}$$

$$Y^t = f(W_{out}X^t) \cdot g(S^t) \tag{1b}$$

where S^t, X^t, Y^t denote the stored memory, input data, and output activation of the network at time t, respectively. Functions $g(*)$ and $f(*)$ refer to the sigmoid function that squashes the data. W_* denotes the weight parameters of the network. In addition, the first term $(W_{forget}X^t)$ is used to control whether to withdraw previous stored memory S^{t-1}.

Bidirectional LSTM [13, 25] is further proposed to predict the current label with past and future contextual information by processing the input sequence in two directions (i.e. from beginning to end and, from end to beginning). It has been applied for handwriting recognition and outperforms the wildly-used Hidden Markov Model (HMM). We introduce the bidirectional LSTM technique into scene text recognition domain, and the powerful model obtains superior recognition performance.

3   Feature Preparation

To apply the RNN model, the input word image needs to be first converted into a sequential feature. In speech recognition, the input signal is already a sequential data and feature can be directly extracted frame by frame. Similarly, a word image can be viewed as a sequential array if we take each column of the word image as a frame. This idea has been applied for handwriting recognition [13] and achieved great success.

However, the same procedure cannot be applied on the scene text recognition problem due to two factors. First, the input data of the handwriting recognition task is usually binary or has a clear bi-modal pattern, where the text pixels can be easily segmented from the background. Second, the handwritten text usually has a much smaller stroke width variation compared with texts in scenes, where features extracted from each column of handwriting images contains more meaningful information for classification.

On the other hand, quite a number of visual features in computer vision such as HOG are extracted in image patches, which perform well in text recognition due to their robustness to illumination variation and invariance to the local geometric and photometric transformations. We first convolutionally partition the input image into patches with step size 1, which is described in Algorithm 1 below.

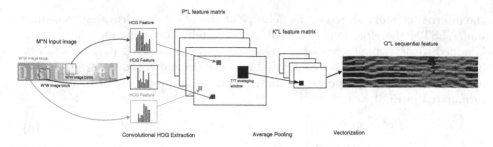

Fig. 4. The overall process of column feature construction. From left to right, HOG features are extracted convolutionally from every image blocks of the input image exhaustively; Average pooling is then performed on each column; Finally, the vectorization process is applied to obtain the sequential feature. It is worth to note that, $P = M - W + 1$, $L = N - W + 1$, $K = P/T$, and $Q = K * H$, where H denotes the length of the HOG feature.

Algorithm 1. Convolutional Image Patch Extraction

1: **procedure** PATCHEXTRACTION(img, W)
2:     M : height of img
3:     N : width of img
4:     $Patches$: (M-W+1) × (N-W+1) matrix, each entry is a $W \times W$ matrix.
5:     **for** i = 1:M-W+1 **do**
6:         **for** j = 1:N-W+1 **do**
7:             $Patches$(i,j) = img(i:i+W-1,j:j+W-1)
8:         **end for**
9:     **end for**
10:     Return $Patches$
11: **end procedure**

---

where img denotes the input word image, W denotes the size of one image patch. The HOG feature is then extracted and normalized for each image patch. After that, the HOG features of the image patches at the same column are linked together. An average pooling strategy is applied to incorporate information of neighbouring blocks by averaging the HOG feature vectors within a neighbouring window as defined in Eq. 2.

$$HOG(i,j) = \sum_{p=i-{}^T/_2}^{i+{}^T/_2} (HOG(p,j))/T \qquad (2)$$

where i, j refer to index, HOG denotes the extracted normalized HOG feature vector of corresponding patch, HOG_{avg} denotes the feature vector after averaging pooling, and T denotes the size of neighbouring window for average pooling. A column feature is finally determined by concatenating the averaged HOG feature vectors at the same column.

Figure 4 shows the overall process of column feature vector construction. To ensure that all the column features have the same length, the input word image needs to be normalized to be of the same height M beforehand. Furthermore, the patch size W and neighbouring windows size T can be set empirically, and will be discussed in the experiment section.

4 Recurrent Neural Network Construction

A word image can thus be recognized by classifying the correspondingly converted sequential column feature vector. We use the RNN [23] instead of the traditional neural network or HMM due to its superior characteristics in several aspects. First, unlike the HMM that generates observations based only on the current hidden state, RNN incorporates the context information including the historical states by using the LSTM structure [13] and therefore outperform the HMM greatly. Second, unlike the traditional neural network, the bidirectional LSTM RNN model [13] does not require explicit labelling of every single column vector of the input sequence. This is very important to the scene text recognition because characters in scenes are often connected, broken, or blurred where the explicit labelling is often an infeasible task as illustrated in Fig. 1. Note that RNNLIB [26] is implemented to build and train the multi-layer RNN.

CTC [13] is applied to the output layer of RNN to label the unsegmented data. In our system, a training sample can be viewed as a pair of input column feature and a target word string $(\mathbf{C}, \mathcal{W})$. The objective function of CTC is then defined as follows:

$$\mathcal{O} = -\sum_{(\mathbf{C},\mathcal{W})\in\mathcal{S}} \ln p(\mathcal{W}|\mathbf{C}) \tag{3}$$

where $\mathcal{S}$ denotes the whole training set and $p(\mathcal{W}|\mathbf{C})$ denotes the conditional probability of word $\mathcal{W}$ given a sequence of column feature $\mathbf{C}$. The target is to minimize $\mathcal{O}$, which is equivalent to maximize the conditional probability $p(\mathcal{W}|\mathbf{C})$.

The output path π of the RNN output activations has the same length of the input sequence $\mathbf{C}$. Since the neighbouring column feature vectors might represent the same character, some column feature vectors may not represent any labels. An additional 'blank' output cell therefore needs to be added into the RNN output layer. In addition, the repeating labels and empty labels also need to be removed to map to the target word $\mathcal{W}$. For example, $('-','a','a','-','-','b','b','b')$ can be mapped to (a, b), where $'-'$ denotes the empty label. So the $p(\mathcal{W}|\mathbf{C})$ is defined as follows:

$$p(\mathcal{W}|\mathbf{C}) = \sum_{V(\pi)=\mathcal{W}} p(\pi|\mathbf{C}) \tag{4}$$

where V denotes the operator that translates the output path π to target word $\mathcal{W}$. It is worth to note that the translation process V is not unique. $p(\pi|\mathbf{C})$ refers to the conditional probability of output path π given input sequence $\mathbf{C}$, which is defined as follows:

$$p(\pi|\mathbf{C}) = \prod_{t=1}^{L} p(\pi_t|\mathbf{C}) = \prod_{t=1}^{L} y_{\pi_t}^t \qquad (5)$$

where L denotes the length of the output path and π_t denotes label of output path π at time t. The term y^t denotes the network output of RNN at time t, which can be interpreted as the probability distribution of the output labels at time t. Therefore $y_{\pi_t}^t$ denotes the probability of π_t at time t.

The CTC forward backward algorithm [13] is then applied to calculate $p(\mathcal{W}|\mathbf{C})$. The RNN network is trained by back-propagating the gradient through the output layer based on the objective function as defined in Eq. 3. Once the RNN is trained, it can be used to convert a sequential feature vector into a probability matrix. In particular, the RNN will produce a $L \times G$ probability matrix $\mathbf{Y}$ given an input sequence of column feature vector, where L denotes the length of the sequence, and G denotes the number of possible output labels. Each entry of $\mathbf{Y}$ can be interpreted as the probability of a label at a time step.

5   Word Scoring with Lexicon

Given a probability matrix $\mathbf{Y}$ and a lexicon $\mathcal{L}$ with a set of possible words, the word recognition can be formulated as searching for the best match word w^* as follows:

$$w^* = \arg\max_{w \in \mathcal{L}} p(w|\mathbf{Y}) = \arg\max_{w \in \mathcal{L}} \sum_{V(\pi)=w} p(\pi|\mathbf{Y}) \qquad (6)$$

where $p(w|\mathbf{Y})$ is the conditional probability of word w given $\mathbf{Y}$. A direct graph can be constructed for the word w so that each node represents a possible label of w. In another word, we need to sum over all the possible paths that can form a word w on the probability matrix $\mathbf{Y}$ to calculate the score of a word w.

A new word w^i can be generated by adding some blank interval into the beginning and ending of w as well as the neighbouring labels of w, where the blank interval denotes the empty label. The length of w^i is $2 * |w| + 1$, where $|w|$ denotes the length of w. A new $|w^i| \times L$ probability matrix $\mathfrak{P}$ can thus be formed, where $|w^i|$ denotes the length of w^i and L denotes the length of the input sequence. $\mathfrak{P}(m, t)$ denotes the probability of label w_m^i at time t, which can be determined by the probability matrix $\mathbf{Y}$. Each path from $\mathfrak{P}(1, 1)$ to $\mathfrak{P}(|w^i|, L)$ denotes a possible output π of word w, where the probability can be calculated using Eq. 5.

The problem thus changes to the score accumulation along all the possible paths in $\mathfrak{P}$. It can be solved with the CTC token pass algorithm [13] using dynamic programming. The computational complexity of this algorithm is $O(L \cdot |w^i|)$. Finally, the word with highest score in the lexicon is determined as the recognized word.

6 Experiments and Discussion

6.1 System Details

In the proposed system, all cropped word images are normalized to be of the same height, i.e., $M = 32$. The patch size W, the HOG bin number, and the averaging window size T are set to 8, 8, and 5, respectively. For RNN, the number of input cells is the same as the length of the extracted column feature at 40. The output layer is 64 including 62 characters ([a...z,A...Z,0...9]), one label for special characters ([+,&,$,...]), and one empty label. 3 hidden layers are used that have 60, 100, and 140 cells, respectively. The system is implemented on Ubuntu 13.10 with 16 GB RAM and Intel 64 bit 3.40 GHz CPU. The training process takes about 1 h on a training set with about 3000 word images. The average time for recognizing a cropped word image is around one second. This is comparable with the state-of-the-art techniques and can be further improved to satisfy the requirement of real-time applications.

6.2 Experiments on ICDAR and SVT Datasets

The proposed method has been tested on three public datasets, including ICDAR 2003[1] dataset, ICDAR 2011[2] dataset, and Street View Text (SVT)[3] dataset. The three datasets consist of 1156 training images and 1110 testing images, 848 training images and 1189 testing images, 257 training images and 647 testing images, respectively.

During the experiments, we add the Char74k character images[4] [27] to form a bigger training dataset. For the Char74k dataset, only English characters are used that consists of more than ten thousands of character images in total. In particular, 7705 characters images are obtained from natural images and the rest are hand drawn using a tablet PC. The trained RNN is applied to the testing images of the three datasets for word recognition.

We compare our proposed method with eight state-of-the-art techniques, including markov random field method (MRF) [5], inverse rendering method (IR) [7], nonlinear color enhancement method (NESP) [6], pictorial structure method (PLEX) [16], HOG based conditional random field method (HOG+CRF) [10], weighted finite-state transducers method (WFST) [11], part based tree structure method (PBS) [9] and convolutional neural network method (CNN) [14].

To make the comparison fair, we evaluate recognition accuracy on testing data with a lexicon created from all the words in the test set (as denoted by ICDAR03(FULL) and ICDAR11(FULL) in Table 1), as well as with lexicon consisting of 50 random words from the test set (as denoted by ICDAR03(50) and ICDAR11(50) in Table 1). For SVT dataset, a lexicon consisting of about 50 words is provided and directly adopted in our experiments.

---

[1] http://algoval.essex.ac.uk/icdar/Datasets.html.
[2] http://robustreading.opendfki.de/wiki/SceneText.
[3] http://vision.ucsd.edu/~kai/grocr/.
[4] http://www.ee.surrey.ac.uk/CVSSP/demos/chars74k/.

Table 1. Word recognition accuracy on the ICDAR 03 testing dataset, the ICDAR 11 testing dataset and the SVT dataset.

Datsets	ICDAR03 (Full)	ICDAR03 (50)	ICDAR11 (Full)	ICDAR11 (50)	SVT
MRF [5]	0.67	0.69	-	-	-
IR [7]	0.75	0.77	-	-	-
NESP [6]	0.66	-	0.73	-	
PLEX [16]	0.62	0.76	-	-	0.57
HOG + CRF [10]	-	0.82	-	-	0.73
PBS [9]	0.79	0.87	0.83	0.87	0.74
WFST [11]	0.83	-	0.56	-	0.73
CNN [14]	0.84	0.90	-	-	0.70
Proposed	**0.82**	**0.92**	**0.83**	**0.91**	**0.83**

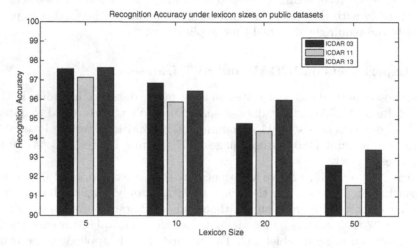

Fig. 5. Recognition accuracy of our proposed method on ICDAR 03, ICDAR 11 and ICDAR 13 datasets when the lexicon size is different.

Table 1 shows word recognition accuracy of the proposed technique and the compared techniques. The text segmentation methods (MRF, IR, and NESP) produce lower recognition accuracy than other methods because robust and accurate scene text segmentation by itself is an very challenging task. Our proposed method produce good recognition results on all the testing datasets. Especially in the SVT data set, our proposed method achieves 83 % word recognition accuracy, which outperforms the state-of-the-art methods significantly. The deep learning technique using convolutional neural network [14] also produces good performances but it requires a much larger training dataset together with a portion of synthetic data which are not available to the public.

We also tested our proposed method on the ICDAR 2011 and 2013 word recognition dataset for Born-Digital Images (Web and Email). It achieves 92 % and 94 % recognition accuracies, respectively, which clearly outperforms other methods as listed on the competition websites (with best recognition accuracy at 82.9 %[5] and 82.21 %[6], respectively). The much higher recognition accuracy also demonstrates the robustness and effectiveness of our proposed word image recognition system.

In addition, the correlation between lexicon size and word recognition accuracy of our proposed method is investigated. Figure 5 shows the experimental results based on the ICDAR03, ICDAR11, and ICDAR13 datasets. In addition, four lexicon sizes are tested that consist of 5, 10, 20, and 50 words, respectively. As illustrated in Fig. 5, the word recognition performance can actually be further improved when some prior knowledge is incorporated and the lexicon size is reduced.

We further apply our proposed method on the recent ICDAR 2013 Rubust Text Reading Competetion dataset [3][7], where 22 algorithms from 13 different research groups have been submitted and evaluated under the same criteria. The data of ICDAR 2013 is a actually subset of ICDAR 2011 dataset where a small number of duplicated images are removed.

The winning PhotoOCR method [8] makes use of a large multi-layer deep neural network and obtains 83 % accuracy on the testing dataset. As a comparison, our proposed method achieved 84 % recognition accuracy. Note that our proposed method incorporates a lexicon with around 1000 words, whereas PhotoOCR method does not use lexicon. The lexicon is generated by including all the ground truth words of ICDAR 2013 test dataset. On the other hand, the PhotoOCR method uses a huge amount of training data that consists of more than five million word images (which are not available to the public).

6.3 Discussion

In our proposed system, we assume that the cropped words are more or less horizontal. This is true in most of the real world cases. However, it might fail when texts in scenes are severely curved or suffer from severe perspective distortion as illustrated in Fig. 6. It partially explains the lower recognition accuracy on SVT dataset, which consists of a certain amount of severely perspectively distorted word images. In addition, the SVT dataset is generated from the Google Street View and so consists of a large amount of difficult images such as shop names, street names, etc. In addition, the proposed technique could fail when the word image has a low resolution or inaccurate text bounding boxes are detected as illustrated in Fig. 6. We will investigate these two issues in our future study.

With a very limited set of training data, our proposed method produces much higher recognition accuracy than the state-of-the-art methods as illustrated in Table 1. The PhotoOCR reports a better word recognition accuracy (90 %) on SVT dataset. The better accuracy is largely due to the usage of a huge amount of training data that is not available to the public. As a comparison, our proposed

---

[5] ICDAR 2011: http://www.cvc.uab.es/icdar2011competition/.

[6] ICDAR 2013: http://dag.cvc.uab.es/icdar2013competition/.

[7] http://dag.cvc.uab.es/icdar2013competition.

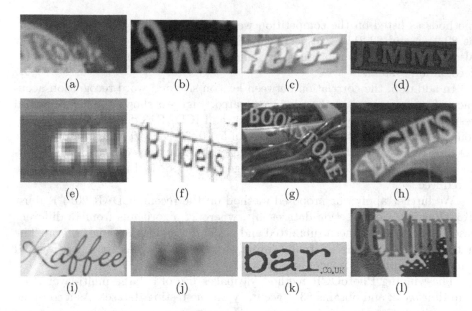

Fig. 6. Examples of falsely recognized word images

method is better in terms of training data size, training time, and computational costs. More importantly, our proposed model is trained by using the publicly available datasets, which provides a benchmarking baseline for the future scene text recognition techniques.

7   Conclusion

Word recognition under unconstrained condition is a difficult task and has attracted increasing research interest in recent years. Many methods have been reported to address this problem. However, there still exists a large gap for computer understanding of texts in natural scene. This paper presents a novel scene text recognition system that makes use of the HOG feature and RNN model.

Compared with state-of-the-art techniques, our proposed method is able to recognize the whole word images without segmentation. It works by integrating two key components. First, it converts a word image into a sequential feature vector and so requires no character-level segmentation and recognition. Second, the RNN is introduced and exploited to classify the sequential column feature vectors into word accurately. Experiments on several public datasets show that the proposed technique obtains superior word recognition accuracy. In addition, the proposed technique is trained and tested over several publicly available datasets which forms a good baseline for future benchmarking of other new scene text recognition techniques.

References

1. Lucas, S.M., Panaretos, A., Sosa, L., Tang, A., Wong, S., Young, R.: ICDAR 2003 robust reading competitions. In: 2003 International Conference on Document Analysis and Recognition (ICDAR), pp. 682–687 (2003)
2. Shahab, A., Shafait, F., Dengel, A.: ICDAR 2011 robust reading competition challenge 2: Reading text in scene images. In: Proceedings of the 2011 International Conference on Document Analysis and Recognition, ICDAR 2011, pp. 1491–1496 (2011)
3. Karatzas, D., Shafait, F., Uchida, S., Iwamura, M., Gomez i Bigorda, L., Robles Mestre, S., Mas, J., Fernandez Mota, D., Almazan Almazan, J., de las Heras, L.P.: ICDAR 2013 robust reading competition. In: 2013 12th International Conference on Document Analysis and Recognition (ICDAR), pp. 1484–1493 (2013)
4. Wang, K., Belongie, S.: Word spotting in the wild. In: Daniilidis, K., Maragos, P., Paragios, N. (eds.) ECCV 2010, Part I. LNCS, vol. 6311, pp. 591–604. Springer, Heidelberg (2010)
5. Mishra, A., Alahari, K., Jawahar, C.V.: An MRF model for binarization of natural scene text. In: 2011 11th International Conference on Document Analysis and Recognition (ICDAR), pp. 11–16 (2011)
6. Kumar, D., Anil Prasad, M.N., Ramakrishnan, A.G.: Nesp: Nonlinear enhancement and selection of plane for optimal segmentation and recognition of scene word images. In: Proceedings of SPIE, vol. 8658 (2013)
7. Zhou, Y., Feild, J., Learned-Miller, E., Wang, R.: Scene text segmentation via inverse rendering. In: 2013 12th International Conference on Document Analysis and Recognition (ICDAR), pp. 457–461 (2013)
8. Bissacco, A., Cummins, M., Netzer, Y., Neven, H.: PhotoOCR: Reading text in uncontrolled conditions. In: 2013 IEEE International Conference on Computer Vision (ICCV) (2013)
9. Shi, C., Wang, C., Xiao, B., Zhang, Y., Gao, S., Zhang, Z.: Scene text recognition using part-based tree-structured character detection. In: 2013 IEEE Conference on Computer Vision and Pattern Recognition (CVPR), pp. 2961–2968 (2013)
10. Mishra, A., Alahari, K., Jawahar, C.: Top-down and bottom-up cues for scene text recognition. In: 2012 IEEE Conference on Computer Vision and Pattern Recognition (CVPR), pp. 2687–2694 (2012)
11. Novikova, T., Barinova, O., Kohli, P., Lempitsky, V.: Large-lexicon attribute-consistent text recognition in natural images. In: Fitzgibbon, A., Lazebnik, S., Perona, P., Sato, Y., Schmid, C. (eds.) ECCV 2012, Part VI. LNCS, vol. 7577, pp. 752–765. Springer, Heidelberg (2012)
12. Graves, A., Schmidhuber, J.: Framewise phoneme classification with bidirectional lstm and other neural network architectures. Neural Netw. 18, 602–610 (2005)
13. Graves, A., Liwicki, M., Fernandez, S., Bertolami, R., Bunke, H., Schmidhuber, J.: A novel connectionist system for unconstrained handwriting recognition. IEEE Trans. Pattern Anal. Mach. Intell. 31, 855–868 (2009)
14. Wang, T., Wu, D., Coates, A., Ng, A.: End-to-end text recognition with convolutional neural networks. In: 2012 21st International Conference on Pattern Recognition (ICPR), pp. 3304–3308 (2012)
15. Dalal, N., Triggs, B.: Histograms of oriented gradients for human detection. In: IEEE Computer Society Conference on Computer Vision and Pattern Recognition, 2005, CVPR 2005, vol. 1, pp. 886–893 (2005)

16. Wang, K., Babenko, B., Belongie, S.: End-to-end scene text recognition. In: 2011 IEEE International Conference on Computer Vision (ICCV), pp. 1457–1464 (2011)

17. Tian, S., Lu, S., Su, B., Tan, C.L.: Scene text recognition using co-occurrence of histogram of oriented gradients. In: 2013 12th International Conference on Document Analysis and Recognition (ICDAR), pp. 912–916 (2013)

18. Epshtein, B., Ofek, E., Wexler, Y.: Detecting text in natural scenes with stroke width transform. In: 2010 IEEE Conference on Computer Vision and Pattern Recognition (CVPR), pp. 2963–2970 (2010)

19. Yao, C., Bai, X., Liu, W., Ma, Y., Tu, Z.: Detecting texts of arbitrary orientations in natural images. In: 2012 IEEE Conference on Computer Vision and Pattern Recognition (CVPR), pp. 1083–1090 (2012)

20. Neumann, L., Matas, J.: Real-time scene text localization and recognition. In: 2012 IEEE Conference on Computer Vision and Pattern Recognition (CVPR), pp. 3538–3545 (2012)

21. Phan, T.Q., Shivakumara, P., Tian, S., Tan, C.L.: Recognizing text with perspective distortion in natural scenes. In: 2013 IEEE International Conference on Computer Vision (ICCV) (2013)

22. Coates, A., Carpenter, B., Case, C., Satheesh, S., Suresh, B., Wang, T., Wu, D., Ng, A.: Text detection and character recognition in scene images with unsupervised feature learning. In: 2011 International Conference on Document Analysis and Recognition (ICDAR), pp. 440–445 (2011)

23. Hochreiter, S., Schmidhuber, J.: Long short-term memory. Neural Comput. **9**, 1735–1780 (1997)

24. Gers, F.A., Schmidhuber, J.A., Cummins, F.A.: Learning to forget: Continual prediction with lstm. Neural Comput. **12**, 2451–2471 (2000)

25. Zhang, X., Tan, C.: Segmentation-free keyword spotting for handwritten documents based on heat kernel signature. In: 2013 12th International Conference on Document Analysis and Recognition (ICDAR), pp. 827–831 (2013)

26. Graves, A.: Rnnlib: A recurrent neural network library for sequence learning problems. (http://sourceforge.net/projects/rnnl/)

27. de Campos, T.E., Babu, B.R., Varma, M.: Character recognition in natural images. In: Proceedings of the International Conference on Computer Vision Theory and Applications (2009)

Massive City-Scale Surface Condition Analysis Using Ground and Aerial Imagery

Ken Sakurada[1]($\boxtimes$), Takayuki Okatani[1], and Kris M. Kitani[2]

[1] Tohoku University, Sendai, Japan
{sakurada,okatani}@vision.is.tohoku.ac.jp
[2] Carnegie Mellon University, Pittsburgh, USA
kkitani@cs.cmu.edu

Abstract. Automated visual analysis is an effective method for under-standing changes in natural phenomena over massive city-scale land-scapes. However, the view-point spectrum across which image data can be acquired is extremely wide, ranging from macro-level overhead (aerial) images spanning several kilometers to micro-level front-parallel (street-view) images that might only span a few meters. This work presents a unified framework for robustly integrating image data taken at vastly different viewpoints to generate large-scale estimates of land surface con-ditions. To validate our approach we attempt to estimate the amount of post-Tsunami damage over the entire city of Kamaishi, Japan (over 4 million square-meters). Our results show that our approach can effi-ciently integrate both micro and macro-level images, along with other forms of meta-data, to efficiently estimate city-scale phenomena. We eval-uate our approach on two modes of land condition analysis, namely, city-scale debris and greenery estimation, to show the ability of our method to generalize to a diverse set of estimation tasks.

1 Introduction

We address the task of estimating large-scale land surface conditions using over-head aerial (macro-level) images and street view (micro-level) images. These two types of images are captured from orthogonal viewpoints and have different res-olutions, thus conveying very different types of information that can be used in a complementary way. Moreover, their integration is necessary to make it possible to accurately understand changes in natural phenomena over massive city-scale landscapes.

Aerial images are an excellent source for collecting wide-area information of land surface conditions. However, it may come at the cost of a lower resolution (i.e., number of pixels per meter) and visiblity may drastically change depending on the weather. For example, clouds may obscure the visibility of the land surface (Fig. 1). A more important limitation of aerial images is that they are limited to

---

Electronic supplementary material The online version of this chapter (doi:10. 1007/978-3-319-16865-4_4) contains supplementary material, which is available to authorized users. Videos can also be accessed at http://www.springerimages.com/ videos/978-3-319-16864-7.

© Springer International Publishing Switzerland 2015
D. Cremers et al. (Eds.): ACCV 2014, Part I, LNCS 9003, pp. 49–64, 2015.
DOI: 10.1007/978-3-319-16865-4_4

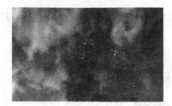 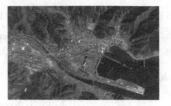

Fig. 1. Aerial images affected by weather condition (Left: March 11, 2011, Right: March 31, 2011). The land surface might be covered by clouds and illumination conditions change drastically in aerial image.

a vertical (top-down) perspective of the ground surface, such that areas occluded by a roof or highway overpass are not visible to the camera (first and second row of Fig. 2) making it difficult to estimate land conditions in covered areas.

Street-view images, on the other hand, captured from the ground-level can obtain higher resolution images of vertical structures and have better access to information about covered areas. They are also less affected by weather conditions. In the same token however, street view images are constrained to the ground plane and a single image has limited physical range. It is also labor intensive to acquire street-level images of large land surface areas (i.e., millions of square meters).

The key technical challenge is devising a method to integrate these two disparate types of image data in an effective manner, while leveraging the wide coverage capabilities of macro-level images and detailed resolution of micro-level images. The strategy proposed in the work uses macro-level imaging to learn land condition correspondences between land regions that share similar visual characteristics (e.g., mountains, streets, buildings, rivers), while micro-level images are used to acquire high resolution statistics of land conditions (e.g., the amount of debris on the ground). By combining the macro and micro level information about region correspondences and surface conditions, our proposed method generates detailed estimates of land surface conditions over the entire city.

The technical contribution of this paper is a novel procedure for generalizing from a sparse set of visual recognition results to a large-scale land condition regression estimate. The proposed system carefully brings together the state-of-the-art algorithms for semantic scene understanding, structure-from-motion and non-parametric regression to generate a massive city-scale land condition probability map (Fig. 3). To the best of our knowledge, this is the first work of its kind to use sparse image-based street-level object recognition results to extrapolate the surface conditions of an entire city (over 4 million square meters).

Although our method can generalize to different types of large-scale phenomena, we ground our proposed approach in a real-world application of post-Tsunami city-scale damage estimation. In regions affected by such disasters, it is extremely hard to efficiently assess the large-scale impact of a natural disaster. Technologies that enable fast and efficient city-scale estimates of damage can be extremely helpful for expediting aid to seriously damages areas. The approach describe in this paper can also be used for long-term analysis by monitoring and tracking recovery efforts.

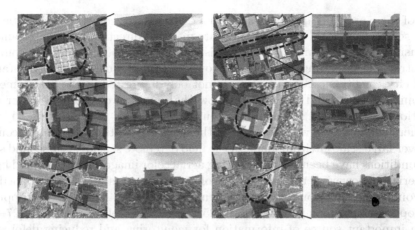

Fig. 2. Example aerial and street-view images. There are many cases in which aerial images and street-view images give complementary information about the land surface condition. For example, the areas covered by the building roof (the top and second row), stacked objects (the bottom row) are best viewed from the street.

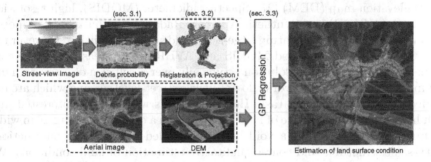

Fig. 3. Data flow diagram of city-scale estimation of land surface condition. Our approach efficiently integrates both micro (street-view) and macro-level (aerial) images along with other forms of meta-data to estimate city-scale land surface condition.

2   Related Work

There has been significant advances in the state-of-the-art techniques for quantitative geometric interpretations of large-scale city scenes. Methods for city-scale 3D reconstruction have been proposed using thousands of images gathered from Internet images [1,2]. Similar techniques have been proposed for images captured by a vehicle-mounted camera [3,4] or aerial images [5–7]. Street-view images have also been combined with aerial images for the purpose of improving 3D reconstruction, where 3D point clouds have been projected to the ground plane and aligned with edges of buildings detected from aerial images [8] or building maps [9]. There has also been work using aerial and street view images taken several months or decades apart [10–14] to understand temporal changes of a scene. The focus of these previous approaches are on a quantitative geometric interpretation of the scene where local visual features are matched directly to estimate camera pose using epipolar geometry [15]. In this work we aim to push beyond a purely geometric understanding of the scene towards a more qualitative understanding of city conditions. For instance, we not only interested in the 3D geometry of a building but would also like to know the condition of the building or the condition of the ground surrounding a building.

There also has been work focused on the qualitative estimation of land condition over large-scale environments. In the field of remote sensing, coarse land surface conditions have been estimated using aerial color images, aerial infrared light and aerial microwave sensing [16–21]. Color aerial images have been applied to land condition estimation for vegetation monitoring [22–24], land cover mapping, and flood risk and damage assessment [25,26]. For example, forest maps [27–29] are an important source of information for monitoring and reducing deforestation, allowing environmental scientists to know how forested areas increase or decrease in over the entire earth.

Apart from aerial imaging using color cameras, many other modes of sensing have been proposed for estimating coarse large-scale land surface conditions. Digital elevation map (DEM) [27], Spectroradiometer (MODIS), high resolution radiometer (AVHRR) and Synthetic Aperture Radar (SAR) have been proposed to improve accuracy of estimating large-scale land surface condition. However the resolution of satellite-mounted MODIS and AVHRR only measure surface conditions over a very rough resolution – typically over a cell size of a several hundred meters. As such, these works do not utilize street-level sensing which are too detailed for their estimation task. However, in this work we are interested in a much high resolution estimate of land conditions on a cell size closer to 20 m wide.

Our proposed work fills a void between detailed geometric reconstructions of city-scale structures and coarse qualitative estimation of land conditions. We use known techniques to provide an accurate geometric model of the city and use state-of-the-art object recognition results carefully registered to the scene geometry to understand the qualitative conditions of the entire city.

3   Large-Scale Estimation of Land Surface Condition

Our framework integrates aerial and street-view images to estimate land surface conditions. In this section, we explain the details of the proposed method contextualized for post-Tsunami debris detection. Although the following explanation takes debris as an example, the method is generally applicable to other types of land surface conditions. The proposed method consists of the following three steps;

(i) Debris detection on perspective street-view image. (Sect. 3.1)
(ii) Projection of debris probabilities on street-view images to the ground using building contours. (Sect. 3.2)
(iii) Estimation of debris over an entire city by integrating the projection result with all other data (e.g. aerial image, DEM) using a Gaussian process. (Sect. 3.3)

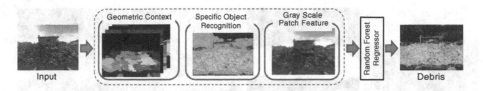

Fig. 4. Data flow diagram of debris detection. As features of debris, the probabilities of geometric context, specific object recognition and patch features are employed.

In the first step, the probability map of debris is calculated for each street-view image. Then, using the camera parameters for the street-view image, the probability map is projected onto the ground plane registered to a corresponding part of the aerial image. This projection method takes the existence of building walls into consideration. Finally in order to complement the estimation results obtained from street-view images, the projected probability map is integrated with the information obtained from aerial images and DEM using Gaussian process regression model.

3.1 Debris Detection

We developed a method to calculate the probability map of debris (Fig. 4). The debris model is learned from a hand-labeled training image. The debris in the images are irregular, complicated in shape and appearance. Therefore, we exploit Geometric Context [30] as geometric feature and pixel-wise object probability [31] as an appearance feature. Geometric Context estimates the probabilities that a super-pixel belongs to seven classes. We chose four of the seven classes, "ground plane", "sky", "porous non-planar" and "solid non-planar", and used the probabilities of them as debris features. The pixel-wise object probability p_{object} is calculated using [31], Lab, HOG [32], BRIEF [33] and ORB [34]. The feature vector of debris is as follows.

$$\mathbf{x} = (p_{ground}, p_{sky}, p_{porous}, p_{solid}, p_{object}, m_{patch}, v_{patch})^{T}, \qquad (1)$$

where p_{ground}, p_{sky}, p_{porous} and p_{solid} are the probabilities of "ground plane", "sky", "porous non-planar" and "solid non-planar", respectively. In addition to these probabilities, mean m_{patch} and variance v_{patch} of grayscale patch (5×5) are added to the features.

We evaluated the accuracy of our debris detector. We made two datasets for the evaluation. Figure 5 shows an example of the datasets and detection results. Each dataset consists of fifty images of debris. The images in two data set were taken in different date and time. We compared random forest [35], logistic regression [36] and support vector machine [37]. Figure 6 shows the F_1-scores of the debris detections. We chose the random forest as our debris detector for all experiments because the score of random forest regressor is the best.

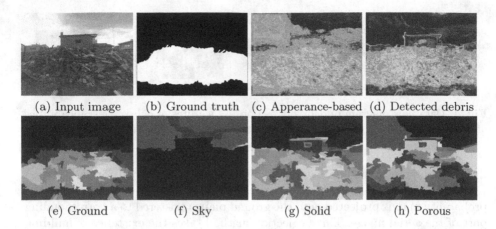

(a) Input image   (b) Ground truth   (c) Apperance-based   (d) Detected debris

(e) Ground   (f) Sky   (g) Solid   (h) Porous

Fig. 5. Inputs and outputs of debris detection. First rows: (a) input image. (b) hand-labeled ground truth of debris. (c) result of specific object recognition. (d) final result of debris detection. Second rows: probability of geometric context (e) ground plane, (f) sky, (g) solid non-planar, (h) porous non-planar. Color denotes probability of each class, with blue corresponding to 0 and red to 1 (Color figure online).

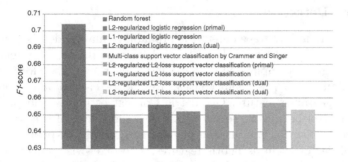

Fig. 6. F_1-score of debris detection.

3.2   Projection of Debris Probabilities onto the Ground

The debris probability explained in the previous section is the probability map on the street-view image. In order to integrate this probability map with the aerial image, the debris probability is projected onto the ground plane. Figure 7 shows the data flow diagram of projection of street-view image to the coordinate of the aerial image. The projection requires camera parameters of each street-view image. First, we performed Structure from Motion (SfM) to acquire the camera trajectories. We employ a standard SfM method [15,38,39] with extensions to deal with omni-directional images [4]. The estimated camera trajectories are fitted to the GPS trajectory by similarity transformations in a least squares sense.

Dividing the ground plane into a grid, we project the debris probability to the grid using projection matrix of each image. In this projection, we use the 3D models of the buildings that are generated from a 2D map of the city (Sect. 4.2).

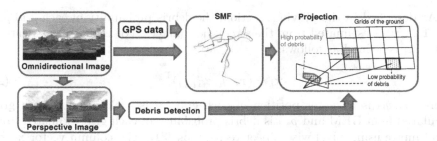

Fig. 7. Data flow diagram of the projection onto the ground plane. SfM is performed using omnidirectional street-view images. The street-view camera poses are registered to a common coordinate with aerial images and other forms of meta-data using the GPS data. After debris detection, the debris probabilities are projected to the ground plane.

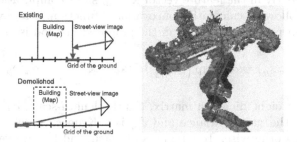

Fig. 8. Projection of probabilities on street-view images to the grids of the ground plane using building information. Left: The probabilities on a street-view image are projected to a building wall if the building is on the projection path, otherwise it is projected to the ground directly. Right: Example of projection results (top-view). The area unobserved from street-view images is shown in white.

To be specific, the debris probability is projected to a building wall if the wall is on the projection path, and otherwise it is directly projected to the ground, as shown in Fig. 8.

3.3   Integration Using Gaussian Process Regression

The projected debris probability map obtained up to now has no information for some areas because of occlusions or the lack of street-level images, as shown in Fig. 8. Estimating debris probability map from only an aerial image is difficult due to its low-resolution, occlusion or weather conditions. To mutually complement the street-view images and the aerial image, we used a Gaussian process regression model [40]. The main idea here is that similar geographical location tend to have similar debris probability. In the case of Tsunami-disaster, Tsunami continuously spreads from seashore to hill side, which means the damage caused by Tsunami has strong correlation with the location, especially with the elevation.

As described in the previous section, the debris probability of each grid $p_{s,i}$ ($i = 1, ..., n$) is estimated from the street-view images. For each grid, its feature vector $\mathbf{x}_i$ is defined as follows.

$$\mathbf{x}_i = (x_i, y_i, z_i, p_{a,i})^{\mathrm{T}} \tag{2}$$

where (x_i, y_i) is a center position of each grid, z_i is a elevation of each grid calculated from DEM and $p_{a,i}$ is debris probability of each grid estimated from aerial image using pixel-wise object recognition [31]. The column vector $\mathbf{x}_i$ for all n grid are aggregated in the $4 \times n$ training inputs matrix X, and the training outputs $p_{s,i}$ are collected in the vector $\mathbf{y}$.

$\mathbf{x}_i$ contains $p_{a,i}$ as the visual feature of the ith grid. Although $p_{a,i}$ is a scalar, due to the pixel-wise object recognition [31], it summarizes the visual information of the ith grid. Compared to using general visual feature descriptors, such as SIFT [38], directly in the feature vector $\mathbf{x}_i$, $p_{a,i}$ saves computational resources required in the following calculation of covariance function. The covariance function for Gaussian process regression in the proposed method is as follows.

$$k(\mathbf{x}_p, \mathbf{x}_q) = \sigma_f^2 \exp\left(-\frac{1}{2l^2} |W(\mathbf{x}_p - \mathbf{x}_q)|^2\right) + \sigma_n^2 \delta_{pq} \tag{3}$$

where W is the weight diagonal matrix, l is the length-scale, σ_f^2 is the signal variance, σ_n^2 is the noise variance and δ_{pq} is a Kronecker delta which is one if $p = q$ and zero otherwise. Test input $\mathbf{x}_\star$ is each grid feature vector and test output is debris probability of each grid $\overline{f}_\star$.

The key insight to note here is that the output of the aerial image regressor $p_{a,i}$ enforces a correlation between parts of the scene that look similar. If two parts of the scene belong to an open field, the per-pixel response of the aerial object detection regressor will produce a similar response. The DEM also works in a similar manner to draw correlations between regions with similar elevation. The location feature enforces local smoothness over the final estimate of debris over the city. When the feature vectors $\mathbf{x}_i$ are used to compute the covariance function, regions that are similar in appearance and elevation will be constrained to have similar target values (debris estimates generated by high resolution debris regressor computed on the street images). In this way, the Gaussian process regression model is able to propagate local estimates of debris to the entire map. This regression mechanism is what allows our model to effectively estimate debris over the entire city from only a sparse set of street view debris estimation results.

4   Experimental Results

In order to evaluate the effectiveness of our proposed approach for estimating large-scale land conditions, we perform two experiments. Our first experiment is a comprehensive ablative analysis to examine the benefit of integrating micro and macro-level imagery for city-scale land condition estimation. In addition to color imaging, we also evaluate the contributions of two other modes of data,

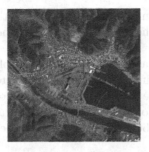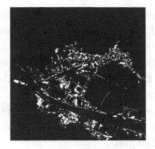

Fig. 9. Estimation target area in Kamaishi on March 31st, 2011 (left) and its hand-labeled ground truth of debris area (right). White area shows debris area.

namely, a digital elevation map (DEM) and building occupancy maps (BOM). In our second experiment, we focus on estimating the amount of greenery and vegetation across the entire city of Kamaishi. We use the exact same approach as the debris estimation described in this paper and apply it to greenery estimation. Our results show that our approach is not limited to post-disaster analysis but can easily be applied to other modes of land condition analysis.

We created the ground truth labels used for the following evaluation by many hours of manual labeling of regions on the aerial images. Ground truth data of debris and greenery were generated by visual inspection by comparing the aerial image against the street-view images available on Google Earth. Many hours of ground truth labeling confirms that the manual inspection of large-scale land conditions is not a practical solution for real-world applications.

4.1 Our Data

Our experiment includes two image-based input modalities and two sources of city-scale meta-data, which are described below.

Street Images. We have been creating image archives of urban and residential areas damaged by Great East Japan Earthquake in 2011. The target area is 500 km long along the northern-east coastal line in Japan. The images were captured every three to four months by a vehicle having an omni-directional camera (Ladybug 3 and 5 of Point Grey Research Inc.) on its roof. The image data accumulated so far amount to about 20 terabytes. The target of this experiment is the entire city of Kamaishi, Japan (over 4 million square-meters). For the experiments, we chose the two image sequences captured on April 26th, 2011 (one month after the Tsunami) and August 17th, 2013 (two years and five months after the Tsunami). The debris can often be seen in the earlier images, while they tend to disappear in the later images as the recovery operation proceeds.

The street images are used for appearance-based recognition of 'stuff' [41] described in Sect. 3.1. The results of pixel-wise regression are then projected onto the ground plane as an input feature for our city-scale GP regressor.

Aerial Images. We downloaded aerial images from Google Earth for March 31st, 2011 and May 13th, 2012. We chose these dates to match up the timestamp of the street images.

We used the aerial images for appearance-based recognition of 'stuff' categories using the same method describe in Sect. 3.1 but applied to the entire aerial image as a comparative baseline. We used the aerial images of May 13th, 2012 as the labeled training data and test on the March 31st, 2011 aerial image. Figure 9 shows an example of the hand-labeled ground truth of the debris area on the aerial images.

Digital Elevation Map (DEM). We obtained the DEM information freely available from the Geospatial Information Authority, under the Ministry of Land, Infrastructure, Transportation and Tourism in Japan. The mesh resolution of the DEM is 5 × 5 square-meters and contains the elevation level for each grid location. The elevation is used directly as a feature for the city-scale GP regression.

Building Occupancy Map (BOM). The BOM provides building contours. We obtained the data from Zenrin Company. The building contour data used for this experiment was made before the earthquake. We used the BOM to prevent 'stuff' from being projected onto the ground over building location.

4.2   Ablative Analysis

We examine the effects of each input data type on the overall performance of our proposed approach. Figure 10 shows the estimation results of the debris amounts in the entire city on April 26th, 2011 and August 17th, 2013, respectively. The lines on the aerial images are the camera trajectories. Figure 11 shows the performance of our debris detection by PR-plot and F1-score using different combination of

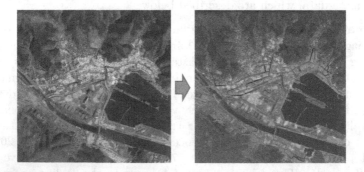

Fig. 10. City-scale **Debris** Probability in Kamaishi before and after the recovery operation (Left: April 26th, 2011, Right: August 17th, 2013). In the earlier images, there are much debris in the entire city, however, most of them have been cleaned up in later images. The city-scale temporal change is estimated and visualized accurately by our approach. Color denotes probability of debris, with blue corresponding to 0 and red to 1 (Color figure online).

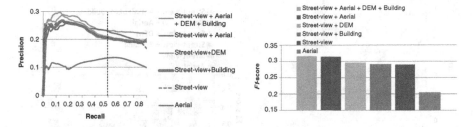

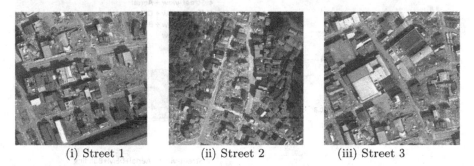

Fig. 11. Precision-recall curve of the debris area detection whose ground truth is Fig. 9. These figures show that the integration of street-view image with aerial image is efficient to estimate city-scale land surface condition.

(i) Street 1   (ii) Street 2   (iii) Street 3

Fig. 12. Target streets of the evaluation of each input data type and different number of street-view images in our proposed approach.

input data. The results indicate that using aerial images alone yields low performance because the appearance of land conditions can change significantly over time due to changes in imaging conditions. When compared to the independent use of aerial images, our results indicate that street images are more accurate for estimating city-scale debris. Furthermore, when both aerial and street images are combined we obtain better performance as the aerial information helps the city-scale GP regression to generalize to across similar looking city regions.

Additionally, we evaluated the effects of each input data type and different number of street-view images in three different streets. Figures 12 (i)–(iii) show input aerial images of target areas. Figure 13 shows precision-recall curve (Left) and $F1$-scores (Right, recall=0.5) of the debris area detection. We examined the detection performance for a specific area. The effect of different input type is different depending on the area-condition. For example, aerial image could cause errors in occluded areas we mentioned in the introduction, and DEM information could cause errors because its elevation includes height of building. However, street-view images basically provide detailed and accurate information of land-surface condition.

We also tested the effect of street coverage. Figure 14 shows the $F1$-score of different number of street-view images. In this experiment, we randomly sampled street-view images. The accuracy improves as we add more images, but it quickly saturates. This indicates our algorithm needs only sparse street-view images. The

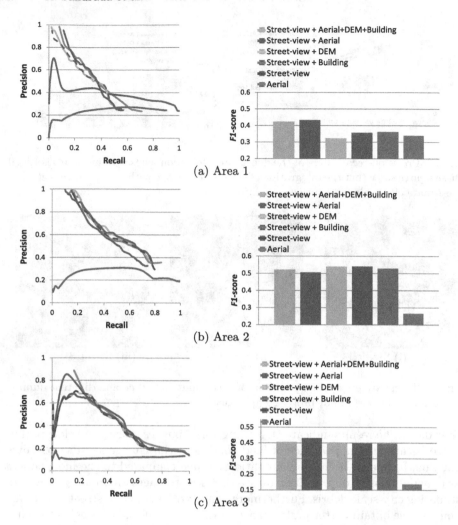

Fig. 13. Precision-recall curve (Left) and F1-scores (Right, recall=0.5) of the debris-area detection. These plots show that the integration of street-view image with aerial image is effective to estimate the condition of land surface.

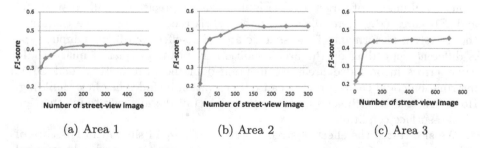

Fig. 14. F1-scores of different number of street-view images. Our algorithm does not require large number of images.

sparse sampling requirement of our algorithm is beneficial in many other applications, for example, large scale citizen science or journalism in which images captured at the scene are sent to cloud computers to analyze city scale condition.

4.3 Extensions to City-Scale Vegetation Estimation

We applied our method to vegetation detection, to show how our approach can generalize to other modes of land condition estimation. Figure 15 shows an example of vegetation estimation in street-level images. The green vegetation detected in the street-view images is estimated using the same pixel-wise object recognition method [31].

Figure 16 shows the results of vegetation estimation for the entire city. By observing the vegetation heat map for the entire city, it is clear that most of the vegetation has been washed away by the Tsunami. There is also a sharp contrast between the wide spread distribution of debris and the lack of vegetation in the time period directly after the Tsunami. By 2013 however, we can see a

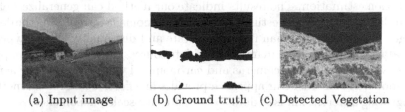

(a) Input image   (b) Ground truth   (c) Detected Vegetation

Fig. 15. Green vegetation detection. (a) input image. (b) hand-labeled ground truth of green vegetation. (c) probability of green vegetation. Color denotes probability of green vegetation, with blue corresponding to 0 and red to 1 (Color figure online).

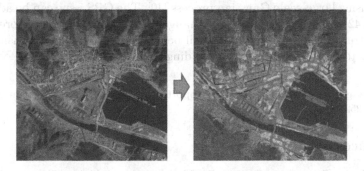

Fig. 16. City-Scale **Vegetation** Probability in Kamaishi before and after the recovery operation (Left: April 26, 2011, Right: August 17, 2013). In contradiction to the debris (Fig. 10), there was no green vegetation due to Tsunami-damage in April, 2011, however, the vegetation in entire city has grown and recovered until August, 2013. Our approach can estimate and visualize such changes in natural phenomena over massive city-scale landscapes. Color denotes probability of green vegetation, with blue corresponding to 0 and red to 1 (Color figure online).

large increase in the number of regions covered by vegetation. Our successful vegetation detection indicates that our proposed method can indeed generalize to different types of targeted estimation of city-scale land conditions.

5   Conclusion

We presented a unified framework for robustly integrating image data taken at vastly different viewpoints to generate large-scale estimates of land surface conditions. The proposed strategy uses macro-level imaging to learn land condition correspondences between land regions that share similar visual characteristics, while micro-level images are used to acquire high resolution statistics of land conditions. For the validation of our approach, we conducted experiments to estimate the amount of post-Tsunami damage over the entire city of Kamaishi, Japan. The experimental results show that our approach can effectively integrate both macro (aerial) and micro-level (street view) images, along with other forms of meta-data, to estimate city-scale phenomena.

Furthermore, we showed that our detection method can be successfully applied to vegetation estimation. The results indicate our method can generalize well to many kinds of applications to estimate city-scale phenomena by replacing the detector target, for example, human flow, real-estate and dirt quality. These types of image data are available from many kinds of data sources, such as camera equipped mobile devices, surveillance cameras and car-mounted video recorders, or aerial-vehicle-mounted cameras. Our approach provides an effective and robust method for integrating different kinds of data to estimate city-scale phenomena.

For future work, we plan to improve the estimation accuracy of our approach. Our method has relatively low absolute precision because (i) the grid size is too large due to limitation of computational resources and (ii) the estimated camera poses have errors due to GPS errors. We believe that we can solve the first problem using large-scale Gaussian process [40]. The GPS issue can be addressed with [8,9,42] while taking temporal changes into account. Furthermore, in the case of extreme calamities, methods will be developed to take into consideration the complete disappearance of the buildings due to disasters.

Acknowledgements. This work was supported by JSPS KAKENHI Grant Numbers 25135701, 25280054.

References

1. Snavely, N., Seitz, S.M., Szeliski, R.: Modeling the world from internet photo collections. IJCV **80**, 189–210 (2007)
2. Agarwal, S., Snavely, N., Simon, I., Seitz, S.M., Szeliski, R.: Building Rome in a day. In: ICCV, pp. 72–79 (2009)
3. Pollefeys, M., Nistér, D., Frahm, J.M., Akbarzadeh, A., Mordohai, P., Clipp, B., Engels, C., Gallup, D., Kim, S.J., Merrell, P., Salmi, C., Sinha, S., Talton, B., Wang, L., Yang, Q., Stewénius, H., Yang, R., Welch, G., Towles, H.: Detailed real-time urban 3D reconstruction from video. IJCV **78**, 143–167 (2008)

4. Torii, A., Havlena, M., Pajdla, T.: From google street view to 3D city models. In: ICCV Workshops, pp. 2188–2195 (2009)
5. Lin, C., Nevatia, R.: Building detection and description from a single intensity image. Comput. Vis. Image Underst. **72**, 101–121 (1998)
6. Suveg, I., Vosselman, G.: Reconstruction of 3D building models from aerial images and maps. ISPRS J. Photogram. Remote Sens. **58**, 202–224 (2004)
7. Zebedin, L., Klaus, A., Gruber-Geymayer, B., Karner, K.: Towards 3D map generation from digital aerial images. ISPRS J. Photogram. Remote Sens. **60**, 413–427 (2006)
8. Kaminsky, R., Snavely, N., Seitz, S., Szeliski, R.: Alignment of 3D point clouds to overhead images. In: CVPR Workshops, pp. 63–70 (2009)
9. Strecha, C., Pylvanainen, T., Fua, P.: Dynamic and scalable large scale image reconstruction. In: CVPR, pp. 406–413 (2010)
10. Huertas, A., Nevatia, R.: Detecting changes in aerial views of man-made structures. In: ICCV, pp. 73–80 (1998)
11. Radke, R.J., Andra, S., Al-Kofahi, O., Roysam, B.: Image change detection algorithms: a systematic survey. Trans. Image Proces. **14**, 294–307 (2005)
12. Pollard, T., Mundy, J.L.: Change detection in a 3-d world. In: CVPR, pp. 1–6 (2007)
13. Schindler, G., Dellaert, F.: Probabilistic temporal inference on reconstructed 3D scenes. In: CVPR, pp. 1410–1417 (2010)
14. Taneja, A., Ballan, L., Pollefeys, M.: City-scale change detection in cadastral 3D models using images. In: CVPR, pp. 113–120 (2013)
15. Hartley, R., Zisserman, A.: Multiple View Geometry in Computer Vision, 2nd edn. Cambridge University Press, Cambridge (2004)
16. Li, F., Jacksona, T.J., Kustasa, W.P., Schmuggea, T.J., Frenchb, A.N., Cosha, M.H., Bindlish, R.: Deriving land surface temperature from Landsat 5 and 7 during SMEX02/SMACEX. Remote Sens. Environ. **92**, 521–534 (2004)
17. Weng, Q., Lu, D., Schubring, J.: Estimation of land surface temperaturevegetation abundance relationship for urban heat island studies. Remote Sens. Environ. **89**, 467–483 (2004)
18. Schowengerdt, R.A.: Remote Sensing: Models and Methods for Image Processing. Academic Press, San Diego (2006)
19. Martinez, J., Letoan, T.: Mapping of flood dynamics and spatial distribution of vegetation in the Amazon floodplain using multitemporal SAR data. Remote Sens. Environ. **108**, 209–223 (2007)
20. Weng, Q.: Remote Sensing of Impervious Surfaces. CRC Press, Boca Raton (2010)
21. Lu, D., Hetrick, S., Moran, E.: Impervious surface mapping with quickbird imagery. Int. J. Remote Sens. **32**, 2519–2533 (2011)
22. Hall, A., Louis, J., Lamb, D.: Characterising and mapping vineyard canopy using high-spatial-resolution aerial multispectral images. Comput. Geosci. **29**, 813–822 (2003)
23. Berni, J.A.J., Member, S., Zarco-tejada, P.J., Suárez, L., Fereres, E.: Thermal and narrowband multispectral remote sensing for vegetation monitoring from an unmanned aerial vehicle. IEEE Trans. Geosci. Remote Sens. **47**, 722–738 (2009)
24. Delenne, C., Durrieu, S., Rabatel, G., Deshayes, M.: From pixel to vine parcel: a complete methodology for vineyard delineation and characterization using remote-sensing data. Comput. Electron. Agric. **70**, 78–83 (2010)
25. van der Sande, C., de Jong, S., de Roo, A.P.J.: A segmentation and classification approach of IKONOS-2 imagery for land cover mapping to assist flood risk and flood damage assessment. Int. J. Appl. Earth Obs. Geoinf. **4**, 217–229 (2003)

26. Herold, M., Liu, X., Clarke, K.C.: Spatial metrics and image texture for mapping urban land use. Photogram. Eng. Remote Sens. **69**, 991–1001 (2003)
27. Gong, P., Pu, R., Chen, J.: Mapping ecological land systems and classification uncertainties from digital elevation and forest-cover data using neural networks. Photogram. Eng. Remote Sens. **62**, 1249–1260 (1996)
28. Solberg, A.H.S.: Contextual data fusion applied to forest map revision. IEEE Trans. Geosci. Remote Sens. **37**, 1234–1243 (1999)
29. Hansen, M.C., Potapov, P.V., Moore, R., Hancher, M., Turubanova, S.A., Tyukavina, A., Thau, D., Stehman, S.V., Goetz, S.J., Loveland, T.R., Kommareddy, A., Egorov, A., Chini, L., Justice, C.O., Townshend, J.R.G.: High-resolution global maps of 21st-century forest cover change. Science **342**, 850–853 (2013)
30. Hoiem, D., Efros, A.A., Hebert, M.: Geometric context from a single image. In: ICCV, pp. 654–661 (2005)
31. Li, C., Kitani, K.M.: Pixel-level hand detection in ego-centric videos. In: CVPR, pp. 3570–3577 (2013)
32. Dalal, N., Triggs, B.: Histograms of oriented gradients for human detection. In: CVPR, pp. 886–893 (2005)
33. Calonder, M., Lepetit, V., Strecha, C., Fua, P.: BRIEF: binary robust independent elementary features. In: Daniilidis, K., Maragos, P., Paragios, N. (eds.) ECCV 2010, Part IV. LNCS, vol. 6314, pp. 778–792. Springer, Heidelberg (2010)
34. Rublee, E., Rabaud, V., Konolige, K., Bradski, G.: ORB: an efficient alternative to SIFT or SURF. In: ICCV, 2564–2571 (2011)
35. Breiman, L.: Random forests. Mach. Learn. **45**, 5–32 (2001)
36. Mitchell, T.M.: Machine Learning. McGraw-Hill, Maidenhead (1997)
37. Vapnik, V.N.: Estimation of Dependences Based on Empirical Data. Springer, New York (2006)
38. Lowe, D.G.: Distinctive image features from scale-invariant keypoints. IJCV **60**, 91–110 (2004)
39. Triggs, B., McLauchlan, P., Hartley, R., Fitzgibbon, A.: Bundle adjustment - modern synthesis. In: ICCV, pp. 298–372 (1999)
40. Rasmussen, C.E., Williams, C.K.I.: Gaussian Processes for Machine Learning (Adaptive Computation and Machine Learning). The MIT Press, Cambridge (2005)
41. Forsyth, D.A., Malik, J., Fleck, M.M., Greenspan, H., Leung, T., Belongie, S., Carson, C., Bregler, C.: Finding pictures of objects in large collections of images. In: Ponce, J., Hebert, M., Zisserman, A. (eds.) ECCV-WS 1996. LNCS, vol. 1144, pp. 335–360. Springer, Heidelberg (1996)
42. Cham, T.J., Ciptadi, A., Tan, W.C., Pham, M.T., Chia, L.T.: Estimating camera pose from a single urban ground-view omnidirectional image and a 2D building outline Map. In: CVPR, pp. 366–373

Can Visual Recognition Benefit from Auxiliary Information in Training?

Qilin Zhang[1], Gang Hua[1]([✉]), Wei Liu[2],
Zicheng Liu[3], and Zhengyou Zhang[3]

[1] Stevens Institute of Technology, Hoboken, NJ, USA
ganghua@gmail.com
[2] IBM Thomas J. Watson Research Center, Yorktown Heights, NY, USA
[3] Microsoft Research, Redmond, WA, USA

Abstract. We examine an under-explored visual recognition problem, where we have a main view along with an auxiliary view of visual information present in the training data, but merely the main view is available in the test data. To effectively leverage the auxiliary view to train a stronger classifier, we propose a collaborative auxiliary learning framework based on a new discriminative canonical correlation analysis. This framework reveals a common semantic space shared across both views through enforcing a series of nonlinear projections. Such projections automatically embed the discriminative cues hidden in both views into the common space, and better visual recognition is thus achieved on the test data that stems from only the main view. The efficacy of our proposed auxiliary learning approach is demonstrated through three challenging visual recognition tasks with different kinds of auxiliary information.

1 Introduction

We explore a new visual recognition problem dealing with visual data of two views, where a main view along with an auxiliary view is present in the training data. This particular vision problem attracts our attention, due to the recent popularity of multi-sensory and multiple spectrum imaging, such as depth-sensing and infrared (IR) sensing cameras, and hence the accumulation of labeled multi-view visual data.

However, a "missing-of-auxiliary view" problem frequently occurs in the test phase. This phenomenon could be incurred by sensor malfunction caused by, for example, an adversarial sensing environment or insufficient bandwidth allowing the transmission of only the main view data. In addition, the "missing view" problem could also arise when processing a backlog of historical data without an auxiliary sensing channel. Then a question naturally emerges: can visual recognition on the main view benefit from such auxiliary information that only exists in the training data?

Electronic supplementary material The online version of this chapter (doi:10.1007/978-3-319-16865-4_5) contains supplementary material, which is available to authorized users.

© Springer International Publishing Switzerland 2015
D. Cremers et al. (Eds.): ACCV 2014, Part I, LNCS 9003, pp. 65–80, 2015.
DOI: 10.1007/978-3-319-16865-4_5

Unlike conventional settings where training and testing data follow similar, if not identical, probability distributions [1], this problem requires techniques which can incorporate the beneficial information from the auxiliary view into the training of a classification model that works only with the main view. We shall emphasize that the problem studied in this paper is different from the domain adaptation and transfer learning problems [2–4] in computer vision. The goal of most domain adaptation/transfer learning problems is to leverage existing abundant labeled data in one domain to facilitate learning a better model in the target domain with scarce labeled data, if at all. Essentially, the knowledge is transferred from one data domain to a related but statistically different one. In contrast, in our problem the data domain in the test phase (*i.e.*, the main view) is a proper subset of the training data domain that contains the auxiliary view other than the main view.

In this sense, the problem we are addressing is more closely related to the multi-view and multi-task learning problems. The previous work in multi-view learning [5–7] has demonstrated that improved performance can be achieved by synergistically modeling all views. As a matter of fact, the existing multi-view recognition methods [5,8,9] emphasize heavily on properly combining per-view information.

We adopt a verification-by-construction approach by showing that there exists at least one method that consistently presents higher recognition accuracy on several multi-view visual datasets under this problem setting. In particular, we propose to seek a common semantic space to capture the relevance between the main and auxiliary views. This is achieved by a new discriminative canonical correlation analysis (DCCA) inspired by [10]. The new DCCA algorithm not only takes supervised label information into consideration, but also concurrently optimizes multiple nonlinear projections with a guaranteed convergence. Our DCCA algorithm is parallel to and even exceeds most previous CCA algorithms which did not explore label information and pursued multiple projections one by one.

With a desirable common semantic space, the auxiliary view information in the training data is carried into a classifier defined in the common space. Subsequent tests are conducted by projecting the only available main view information of the test data onto the common space and then applying the classifier obtained in the training phase.

The primary contributions of this paper are: (1) we focus on an under-explored visual recognition problem, *i.e.*, the "missing-view-in-test-data" problem with real-world multisensory visual datasets; (2) we propose a new discriminative canonical correlation algorithm together with a rigorous convergence proof, and its efficacy is validated on three benchmarks.

The rest of the paper is organized as follows. Section 2 briefly summarizes the related work. Section 3 formally defines the "missing-view-in-test-data" problem. Section 4 formulates the proposed DCCA algorithm. Section 5 gives a solution to the DCCA algorithm. Section 6 presents the experiments. Section 7 concludes the paper.

2   Related Work

Here we summarize the related work in domain adaptation, transfer learning, and multi-view learning, and also highlight their differences from the "missing-view-in-test-data" problem we investigate in the paper.

Recently, metric learning has been successfully applied to domain adaptation/transfer learning problems [1,3]. These methods attempt to transfer discriminative information from a source domain to a related but statistically different target domain. Metric learning based domain transfer methods can be applied to various problems such as machine translation [2,5], multimedia information retrieval [11], and visual recognition [3,4].

It is noted that these methods assume abundant labeled training samples present in the source domain. While in the target domain, there are a limited number of labeled training samples. Therefore, it is difficult to directly train an effective classifier using the scarce labeled data in the target domain. Then the recent approaches such as [3,4] exploit the corresponding relationship between the two domains to build a regularized cross-domain transform via techniques such as metric learning and kernel learning [12] to fulfill knowledge transferring. However, these domain transfer problems are different from the "missing-view-in-test-data" problem we are tackling in the paper. In our problem, there exists a bijection between every corresponding pair of the (main,auxiliary)-view observations in the training set, due to the intrinsic semantic consistency between the two views.

The multi-view/multi-task learning, e.g., [5,8,9], endeavors to learn a principled fusion which combines information from two or more related but statistically different views/tasks to achieve certain goals. It was demonstrated in [5] that the learning performance does benefit from explicitly leveraging the underlying semantic consistency between two views or among multiple views, which also motivates us to leverage this cross-view semantic consistency appearing in our problem. In our experiments shown in Sect. 6, a simple modification of the SVM2K algorithm [5] is implemented and treated as a competing baseline.

Another line of related work which can benefit from the multi-view data may be the co-training framework [13] proposed by Blum and Mitchell. Nevertheless, it falls into semi-supervised learning, and cannot deal with missing views. In [14], both the missing view and the domain transfer problem are considered, however, the objective function ignores the discriminative label information. A different RGBD-RGB data based object detection problem is addressed in [15] where explicit 3D geometry information is modeled. Tommasi et al. [16] focus on the dataset bias problem with a similar latent space model. In [17], a different missing feature problem is addressed, where the features are missing randomly in all dimensions, instead of the systematic absence of views in the multi-view settings considered in this paper. In the deep learning community, multi-modal deep learning systems such as [18] also show the robustness against missing views. In another related field, Chen et al. [19] suggest boosting-based learning with side information. Unlike our proposed latent space model, this method is not straightforward in terms of handling multiple sets of side information. In the area of human perception and psychology, Shams et al. [20] show that humans recognize better in unisensory tests with previous multisensory experiences than with the unisensory counterparts. Through establishing our proposed auxiliary learning framework, we show that this benefit also exists in the context of visual recognition. We also note that there exists a discriminative CCA [21] proposed for image set recognition where each sample consists of many observations/views. However, this CCA method exploits the correlations between sets of observations, which require abundant views for the robust estimation of sample covariance matrices. In contrast, our missing-view-in-test-data problem involves many observations but only a few views and even a single view in the test phase, so we are able to more easily exploit the correlations between views.

3   A Latent Space Model: Addressing Missing-View-in-Test-Data

Suppose that m view observations $\mathbf{z}(i) \overset{\text{def}}{=} (\mathbf{x}_1(i), \mathbf{x}_2(i))$ $(i = 1, 2, \cdots, m)$ are generated. Let $\mathbf{x}_1(i) \in \mathcal{X}_1$ and $\mathbf{x}_2(i) \in \mathcal{X}_2$ denote observations from the main view and auxiliary view, respectively. We assume $\mathcal{X}_1 \subset \mathbb{R}^{n_1}$ and $\mathcal{X}_2 \subset \mathbb{R}^{n_2}$, and define $\mathcal{Z} \overset{\text{def}}{=} \mathcal{X}_1 \times \mathcal{X}_2$, so $\mathbf{z}(i) \in \mathcal{Z}$. Within the training dataset, there comes with a label $l(i) \in \mathcal{L}$ for each observation $\mathbf{z}(i)$.

Unlike a conventional visual object recognition problem whose classifier $f_{\boldsymbol{\theta}}: \mathcal{Z} \to \mathcal{L}$ is obtained by the identification of the parameters $\boldsymbol{\theta} = \boldsymbol{\theta}(\mathbf{z}(1), \mathbf{z}(2), \cdots, \mathbf{z}(m))$ based on the training set, the "missing-view-in-test-data" problem requires a classifier in the form of $\tilde{f}_{\tilde{\boldsymbol{\theta}}}: \mathcal{X}_1 \to \mathcal{L}$ due to the missing auxiliary view in the test data. To effectively incorporate the available information in the entire training set $\{\mathbf{z}(i), l(i)\}_{i=1}^m$, this paper focuses on constructing the classifier $\tilde{f}_{\tilde{\boldsymbol{\theta}}}$, where $\tilde{\boldsymbol{\theta}} = \tilde{\boldsymbol{\theta}}(\mathbf{z}(1), \mathbf{z}(2), \cdots, \mathbf{z}(m), l(1), l(2), \cdots, l(m))$. To capture the information hidden in the auxiliary view $\mathbf{x}_2(j)$ and training labels $l(j)$, an intermediate space $\mathcal{S}$ is constructed to maximally retain the discriminative information from both views.

During this process, we construct projections $p_1(\cdot)$ and $p_2(\cdot)$ that map $\{\mathbf{x}_1(i)\}_{i=1}^m$ and $\{\mathbf{x}_2(i)\}_{i=1}^m$ to $p_1(\mathbf{x}_1(i)) \in \mathcal{S}$ and $p_2(\mathbf{x}_2(i)) \in \mathcal{S}$, respectively. In $\mathcal{S}$, the classification problem becomes easier: a discriminative classifier $f: \mathcal{S} \to \mathcal{L}$ (e.g., the SVM classifier [22]) is trained based on $\{p_1(\mathbf{x}_1(i)), l(i)\}_{i=1}^m \cup \{p_2(\mathbf{x}_2(i)), l(i)\}_{i=1}^m$. The training process is shown in blue arrows in Fig. 1(a). In the test phase, the test samples $\{\hat{\mathbf{x}}_1(j)\}_{j=1}^k$ are first projected to $p_1(\hat{\mathbf{x}}(j)) \in \mathcal{S}$ and subsequently fed to the trained classifier $f: \mathcal{S} \to \mathcal{L}$. The test process is shown in yellow arrows in Fig. 1(a).

The success of the aforementioned latent space based approach depends on not only the maximal preservation of the congruent information among views, but also the discriminative label information acquired in constructing $\mathcal{S}$. To achieve this, we propose a discriminative canonical correlation analysis (DCCA) algorithm, which simultaneously extracts multiple CCA projections and also incorporates the label information. In the following section, we formally formulate the optimization problem of DCCA and compare our proposed optimization method against previous ones.

4   DCCA: Formulation

In this section, we formulate the DCCA algorithm and compare it with previous related work. The classical Canonical Correlation Analysis (CCA) (see [11,23,24]) and its variants have been popular among practitioners for decades. In its basic form, the CCA algorithm finds a pair of linear projection vectors that maximize the linear correlation:

$$\max_{\alpha_j, \alpha_k} \alpha_j^T \Sigma_{jk} \alpha_k$$

$$\text{s.t. } \alpha_j^T \Sigma_{jj} \alpha_j = 1 \quad (j, k = 1, 2, \cdots, J) \tag{1}$$

where $\Sigma_{jk} = \mathcal{E}(\mathbf{x}_j \mathbf{x}_k^T)$, $\mathcal{E}$ denotes the mathematical expectation, and $\mathbf{x}_j$ denotes the observations in the jth view ($j = 1, 2, \cdots, J$, J denotes the number of distinct views in the multi-view data). In this way, α_j and α_k project the jth and kth views to a one-dimensional space by computing the inner products $\alpha_j^T \hat{\mathbf{x}}_j$ and $\alpha_k^T \hat{\mathbf{x}}_k$, respectively. In practice, a latent space of more of dimension d ($d > 1$) is often desired, hence this procedure in Eq. (1) needs to be repeated d times. Alternatively, as shown in [11], the following formulation can be used equivalently:

$$\max_{A_j, A_k} \text{tr}(A_j^T \Sigma_{jk} A_k)$$

$$\text{s.t. } A_j^T \Sigma_{jj} A_j = \mathbf{I} \quad (j, k = 1, 2, \cdots, J) \tag{2}$$

where $A_j - [\alpha_j(1), \cdots, \alpha_j(d)]$ contains all d projection vectors to form a d-dimensional latent space. The projections are computed as $A_j^T \hat{\mathbf{x}}_j$ and $A_k^T \hat{\mathbf{x}}_k$. To preserve the semantic consistency between the jth and kth views, we strive to make sure that $A_j^T \hat{\mathbf{x}}_j$ and $A_k^T \hat{\mathbf{x}}_k$ are as similar as possible, therefore maximizing $\text{tr}(A_j^T \Sigma_{jk} A_k)$ as Eq. (2).

These CCA algorithms are extended to handle more than two views, which are generally termed as the generalized CCA (gCCA) [11,25]. However, among the gCCA algorithms where per-view "correlations" are combined nonlinearly, most of them cannot be solved in a closed form and require a computing scheme to optimize the projections one by one. Also, the naive version of gCCA ignores the discriminative information in the class labels provided in the training process.

To address these two potential issues, we propose a new algorithm, named as *Discriminative CCA* (DCCA), which is inspired by [10]. It not only inherits the guaranteed optimization convergence property, but also has two extended properties: (1) the simultaneous optimization of multiple CCA projections contributes to better projection coefficients even in a kernelized version; (2) the pursuit of DCCA incorporates the label view information. Empirically, we find that the combination of (1) and (2) leads to performance gains across three challenging visual datasets, as shown in Sect. 6.

Starting from leveraging discriminative information like Loog *et al.* [26], we first encode the training labels as the Jth view based on k-nearest neighbors (k-NNs) of the training samples, where observations from all views are normalized and concatenated and then used in computing k-NNs. Suppose that there are C classes. For each labeled training sample $\mathbf{x}(0) \overset{\text{def}}{=} [\mathbf{x}_1(0)^T, \cdots, \mathbf{x}_J(0)^T]^T$, we consider its k-NNs $\mathbf{x}(i) \overset{\text{def}}{=} [\mathbf{x}_1(i)^T, \cdots, \mathbf{x}_J(i)^T]^T$ ($i = 0, \cdots, k$, including itself $\mathbf{x}(0)$). We record their labels as $\mathbf{L}_{(i)}$ ($i = 0, \cdots, k$) accordingly. The encoded label view for this training sample is a binary vector consisting of $k + 1$ length-C blocks.

After obtaining the label view, we can simultaneously optimize all d projections in the form of A_j ($j = 1, 2, \cdots, J$) as follows:

$$\arg \max_{\mathbf{A}} \sum_{j,k=1, j \neq k}^{J} c_{jk} g \left(\text{tr}(A_j^T \Sigma_{jk} A_k) \right)$$

$$\text{s.t.} \quad A_j^T \Sigma_{jj} A_j = \mathbf{I} \quad (j = 1, 2, \cdots, J) \tag{3}$$

where $\mathbf{A} \overset{\text{def}}{=} [A_1, \cdots, A_J]$, $A_j \overset{\text{def}}{=} [\boldsymbol{\alpha}_j(1), \cdots, \boldsymbol{\alpha}_j(d)]$ projects $\mathbf{x}_j$ to the d-dimensional common semantic space, c_{jk} is the selecting weights (either 0 or 1), and function $g(\cdot)$ is the view combination function (e.g., direct combination $g(x) = x$, or squared combination $g(x) = x^2$). The space dimension d is chosen such that each diagonal element of $A_j^T \Sigma_{jk} A_k$ is positive, which implies that the observations from all views are positively correlated. The Lagrangian of Eq. (3) is

$$F(\mathbf{A}, \mathbf{\Lambda}) = \sum_{k \neq j} c_{jk} g \left(\text{tr}(A_j^T \Sigma_{jk} A_k) \right) - \phi \sum_j \frac{1}{2} \text{tr} \left(\mathbf{\Lambda}_j^T (A_j^T \Sigma_{jj} A_j - \mathbf{I}) \right) \tag{4}$$

where $\mathbf{\Lambda} \overset{\text{def}}{=} [\mathbf{\Lambda}_1, \cdots, \mathbf{\Lambda}_J]$, $\mathbf{\Lambda}_j \in \mathcal{R}^{d \times d}$ is the multiplier, and ϕ is a scalar which is equal to 1 if $g(x) = x$ and 2 if $g(x) = x^2$. The derivative of $g(x)$ is denoted as $g'(x)$.

From Eq. (4), the following stationary equations hold:

$$\frac{1}{\phi} \sum_{k \neq j} c_{jk} g' \left(\text{tr}(A_j^T \Sigma_{jk} A_k) \right) \Sigma_{jk} A_k = \Sigma_{jj} A_j \mathbf{\Lambda}_j; \quad A_j^T \Sigma_{jj} A_j = \mathbf{I} \tag{5}$$

In practice, a kernelized version of DCCA is often favored, because linear correlations are not sufficient in modeling the nonlinear interplay among different views. Suppose that $\boldsymbol{K}_j$ is the Gram matrix of the centered data points $[\mathbf{x}_1, \cdots, \mathbf{x}_J]$. The empirical covariance is $\frac{1}{n} \boldsymbol{\alpha}_j^T \boldsymbol{K}_j \boldsymbol{K}_k \boldsymbol{\alpha}_k$, where $\boldsymbol{\alpha}_j$ is the coefficient vector and n is the number of training samples. Let $A_j = [\boldsymbol{\alpha}_j(1), \cdots, \boldsymbol{\alpha}_j(d)]$ and the empirical covariance matrix be $\frac{1}{n} A_j^T \boldsymbol{K}_j \boldsymbol{K}_k A_k$. Suppose that $\boldsymbol{K}_j$ can be decomposed as $\boldsymbol{K}_j = \boldsymbol{R}_j^T \boldsymbol{R}_j$. We define the projection matrix $\mathbf{W}_j = \boldsymbol{R}_j A_j$, and similarly define $\mathcal{W} \overset{\text{def}}{=} [\mathbf{W}_1, \cdots, \mathbf{W}_J]$. The optimization objective function of the kernelized DCCA is

$$\arg \max_{\mathcal{W}} \sum_{j,k=1, j \neq k}^{J} c_{jk} g \left(\text{tr}(\frac{1}{n} \mathbf{W}_j^T \boldsymbol{R}_j \boldsymbol{R}_k^T \mathbf{W}_k) \right)$$

$$\text{s.t.} \quad \mathbf{W}_j^T \left[(1 - \tau_j) \frac{1}{n} \boldsymbol{R}_j \boldsymbol{R}_j^T + \tau_j \mathbf{I}_n \right] \mathbf{W}_j = \mathbf{I} \tag{6}$$

Let us define $N_j = (1 - \tau_j)\frac{1}{n}R_j R_j^T + \tau_j I_n$, where $0 < \tau < 1$ is a pre-specified regularization parameter. Similar to Eq. (5), the following stationary equations hold

$$\frac{1}{\phi}\sum_{k \neq j} c_{jk}g'\left(\text{tr}(\frac{1}{n}\mathbf{W}_j^T R_j R_k^T \mathbf{W}_k)\right)\frac{1}{n}R_j R_k^T \mathbf{W}_k = N_j \mathbf{W}_j \Lambda_j \qquad (7)$$

$$\mathbf{W}_j^T N_j \mathbf{W}_j = I \qquad (8)$$

whose solution[1] is presented in Sect. 5.

5 DCCA: Solution

In this section, a monotonically convergent iterative algorithm to solve the DCCA problem is presented. For generic $g(\cdot)$ and c_{jk} value assignments, there is no closed-form solution to Eqs. (5) or (7). However, following [10], a similar "PLS-type", monotonically convergent iterative algorithm can be formulated. For conciseness, we only present the details of this algorithm with the solution to the problem in Eq. (7). Define the outer component $\mathbf{Y}_j$ and inner component $\mathbf{Z}_j$, respectively, as

$$\mathbf{Y}_j \stackrel{\text{def}}{=} R_j^T \mathbf{W}_j \qquad (9)$$

$$\mathbf{Z}_j \stackrel{\text{def}}{=} \frac{1}{\phi}\sum_{k \neq j} c_{jk}g'\left(\text{tr}(\frac{1}{n}\mathbf{W}_j^T R_j R_k^T \mathbf{W}_k)\right)\mathbf{Y}_k \qquad (10)$$

Differentiating the Lagrangian with respect to $\mathbf{W}_j$ and setting the gradient to zero, we obtain

$$R_j \mathbf{Z}_j = N_j \mathbf{W}_j \Lambda_j; \quad \mathbf{W}_j^T N_j \mathbf{W}_j = I \qquad (11)$$

From Eqs. (11) and (10), we have

$$\Lambda_j = \mathbf{W}_j^T R_j \mathbf{Z}_j = \frac{1}{\phi n}\sum_{k \neq j} c_{jk}g'\left(\text{tr}(\frac{1}{n}\mathbf{W}_j^T R_j R_k^T \mathbf{W}_k)\right)\mathbf{W}_j^T R_j R_k^T \mathbf{W}_k \qquad (12)$$

where $\text{tr}(\frac{1}{n}\mathbf{W}_j^T R_j R_k^T \mathbf{W}_k)$ is assumed to be positive, $c_{jk} = 0$ or 1, and due to the definition of g', Λ_j is a positive semi-definite matrix. From Eqs. (11) and (12), we have $\Lambda_j^T \Lambda_j = \mathbf{Z}_j^T R_j^T N_j^{-1} R_j \mathbf{Z}_j$. Since Λ_j has non-negative eigenvalues, Λ_j can be obtained via the matrix square root $[\mathbf{Z}_j^T R_j^T N_j^{-1} R_j \mathbf{Z}_j]^{1/2}$. Therefore,

$$\mathbf{W}_j = N_j^{-1} R_j \mathbf{Z}_j \left(\left[\mathbf{Z}_j^T R_j^T N_j^{-1} R_j \mathbf{Z}_j\right]^{1/2}\right)^{\dagger} \qquad (13)$$

where $\dagger$ denotes the pseudoinverse of a matrix.

---

[1] Note that Eq. (5) is a linear version of Eq. (7) and has a very similar solution. For conciseness, the solution to Eq. (5) is omitted.

A monotonically convergent iterative algorithm is described in Algorithm 1. Let $f(\mathcal{W}) \overset{\text{def}}{=} \sum_{k \neq j} c_{jk} g\left(\text{tr}(\frac{1}{n}\mathbf{W}_j^T \mathbf{R}_j \mathbf{R}_k^T \mathbf{W}_k)\right)$. Importantly, we have the following proposition:

Proposition 1. $f(\mathcal{W}(s=1)) \leq f(\mathcal{W}(s=2)) \leq f(\mathcal{W}(s=3)) \leq \ldots \leq C_u < \infty$ holds for all $s \in \mathcal{N}$, where s denotes the iteration index and C_u is a constant bound. This guarantees Algorithm 1 to converge monotonically.

Proof. Due to space limit, we defer the proof to the supplemental material. □

Algorithm 1. A monotonically convergent iterative algorithm for DCCA

Input: Observations from all J views: $\mathbf{x}_j, j = 1, \cdots, J$.
Output: J projection matrices $\mathbf{W}_j, j = 1, \cdots, J$.
Initialization:
Randomly initialize $\mathbf{W}_j(0)$, normalize them by
$\mathbf{W}_j(0) \leftarrow N_j^{-1}\mathbf{W}_j(0) \left([\mathbf{W}_j(0)^T N_j^{-1}\mathbf{W}_j(0)]^{1/2}\right)^\dagger$, and compute the initial outer components $\mathbf{Y}_j(0)$ by Eq. (9).
for $s = 0, 1, \cdots$ *until the convergence of* $\mathbf{W}_j$ **do**
    for $j = 1, 2, \cdots J$ **do**
        update the inner components by Eq. (10):
        $\mathbf{Z}_j(s) \leftarrow \frac{1}{\phi}\sum_{k=1}^{j-1} c_{jk} g'(\text{tr}(\frac{1}{n}\mathbf{Y}_j^T(s)\mathbf{Y}_k(s+1)))\mathbf{Y}_k(s+1) +$
        $\frac{1}{\phi}\sum_{k=j+1}^{J} c_{jk} g'(\text{tr}(\frac{1}{n}\mathbf{Y}_j^T(s)\mathbf{Y}_k(s)))\mathbf{Y}_k(s);$
        update the outer weighs by Eq. (13):
        $\mathbf{W}_j(s+1) \leftarrow N_j^{-1}\mathbf{R}_j\mathbf{Z}_j(s) \left([\mathbf{Z}_j(s)^T \mathbf{R}_j^T N_j^{-1} \mathbf{R}_j\mathbf{Z}_j(s)]^{1/2}\right)^\dagger;$
        update the outer components by Eq. (9): $\mathbf{Y}_j(s+1) \leftarrow \mathbf{R}_j^T\mathbf{W}_j(s+1);$
    end
end
return

---

6   Experiments

6.1   Compared Methods and Datasets

We compare the performances of the kernelized DCCA algorithm (paired with the RBF SVM classifier) against the following algorithms: A vanilla "SVM": that is trained on the main view of the visual information only. A variant of "SVM2K" [5]: which we train with two views in the train phase but only use one of the classifier due to the missing auxiliary view in the test phase[2]. The "KCCA": a kernel CCA based on the main view and the auxiliary view. The "KCCA+L": a kernel CCA based on the main view and the encoded label view, it ignores the auxiliary view. The "RGCCA": a kernel variant of the regularized generalized CCA [10] based on the main view and the auxiliary view. As an

---

[2] The original form of SVM2K is not directly applicable to the missing view problem.

extended version of gCCA, it iteratively optimizes each one-dimensional projection vectors (one column of $\mathbf{W}_j$), and all d columns of $\mathbf{W}_j$ are pursued one by one, similar to the algorithm presented in [24]. The "RGCCA+L": similar to "RGCCA", except it is based on the main view and the encoded label view. The "RGCCA+AL": similar to the proposed DCCA, except it iteratively optimizes each one-dimensional projection vectors (one column of $\mathbf{W}_j$).

In selecting the competing algorithms, we choose the "SVM2K" to represent a variant of multi-view learning algorithm. We select "KCCA" and "RGCCA" to represent classical and recent implementations of the CCA algorithms, both of which ignore the encoded label view. To isolate the effects of the auxiliary view and encoded train label view, we have included a series of combinations "KCCA+L", "RGCCA+L" and "RGCCA+AL". In the following experiments, the RBF kernel is applied in both the KCCA algorithm and the SVM algorithms. Parameters such as c_{jk}, $g(\cdot)$, the bandwidth parameter in the RBF kernel, and those parameters in the SVM2K algorithm, are all selected by a 4-fold cross validation. The experiments are conducted on three different datasets, $i.e.$, the "NYU Depth V1" Indoor Scenes dataset [27], the RGBD Object dataset [28], and the multi-spectral scene dataset [29]. The NYU Depth V1 dataset consists of RGBD images of indoor scenes collected by a modified Kinect sensor [27]. With this dataset, we demonstrate that the depth information in the train phase can benefit the scene classification based solely on the RGB images. The RGBD object dataset [28] consists of a large collection of paired RGB images and depth maps of common objects. We focus on the instance level object recognition, and demonstrate that the additional depth information during the train phase can facilitate better recognition based on the RGB information only. The multi-spectral scene dataset [29] consists of 477 registered and aligned RGB and near-infrared (IR) images from 9 different scene categories, $i.e.$, country, field, forest, indoor, mountain, old-building, street, urban and water. In this experiment, we demonstrate that the auxiliary information hidden in the IR channel can help to train a better scene recognition model that operates only on the main view.

6.2 NYU-Depth-V1-Indoor Scene Dataset

On the NYU Depth V1 indoor scenes dataset [27], we carry out the multi-spectral scene recognition task. Following [27], the scene observations are randomly split into 10 folds with equal size of the train set and the test set. Subsequently, we extract both the GIST [30] features and the spatial pyramid bag-of-feature representation [31] independently from each channel. For the latter, we densely extract SIFT descriptors from 40×40 patches with a stride of 10 pixels, and use two k-means dictionaries of sizes 200 and 800 to build the representation, which are shorted as SP200 and SP800, respectively. While grouping the imaging channels into views, we investigate the following two settings: (1) $\mathbf{L+D}$: Grayscale image features are assigned as the main view, while the depth features are assigned as the auxiliary view. (2) $\mathbf{RGB+D}$: RGB image features are concatenated and assigned as the main view, while the depth features are assigned as the auxiliary view.

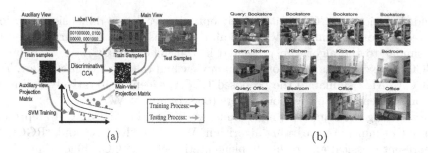

(a)   (b)

Fig. 1. (a) A latent space model to address the "missing-view-in-test-data" problem. The training and test processes are displayed in blue and yellow arrows, respectively. (b) k-NN retrieval from the NYU depth Indoor scenes data base. Actual scene class labels are listed above each image.

Table 1. NYU Depth V1 Indoor Scenes Classification, the highest and second highest values are colored red and blue, respectively.

Features	GIST		SP200		SP800	
Views	L+D	RGB+D	L+D	RGB+D	L+D	RGB+D
SVM	59.57±3.31	60.79±3.12	64.11±3.11	64.71±3.95	64.73±2.79	65.34±3.18
SVM2K	57.52±3.88	60.01±3.71	59.62±3.23	60.42±4.55	58.00±3.58	60.64±3.84
KCCA	58.16±6.55	62.58±3.55	64.94±4.58	64.00±4.92	64.77±4.69	65.01±4.86
KCCA+L	58.48±3.37	59.95±3.62	62.99±3.80	60.67±4.23	62.26±3.56	60.55±4.40
RGCCA	58.66±5.93	59.75±4.11	60.49±5.21	60.31±5.75	61.70±4.00	60.42±3.68
RGCCA+L	59.12±4.11	59.82±4.50	63.34±4.18	62.48±3.49	63.81±4.51	61.04±4.99
RGCCA+AL	59.82±6.10	62.85±4.24	65.61±4.22	65.31±4.23	65.38±4.22	65.66±3.04
DCCA	60.26±3.86	63.60±3.43	66.20±3.69	65.35±4.72	66.09±4.18	66.28±4.16

We first demonstrate the k-NN retrieval results in Fig. 1(b) to visualize some typical images from this dataset. The query images (from the test set) are displayed on the left and the corresponding 3 nearest neighbors (in the train set) are displayed on the right. Clearly, this dataset consists of highly cluttered indoor scenes, making this scene recognition task a challenging one.

In Table 1, the means and standard deviations of the recognition accuracy (in percentage) are reported. we observe that higher dimensional features offer better accuracy and the color information also helps recognition slightly. Generally, experiments based on "RGB+D" features achieve slightly higher accuracies than their "L+D" counterparts.

In Table 1, the SVM2K-variant gives lower accuracies than the SVM baseline, we speculate that the loose "prediction consistency" regularization of SVM2K-variant is only helpful when two views satisfy certain distributions. In addition, neither the KCCA nor the RGCCA approach sees significant performance improvements.

With the Label view alone, neither the "KCCA+L" nor the "RGCCA+L" algorithm achieves any advantage over the baseline. Intuitively, the information embedded in the label view is far less significant than that in the auxiliary view. However, with both the label view and the auxiliary view, the "RGCCA+AL" algorithm is capable of achieving a small advantage over the baseline, though not as significant as the proposed DCCA algorithm, whose projections are optimized and computed simultaneously and more accurately.

The large standard deviation in Table 1 stem from the difficult nature of the datasets, which can be seen in the baseline SVM performance in Table 1.

6.3 RGBD Object Dataset

With this RGBD Object dataset from [28], we focus on the instance level object recognition. There are multiple instances of objects across all the 51 categories, the target is to correctly recover the object instance labels in the test set. We follow the "leave-one-sequence-out" scheme in [28] and split recordings with camera mounting angle of 30° and 60° as the train set and the remaining recordings as the test set (the train/test sets are fixed, hence the standard deviation are not defined). In this section, we present the results with the EMK-based features [28] extracted from the RGB channels as the main view, and depth channel as the auxiliary view. In addition, we have also verified the efficacy of the proposed method with the state-of-the-art HMP-based features [32], but we defer the detailed results and comments to the supplemental material due to limited space.

As is seen in Tables 2 and 3(too many entries to fit in a single page), the recognition accuracy (in percentage) within each category fluctuates significantly. With some of the easy categories (*e.g.*, "pitcher"), the baseline SVM algorithm already achieves perfect recognition. However, with some of the challenging categories (*e.g.*, "food bag" and "lime"), the proposed DCCA offers the most significant performance boost. Overall, the "KCCA | L" and the "RGCCA+L" algorithms achieve a small advantage over the SVM baseline, both of which are inferior to the RGCCA algorithm that only maximizes the main view and auxiliary view correlation. However, the "RGCCA+AL" algorithm performs much better, though not as good as the proposed DCCA algorithm. Among the 51 categories in Tables 2 and 3, the "RGCCA+AL" algorithm achieves the best and second best accuracies in 8 and 24 categories, earning itself an overall average accuracy of 85.7 %. The proposed DCCA achieves the best and second best recognition accuracies in 28 and 19 categories, acquiring an average accuracy of 86.6 % across all categories, highest among all algorithms.

6.4 Multi-Spectral Scene Dataset

Following [29], we construct 10 random training/testing splits. For each split, 99 RGB images (11 per category) are used as the test set while the remaining 378 pairs as the train set. Before the feature extraction, each RGB image is converted to the **LAB** color space (similarly to [29]). Then the GIST [30] features are computed independently on each of the channels. Of these four channels, we choose the following two view assignment schemes: (1) **L+I**: Grayscale GIST features and the IR channel GIST features are assigned as the main view and the auxiliary view, respectively. (2) **LAB+I**: GIST features extracted independently from the L,A and B channels are concatenated as the main view, while those

Table 2. Accuracy Table Part 1 for the Multi-View RGBD Object Instance recognition, the highest and second highest values are colored red and blue, respectively. The remaining part is in Table 3.

Category	SVM	SVM2K	KCCA	KCCA +L	RGCCA	RGCCA +L	RGCCA +AL	DCCA
apple	65.2	72.4	77.6	64.8	79.0	68.1	76.7	77.6
ball	95.9	97.3	97.8	99.5	94.2	95.3	97.8	98.4
banana	74.2	61.1	80.3	71.7	77.3	77.3	80.3	80.3
bell pepper	71.3	59.8	69.3	65.7	66.1	68.9	69.3	69.3
binder	67.3	36.7	74.1	52.4	75.5	68.7	74.1	74.8
bowl	85.0	85.8	87.7	81.2	90.0	86.2	88.1	88.1
calculator	99.4	88.3	99.4	100	97.8	99.4	99.4	99.4
camera	91.7	49.6	97.5	90.1	96.7	95.9	97.5	97.5
cap	91.8	88.9	95.9	91.2	96.5	93.0	95.9	95.9
cellphone	93.2	81.7	96.3	93.2	94.2	95.3	96.3	96.3
cereal box	77.4	75.7	82.5	89.8	82.5	80.8	81.9	82.5
coffee mug	82.7	81.7	89.2	62.5	81.7	82.7	87.3	89.2
comb	97.3	96.0	99.3	100	98.7	98.7	99.3	100
dry battery	90.3	79.3	86.3	87.7	92.5	86.3	88.1	87.7
flashlight	77.1	75.0	80.3	74.5	78.2	77.7	81.4	82.4
food bag	72.7	69.1	80.8	82.5	84.9	77.7	86.6	89.2
food box	75.1	72.6	78.0	83.8	84.1	76.1	84.4	86.4
food can	70.0	63.7	70.7	78.2	73.7	66.2	81.0	83.7
food cup	87.1	86.4	84.9	94.5	83.8	84.2	90.1	91.5
food jar	84.5	81.0	88.6	86.1	85.8	85.4	88.3	88.9
garlic	95.5	93.3	92.2	95.5	89.0	91.2	92.8	93.3
glue stick	100	89.3	99.4	95.6	100	93.7	99.7	99.4
greens	75.7	70.3	82.2	84.9	74.6	80.5	81.1	82.2
hand towel	80.1	74.5	80.9	82.4	79.0	78.7	83.9	85.4
instant noodles	83.1	78.7	97.1	88.8	89.5	88.5	95.4	97.1
keyboard	88.1	82.7	90.6	88.1	93.6	88.1	95.0	95.0
kleenex	96.6	90.9	95.1	89.8	94.7	93.6	95.8	95.8
lemon	45.8	44.2	43.4	45.0	44.2	43.0	51.8	53.0
light bulb	93.2	92.5	95.9	98.6	95.9	95.2	95.2	95.9
lime	37.8	38.3	42.2	37.2	45.0	40.0	48.3	50.0
marker	48.4	39.3	46.0	48.4	49.9	46.2	46.6	46.9
mushroom	100	99.4	100	100	100	99.4	100	100
notebook	80.5	73.3	86.5	82.0	85.7	82.7	85.7	86.5
onion	91.5	86.4	88.6	94.0	93.1	88.6	93.4	93.4
orange	41.1	42.0	57.0	49.8	19.3	48.3	51.7	57.0
peach	100	74.2	100	97.4	99.3	98.7	100	100
pear	68.7	61.6	79.0	70.1	79.0	74.0	81.9	84.0
pitcher	100	100	100	100	100	98.3	100	100
plate	89.8	74.2	96.3	85.8	96.9	91.9	97.6	98.0
pliers	78.2	62.4	86.5	79.5	72.1	80.8	84.7	87.3
potato	62.9	65.6	70.3	71.8	64.5	67.6	69.1	70.3
rubber eraser	99.0	75.5	95.1	96.6	93.1	96.1	97.5	98.5
scissors	87.5	84.9	96.7	96.7	96.1	92.8	96.1	96.7
shampoo	84.5	82.9	94.5	82.3	95.5	89.0	94.2	94.8
soda can	89.6	87.8	91.0	97.7	92.8	88.7	95.5	96.8

Table 3. Continued from Table 2: Accuracy Table Part 2 for the Multi-View RGBD Object Instance recognition, the highest and second highest values are colored red and blue, respectively.

Category	SVM	SVM2K	KCCA	KCCA+L	RGCCA	RGCCA+L	RGCCA+AL	DCCA
sponge	76.4	64.8	75.2	69.4	78.6	72.8	76.4	77.4
stapler	71.8	67.7	73.3	70.6	74.2	71.5	77.4	78.0
tomato	81.9	70.0	79.6	76.8	82.2	77.1	85.0	85.0
tooth brush	78.4	69.6	76.8	70.1	79.4	74.7	77.8	77.8
tooth paste	84.5	68.3	90.0	86.0	81.9	87.1	88.9	90.4
water bottle	88.2	88.2	90.6	82.6	80.2	87.4	89.3	90.6
average	81.3	74.4	84.5	81.6	83.0	81.8	85.7	86.6

Table 4. Multi-Spectral Scene recognition, the highest and second highest values are colored red and blue, respectively.

Views	SVM	SVM2K	KCCA	KCCA+L
LAB+I	67.78±5.25	67.17±5.58	66.87±4.76	66.46±2.83
L+I	61.82±3.77	61.82±4.59	62.32±4.81	61.92±3.64

Views	RGCCA	RGCCA+L	RGCCA+AL	DCCA
LAB+I	68.59±3.94	67.27±4.88	69.90±3.16	70.51±2.37
L+I	62.22±3.96	62.42±4.45	64.55±3.44	65.66±4.57

extracted from the IR channel are considered as the auxiliary view. In Table 4, the mean and the standard deviation (both in percentage) of the recognition accuracies are reported. We observe that under either view assignment, neither the KCCA nor the SVM2K algorithm achieves a significant advantage over the SVM baseline. With the label view alone, "KCCA+L" and "RGCCA+L" achieve recognition accuracy on a par with the baseline SVM. We speculate that the auxiliary view is more informative in this dataset: with the auxiliary view, the RGCCA algorithm is capable of outperform the baseline by a small margin. Furthermore, with the additional label view information in "RGCCA+AL", this margin is enlarged. Overall, the proposed DCCA still outperforms all other competing algorithms. The large standard deviations in Table 4 could stem from the nature of this dataset. Indeed, in [29], Brown and Susstrunk also report large standard deviations on a par with ours.

6.5 Discussion

Overall, based on the aforementioned empirical results, we have the following observations. The latent space-based model is capable of leveraging the information from the auxiliary view in training, and hence effectively address the missing-view-in-test-data problem. Without the auxiliary view, the encoded label view alone is not significant enough to evidently boost the recognition performance. Incorporating the encoded label view with the auxiliary view yields some additional boost in recognition performance. DCCA consists of three components: the incorporation of the auxiliary view, the encoded label view, and the simultaneous optimization. They jointly contribute to the performance gains.

7   Conclusions

In this paper, we explored a practical visual recognition problem, where we have multi-view data in the train phase but only the single-view data in the test phase. We have verified that information from the auxiliary view in the train data can indeed lead to better recognition in the test phase even when the auxiliary view is entirely missing. As a part of our verification-by-construction proof, we have proposed a new discriminative canonical correlation analysis to integrate and map the semantic information from all views to a common latent space, over which all subsequent classification is conducted. We also investigated and isolated the effects of the encoded label view and the auxiliary view. The experimental results demonstrate that the proposed approach achieves performance advantages on all three benchmarks.

Acknowledgement. Research reported in this publication was partly supported by the National Institute Of Nursing Research of the National Institutes of Health under Award Number R01NR015371. The content is solely the responsibility of the authors and does not necessarily represent the official views of the National Institutes of Health. This work is also partly supported by US National Science Foundation Grant IIS 1350763, China National Natural Science Foundation Grant 61228303, GH's start-up funds form Stevens Institute of Technology, a Google Research Faculty Award, a gift grant from Microsoft Research, and a gift grant from NEC Labs America.

References

1. Quanz, B., Huan, J.: Large margin transductive transfer learning. In: Proceedings of the 18th ACM Conference on Information and Knowledge Management, pp. 1327–1336. ACM (2009)
2. Davis, J.V., Kulis, B., Jain, P., Sra, S., Dhillon, I.S.: Information-theoretic metric learning. In: Proceedings of the 24th International Conference on Machine Learning, pp. 209–216. ACM (2007)
3. Saenko, K., Kulis, B., Fritz, M., Darrell, T.: Adapting visual category models to new domains. In: Daniilidis, K., Maragos, P., Paragios, N. (eds.) ECCV 2010, Part IV. LNCS, vol. 6314, pp. 213–226. Springer, Heidelberg (2010)
4. Kulis, B., Saenko, K., Darrell, T.: What you saw is not what you get: Domain adaptation using asymmetric kernel transforms. In: 2011 IEEE Conference on Computer Vision and Pattern Recognition (CVPR), pp. 1785–1792. IEEE (2011)
5. Farquhar, J., Hardoon, D., Meng, H., Shawe-taylor, J.S., Szedmak, S.: Two view learning: Svm-2k, theory and practice. In: Advances in Neural Information Processing Systems, pp. 355–362 (2005)
6. Zhang, D., He, J., Liu, Y., Si, L., Lawrence, R.D.: Multi-view transfer learning with a large margin approach. In: Proceedings of the 17th ACM SIGKDD International Conference on Knowledge Discovery and Data Mining, pp. 1208–1216 (2011)

7. Qi, Z., Yang, M., Zhang, Z.M., Zhang, Z.: Mining noisy tagging from multi-label space. In: Proceedings of the 21st ACM International Conference on Information and Knowledge Management, pp. 1925–1929. ACM (2012)
8. Vapnik, V., Vashist, A., Pavlovitch, N.: Learning using hidden information (learning with teacher). In: International Joint Conference on Neural Networks, IJCNN 2009, pp. 3188–3195. IEEE (2009)
9. Argyriou, A., Evgeniou, T., Pontil, M.: Convex multi-task feature learning. Mach. Learn. **73**, 243–272 (2008)
10. Tenenhaus, A., Tenenhaus, M.: Regularized generalized canonical correlation analysis. Psychometrika **76**, 257–284 (2011)
11. Hardoon, D.R., Szedmak, S., Shawe-Taylor, J.: Canonical correlation analysis: an overview with application to learning methods. Neural Comput. **16**, 2639–2664 (2004)
12. Kulis, B., Sustik, M., Dhillon, I.: Learning low-rank kernel matrices. In: Proceedings of the 23rd International Conference on Machine Learning, pp. 505–512. ACM (2006)
13. Blum, A., Mitchell, T.: Combining labeled and unlabeled data with co-training. In: Proceedings of the Eleventh Annual Conference on Computational Learning Theory, pp. 92–100. ACM (1998)
14. Chen, L., Li, W., Xu, D.: Recognizing rgb images by learning from rgb-d data. In: 2014 IEEE Conference on Computer Vision and Pattern Recognition (CVPR). IEEE (2014)
15. Shrivastava, A., Gupta, A.: Building part-based object detectors via 3d geometry. In: 2013 IEEE International Conference on Computer Vision (ICCV), pp. 1745–1752. IEEE (2013)
16. Tommasi, T., Quadrianto, N., Caputo, B., Lampert, C.H.: Beyond dataset bias: multi-task unaligned shared knowledge transfer. In: Lee, K.M., Matsushita, Y., Rehg, J.M., Hu, Z. (eds.) ACCV 2012, Part I. LNCS, vol. 7724, pp. 1–15. Springer, Heidelberg (2013)
17. Globerson, A., Roweis, S.: Nightmare at test time: robust learning by feature deletion. In: Proceedings of the 23rd International Conference on Machine Learning, pp. 353–360. ACM (2006)
18. Srivastava, N., Salakhutdinov, R.: Multimodal learning with deep boltzmann machines. In: Advances in Neural Information Processing Systems, pp. 2222–2230 (2012)
19. Chen, J., Liu, X., Lyu, S.: Boosting with side information. In: Lee, K.M., Matsushita, Y., Rehg, J.M., Hu, Z. (eds.) ACCV 2012, Part I. LNCS, vol. 7724, pp. 563–577. Springer, Heidelberg (2013)
20. Shams, L., Wozny, D.R., Kim, R., Seitz, A.: Influences of multisensory experience on subsequent unisensory processing. Front. Psychol. **2**, 264 (2011)
21. Kim, T.K., Kittler, J., Cipolla, R.: Discriminative learning and recognition of image set classes using canonical correlations. IEEE Trans. Pattern Anal. Mach. Intell. **29**, 1005–1018 (2007)
22. Chang, C.C., Lin, C.J.: Libsvm: a library for support vector machines. ACM Trans. Intell. Syst. Technol. (TIST) **2**, 27 (2011)
23. Hotelling, H.: Relations between two sets of variates. Biometrika **28**, 321–377 (1936)
24. Witten, D.M., Tibshirani, R., et al.: Extensions of sparse canonical correlation analysis with applications to genomic data. Stat. Appl. Genet. Mol. Biol. **8**, 1–27 (2009)

25. Rupnik, J., Shawe-Taylor, J.: Multi-view canonical correlation analysis. In: Conference on Data Mining and Data Warehouses (SiKDD 2010), pp. 1–4 (2010)
26. Loog, M., van Ginneken, B., Duin, R.P.: Dimensionality reduction of image features using the canonical contextual correlation projection. Pattern Recogn. **38**, 2409–2418 (2005)
27. Silberman, N., Fergus, R.: Indoor scene segmentation using a structured light sensor. In: 2011 IEEE International Conference on Computer Vision Workshops (ICCV Workshops), pp. 601–608. IEEE (2011)
28. Lai, K., Bo, L., Ren, X., Fox, D.: A large-scale hierarchical multi-view rgb-d object dataset. In: 2011 IEEE International Conference on Robotics and Automation (ICRA), pp. 1817–1824. IEEE (2011)
29. Brown, M., Susstrunk, S.: Multi-spectral sift for scene category recognition. In: 2011 IEEE Conference on Computer Vision and Pattern Recognition (CVPR), pp. 177–184. IEEE (2011)
30. Oliva, A., Torralba, A.: Modeling the shape of the scene: a holistic representation of the spatial envelope. Int. J. Comput. Vis. **42**, 145–175 (2001)
31. Lazebnik, S., Schmid, C., Ponce, J.: Beyond bags of features: Spatial pyramid matching for recognizing natural scene categories. In: 2006 IEEE Computer Society Conference on Computer Vision and Pattern Recognition, vol. 2, pp. 2169–2178. IEEE (2006)
32. Bo, L., Ren, X., Fox, D.: Unsupervised feature learning for rgb-d based object recognition. ISER, June 2012

Low Rank Representation on Grassmann Manifolds

Boyue Wang[1], Yongli Hu[1], Junbin Gao[2]([✉]), Yanfeng Sun[1], and Baocai Yin[1]

[1] Beijing Key Laboratory of Multimedia and Intelligent Software Technology, College of Metropolitan Transportation, Beijing University of Technology, Beijing, China
boyue.wang@gmail.com, {huyongli,yfsun,ybc}@bjut.edu.cn
[2] School of Computing and Mathematics, Charles Sturt University, Bathurst, NSW 2795, Australia
jbgao@csu.edu.au

Abstract. Low-rank representation (LRR) has recently attracted great interest due to its pleasing efficacy in exploring low-dimensional subspace structures embedded in data. One of its successful applications is subspace clustering which means data are clustered according to the subspaces they belong to. In this paper, at a higher level, we intend to cluster subspaces into classes of subspaces. This is naturally described as a clustering problem on Grassmann manifold. The novelty of this paper is to generalize LRR on Euclidean space into the LRR model on Grassmann manifold. The new method has many applications in computer vision tasks. The paper conducts the experiments over two real world examples, clustering handwritten digits and clustering dynamic textures. The experiments show the proposed method outperforms a number of existing methods.

1 Introduction

In recent years, sparse representation and dictionary learning gain much attention in signal processing and machine learning applications. The sparse representation is based on the principle that a signal can normally be represented as a linear combinations of few atoms of a dictionary. And plenty of efforts are dedicated to constructing dictionaries with desired properties [1]. The sparse representation model has achieved great success in various application areas such as face recognition [2], image denoising [3], inpainting [4], image super-resolution reconstruction [5], and so on. In most of sparse representation methods, one mainly focuses on independent sparse representation for data objects, and the relation among data objects or the underlying structure of subspaces that the subsets of group data generated is usually not well considered. While this intrinsic property is very important in some learning tasks, especially in classification and clustering applications.

Electronic supplementary material The online version of this chapter (doi:10.1007/978-3-319-16865-4_6) contains supplementary material, which is available to authorized users.

© Springer International Publishing Switzerland 2015
D. Cremers et al. (Eds.): ACCV 2014, Part I, LNCS 9003, pp. 81–96, 2015.
DOI: 10.1007/978-3-319-16865-4_6

Some researchers have introduced holistic constraints such as the low rank or nuclear norm $\| \cdot \|_*$ constraints as favoured sparse representation conditions. The good example in the new trend is the Low Rank Representation (LRR) model [6] which has been successfully used in many applications such as motion segmentation [7], image segmentation [8], and salient object detection [9]. In fact, the low rank criterion as one special type of sparsity measure has long been utilized in matrix completion from corrupted or missing data [10,11]. Low rank representation tries to reveal the latent sparse property embedded in a data set in high dimensional space. Specifically, it has been proved that when the high-dimensional data set is actually composed of a union of several low dimension subspaces, then the LRR model can reveal this structure through subspace clustering [6].

The current LRR method originates from the subspace clustering [12], based on the hypothesis that the data can be represented by the space spanned by a set of samples. However, this hypothesis may not be always true for many high-dimensional data in practices. It has been proved that many high-dimensional data have their embedded low manifold structures. For example, the human face images are considered as samples from a non-linear submanifold [13]. To deal with this type of data, one has to respect the local geometry existed in the data, i.e., manifold learning, or use a non-linear mapping to "flat" the data, like kernel methods. The classical embedding algorithms such as LLE [14], ISOMAP [15], LLP [16] and LE [17] are the examples of manifold learning from data.

On the other hand, in computer vision, there are many cases where we clearly know what the manifold is, but we want to analyze these manifolds for some practical tasks. For example, a short video clip of dynamic texture can be represented by a subspace, and all such clips together make up the so-called Grassmann manifold. Thus the problem of clustering dynamic textures becomes clustering the points on Grassmann manifold, in other words, to cluster many subspaces into subgroups of subspaces.

Most manifolds can be considered as low dimensional smooth "surfaces" embedded in a higher dimensional Euclidean space. At each point of the manifold, it is locally similar to Euclidean space. In recent years, Grassmann manifold has attracted great interest in research community. Its Riemannian geometry has been recently investigated [18]. Grassmann manifold has a nice property that it can be embedded into the space of symmetric matrices via the projection embedding, referring to Sect. 2.2 below. This property was used in subspace tracking [19], clustering [20], discriminant analysis [21], and sparse coding [22,23]. Harandi et al. [23] address the problem of kernel sparse coding and dictionary learning within the space of symmetric positive definite matrices. In this paper, we will establish an LRR model on Grassmann manifold based on the similar approach used in the above work and further explore the model performance in clustering subspaces, i.e., grouping a number of subspaces into subgroups of subspaces. The contributions of this work are listed as follows:

- Formulating the LRR model on Grassmann Manifold;
- Exploring the link between the proposed LRR model and kernelization; and
- Providing a practical and effective algorithm for the formulated LRR model.

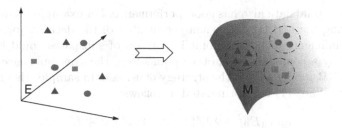

Fig. 1. The points on the Grassmannian manifold and its GLRR representation for clustering.

The rest of the paper is organized as follows. In the next Section, we describe the proposed low-rank representation on Grassmann Manifold in detail. Section 3 gives the optimization algorithms to resolve the proposed LRR model on Grassmann Manifold. In Sect. 4, the performance of the proposed method is evaluated by clustering application on two public databases. Finally, conclusions and suggestions for future work are provided in Sect. 5.

2 LRR on Grassmann Manifold

2.1 Low-Rank Representation (LRR)

LRR model represents a group of signals on a dictionary with low rank constraint which reveals the intrinsical low rank structure in the signals. The general LRR model can be formulated as the following optimization problem:

$$\min_{E,Z} \|E\|_l^2 + \lambda \|Z\|_* \quad \text{s.t.} \quad Y = DZ + E \tag{1}$$

where $Y \in \mathbb{R}^{d \times N}$ is a set of N signals with d dimensions and Z is the correspondent low rank representation of Y under the dictionary D, which could be trained or constructed from data samples, and E represents the error between the signals and its reconstructed values on D. $\|\cdot\|_*$ is the nuclear norm which is defined as the sum of singular values of a matrix and is the low envelop of the rank function of a matrix [24]. $\|\cdot\|_l$ is the reconstruction error measurement. We may choose one of different error measurements, depending on the properties of the signals and the aim of applications. For example, in the LRR clustering applications [6,7], $\|\cdot\|_{2,1}$ is used to cope with columnwise gross errors in signals. Finally $\lambda > 0$ is a penalty parameter to balance the rank term and the reconstruction error.

In the above LRR model, it is critical to use an appropriate dictionary D to represent signals. Generally, a dictionary can be learned from some training data by using one of many dictionary learning methods, such as the K-SVD method [1]. However, a dictionary learning procedure is usually time-consuming and so should be done in an offline manner. So many researchers adopt a simple and direct way to construct a dictionary, i.e. using the original signals themselves as the dictionary. In practice, if there are sufficient data samples, the dictionary composed of original data also has good performance. For example, as in the subspace clustering method [12,25], when the number of the data samples in each subspace is sufficient, each data point in a union of subspaces could be reconstructed well by a combination of other points from the same subspace. In fact, the original LRR model adopts the strategy of using data samples themselves as the dictionary. Thus (1) is reformulated as follows:

$$\min_{E,Z} \|E\|_l^2 + \lambda\|Z\|_* \quad \text{s.t.} \quad Y = YZ + E \tag{2}$$

2.2　LRR on Grassmann Manifolds

In most of cases, the reconstruction error of LRR model in (2) is computed in the original data domain. For example, the common form of the reconstruction error is Frobenius norm with Euclidian distance in original data space, i.e. the error term can be chosen as $\|Y - YZ\|_F$. In practice, many high dimension data have its intrinsic manifold structure, for example, the human faces in images are proved to have an underlying manifold structure [26]. In the ideal scenarios, the error should be measured according to the manifold's geometry[1]. So we consider signal representation for the data with manifold structure and formulate the error measurement in LRR model based on the distance defined on manifold spaces. Consequently, the LRR model in (2) can be changed as the following manifold form:

$$\min_{E,Z} \|E\|_{\mathcal{G}}^2 + \lambda\|Z\|_* \quad \text{s.t.} \quad Y = YZ + E \tag{3}$$

where $\|\cdot\|_{\mathcal{G}}$ is the distance (geodesics) on the manifold. Problem (3) is highly nonlinear and it is hard to design a practical algorithm. However when the underlying manifold is Grassmannian, we can use the distance over its embedded space to replace the manifold distance, as detailed below.

　　Grassmann manifold $\mathcal{G}(p, d)$ [27] is the space of all p-dimensional linear subspaces of $\mathbb{R}^d$ for $0 < p < d$. A point on Grassmann manifold is a subspace of $\mathbb{R}^d$ which can be represented by any of orthonormal basis $X = [\mathbf{x}_1, \mathbf{x}_2, \ldots, \mathbf{x}_p] \in \mathbb{R}^{d \times p}$. The chosen orthonormal basis is called a representative of a subspace $\mathcal{S}$. Grassmann manifold $\mathcal{G}(p, d)$ has one-to-one correspondence to a quotient manifold of $\mathbb{R}^{d \times p}$, see [27]. On the other hand, we can embed Grassmann manifold $\mathcal{G}(p, d)$ into the space of d order symmetric matrices $\text{Sym}(d)$ by mapping

$$\Pi : \mathcal{G}(p, d) \rightarrow \text{Sym}(d), \quad \Pi(X) = XX^T \tag{4}$$

　　This process can be demonstrated in Fig. 1. The embedding $\Pi(X)$ is diffeomorphism [28] (a one-to-one, continuous, differentiable mapping with a continuous, differentiable inverse). Then it is reasonable to replace the distance on

---

[1] As the manifold is generally no longer linear, so the linear combination on the manifold should be implemented via exp and log operations on the manifold. We ignore this for the simplicity of presenting our idea.

Grassmann manifold by the following distance defined on the symmetric matrix space under this mapping,

$$\delta(X_1, X_2) = \|\Pi(X_1) - \Pi(X_2)\|_F = \|X_1 X_1^T - X_2 X_2^T\|_F \qquad (5)$$

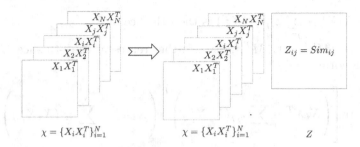

Fig. 2. The GLRR Model. The mapping of the points on Grassmann manifold, the tensor $\mathcal{X}$ with each slice being a symmetric matrix can be linearly represented by itself. The element z_{ij} of Z represents the similarity between slice i and j.

Given a set of data points $\{X_1, X_2, \ldots, X_N\}$ on Grassmann manifold, i.e., a set of subspaces $\{\mathcal{S}_1, \mathcal{S}_2, \ldots, \mathcal{S}_N\}$ of dimension p accordingly, we have their mapped symmetric matrices $\{X_1 X_1^T, X_2 X_2^T, \ldots, X_N X_N^T\} \subset \mathrm{Sym}(d)$. Similar to the LRR model in (3), we represent these symmetric matrices by itself and use the error measurement defined in (5) to construct the LRR model on Grassmann manifold as follows:

$$\min_{E,Z} \|E\|_F^2 + \lambda \|Z\|_* , \text{ s.t. } \mathcal{X} = \mathcal{X} \times_3 Z + E \qquad (6)$$

where $\mathcal{X}$ is a 3-order tensor by stacking all mapped symmetric matrices $\{X_1 X_1^T, X_2 X_2^T, \ldots, X_N X_N^T\}$ along the 3rd mode and $\times_3$ means the mode-3 multiplication of a tensor and a matrix, see [29]. The representation of $\mathcal{X}$ and the 3-order product operation are illustrated in Fig. 2. E is the reconstruction error in the 3-order tensorial form and $\|\cdot\|_F$ is the Frobenius norm of a tensor, which can be defined as the square root of the sum of the absolute squares of all elements in E.

To provide a practical algorithm to the optimization problem in (6), we further investigate the structure of tensor used in the problem. Intuitively, the tensor calculation can be converted to matrix operation by tensorial matricization, see [29]. For example, we can matricize the tensor $\mathcal{X} \in \mathbb{R}^{d \times d \times N}$ in mode-3 and obtain a matrix $\mathcal{X}_{(3)} \in \mathbb{R}^{N \times (d*d)}$ of N data points (in rows). So the problem seems be solved using the method of the standard LRR model. However, as the dimension $d * d$ is often too large in practical problems, the existing LRR algorithm could break down. To avoid this scenario, we carefully analyze the representation of the construction tensor error E and convert the optimization problem to an equivalent and readily solvable optimization model.

Consider the construction error term $\|E\|_F^2 = \|\mathcal{X} - \mathcal{X} \times_3 Z\|_F^2$ in (6). First we write it into a sum of slices of E as follows:

$$\|E\|_F^2 = \sum_{i=1}^{N} \|E_i\|_F^2 \tag{7}$$

where $E_i = X_i X_i^T - \sum_{j=1}^{N} z_{ij}(X_j X_j^T)$ is the i-th slice of E.

Using that $\|M\|_F^2 = \text{tr}(M^T M)$, we further represent the i-th slice $\|E_i\|_F^2$ in the following form:

$$\|E_i\|_F^2 = \text{tr}\left[\left(X_i X_i^T - \sum_{j=1}^{N} z_{ij}(X_j X_j^T)\right)^T \left(X_i X_i^T - \sum_{j=1}^{N} z_{ij}(X_j X_j^T)\right)\right]$$

$$= \text{tr}\left[(X_i X_i^T)^T(X_i X_i^T)\right] - 2\sum_{j=1}^{N} z_{ij}\text{tr}\left[(X_i X_i^T)^T(X_j X_j^T)\right] \tag{8}$$

$$+ \sum_{j_1=1}^{N}\sum_{j_2=1}^{N} z_{ij_1} z_{ij_2}\text{tr}\left[(X_{j_1} X_{j_1}^T)(X_{j_2} X_{j_2}^T)\right]$$

It is easy to show that

$$\text{tr}\left[(X_i X_i^T)^T(X_i X_i^T)\right] = \text{tr}\left[(X_i^T X_i)(X_i^T X_i)\right] = \text{tr}[I_p] = p \tag{9}$$

and

$$\text{tr}\left[(X_j X_j^T)^T(X_i X_i^T)\right] = \text{tr}\left[(X_j^T X_i)^T(X_i^T X_j)\right]. \tag{10}$$

Substituting (9) and (10) into (8), we have

$$\|E_i\|_F^2 = p - 2\sum_{j=1}^{N} z_{ij}\text{tr}\left[(X_j^T X_i)(X_i^T X_j)\right]$$

$$+ \sum_{j_1=1}^{N}\sum_{j_2=1}^{N} z_{ij_1} z_{ij_2}\text{tr}\left[(X_{j_1}^T X_{j_2})(X_{j_2}^T X_{j_1})\right] \tag{11}$$

We note that $(X_j^T X_i)$ has a small dimension $p \times p$ which is easy to handle. To simplify expression (11), we denote

$$\Delta_{ij} = \text{tr}\left[(X_j^T X_i)(X_i^T X_j)\right] \tag{12}$$

Clearly $\Delta_{ij} = \Delta_{ji}$. So we construct an $N \times N$ symmetrical matrix

$$\Delta = (\Delta_{ij})_{i=1, j=1}^{N} \tag{13}$$

Substituting (12) and (13) into (11), we have

$$\|E_i\|_F^2 = p - 2\sum_{j=1}^{N} z_{ij}\Delta_{ij} + \sum_{j_1=1}^{N}\sum_{j_2=1}^{N} z_{ij_1}z_{ij_2}\Delta_{j_1 j_2}$$
$$= p - 2\sum_{j=1}^{N} z_{ij}\Delta_{ij} + \mathbf{z}_i\Delta\mathbf{z}_i^T \tag{14}$$

where $\mathbf{z}_i$ is the i-th row of Z. Substituting (14) into (7), we have a simplified reconstruction error representation:

$$\|E\|_F^2 = Np - 2\text{tr}[Z\Delta] + \text{tr}[Z\Delta Z^T] \tag{15}$$

It can be proved that Δ is semi-definite positive (see supplementary materials), so we have $\Delta = LL^T$ by Cholesky decomposition [30], where L is a $N \times N$ matrix. So the above representation can be further written as:

$$\|E\|_F^2 = Np - 2\text{tr}[ZLL^T] + \text{tr}[ZL(ZL)^T]$$
$$= \|ZL - L\|_F^2 + \text{const.} \tag{16}$$

Combining (16) and (6), we have an equivalent problem to the LRR model on Grassmann manifold in (6):

$$\min_{Z} \|ZL - L\|_F^2 + \lambda\|Z\|_* \tag{17}$$

The final LRR model on Grassmann manifold resembles the original LRR model. We would like to give a remark here. In fact, the LRR model on Grassman manifold (6) can be regarded a kernelized LRR with a kernel feature mapping defined by (4). It is not surprised that Δ semi-definite positive as it serves as a kernel matrix. Finally it is natural that we can further generalize the LRR model on Grassmann manifold based on other kernel functions.

3   Solution to LRR on Grassmann Manifold

In this section, we consider an algorithm to solve the optimization problem in (17) with a combination of nuclear and Frobenius norm about Z. We can easily solve it by using linearization technique to deal with the quadratic term $\|ZL - L\|_F^2$. However, to sufficiently take advantage of the existing algorithm for the original LRR, we employ the Augmented Lagrangian Multiplier (ALM) [31]

So we let $J = Z$ to separate the terms of variable Z and the problem in (17) can be formulated as follows:

$$\min_{Z} \frac{1}{\lambda}\|ZL - L\|_F^2 + \|J\|_* \quad \text{s.t.} \quad J = Z \tag{18}$$

Its Augmented Lagrangian Multiplier formulation can be defined as the following unconstrained optimization:

$$\min_{Z,J} \frac{1}{\lambda}\|ZL - L\|_F^2 + \|J\|_* + \langle A, Z - J \rangle + \frac{\mu}{2}\|Z - J\|_F^2 \tag{19}$$

where A is the Lagrangian Multiplier and μ is a weight to tune the error term of $\|Z - J\|_F^2$.

In fact, the above problem can be solved by the following two subproblems in an alternative manner fixing Z or J to optimize the other, respectively.

When fixing Z, the following subproblem is solved to update J:

$$\min_J(\|J\|_* + \langle A, Z - J \rangle + \frac{\mu}{2}\|Z - J\|_F^2) \tag{20}$$

When fixing J, the following subproblem should be solved to update Z:

$$\min_Z(\frac{1}{\lambda}\|ZL - L\|_F^2 + \langle A, Z - J \rangle + \frac{\mu}{2}\|Z - J\|_F^2) \tag{21}$$

For the subproblem in (20), it can be solved by the following steps. Firstly, the optimization is revised as follows:

$$\min_J(\|J\|_* + \frac{\mu}{2}\|J - (Z + \frac{A}{\mu})\|_F^2) \tag{22}$$

(22) has a closed-form solution given by,

$$J^* = \Theta_{\mu^{-1}}(Z + \frac{A}{\mu})$$

where $\Theta(\cdot)$ denotes the singular value thresholding operator (SVT), see [32].

The subproblem in (21) is a quadratic optimization problem about Z. The closed-form solution is given by

$$Z = (\lambda\mu J - \lambda A + 2LL^T)(2LL^T + \lambda\mu I)^{-1} \tag{23}$$

Once solving the former two subproblems about J and Z respectively, we achieve a complete solution to LRR on Grassmann manifold. The whole procedure of LRR on Grassmann manifold is summarized in Algorithm 1.

4   Experiments

4.1   Data Preparation and Experiment Settings

To evaluate the proposed LRR model on Grassmann Manifold, we apply it to image signals representation and then the representation results are used for image clustering by Ncut method [33]. We choose two widely used public databases to test our method. One is the MNIST handwriting digits [34] image set, in which there are more than 70000 digit images written by different persons. The other is the DynTex++ database [35]. This database is a collection of videos from different classes.

To apply our method for image clustering, we use three steps to set up experiments: (a) Mapping the raw signals onto the points on Grassmann Manifold;

Algorithm 1. Low-Rank Representation on Grassmann Manifold.

Input: The Grassmann sample set $\{X_i\}_{i=1}^N, X_i \in \mathcal{G}(p,d)$, the cluster number k and the balancing parameter λ.

Output: The Low-Rank Representation Z

1: Initialize:$J = Z = 0, A = B = 0, \mu = 10^{-6}, \mu_{max} = 10^{10}$ and $\varepsilon = 10^{-8}$
2: **for** i=1:N **do**
3:    **for** j=1:N **do**
4:        $\Delta_{ij} \leftarrow \text{tr}[(X_j^T X_i)(X_i^T X_j)]$;
5:    **end for**
6: **end for**
7: Computing L by Cholesky Decomposition $\Delta = LL^T$;
8: **while** not converged **do**
9:    fix Z and update J by
      $J \leftarrow \min_J(||J||_* + < A, Z - J > + \frac{\mu}{2}||Z - J||_F^2)$;
10:   fix J and update Z by
      $Z \leftarrow (\lambda\mu J - \lambda A + 2LL^T)(2LL^T + \lambda\mu I)^{-1}$;
11:   update the multipliers:
      $A \leftarrow A + \mu(Z - J)$
12:   update the parameter μ by $\mu \leftarrow \min(\rho\mu, \mu\text{max})$
13:   check the convergence condition:
      $||Z - J||_\infty < \varepsilon$
14: **end while**

(b) Applying the low-rank representation on Grassmann Manifold and (c) Conducting Ncut over the representation results from LRR. Note that our LRR model is designed to cluster points on Grassmann manifold (i.e., clustering subspaces), while most existing clustering algorithms are designed for clustering raw object/signal points. In essence, all the existing algorithms are only considered as benchmarks in assessing our new method.

The raw data in our experiments are image sets with huge volume, for example, the digit image sets for clustering have 3495 image sets and each set is formulated as a high-dimensional vector of size $28 \times 28 \times 20 = 15680$. It is difficult to process this high-dimensional data set on a common machine. So we use PCA (Principal Component Analysis) to reduce the dimension of raw data. Then the data with reduced dimension is represented by LRR model and used for final clustering. For the purpose of clustering comparison, the Ncut method is compared with K-means method for different data representation. Table 1 shows the methods to be compared with our method in our experiments. Under the LRR model, the performance of K-means is bad, so we give up the 4th and the last experiments. All the algorithms are coded by matlab R2011b and implemented on an Xeon-X5675 3.06 GHz CPU machine with 12G RAM.

Mapping a sub-group of raw signals onto the points on Grassmann Manifold is a key step in our method. As a point on Grassmann Manifold is represented by an orthonormal basis of a subspace, given the samples from a subspace we should construct its basis representation. According to the work of Harandi [22,36], we simply adopt Singular Value Decomposition(SVD) to construct the subspace

Table 1. Different combining clustering methods with variety in data processing, data representation and clustering methods.

Data processing method	Data representation method	Clustering method	Combining method
PCA	-	Ncut	PNcut
PCA	-	K-mean	PK-mean
PCA	LRR	Ncut	PLRRNcut
PCA	LRR	K-mean	-
Grassmann manifold	-	Ncut	GNcut
Grassmann manifold	-	K-mean	GKmean
Grassmann manifold	LRR	Ncut	GLRRNcut (our method)
Grassmann manifold	LRR	K-mean	-

basis. Concretely, given a subset of images from a class, e.g., the same digits written by the same person, denoted by $\{Y_i\}_{i=1}^M$ and each Y_i is a grey-scale image with dimension $m \times n$, we can construct a matrix $\Gamma = [\text{vec}(Y_1), \text{vec}(Y_2), \ldots, \text{vec}(Y_m)]$ of size $(m \times n) \times M$ by vectorizing each image Y_i. Then Γ is decomposed by SVD as $\Gamma = U\Sigma V$. We can pick the first p singular-vectors of U as the representative of a point on Grassmann manifold $\mathcal{G}(p, m \times n)$ with size $(m \times n) \times p$. In the following experiments, the points on Grassmann Manifold of MNIST handwriting digits images are constructed by the above method.

4.2   MNIST Handwritten Digits Clustering

The MNIST database [34] has been widely used in pattern recognition field. The digit images in this database are written by about 250 volunteers and for each digit are different number of samples. In recognition application, 60,000 digit images in the database are often used as training data and 10,000 images are used as testing data. All the digit images in this databse have been size-normalized and centered in a fixed size of 28×28, so it does not need much efforts for preprocessing and formatting. Figure 3(a) shows some digit samples of this database. As the proposed LRR model on Grassmann Manifold dose not need training, we merge the training set and testing set into a single sample set to do clustering experiment.

In our experiment, we created subgroups randomly according to their classes so that the each subgroup consists of 20 images, i.e. $M = 20$. The subspace generated by each subgroup will be considered as a point on Grassmann manifold. Our task is to cluster all the available $N = 3495$ image subgroups into ten categories. Please note that we are clustering subgroups, not single digits. As mentioned above, for each subgroup of 20 images, we form them as vectors and then stack them into a matrix Γ. Then SVD decomposition is applied on Γ and the front $p = 10$ singular-vectors of its left singular matrix are used as the subspace basis, the point on Grassmann Manifold [22,36]. Finally the algorithm of

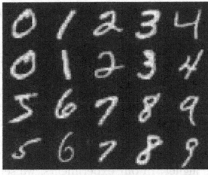

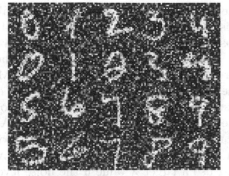

(a) The origin digit images   (b) The digit images with noise

Fig. 3. The MNIST digit samples for experiments

the proposed LRR model on Grassmann Manifold is conducted on these points on Grassmann manifold and the result of Z is pipelined to the Ncut algorithm. As a benchmark comparison, we mimic a point in Euclidean for each subgroup of 20 images by stacking them into a vector of dimension $28 \times 28 \times 20$. For PCA based method, the size $28 \times 28 \times 20 = 15680$ of each vector is reduced to 1566 by PCA.

The experimental results are reported in Table 2. It is shown that our proposed algorithm has the highest accuracy of 99 %, outperforming other methods more than 10 percents. The two worse results are for GNcut and GK-means methods. This can be explained that, after the Grassmann Manifold mapping, it is not a proper way to measure the Enclidean distance between the points on the manifold space. As our LRR model use the Grassmann distance measurement in a transformed space, the clustering results of our method are better than that of PNcut or PLRRNcut, in which the Euclidean distance is used to measure the relation of data reduced by PCA. The manifold mapping extracts more useful information about the differences among sample data. Then the combination of Grassmann distance and LRR model brings good accuracy for Ncut clustering.

Table 2. Subspace clustering results on the MINST database.

	PK-means	PNcut	PLRRNcut	GK-means	GNcut	our method
Accuracy	0.8638	0.9013	0.8552	0.4103	0.3339	0.99

We further tested the robustness of the proposed algorithm by adding noise to the digit images. We added a Gaussian noise $N(0, \sigma^2)$ onto all the digit images. Figure 3(b) shows the digit images with noise $\sigma = 0.45$. Generally, the noises will effect the performance of the clustering algorithm, especially when the noise is heavy. Figure 4 shows the clustering performance of different methods with the noise standard deviation σ ranging from 0.05 to 0.55. It indicates that our algorithm keeps over 99 % accuracy for the standard deviation up to 0.45, while the accuracy of other methods is generally lower than our method and behaves unstable when the noise standard deviation varies. This indicates that our proposed algorithm is robust for certain level of noises.

λ is an important parameter for balancing the error term and the low-rank term of the LRR model on Grassmann Manifold in (6). This is the same case for the PLRRncut method. We studied the effectiveness of λ for the final clustering result in several experiments. It can be observed that the noise level will change the rank of low-rank representation Z. A larger noise level will increase the rank of the represented coefficient matrix. So a proper way to tune λ is dependent on noise level. Generally we can make λ small when the noise of data is lower and use a larger λ value if the noise level is higher. In our experiments, we set $\lambda = 0.1$ for the our LRR model and set $\lambda = 0.5$ for PLRR method.

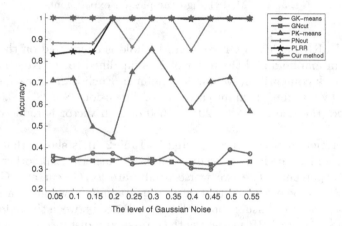

Fig. 4. Clustering on MNIST database with different level of noise.

4.3 Dynamic Texture Clustering

DynTex++ database [35] is derived from a total of 345 video sequences in different scenarios which contains river water, fish swimming, smoke, cloud and so on. These videos are labeled as 36 classes and each class has 100 subsequences (totally 3600 subsequences) with a fixed size of $50 \times 50 \times 50$ (50 gray frames). Some samples of DynTex++ are shown in Fig. 5. This is a challenge database for clustering because most of texture from different class is fairly similar.

Our method uses a set of samples to construct points on Grassmann Manifold, it is suitable to process video sequence data as a clip of continuous frames can be naturally collected as an image set. Moreover, as video sequence contain useful space and time context information for clustering, in order to utilize these information, instead of using SVD method, we use Local Binary Patterns from Three Orthogonal Plans (LBP-TOP) model [37] to construct points on Grassmann Manifold. The LBP-TOP method extract LBP features from three orthogonal planes and concatenate a number of neighbour points' features to

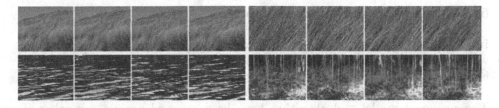

Fig. 5. DynTex++ samples. Each row includes frames from same video sequence and each four frames is a continuous clip.

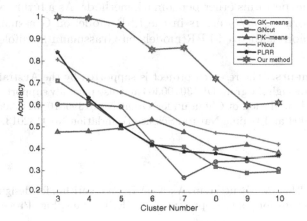

Fig. 6. Clustering results on DynTex++ database with the number of classes ranging from 3 to 10.

form a co-occurrence feature. After extracting LBP-TOP features for the 3600 subsequences, we get 3600 matrices of size 177×14 as the points on Grassmann Manifold. Then these features are represented by LRR model on Grassmann Manifold and its representation Z is used for Ncut clustering. As the data volume of all the 3600 subsequence is huge, we randomly pick K classes from 36 chesses and use these classes data for clustering experiments. The experiments is repeated several times for each K. In the experiments, λ is also set to 0.1. For the PCA based method, the prototype $50 \times 50 \times 50$ subsequence is reduced to 2478 and λ for the PLRRNcut is set to 0.5.

The clustering results for the DynTex++ database are shown in Fig. 6. For different number of classes, the accuracy of the proposed LRR model on Grassmann Manifold are superior to the other methods more than 10 percents, due to information extraction capability in Grassmann Manifold mapping over the LBP-TOP features. We also observed that all of accuracies decreases as the number of classes increases. This may be caused by the clustering challenge when more similar texture images are added into the data set.

5   Conclusion and Future Work

In this paper, we propose a novel LRR model on Grassmann manifold, in which we exploit the property of Grassmann manifold. To resolve the high-dimension issue in the resulting LRR model, we further explore the structured embedding mapping and derive an equivalent optimization problem which is easily solvable. The proposed model and algorithm have been assessed against a number of existing clustering algorithms. The experimental results show the efficiency and robustness of the proposed model. In most of the experimental cases, the proposed method outperforms other benchmark methods. As a future work, we will consider incorporating ℓ_1/ℓ_2 errors in the LRR model on Grassmann manifold and further explore kernelized LRR models on Grassmann manifold.

Acknowledgements. The research project is supported by the Australian Research Council (ARC) through the grant DP130100364 and also partially supported by National Natural Science Foundation of China under Grant No.61390510, 61133003, 61370119, 61171169, 61227004 and Beijing Natural Science Foundation No.4132013.

References

1. Aharon, M., Elad, M., Bruckstein, A.: K-SVD: an algorithm for designing overcomplete dictionaries for sparse representation. IEEE Trans. Sig. Process. **54**, 4311–4322 (2006)
2. Wright, J., Yang, A., Ganesh, A., Sastry, S., Ma, Y.: Robust face recognition via sparse representation. IEEE Trans. Pattern Anal. Mach. Intell. **31**, 210–227 (2009)
3. Elad, M., Aharon, M.: Image denoising via sparse and redundant representations over learned dictionaries. IEEE Trans. Image Process. **15**, 3736–3745 (2006)
4. Mairal, J., Elad, M., Sapiro, G.: Sparse representation for color image restoration. IEEE Trans. Image Process. **17**, 53–69 (2008)
5. Yang, J., Wang, Z., Lin, Z., Huang, T.: Coupled dictionary training for image super-resolution. IEEE Trans. Image Process. **21**, 3467–3478 (2012)
6. Liu, G., Lin, Z., Yu, Y.: Robust subspace segmentation by low-rank representation. In: International Conference on Machine Learning, pp. 663–670 (2010)
7. Liu, G., Lin, Z., Sun, J., Yu, Y., Ma, Y.: Robust recovery of subspace structures by low-rank representation. IEEE Trans. Pattern Anal. Mach. Intell. **35**, 171–184 (2013)
8. Cheng, B., Liu, G., Wang, J., Huang, Z., Yan, S.: Multi-task low-rank affinity pursuit for image segmentation. In: International Conference on Computer Vision, pp. 2439–2446 (2011)
9. Lang, C., Liu, G., Yu, J., Yan, S.: Saliency detection by multitask sparsity pursuit. IEEE Trans. Image Process. **21**, 1327–1338 (2012)
10. Wright, J., Ganesh, A., Rao, S., Peng, Y., Ma, Y.: Multi-task low-rank affinity pursuit for image segmentation. In: Advances in Neural Information Processing Systems, vol. 22 (2009)
11. Candés, E.J., Li, X., Ma, Y., Wright, J.: Robust principal component analysis? J. ACM **58**, 11 (2011). Article 11
12. Elhamifar, E., Vidal, R.: Subspace clustering. IEEE Sig. Process. Mag. **28**, 52–68 (2011)

13. Wang, R., Shan, S., Chen, X., Gao, W.: Manifold-manifold distance with application to face recognition based on image set. In: Computer Vision and Pattern Recognition, pp. 1–8 (2008)
14. Roweis, S., Saul, L.: Nonlinear dimensionality reduction by locally linear embedding. Science **290**, 2323–2326 (2000)
15. Tenenbaum, J., Silva, V., Langford, J.: A global geometric framework for nonlinear dimensionality reduction. Optim. Methods Softw. **290**, 2319–2323 (2000)
16. He, X., Niyogi, P.: Locality Preserving Projections. Advances in Neural Information Processing Systems, vol. 16. MIT Press, Cambridge (2003)
17. Belkin, M., Niyogi, P.: Laplacian eigenmaps and spectral techniques for embedding and clustering. Advances in Neural Information Processing Systems, vol. 14. MIT Press, Cambridge (2001)
18. Absil, P.A., Mahony, R., Sepulchre, R.: Riemannian geometry of Grassmann manifolds with a view on algorithmic computation. Acta Appl. Math. **80**, 199–220 (2004)
19. Srivastava, A., Klassen, E.: Bayesian and geometric subspace tracking. Adv. Appl. Probab. **36**, 43–56 (2004)
20. Cetingul, H., Vidal, R.: Intrinsic mean shift for clustering on Stiefel and Grassmann manifolds. In: IEEE Conference on Computer Vision and Pattern Recognition, pp. 1896–1902 (2009)
21. Hamm, J., Lee, D.: Grassmann discriminant analysis: a unifying view on sub-space-based learning. In: International Conference on Machine Learning, pp. 376–383 (2008)
22. Harandi, M., Shirazi, S., Sanderson, C., Lovell, B.: Graph embedding discriminant analysis on Grassmannian manifolds for improved image set matching. In: Computer Vision and Pattern Recognition. pp. 2705–2712 (2011)
23. Harandi, M., Sanderson, C., Shen, C., Lovell, B.: Dictionary learning and sparse coding on grassmann manifolds: an extrinsic solution. In: International Conference on Computer Vision, vol. 14, pp. 3120–3127 (2013)
24. Fazel, M.: Matrix rank minimization with applications. Ph.D. thesis, Stanford University (2002)
25. Elhamifar, E., Vidal, R.: Sparse subspace clustering: algorithm, theory, and applications. IEEE Trans. Pattern Anal. Mach. Intell. **35**, 2765–2781 (2013)
26. Xu, C., Wang, T., Gao, J., Cao, S., Tao, W., Liu, F.: An ordered-patch-based image classification approach on the image Grassmannian manifold. IEEE Trans. Neural Networks Learn. Syst. **25**, 728–737 (2014)
27. Absil, P., Mahony, R., Sepulchre, R.: Optimization Algorithms on Matrix Manifolds. Princeton University Press, Princeton (2008)
28. Helmke, J.T., Hüper, K.: Newtons's method on Grassmann manifolds. Technical report (2007). Preprint: [arXiv:0709.2205]
29. Kolda, G., Bader, B.: Tensor decomposition and applications. SIAM Rev. **51**(3), 455–500 (2009)
30. Gentle, J.E.: Numerical Linear Algebra for Applications in Statistics. Springer, New York (1998)
31. Shen, Y., Wen, Z., Zhang, Y.: Augmented Lagrangian alternating direction method for matrix separation based on low-rank factorization. Optim. Methods Softw. **29**, 239–263 (2014)
32. Cai, J.F., Candès, E.J., Shen, Z.: A singular value thresholding algorithm for matrix completion. SIAM J. Optim. **20**, 1956–1982 (2008). http://www-stat.stanford.edu/candes/papers/SVT.pdf

33. Shi, J., Malik, J.: Normalized cuts and image segmentation. IEEE Trans. Pattern Anal. Mach. Intell. **22**, 888–905 (2000)
34. Lecun, Y., Bottou, L., Bengio, Y., Haffner, P.: Gradient-based learning applied to document recognition. Proc. IEEE **86**, 2278–2324 (1998)
35. Ghanem, B., Ahuja, N.: Maximum margin distance learning for dynamic texture recognition. In: Daniilidis, K., Maragos, P., Paragios, N. (eds.) ECCV 2010, Part II. LNCS, vol. 6312, pp. 223–236. Springer, Heidelberg (2010)
36. Harandi, M.T., Sanderson, C., Hartley, R., Lovell, B.C.: Sparse coding and dictionary learning for symmetric positive definite matrices: a kernel approach. In: Fitzgibbon, A., Lazebnik, S., Perona, P., Sato, Y., Schmid, C. (eds.) ECCV 2012, Part II. LNCS, vol. 7573, pp. 216–229. Springer, Heidelberg (2012)
37. Zhao, G., Pietikäinen, M.: Dynamic texture recognition using local binary patterns with an application to facial expressions. IEEE Trans. Pattern Anal. Mach. Intell. **29**, 915–928 (2007)

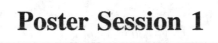

Poster Session 1

Learning Detectors Quickly
with Stationary Statistics

Jack Valmadre[1,2](✉), Sridha Sridharan[1], and Simon Lucey[3]

[1] Queensland University of Technology, Brisbane, Australia
[2] CSIRO, Brisbane, Australia
{j.valmadre,s.sridharan}@qut.edu.au
[3] Carnegie Mellon University, Pittsburgh, PA, USA
slucey@cs.cmu.edu

Abstract. Computer vision is increasingly becoming interested in the rapid estimation of object detectors. The canonical strategy of using Hard Negative Mining to train a Support Vector Machine is slow, since the large negative set must be traversed at least once per detector. Recent work has demonstrated that, with an assumption of signal stationarity, Linear Discriminant Analysis is able to learn comparable detectors without ever revisiting the negative set. Even with this insight, the time to learn a detector can still be on the order of minutes. Correlation filters, on the other hand, can produce a detector in under a second. However, this involves the unnatural assumption that the statistics are periodic, and requires the negative set to be re-sampled per detector size. These two methods differ chiefly in the structure which they impose on the covariance matrix of all examples. This paper is a comparative study which develops techniques (i) to assume periodic statistics without needing to revisit the negative set and (ii) to accelerate the estimation of detectors with aperiodic statistics. It is experimentally verified that periodicity is detrimental.

1 Introduction

Historically in computer vision, the time required to train a detector has been considered of minimal consequence because it only needs to be performed once. However, a number of vision algorithms for modern tasks involve learning a multitude of detectors, sometimes even in online settings. Examples include adaptive tracking [1,2], object detection with a large number of classes [3,4], algorithms for discovering discriminable clusters [5–7] and exemplar-based methods which train a detector per example [8]. An algorithm which drastically reduces the time and memory in which an effective detector can be trained has a big potential impact on these higher-level tasks.

Detectors are generally trained using machine learning algorithms for classification. One of the immediate and fundamental questions is: how to treat

---

Electronic supplementary material The online version of this chapter (doi:10. 1007/978-3-319-16865-4_7) contains supplementary material, which is available to authorized users.

© Springer International Publishing Switzerland 2015
D. Cremers et al. (Eds.): ACCV 2014, Part I, LNCS 9003, pp. 99–114, 2015.
DOI: 10.1007/978-3-319-16865-4_7

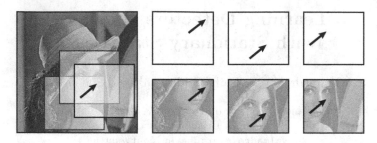

Fig. 1. The set of all translated windows exhibits stationarity since a single pair of pixels (indicated by the arrow) contributes to the statistics of all pairs with the same relative displacement. This results in a covariance matrix with Toeplitz structure, which Hariharan et al. [9] enforce to make estimation of the statistics of all windows feasible.

the enormous negative set? Any image which does not contain the object can contribute all of its sub-images, quickly generating myriad negative examples. Support Vector Machines (SVMs) are attractive in this regard, as they seek a solution which depends on only a sparse subset of the examples (i.e. the support vectors). Finding this set is, however, no easier than solving the original problem. A popular heuristic is Hard Negative Mining (HNM), which alternates between training a detector and adding possible support vectors to the training set. New examples are found by using the current detector to exhaustively search a large negative set for false positives, making HNM poorly suited to the aforementioned tasks.

An alternative to SVMs is to entertain simple approaches which obtain a detector as the solution to a system of linear equations $\mathbf{w} = \mathbf{S}^{-1}\mathbf{r}$ whose dimension is independent of the number of examples. These include Linear Discriminant Analysis (LDA) and linear least-squares regression, in both of which $\mathbf{S}$ is a covariance matrix. Forming this system, however, tends to be computationally prohibitive without some additional knowledge of the problem. This paper examines two algorithms which make different assumptions regarding the structure of the covariance matrix, each with its own distinct motivation.

The first is the method of Hariharan et al. [9], in which the set of examples is assumed to be stationary, resulting in a Toeplitz covariance matrix

$$S_{ui} = g[i - u]. \tag{1}$$

This redundant structure imposes the assumption that the covariance of samples $x[u]$ and $x[i]$ is governed exclusively by their relative position, independent of their absolute position. This is motivated by the observation that any sub-image or "window" of a natural image also belongs to the set of natural images, therefore the statistics of the set of all natural images must be translation invariant (see Fig. 1). The redundancy is sufficient to make estimation of the covariance matrix computationally tractable. Adopting this assumption within an LDA framework, comparable detection performance to HNM has been demonstrated [9].

The second method is that of correlation filters [10,11], in which all circular shifts of each example are incorporated into the training set (see Fig. 2).

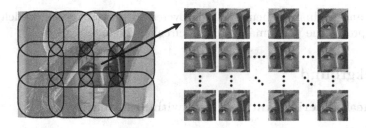

Fig. 2. Henriques et al. approximated the set of all translated windows in an image with all circular shifts (right) of a coarsely-sampled set of windows which cover the image (left). This results in a circulant covariance matrix which can be inverted in closed form. Rounded rectangles illustrate overlap.

This manifests in a covariance matrix which is not only Toeplitz, but circulant

$$S_{ui} = h[(i - u) \bmod m] \tag{2}$$

for example signals of length m. The mod operator extends the assumption of stationarity beyond the boundary of the signal, under periodic extension. We refer to this stronger assumption as "periodic stationarity." The set of all circular shifts seems like an unnatural set to want to include, and indeed, the motivation is entirely computational. The discrete Fourier basis constitutes eigenvectors for any circulant matrix, meaning that efficient inversion can be performed using the Fast Fourier Transform (FFT). Thus, while the Toeplitz covariance more closely reflects the nature of the problem, the circulant system can be solved in much less time and memory.

Another critical difference is that the elements of the circulant covariance matrix depend on the signal size m, whereas those of the Toeplitz covariance matrix do not. This is due to the difference between (1) and (2). Therefore the Toeplitz covariance can be used to train detectors of arbitrary size and only needs to be computed once. It can also be elegantly estimated from signals of arbitrary size. In the circulant case, on the other hand, it is necessary to know the size of the examples *a priori*, and then to choose and sample a representative subset of windows of this size as in [12]. To train a detector of a different size, the entire process must be repeated.

The first contribution of this paper is to develop a simple expression for the (circulant) covariance matrix of all circular shifts of a set of windows of arbitrary size with known Toeplitz covariance. This enables correlation filters to be learnt from the stationary distribution alone, without the need to ever re-visit the negative set.

The second contribution is to investigate methods for efficiently solving the Toeplitz system, particularly in the case of two-dimensional signals such as images. While Toeplitz matrices are shown to produce higher quality detectors, the raw speed of the non-iterative algorithm for circulant matrix inversion may make it an attractive option despite the degradation of performance. We additionally elucidate and evaluate a heuristic, discovered in previous work, which significantly improves the performance of the circulant regime.

2   Background

2.1   Linear Discriminant Analysis with Stationarity

Linear Discriminant Analysis (LDA) is a generative approach to binary classification which models both classes with a Gaussian distribution, assuming that the two distributions have the same covariance matrix to ensure that the discriminant is an affine function $f(\mathbf{x}) = \mathbf{w}^T\mathbf{x} + b$. The optimal template $\mathbf{w}$ is obtained in closed form $\mathbf{w} = \mathbf{S}^{-1}\mathbf{r}$, where $\mathbf{r} = \bar{\mathbf{x}}_+ - \bar{\mathbf{x}}_-$ is the difference between the means of the positive and negative classes and $\mathbf{S}$ is the covariance of all examples. Typically when training a detector, the positive class is "object" and the negative class is "not object."

Let $\mathbf{x}_1, \ldots, \mathbf{x}_n \in \mathcal{R}^m$ denote n examples, each with m elements. It can be assumed without loss of generality that the examples are zero-mean. The covariance of these examples would typically be estimated

$$\mathbf{S} = \frac{1}{n} \sum_{k=1}^{n} \mathbf{x}_k \mathbf{x}_k^T. \tag{3}$$

This computation requires $\mathcal{O}(nm^2)$ time and $\mathcal{O}(m^2)$ memory. Clearly it is impractical to evaluate this on the set of all windows in a collection of images, where n numbers thousands per image and m is the number of pixels in a window.

Hariharan et al. [9] recognised that the set of natural images exhibits stationarity. This is motivated by observing that all sub-images of a natural image also belong to the set of natural images, therefore the statistics of the set of *all* natural images must be translation invariant (see Fig. 1).

Let us first consider each vector $\mathbf{x}_k$ to be a scalar-valued time-series of length m with samples $x_k[0], \ldots, x_k[m-1]$, before later generalising to feature images. If the set of examples is drawn from a stationary distribution, then the covariance matrix possesses a highly redundant Toeplitz structure $S_{ui} = g[i - u]$, which encodes that the correlation of samples $x[u]$ and $x[i]$ depends only on their relative position. For signals of length m, this $m \times m$ matrix is fully specified by the $2m - 1$ elements in $g[\delta]$, which is defined for $\delta = -m + 1, \ldots, m - 1$. The symmetry of the covariance matrix further implies $g[\delta] = g[-\delta]$ and therefore m elements are sufficient. The zero-mean assumption in this context is discussed in Appendix B.1.

When considering detection problems in which the negative class is "not object," the covariance and mean are dominated by the negative set. Typically a set of large signals $\phi_1[t], \ldots, \phi_N[t]$ of length $M \geq m$ is available from which every window of length m constitutes a negative example (as in the canonical HNM problem). Under stationarity, the expected covariance is computed per relative displacement δ from all instances of that displacement in the large signals

$$g[\delta] = \frac{1}{N\rho(\delta)} \sum_{k=1}^{N} \sum_{t=a(\delta)}^{b(\delta)-1} \phi_k[t] \cdot \phi_k[t+\delta] \qquad (4)$$

where the limits $a(\delta) = \max(0, -\delta)$ and $b(\delta) = M - \max(0, \delta)$ ensure that both t and $t+\delta$ lie within the domain of the signal $\{0, \ldots, M-1\}$. The normalisation factor $\rho(\delta) = b(\delta) - a(\delta) = M - |\delta|$ counts the number of occurrences of the displacement δ in each signal (shorter displacements are observed more times). Unlike the true covariance matrix, which is a sum of outer products, a Toeplitz matrix obtained in this fashion is not guaranteed to be positive semidefinite. Given enough data, however, the eigenvalues converge to non-negativity.

If the covariance matrix were computed naively from the full set of $M - m + 1$ overlapping windows contained in each signal, its estimation would take $\mathcal{O}(Mm^2)$ time. Using the above expression, statistics can instead be gathered directly from each large signal in $\mathcal{O}(Mm)$ time. Furthermore, this method only requires $\mathcal{O}(m)$ memory instead of $\mathcal{O}(m^2)$.

Hariharan et al. [9] applied this technique to the problem of computing the covariance of every translated window in a set of larger images, which would otherwise have been intractable. To obtain a detector, they finally instantiated the full covariance matrix and employed a direct method such as Cholesky decomposition, noting that it was necessary to add some small regularisation $\lambda\mathbf{I}$. Since the negative examples dominate the statistics, the mean of the negative class is taken to be that of the stationary distribution so that $\mathbf{r} = \bar{\mathbf{x}}_+ - \bar{\mathbf{x}}$.

2.2 Correlation Filters

The algorithm of correlation filters [10] in its unconstrained form [11] is simply linear least-squares regression applied to the set of all circular shifts of every example. While including circular shifts in the training set may seem peculiar, it leads to a system of equations which can be constructed and solved in the Fourier domain.

It is a famous result that LDA is equivalent to linear least-squares regression when the desired outputs of the regression problem take on exactly two distinct values, corresponding to the two classes [13]. Given a set of general vectors $\mathbf{x}_1, \ldots, \mathbf{x}_n \in \mathcal{R}^m$ with desired outputs $y_1, \ldots, y_n \in \mathcal{R}$, the regularised problem, also known as ridge regression, finds the solution to

$$\min_{\mathbf{w}, b} \quad \frac{1}{2n} \sum_{k=1}^{n} \left(\mathbf{w}^T \mathbf{x}_k + b - y_k \right)^2 + \frac{\lambda}{2} \|\mathbf{w}\|^2 . \qquad (5)$$

If the examples are assumed to be zero-mean, then the solution is obtained by taking the bias to be the mean label $b = \bar{y}$, and solving for the template in

$$\min_{\mathbf{w}} \quad \frac{1}{2n} \sum_{k=1}^{n} \left(\mathbf{w}^T \mathbf{x}_k - y_k \right)^2 + \frac{\lambda}{2} \|\mathbf{w}\|^2 . \qquad (6)$$

The optimal template is obtained in closed form $\mathbf{w} = (\mathbf{S} + \lambda \mathbf{I})^{-1} \mathbf{r}$ with $\mathbf{S}$ defined as in (3) and the right-hand side given

$$\mathbf{r} = \frac{1}{n} \sum_{k=1}^{n} y_k \mathbf{x}_k. \tag{7}$$

See Appendix B.2 for the derivation. Note that if we choose $y_k = 0$ for negative examples, then they do not appear in the solution beyond their contribution to the covariance and the mean.

Let us again consider each $\mathbf{x}_k$ to be a scalar-valued time-series of length m. Computing the expected covariance of all circular shifts of these examples generates a circulant matrix $S_{ui} = h[(i - u) \bmod m]$. This $m \times m$ matrix is defined by only m unique elements, or $\lceil m/2 \rceil$ accounting for symmetry. These are estimated from data according to

$$h[\delta] = \frac{1}{mn} \sum_{k=1}^{n} \sum_{t=0}^{m-1} x_k[t] \cdot x_k[(t + \delta) \bmod m]. \tag{8}$$

See Appendix B.3 for the derivation. This means that the covariance of two samples $x[u]$ and $x[i]$ is estimated from all pairs of samples which have relative displacement $(i - u) \bmod m$, including some displacements which cross the boundary of the signal and wrap around.

Circulant matrices can be inverted efficiently in the Fourier domain because a matrix-vector product amounts to periodic cross-correlation. Let $\star$ denote the periodic cross-correlation operator such that

$$(w \star x)[u] = \sum_{t=0}^{m-1} w[t] \cdot x[(u + t) \bmod m] \tag{9}$$

for $u = 0, \ldots, m - 1$, and recall that this is equivalent to element-wise multiplication in the Fourier domain $\mathcal{F}\{\mathbf{w} \star \mathbf{x}\} = \mathrm{conj}(\hat{\mathbf{w}}) \circ \hat{\mathbf{x}}$, where we denote the Fourier transform of a signal $\mathcal{F}\{\mathbf{x}\} = \hat{\mathbf{x}}$. Multiplication by the circulant covariance matrix $\mathbf{z} = \mathbf{S}\mathbf{w}$ computes the cross-correlation $\mathbf{z} = \mathbf{h} \star \mathbf{w}$ or equivalently $\hat{\mathbf{z}} = \mathrm{conj}(\hat{\mathbf{h}}) \circ \hat{\mathbf{w}}$. This enables the re-expression of $\mathbf{w} = (\mathbf{S} + \lambda \mathbf{I})^{-1} \mathbf{r}$ as a diagonal system of equations

$$\hat{\mathbf{w}} = \left[\mathrm{diag}(\mathrm{conj}(\hat{\mathbf{h}})) + \lambda \mathbf{I} \right]^{-1} \hat{\mathbf{r}}. \tag{10}$$

Whereas a general $m \times m$ system of equations requires $\mathcal{O}(m^3)$ time to solve via factorisation, the solution to this system is obtained in $\mathcal{O}(m)$ time, with $\mathcal{O}(m \log m)$ additional time required to compute the FFT. Further, while factorisation algorithms generally require $\mathcal{O}(m^2)$ space to store the full matrix, this system can be solved in $\mathcal{O}(m)$ space.

The system in (10) can also be constructed in the Fourier domain since

$$h[\delta] = \frac{1}{mn} \sum_{k=1}^{n} (x_k \star x_k)[\delta], \qquad r[u] = \frac{1}{mn} \sum_{k=1}^{n} (y_k \star x_k)[u]. \tag{11}$$

See Appendix B.4 for the derivation. This can be performed in $\mathcal{O}(nm \log m)$ time. Taking the desired response function $y_k[t]$ to be zero everywhere for negative examples and an impulse function (1 at the origin, 0 everywhere else) for positive examples results in the same right-hand side $\mathbf{r} = \bar{\mathbf{x}}_+ - \bar{\mathbf{x}}$ as in LDA.

Henriques et al. [12] proposed correlation filters as an alternative to HNM. They approximated the set of all windows in an image by the set of all circular shifts of a subset of windows which was sufficient to cover the image with significant overlap (see Fig. 2). This subset would need to be re-sampled to train a detector of a different size.

2.3   Related Work

A number of other works have used fast correlation in the Fourier domain to accelerate the process of training a detector. Anguita et al. [14] used it to efficiently compute subgradients when training an SVM across all windows in a set of images. However, this is liable to be even slower than HNM, since the negative set must be traversed per gradient descent iteration. Dubout and Fleuret [15] treated images as mini-batches within stochastic descent and used the FFT to efficiently compute the subgradient of the objective function across all windows in an image. While this is undoubtedly more efficient than naively computing inner products, it cannot rival the closed-forms solution of correlation filters.

Rodríguez et al. [16] proposed an objective function which comprises a hinge loss on each un-shifted example plus a least-squares loss on all circular shifts, and showed that it can be solved in a canonical SVM framework. They noted that the loss over circular shifts can be considered a linear transformation of the space in which the margin is measured as in [17]. Our paper provides a method to obtain such a transformation from a large training set, without the need to re-compute it for different sizes. It would also be possible to adopt the Toeplitz matrix in their framework to eliminate periodic effects.

Henriques et al. [18] showed that the kernel matrix of circularly shifted examples also exhibits block-circulant structure, where the size of the blocks is the number of base examples rather than of the number of feature channels. We restrict discussion to the primal form in this paper, since we are primarily interested in learning from a large number of examples. In addition to ridge regression, the same authors used the dual formulation to approximately solve Support Vector Regression (SVR) in a canonical co-ordinate descent framework [12].

3   Fast Estimation of the Toeplitz Covariance

The previous section established that the circulant system is not only solved but also constructed efficiently in the Fourier domain. In this section, we briefly demonstrate that the FFT can likewise be used to construct the Toeplitz system.

It's clear on inspection of (4) that the elements of the Toeplitz matrix $S_{ui} = g[i - u]$ are computed by a sum of (non-periodic) auto-correlations. Let us introduce ψ_k to denote ϕ_k padded from length M to length $P = M + m - 1$ with zeros. Then g can be obtained via *periodic* auto-correlation

$$g[\delta] = \frac{1}{N\rho(\delta)} \sum_{k=1}^{N} (\psi_k \star \psi_k)[\delta \bmod P], \qquad (12)$$

taking only the subset $\delta = -m+1, \ldots, m-1$ of each output. See Appendix B.5 for details. Comparing this expression to (11), the unique elements of the Toeplitz matrix $g[\delta]$ can be obtained in almost exactly the same manner as those of the circulant matrix $h[\delta]$.

This can be performed using the FFT in $\mathcal{O}(M \log M)$ time per signal. This implies that the statistics can be gathered for any window size $m \leq M$ without affecting the asymptotic computational complexity. As far as we know, the original authors did not take advantage of this aspect of the problem.

4   From Toeplitz to Circulant

We have now established that the Toeplitz and circulant covariance matrices can be estimated with similar computational effort, and that the circulant system can be solved very efficiently. However, a distinct advantage of adopting the Toeplitz covariance is that, comparing (4) and (8), its elements do not depend on the length m of the template $\mathbf{w}$. This means that the same covariance $g[\delta]$ could be used to learn affine functions $f(\mathbf{x}) = \mathbf{w}^T \mathbf{x} + b$ of different sizes.

It also provides a far more elegant way to obtain statistics from a set of larger signals, of which every sub-signal could be considered a negative example. Unlike correlation filters, where it is necessary to sample windows of size m, the stationary covariance can be estimated from the whole signal as in (4).

This section formulates an expression for the elements of the circulant matrix $h[\delta]$ from those of the Toeplitz matrix $g[\delta]$. This is performed in the same way that a circulant matrix is obtained in correlation filters: by incorporating all circular shifts of all signals in some set. The set which we consider is one which possesses stationarity.

Theorem 1. *If a set of length-m signals is stationary with Toeplitz covariance matrix $S_{ij} = g[j - i]$, then the covariance of the set of all circular shifts of these signals is circulant $S_{ij} = h[(j - i) \bmod m]$ with elements*

$$h[\delta] = (1 - \theta)\, g[\delta \bmod m] + \theta\, g[-(-\delta \bmod m)] \qquad (13)$$

for $\delta = 0, \ldots, m - 1$ with $\theta = (\delta \bmod m)/m$.

Proof. See Appendix A.

This is a convex combination of the Toeplitz covariance for the relative displacements of $(\delta \bmod m)$ and $-(-\delta \bmod m)$, with greater weight given to the smaller of the two. The intuition behind this is that, under periodic extension, a given

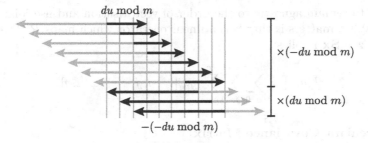

Fig. 3. Under periodic extension, a relative displacement $\delta \neq 0$ from every position in the signal is more often observed as the smaller displacement of the two modulo complements. For example, a small positive and a large negative displacement are both predominantly observed as a small positive displacement.

displacement from every position in the signal is more often observed as the smaller of it and its modulo complement (see Fig. 3). This expression enables correlation filters of arbitrary size to be trained from a stationary distribution, without having to choose explicit negative examples. The result is generalised to two-dimensional vector-valued signals in the following section.

5   Multi-channel, Two-Dimensional Signals

This section generalises the results thus far from time-series to feature images, or from single-channel, one-dimensional signals to multi-channel, two-dimensional signals. We denote elements samples of a feature image $x^p[u, v]$ for channel p at position (u, v).

5.1   Toeplitz Covariance Matrix

For the covariance matrix of two-dimensional signals of size $m \times \ell$ with c channels, we replace $u \leftarrow (u, v, p)$ and $i \leftarrow (i, j, q)$, using (u, v) and (i, j) to denote 2D positions and p and q denote feature indices. Stationarity of such signals is expressed in the constraint

$$S_{(u,v,p),(i,j,q)} = g_{pq}[i - u, j - v], \tag{14}$$

where the four-dimensional array $g_{pq}[du, dv]$ has $c^2(2m - 1)(2\ell - 1)$ elements. We refer to the structure of this covariance matrix as "block two-level Toeplitz." The symmetry of $\mathbf{S}$ gives the further redundancy $g_{pq}[du, dv] = g_{qp}[-du, -dv]$. Note that there is no assumption of stationarity across channel indices p and q. This matrix can also be efficiently estimated in the Fourier domain with appropriate zero-padding as in Sect. 3 (see Appendix B.6). The multi-channel stationary mean is constant per-channel $\bar{x}^p[u, v] = \mu_p$.

For a particular vectorisation of the feature image, this $m\ell c \times m\ell c$ matrix is an $m \times m$ Toeplitz matrix of $\ell \times \ell$ Toeplitz matrices of $c \times c$ blocks. However, we prefer to remain agnostic to the order of vectorisation and use joint indices (u, v, p). What matters is that $\mathbf{S}$ is a linear operator which maps $\mathcal{R}^{m\ell c} \to \mathcal{R}^{m\ell c}$ such that $\mathbf{z} = \mathbf{Sx}$ implies

$$z^p[u, v] = \sum_{i=0}^{m-1} \sum_{j=0}^{\ell-1} \sum_{q=1}^{c} g_{pq}[i - u, j - v] \cdot x^q[i, j]. \tag{15}$$

5.2 Circulant Covariance Matrix

Variously known as Vector Correlation Filters or Multi-Channel Correlation Filters, the periodic case is similar to the pure stationary case, with elements of the covariance matrix defined

$$S_{(u,v,p),(i,j,q)} = h_{pq}[(i - u) \bmod m, (j - v) \bmod \ell]. \tag{16}$$

The only difference is the introduction of the modulo operators. The four-dimensional array $h_{pq}[du, dv]$ has $c^2 m\ell$ elements, with the symmetry of the matrix yielding the further redundancy $h_{pq}[du, dv] = h_{qp}[-du \bmod m, -dv \bmod \ell]$.

Rather than being diagonalised by the 1D Fourier transform, this "block two-level circulant" matrix is block-diagonalised by applying the 2D Fourier transform to each channel independently, a fact which a slew of recent vision papers have taken advantage of [12, 19–21]. After transforming each channel, the problem decomposes into a $c \times c$ complex linear system of equations per sample. See Appendix B.7 for the form of these equations.

Introducing $d = m\ell$ to denote the number of pixels, the time required to compute necessary transforms and then solve these systems of equations is $\mathcal{O}(c^2 d \log d + c^3 d)$. Once the system has been constructed and each block factorised, subsequent solutions can be be obtained in $\mathcal{O}(c^2 d + cd \log d)$ time for back-substitution and inverse transforms. The memory required is the same as to store $h_{pq}[du, dv]$. In contrast, to solve this system using factorisation would take $\mathcal{O}(c^3 d^3)$ time and $\mathcal{O}(c^2 d^2)$ memory, with subsequent solutions obtained in $\mathcal{O}(c^2 d^2)$ time. For even modest template sizes, this makes an enormous difference. Furthermore, transforms of each channel and inversions of each block can be performed in parallel.

5.3 From Toeplitz to Circulant

The case for 2D signals is more involved since displacements can wrap around horizontal and/or vertical boundaries. Elements of the circulant matrix are given

$$\begin{aligned}
h_{pq}[du, dv] = &\ (1 - \alpha)(1 - \beta)\, g_{pq}[& du \bmod m, & & dv \bmod \ell] \\
&+ (1 - \alpha) & \beta\, g_{pq}[& du \bmod m, & -(-dv \bmod \ell)] \\
&+ & \alpha(1 - \beta)\, g_{pq}[-(-du \bmod m), & & dv \bmod \ell] \\
&+ & \alpha & \beta\, g_{pq}[-(-du \bmod m), & -(-dv \bmod \ell)] \tag{17}
\end{aligned}$$

with $\alpha = (du \bmod m)/m$, $\beta = (dv \bmod \ell)/\ell$. The derivation follows the same technique as the one-dimensional case.

6   Solving Toeplitz Systems

Unfortunately, Toeplitz matrices are not diagonalised by the Fourier transform as circulant matrices are. There is, however, an extensive and varied body of literature surrounding the solution of Toeplitz systems, and we briefly review some key results.

6.1   Direct Methods

Recall that a general $m \times m$ system of equations can be factorised in $\mathcal{O}(m^3)$ time with subsequent solutions obtained in $\mathcal{O}(m^2)$ time. Levinson recursion [22,23] allows Toeplitz systems to instead be factorised in $\mathcal{O}(m^2)$ time, with the Gohberg-Semencul formula [24] enabling solutions to then be obtained in $\mathcal{O}(m \log m)$ time. This is entirely without inflicting the $\mathcal{O}(m^2)$ memory requirement of instantiating the explicit matrix or its inverse. There also exist "superfast" or "asymptotic" algorithms [25,26] which solve a system in $\mathcal{O}(m \log^2 m)$ time without factorisation, although the hidden coefficients can be large. Levinson recursion has been generalised to solve $mc \times mc$ block Toeplitz systems, comprising an $m \times m$ Toeplitz structure of arbitrary $c \times c$ blocks, in an algorithm that takes $\mathcal{O}(c^3 m^2)$ time [27]. This is useful for multi-channel, *one*-dimensional signals.

Unfortunately, in the extension to two-level Toeplitz matrices, which are our primary interest in vision, algorithms based on Levinson recursion cannot do better than to treat one level as a general matrix [28,29]. For $m \times \ell$ images with c feature channels, this only enables inversion of the Toeplitz covariance matrix in $\mathcal{O}(c^3 \min(m^2 \ell^3, m^3 \ell^2))$ time. A handful of obscure exceptions have been identified [29,30], although they do not seem pertinent to us.

6.2   Iterative Methods

While the Fourier transform cannot be used directly to invert a Toeplitz matrix, it does enable fast evaluation of matrix-vector products. This is achieved by extending an $m \times m$ Toeplitz matrix to form a $(2m-1) \times (2m-1)$ circulant matrix. This *does* extend to block two-level Toeplitz matrices, as $\mathbf{z} = \mathbf{S}\mathbf{x}$ gives

$$z^p[u,v] = \sum_{q=1}^{c} \sum_{i=0}^{m-1} \sum_{j=0}^{\ell-1} g_{pq}[i-u, j-v]\, x^q[i,j] = \sum_{q=1}^{c} (g_{pq} \star \tilde{x}^q)[u,v] \qquad (18)$$

where $\tilde{x}^q[u,v]$ denotes a zero-padded version of $x^q[u,v]$. For images with d pixels and c channels, this allows multiplication to be performed in $\mathcal{O}(c^2 d \log d)$ time, all without instantiating the full matrix.

The existence of a fast multiplication routine suggests iterative first-order methods. In fact, a number of past works have proposed to solve Toeplitz systems using the Preconditioned Conjugate Gradient (PCG) method. The convergence rate of this algorithm depends on the condition number of the matrix and how tightly clustered its eigenvalues are [31]. PCG considers the equivalent problem

$\mathbf{MSw} = \mathbf{Mr}$, where the preconditioner $\mathbf{M}$ must be full rank and $\mathbf{MS}$ has more desirable spectral properties than $\mathbf{S}$ alone. Most works have centered around the choice of preconditioner, with Chan and Ng [32] in particular arguing that an effective preconditioner renders the number of iterations a small constant, yielding the solution to an $m \times m$ Toeplitz system in $\mathcal{O}(m \log m)$ time.

The ideal choice is $\mathbf{M} = \mathbf{S}^{-1}$, however to obtain this matrix is to solve the original problem. Inverse circulant matrices make attractive preconditioners because they are easily computed and circulant matrices are in some sense "close" to Toeplitz matrices. Strang [33] originally proposed a circulant matrix which used only the inner diagonals of the Toeplitz matrix and was shown to guarantee superlinear convergence for a large class of problems [34]. Chan [35] instead considered the nearest circulant matrix and observed empirically that it was more effective at reducing the condition number and producing a clustered spectrum. Two-level circulant preconditioners have previously been explored for block Toeplitz [36] and two-level Toeplitz systems [32], but to our knowledge not for block two-level Toeplitz systems. Serra Capizzano and Tyrtyshnikov [37] presented the theoretical result that multi-level circulant preconditioners are not guaranteed superlinear convergence for multi-level Toeplitz matrices by the same mechanism as one-level, noting that fast convergence is still possible in practice.

Somewhat surprisingly, the circulant covariance matrix which we obtained in Sect. 4 is in fact the nearest (block multi-level) circulant matrix, analogous to the preconditioner in [35]. Therefore we can optionally employ the circulant solution (i.e. learn a correlation filter) as a preconditioner within conjugate gradient. This preconditioner results in significantly faster convergence (see Fig. 6).

To summarise, this leaves us with several options to learn a detector. Firstly, we can choose to solve either the Toeplitz or the circulant system. If we choose to solve the circulant system, it is done in closed form. If we instead decide to solve the Toeplitz system, then we can either solve it directly by Cholesky decomposition or iteratively using conjugate gradient, with or without the circulant inverse as a preconditioner.

6.3   An Effective Heuristic

The performance of the detector learnt using circulant covariance can be greatly increased with a simple heuristic, which is to train a larger detector than desired and then crop it *after* training. This was discovered in a subset of the experiments of [12], although as far as we are aware, it has not previously been discussed. Figure 4 shows that nearly identical performance to the Toeplitz method is achieved. One extra feature pixel on all sides was found to be sufficient.

While we do not have a theoretical analysis of the cropping heuristic, it at least makes intuitive sense. The most highly correlated feature pixels are those which are adjacent. A circulant matrix considers two pixels on opposite edges to be adjacent. The probable discontinuity between these elements in the mean positive image is likely to be something which the detector learns about the positive set. That one feature pixel is sufficient suggests that the correlation of samples decays rapidly with increasing distance.

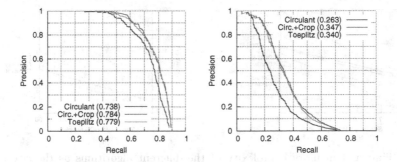

Fig. 4. Precision versus recall for INRIA (left) and Caltech (right) pedestrian detection datasets. Average precision is shown in parentheses.

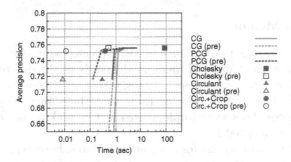

Fig. 5. Average precision versus training time for pedestrian detection on the INRIA dataset. Iterative methods trace a path, closed-form methods mark a single point. Timing shown for full computation and to obtain subsequent detectors (after *pre-computation*). The template was 12×33 features with 31 channels.

7 Empirical Study

Experiments were conducted on HOG images [38] using the 31-channel implementation of [39]. The stationary statistics were estimated once from four million random images from ImageNet [3] to illustrate that all techniques can draw on a huge number of negative examples. Regularisation $\lambda \mathbf{I}$ was added with $\lambda = 10^{-2}$. Further practical details are found in Appendix C.

7.1 Detection Performance

The detectors learnt under Toeplitz and circulant assumptions were compared for the task of pedestrian detection (see Fig. 4). Toeplitz was found to consistently outperform circulant. Surprisingly, learning with a circulant matrix and using the extend-and-crop heuristic rivals the performance of the Toeplitz method. The detectors were evaluated on the ETHZ Shape Classes dataset [40], although the results were found to be noisy and less conclusive due to its insufficient size (see Appendix D).

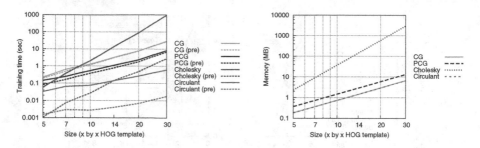

Fig. 6. Time and memory complexity of the different algorithms as the size of the template increases. These specific results are for 31-channel HOG images. Training time is empirical and memory is theoretical.

7.2   Time and Memory

Figure 5 plots the average performance of each detector against its training time. Figure 6 shows how the time and memory demands of the different algorithms grow with template size. We present times with and without pre-computable factorisations and transforms included (note that these must be performed per detector size). Algorithms were implemented in Go, making use of FFTW and LAPACK where appropriate.

Cholesky factorisation is fast for compact templates. However, as the template size grows, it becomes relatively slow unless the factorisation can be pre-computed. The memory required to store such a factorisation also grows rapidly with the template size, soon reaching gigabytes. This makes it impractical to cache and load factorisations for several detector sizes, and may simply be infeasible or restrictive in some scenarios. For the problem of pedestrian detection, conjugate gradient offers a speed increase of nearly two orders of magnitude over computing the factorisation. The direct circulant method is several times faster again, however this requires one to either accept diminished performance or employ the cropping heuristic, the behaviour of which is not yet well understood.

8   Conclusion

Toeplitz and circulant covariance matrices have both previously been employed, within simplistic classifiers, to avoid Hard Negative Mining when learning from a large negative set. This paper has elucidated commonalities between these two techniques and proposed improvements to each. Compared to existing methods which use Toeplitz structure, identical detectors are obtained in orders of magnitude less time and memory. Circulant methods were shown to offer a further order of magnitude increase in speed for a small degradation of performance. Compared to existing methods which use circulant structure, the negative set does not need to be revisited per detector size. These are exciting developments for higher-level vision algorithms which involve learning linear templates.

Acknowledgement. This research was supported by Australian Research Council (ARC) Discovery Grant DP140100793.

References

1. Kalal, Z., Matas, J., Mikolajczyk, K.: P-N learning: Bootstrapping binary classifiers by structural constraints. In: CVPR, pp. 49–56. IEEE (2010)
2. Bolme, D.S., Beveridge, J.R., Draper, B.A., Lui, Y.M.: Visual object tracking using adaptive correlation filters. In: CVPR, pp. 2544–2550. IEEE (2010)
3. Deng, J., Dong, W., Socher, R., Li, L.J., Li, K., Fei-Fei, L.: ImageNet: A large-scale hierarchical image database. In: CVPR, pp. 248–255. IEEE (2009)
4. Dean, T., Ruzon, M., Segal, M., Shlens, J., Vijayanarasimhan, S., Yagnik, J.: Fast, accurate detection of 100,000 object classes on a single machine. In: CVPR (2013)
5. Bourdev, L., Malik, J.: Poselets: Body part detectors trained using 3D human pose annotations. In: ICCV, pp. 1365–1372. IEEE (2009)
6. Singh, S., Gupta, A., Efros, A.A.: Unsupervised discovery of mid-level discriminative patches. In: Fitzgibbon, A., Lazebnik, S., Perona, P., Sato, Y., Schmid, C. (eds.) ECCV 2012, Part II. LNCS, vol. 7573, pp. 73–86. Springer, Heidelberg (2012)
7. Doersch, C., Singh, S., Gupta, A., Sivic, J., Efros, A.A.: What makes Paris look like Paris? In: ACM Transactions on Graphics, vol. 31 (2012)
8. Malisiewicz, T., Gupta, A., Efros, A.A.: Ensemble of exemplar-SVMs for object detection and beyond. In: ICCV, pp. 89–96 (2011)
9. Hariharan, B., Malik, J., Ramanan, D.: Discriminative decorrelation for clustering and classification. In: Fitzgibbon, A., Lazebnik, S., Perona, P., Sato, Y., Schmid, C. (eds.) ECCV 2012, Part IV. LNCS, vol. 7575, pp. 459–472. Springer, Heidelberg (2012)
10. Mahalanobis, A., Vijaya Kumar, B.V.K., Casasent, D.: Minimum average correlation energy filters. Appl. Opt. **26**, 3633–3640 (1987)
11. Mahalanobis, A., Vijaya Kumar, B.V.K., Song, S., Sims, S.R.F., Epperson, J.F.: Unconstrained correlation filters. Appl. Opt. **33**, 3751–3759 (1994)
12. Henriques, J.F., Carreira, J., Caseiro, R., Batista, J.: Beyond hard negative mining: efficient detector learning via block-circulant decomposition. In: ICCV. IEEE (2013)
13. Fukunaga, K.: Introduction to Statistical Pattern Recognition, 2nd edn. Academic Press, London (1990)
14. Anguita, D., Boni, A., Pace, S.: Fast training of support vector machines for regression. In: International Joint Conference on Neural Networks, vol. 5, pp. 210–214. IEEE (2000)
15. Dubout, C., Fleuret, F.: Accelerated training of linear object detectors. In: CVPR Workshop on Structured Prediction, pp. 572–577. IEEE (2013)
16. Rodriguez, A., Boddeti, V.N., Vijaya Kumar, B.V.K., Mahalanobis, A.: Maximum margin correlation filter a new approach for localization and classification. Trans. Image Process. **22**, 631–643 (2013)
17. Ashraf, A.B., Lucey, S., Chen, T.: Reinterpreting the application of Gabor filters as a manipulation of the margin in linear support vector machines. PAMI **32**, 1335–1341 (2010)
18. Henriques, J.F., Caseiro, R., Martins, P., Batista, J.: High-speed tracking with kernelized correlation filters. PAMI (2015). doi:10.1109/TPAMI.2014.2345390

19. Boddeti, V.N., Kanade, T., Vijaya Kumar, B.V.K.: Correlation filters for object alignment. In: CVPR, pp. 2291–2298 (2013)
20. Bristow, H., Eriksson, A., Lucey, S.: Fast convolutional sparse coding. In: CVPR, pp. 391–398. IEEE (2013)
21. Kiani Galoogahi, H., Sim, T., Lucey, S.: Multi-channel correlation filters. In: ICCV. IEEE (2013)
22. Levinson, N.: The Wiener RMS error criterion in filter design and prediction. J. Math. Phys. **25**, 261–278 (1947)
23. Trench, W.F.: An algorithm for the inversion of finite Toeplitz matrices. J. Soc. Ind. Appl. Math. **12**, 515–522 (1964)
24. Gohberg, I., Semencul, A.: On the inversion of finite Toeplitz matrices and their continuous analogs. Mat. Issled. **2**, 201–233 (1972)
25. Brent, R.P., Gustavson, F.G., Yun, D.Y.Y.: Fast solution of Toeplitz systems of equations and computation of Padé approximants. J. Algorithms **295**, 259–295 (1980)
26. Ammar, G.S., Gragg, W.B.: Superfast solution of real positive definite Toeplitz systems. SIAM J. Matrix Anal. Appl. **9**, 61–76 (1988)
27. Akaike, H.: Block Toeplitz matrix inversion. SIAM J. Appl. Math. **24**, 234–241 (1973)
28. Wax, M., Kailath, T.: Efficient inversion of Toeplitz-block Toeplitz matrix. IEEE Trans. Acoust. Speech Signal Process. **31**, 1218–1221 (1983)
29. Yagle, A.E.: A fast algorithm for Toeplitz-block-Toeplitz linear systems. In: ICASSP, vol. 3, pp. 1929–1932. IEEE (2001)
30. Turnes, C.K., Balcan, D., Romberg, J.: Image deconvolution via superfast inversion of a class of two-level Toeplitz matrices. In: ICIP, pp. 3073–3076. IEEE (2012)
31. Nocedal, J., Wright, S.J.: Numerical Optimization, 2nd edn. Springer, Heidelberg (2006)
32. Chan, R.H., Ng, M.K.: Conjugate gradient methods for Toeplitz systems. SIAM Rev. **38**, 427–482 (1996)
33. Strang, G.: A proposal for Toeplitz matrix calculations. Stud. Appl. Math. **4**, 171–176 (1986)
34. Chan, R.H.: Circulant preconditioners for Hermitian Toeplitz systems. SIAM J. Matrix Anal. Appl. **10**, 542–550 (1989)
35. Chan, T.F.: An optimal circulant preconditioner for Toeplitz systems. SIAM J. Sci. Stat. Comput. **9**, 766–771 (1988)
36. Chan, T.F., Olkin, J.A.: Circulant preconditioners for Toeplitz-block matrices. Numer. Algorithms **6**, 89–101 (1994)
37. Capizzano, S.S., Tyrtyshnikov, E.E.: Any circulant-like preconditioner for multi-level matrices is not superlinear. SIAM J. Matrix Anal. Appl. **21**, 431–439 (2000)
38. Dalal, N., Triggs, B.: Histograms of oriented gradients for human detection. In: CVPR, vol. 1, pp. 886–893. IEEE (2005)
39. Felzenszwalb, P.F., Girshick, R.B., McAllester, D.A., Ramanan, D.: Object detection with discriminatively trained part based models. PAMI **32**, 1627–1645 (2010)
40. Ferrari, V., Tuytelaars, T., Van Gool, L.: Object detection by contour segment networks. In: Leonardis, A., Bischof, H., Pinz, A. (eds.) ECCV 2006. LNCS, vol. 3953, pp. 14–28. Springer, Heidelberg (2006)

Age Estimation Based on Complexity-Aware Features

Haoyu Ren$^{(\boxtimes)}$ and Ze-Nian Li

Vision and Media Lab School of Computing Science,
Simon Fraser University, 8888 University Drive,
Vancouver, BC, Canada
hra15@sfu.ca

Abstract. The research related to age estimation using face images has become increasingly important. We propose an age estimator using two kinds of local features, the gradient features which well describe the local characteristic, and the Gabor wavelets which reflect the multi-scale directional information. The RealAdaBoost algorithm with a complexity penalty term in the feature selection module is applied to choose meaningful regions from human face for feature extraction, while balancing the discriminative capability and the computation cost at the same time. Furthermore, the hierarchical classifier, which is composed of an age group classification (e.g., 15–39 years old, 40–59 years old etc.) and a detailed age estimation (e.g. 19, 53 years old, etc.) are utilized to get the final age. Experimental results show that the proposed approach outperforms the methods using single feature on PAL and FG-NET database. It also achieves competitive accuracy with the state-of-the-art algorithms.

1 Introduction

Systems based pattern recognition have been proven to be very useful in many areas such as security and access control, human detection, human computer interaction, and brain computer interface. Recently, the research related to age estimation using face images is more important than ever. The potential applications include automatic guest enrollment, parent TV program control, video surveillance, etc.

In general, age estimation systems consist of two steps: feature extraction and classification/regression [25]. The features used in age estimation can be categorized into the local features and the global features. The local features are extracted on some regions which might contain specific facial characteristic, such as wrinkles and freckles. They have been used to classify people into age groups. Conversely, the global features are extracted based on whole face shape or all facial feature points. They are generally used to estimate the exact age. Some researchers also use hybrid features to improve the estimation accuracy, which is the combination of local features and global features.

After feature extraction, the classification/regression module is utilized to train the age estimator. The commonly-used algorithms include the age group

© Springer International Publishing Switzerland 2015
D. Cremers et al. (Eds.): ACCV 2014, Part I, LNCS 9003, pp. 115–128, 2015.
DOI: 10.1007/978-3-319-16865-4_8

classification, single-level estimation and the hierarchical age estimation. Age group classification is an approach that roughly predicts an age group, whereas single-level method focuses on detailed age prediction. The hierarchical method is a coarse-to-fine method which integrates the single-level and age group methods together.

Regarding the efficiency issue, local features based methods perform better compared to global features based methods utilizing ASM [1] or AAM [2]. Unfortunately, the use of the local features for age estimation has not been well investigated. The methods extracting a dense feature vector for each local region in the aligned face might lead to dimension redundant. In addition, using dense feature is relatively slow. Some other algorithms use AdaBoost to select key dimensions [3] from the dense features. But it is difficult to describe a specific pattern using single dimensional feature in complicate recognition tasks. It also leads to potential risk of weakening the discriminative power of the resulting classifier.

To solve this problem, we focus on selecting the meaningful regions in human face for feature extraction, while dealing with the accuracy and efficiency at the same time. This paper has two contributions. Firstly, we integrate two kinds of localized features together for age estimation, including SIFT, HOG, and Gabor. In addition, different from simply mixing or concatenating these features, we use the complexity-aware RealAdaBoost algorithm, which includes a complexity penalty term in the process of feature selection. As a result, both the discriminative power and the computation cost of the features are evaluated in the training procedure. We divide the training samples into 4 age groups, 0–15, 16–40, 41–59, and 60+. The above complexity-aware RealAdaBoost is applied to select the meaningful regions on each age group respectively. Then the support vector machine is utilized to train a hierarchical age estimator based on these selected features. Plenty of experiments on public datasets are used to evaluate our method. The experimental results show that our approach achieves significant improvement on the estimation accuracy compared to using single features. The result is also competitive with the state-of-the-arts approaches in PAL and FG-NET database.

The rest of this paper is organized as follows. Section 2 is the related work. Section 3 presents the features used in this paper. Section 4 introduces the RealAdaBoost algorithm with the complexity-aware criterion. Section 5 shows our experimental results. Conclusion is given in the last section.

2   Related Work

There has been a great number of work about feature extraction for age estimation. Kwon and Lobo [4] classify facial images into three age groups using the distance ratio of facial components and the wrinkles. Hayashi et al. [5] use histogram equalization and Hough transform for skin extraction and wrinkle detection. A lookup table containing the wrinkle state against appearance at a given age and gender is utilized for age estimation. Fukai et al. [6] adopt fast

Fourier transform to extract features from a face image by genetic algorithms. Gao et al. [7] integrate Gabor features and a fuzzy version of Linear Discriminant Analysis (LDA) to classify face into various age classes. Mu et al. [8] use biologically inspired features and introduced a new operator to model the aging process. Yan et al. [9] combine the local feature and global feature together and utilize a hierarchical classifier to improve the performance.

The problem of age estimation can be converted into a classification/regression problem. Classification can be in groups such as babies, teens, adults or 1–5, 5–10, 10–15, while the regression method predicts the exact age based on a set of coefficients learnt by using suitable loss functions. Lanitis et al. [10] approach the problem of age estimation in a regression way. They propose a quadratic function where age is dependent on feature vector extracted from the face. Ueki et al. [11] introduce a two phased approach based on LDA and 2D-LDA and have used only the first four dimensions of the extracted features to make Gaussian classifier to classify images in various age groups. Wang et al. [20] propose a novel data selection of the Furthest Nearest Neighbour (FNN) that generalizes the margin-based uncertainty to the multi-class case to handle large data efficiently in age classification. Guo et al. [23] and Liu et al. [15] solve the problem by Support Vector Machines (SVM) and Support Vector Regression(SVR). Ni et al. [24] utilize a robust multi-instance regression learning algorithm to learn the kernel regression-based human age estimator in the presence of bag label noises. Kohli et al. [13] propose a technique which extracts features based on AAM and use a global classifier to obtain a rough estimate distinguishing between child/teen-hood and adulthood. An improved version of their work based on hierarchical classifier is published in [14]. Geng et al. [26] develop two algorithms, named IIS-LLD and CPNN, which make single face image not only contribute to the learning of its chronological age, but also to the learning of its adjacent ages.

3 Features Used for Face Description

In this section, we will introduce the three localized features used in our method, SIFT, HOG, and Gabor wavelets.

3.1 Gradient Features

Scale Invariant Feature Transform (SIFT) is invariant to scaling, translation and rotation, and partially invariant to illumination changes and affine projection. Using these descriptors, objects can be reliably recognized even in the case of different views, low illumination or occlusion. In SIFT feature extraction, we first build a scale space by convolving it with multi-scale Gaussian kernels and then calculate the Difference of Gaussian (DoG) between each two adjacent scale spaces. The maximum and minimum of the DoG are selected as candidate interest points, from which elements with low contrast and edge responses are excluded.

After key points detection, we summarize information about local gradient around each key point, as shown in Fig. 1. The histogram of gradient orientation is computed as the resulting feature vector. 4×4 histograms with 8 orientation bins are extracted for each candidate region. The final dimension of SIFT feature is $4 \times 4 \times 8 = 128$.

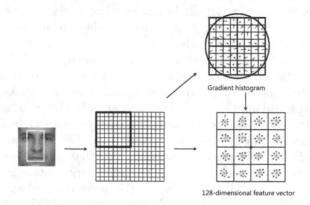

Gradient histogram

128-dimensional feature vector

Fig. 1. SIFT feature extraction

Histogram of Oriented Gradient (HOG) divides the image region into a cell-block structure and generates histogram based on the gradient orientation and spatial location. The input region (block) is divided into small connected regions, called cells, and for each cell a histogram of edge orientations is computed. The histogram channels are evenly spread from 0 to 180 degrees. The histogram counts are normalized for illumination compensation. This can be done by accumulating a measure of local histogram energy over the somewhat larger connected regions and using the results to normalize all cells in the block. The concatenation of these histograms yields the final HOG descriptor. We extract 4 cells and 8 gradient orientation bins for each candidate block, as shown in Fig. 2. The dimension of HOG is $4 \times 8 = 32$.

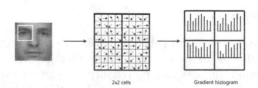

2x2 cells   Gradient histogram

Fig. 2. HOG feature extraction

HOG is not invariant to rotation, but the computation cost is only 1/5 compared to SIFT. This will be considered in the complexity-aware process of the RealAdaBoost procedure.

3.2 Gabor Filters

The Gabor wavelets, whose kernels are similar to the 2D receptive field profiles of the mammalian cortical simple cells, exhibit desirable characteristics of spatial locality and orientation selectivity, and are optimally localized in the space and frequency domains. The Gabor wavelets are defined in Eq. (1)

$$\phi_k(z) = \frac{k^2}{\sigma^2} e^{\frac{k^2 z^2}{2\sigma^2}} [e^{ikz} - e^{-\frac{\sigma^2}{2}}], \quad \ldots \tag{1}$$

where σ decides the ratio of the window width and the wave length, z is the normalization vector, k controls the width of the Gaussian function, the wave length and direction of the shocking part, defined as follows:

$$k = k_v e^{i\phi_u},$$

where $k_v = k_{max}/f_v$ and $\phi_u = \pi u/n$. k_{max} is the maximum frequency, f is the spacing factor between kernels in the frequency domain, n is the maximum orientation number.

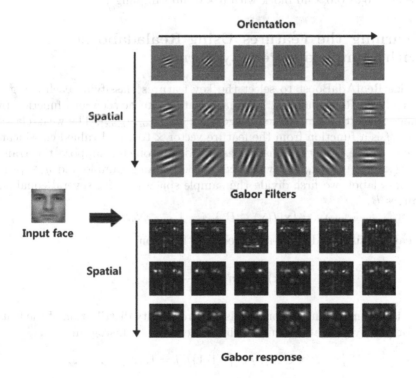

Fig. 3. Gabor filters using 3 scales and 6 orientations

The Gabor wavelets in (1) can be generated from the mother wavelet, by scaling and rotation via the wave vector k. Each kernel is a product of a Gaussian envelope and a complex plane wave, while the first term in the square brackets in (1) determines the oscillatory part of the kernel and the second term compensates for the DC value. The effect of the DC term becomes negligible when the parameter σ, which determines the ratio of the Gaussian window width to wavelength, has sufficiently large values. In our case, we utilize three scales and six orientations to represent the components. And we set

$$\sigma = 2\pi \quad k_{max} = \frac{\pi}{2} \quad f = \sqrt{2}.$$

An example of the extracted Gabor features of an input face are illustrated in Fig. 3.

The feature dimension of dense Gabor feature depends on the size of the block, it will be quite high if we want to extract features in a large region. So we utilize a sub-sampling strategy, which applies a 2×2 to 6×6 sub-sampling based on the block size. The Gabor features are extracted only on the sub-sampled pixels. Using this strategy, the minimum feature dimension of Gabor is $3 \times 6 \times 16 = 256$ (8×8 block with 2×2 sub-sampling), and the maximum is $3 \times 6 \times 36 = 648$ (40×40 block with 6×6 sub-sampling).

4   Learning the Features Using Realadaboost with Complexity Penalty Terms

We utilize RealAdaBoost to select the key features classifying each age group respectively. In RealAdaBoost, an image feature can be seen as a function from the image space to a real valued range $f : \mathbf{x} \rightarrow [f_{min}, f_{max}]$. The weak classifier based on f is a function from the feature vector $\mathbf{x}$ to a real valued classification confidence space. For the binary classification problem, suppose the training data as $(\mathbf{x_1}, y_1), \ldots, (\mathbf{x_n}, y_n)$ where $\mathbf{x}_i$ is the training sample and $y \in \{-1, 1\}$ is the class label, we first divide the sample space into N_b several equal sized sub-ranges B_j

$$X_j = \{\mathbf{x}|f(\mathbf{x}) \in B_j\}, j = 1, \ldots, N_b. \quad \ldots \tag{2}$$

The weak classifier is defined as a piecewise function

$$h(\mathbf{x}) = \frac{1}{2}ln(\frac{W_+^j + \epsilon}{W_-^j + \epsilon}), \quad \ldots \tag{3}$$

where ϵ is the smoothing factor, $W_\pm$ is the probability distribution of the feature value for positive/negative samples, implemented as a histogram

$$W_\pm^j = P(\mathbf{x} \in X_j, y \in \{-1, 1\}), j = 1, \ldots, N_b. \quad \ldots \tag{4}$$

The best weak classifier is selected according to the classification error Z of the piecewise function in Eq. (5)

$$Z = 2\sum_j \sqrt{W_+^j W_-^j}. \quad \ldots \tag{5}$$

We adopt RealAdaBoost to learn the key regions and the type of feature extraction methods. In consideration of the efficiency, we add a complexity-aware criteria into the decision term of RealAdaBoost, as shown in Eq. (6)

$$Z = 2 \sum_j \sqrt{W_+^j W_-^j} + a \cdot fp \cdot C, \quad \ldots \tag{6}$$

where C is the computation cost of the features, a is the complexity-aware factor to balance the discriminative capability and the computation complexity, fp is the false positive rate of current stage. In the training procedure, features with minimum Z are selected.

The Eq. (6) could be explained as follows, in the first stages of RealAdaBoost, the age group of faces are still easy to be classified, so efficient features are preferred. In the following stages, the patterns of the training samples are complicated. Then the features with high computation cost are considered.

We apply the above RealAdaBoost on the 4 age group classification tasks respectively. In each task, the positive samples are the samples in that age group, while the negative samples are the combination of all samples in other 3 groups. To evaluate the computation cost, we test the execution time of different feature extraction modules and set the C of SIFT to 10, HOG to 2, and Gabor to 3–6 based on its dimension. The complexity-aware factor a is set to 0.15 in our experiment. The diagram of the whole complexity-aware RealAdaBoost is illustrated in Fig. 4.

5   Experiments

5.1   Experiments Setup

In the experiments, two databases are used to evaluate the performance of the proposed method: the PAL aging database and the FG-NET aging database. The PAL aging database contains 430 Caucasians with age range 18–93 years old [16]. The images in the database were captured using a digital camera with fixed light and position conditions. The resolution of the images is 640 × 480 pixels. This database includes various expressions such as smiling, sadness, anger, or neutral faces. In the experiments, we used only neutral faces in order to exclude the facial expression effect. Sample images used in our experiments are shown in Fig. 5.

The FG-NET aging database [19] is one of the most frequently used database for estimating age in the previous works. The database has 1,002 images composed of 82 Europeans in the age range 0–69 years old. Individuals in the database have one or more images included at different ages. These Images were obtained by scanning. Therefore, there are extreme variations in lighting, expression, background, pose, resolution and noise from scanning. Sample images of the FG-NET aging database are shown in Fig. 6.

With the PAL aging databases, five-folds cross validations are performed to evaluate the performance, which is similar to [17]. The age and gender are evenly

Parameters

   N number of training samples

   M number of evaluated features each iteration

   T maximum number of weak classifiers

Input: Training set

   $\{(\mathbf{x}_i, y_i)\}, i = 1, \ldots, N, \mathbf{x}_i \in R^d, y_i \in \{-1, 1\}$

1. Initialize sample weight, classifier output, and false positive rate

   $w_i = \frac{1}{N}, F(\mathbf{x}_i) = 0, i = 1, \ldots, N, fp_0 = 1$

2. Repeat for $t = 1, 2, \ldots, T$

  2.1 Update the sample weight w_i using the hth weak classifier output

  $w_i = w_i e^{-y_i h_i(\mathbf{x}_i)}$

  2.2 For $m = 1$ to M

    2.2.1 Generate a random region with a specific feature extraction method (SIFT, HOG, or Gabor)

    2.2.2 Extract features and do least square to $y_i \in \{-1, 1\}$

    2.2.3 Build the predict distribution function W_+ and W_-

    2.2.4 Select the best feature which minimizes Z in equation (6)

  2.3 Update weak classifier using (3)

  2.4 Update strong classifier $F_{t+1}(\mathbf{x}_i) = F_t(\mathbf{x}_i) + h_t(\mathbf{x}_i)$

  2.5 Calculate current false positive rate fp_t

3. Output classifier $F(\mathbf{x}) = sign[\sum_{j=1}^{T} h_j(\mathbf{x})]$

Fig. 4. Learning the features using RealAdaBoost with complexity penalty term

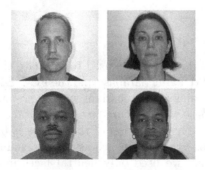

Fig. 5. Sample images in PAL aging database

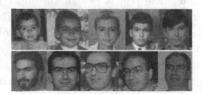

Fig. 6. Sample images in FG-NET aging database

distributed each fold. With the FG-NET aging database, Leave-One-Person-Out (LOPO) is performed because it contains a number of images of the same person. That means, 82-folds are used on the FG-NET aging database.

We divide the training samples into 4 age groups, 0–15, 16–40, 41–59, and 60+. All the faces are resized to 100×100. The complexity-aware RealAdaBoost is applied on each group classification to select the meaningful features. Moreover, a two-steps hierarchical classifier is further adopted to generate the final age estimator. Firstly, linear support vector machine based age group classification is trained based on the selected features. Then we use the support vector regression to estimate the exact age in each age group.

The evaluation is based on the Mean Absolute Error (MAE) and the Cumulative Score (CS). The MAE is defined as the mean of the absolute difference between the estimated age and the real age, as

$$MAE = \frac{\sum_{i=1}^{N} |e_i - g_i|}{N},$$

where N is the number of the test images, e_i is the estimated age of the test image i and g_i is the ground-truth age. The Cumulative Score(CS) is defined as the ratio of the number of data whose errors are lower than a threshold, as

$$CS = \frac{N_{error \leq threshold}}{N}.$$

5.2 Experimental Results

We train 7 age estimators using the proposed framework, which includes the classifiers utilizing single feature (SIFT, HOG, and Gabor), the combination of two features, and all of the three features. There are no complexity-aware procedure

Table 1. MAE in PAL database. Units: years old

Approach	Mean Absolute Error (MAE)
SIFT	5.98
HOG	6.14
Gabor	5.88
SIFT + HOG	5.54
SIFT + Gabor	5.05
HOG + Gabor	5.57
All three features	**4.29**
[17]	5.36
[9]	4.33
[18]	4.52

if single feature is adopted. Tables 1 and 2 present the MAE of these age estimators in the PAL database and FG-NET database. It can be seen that using the complexity-aware feature combination, the estimation accuracy is significantly improved compared to using SIFT, HOG, or Gabor independently. Using all three features, the MAE is further reduced. The accuracy is also comparable with the state-of-the-art algorithms in both of the two datasets. This result show that the features evaluated by complexity-aware RealAdaBoost might be more effective than some artificial designed features.

Table 2. MAE in FG-NET database. Units: years old

Approach	Mean Absolute Error (MAE)
SIFT	5.97
HOG	5.86
Gabor	5.68
SIFT + HOG	5.27
SIFT + Gabor	5.09
HOG + Gabor	5.10
All three features	**4.49**
[21]	5.05
[9]	4.66
[22]	4.67

We also plot the curve of the cumulative scores for the above 7 age estimators in Fig. 7. It can been seen that the cumulative score moved up at a clear border on the PAL database and FG-NET database using the proposed complexity-aware method (black curve). This result also shows the effectiveness of our method.

5.3   Analysis

We draw the first 7 features selected by the RealAdaBoost algorithm in LFW database. The LFW is used instead of any age databases because LFW contains a large number of faces in variable illuminations, ages, emotions, and ethnics. As shown in Fig. 8, there are 2 SIFT features, 3 HOG features, and 2 Gabor features. It could be seen that these features lay on the eyes, forehead and mouth region. This result is reasonable, because it is much easier to estimate the age from these regions rather than other face regions such as nose or eyebrow. For example, the wrinkles in the forehead and the shape of month describe the key characteristic for human ages.

We test the resulting classifiers on a desktop PC with a 2.5 GHz I3 PC and 2 GB memory. The execution speed is shown in Table 3. We find that the estimator based on SIFT is relatively slow compared to the one using HOG or Gabor.

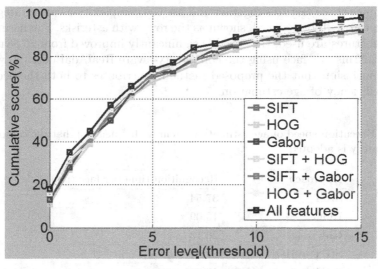

(a) CS on PAL dataset

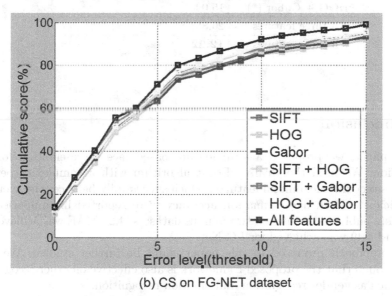

(b) CS on FG-NET dataset

Fig. 7. CS on PAL and FG-NET database

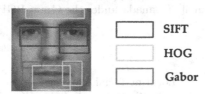

Fig. 8. The first 7 features selected by RealAdaBoost in human face

If we combine these features together and use the complexity-aware strategy, the execution time will be reduced, shown as the rows with asterisks. Furthermore, if all three features are used, the speed is significantly improved from 26.88 ms per face to 12.22 ms per face using the complexity-aware RealAdaBoost. So we can get the conclusion that the proposed method contributes to both the accuracy and the efficiency of age estimation.

Table 3. Execution speed of age estimators. Item with * denotes that the complexity-aware strategy is adopted.

Approach	Recognition time per face (ms)
SIFT	37.54
HOG	13.09
Gabor	20.13
SIFT + HOG (*)	22.11
SIFT + Gabor (*)	16.22
HOG + Gabor (*)	15.09
All three features	26.88
All three features (*)	**12.22**

6   Conclusion

In this paper, we proposed a local feature based face representation for age estimation. We used the RealAdaBoost algorithm with a complexity penalty term to select the meaningful features, which successfully balances the accuracy and efficiency. High age estimation accuracy were reported in comparison to previously published results on two famous datasets. 4.29 MAE was achieved for PAL, and 4.49 was achieved for FG-Net.

The approach proposed in this paper could be further studied. We have already found that the proposed framework is also effective on other recognition tasks, such as gender recognition and emotion recognition.

Acknowledgement. This work was supported in part by the Natural Sciences and Engineering Research Council of Canada under the Grant RGP36726.

References

1. Milborrow, S., Nicolls, F.: Locating facial features with an extended active shape model. In: Forsyth, D., Torr, P., Zisserman, A. (eds.) ECCV 2008, Part IV. LNCS, vol. 5305, pp. 504–513. Springer, Heidelberg (2008)

2. Cootes, T.F., Edwards, G.J., Taylor, C.J., et al.: Active appearance models. IEEE Trans. Pattern Anal. Mach. Intell. **23**, 681–685 (2001)
3. Shan, C.: Learning local features for age estimation on real-life faces. In: Proceedings of the 1st ACM International Workshop on Multimodal Pervasive Video Analysis, pp. 23–28 (2010)
4. Kwon, Y.H., da Vitoria Lobo, N.: Age classification from facial images. In: Computer Vision and Pattern Recognition, pp. 762–767 (1994)
5. Hayashi, J., Yasumoto, M., Ito, H., Koshimizu, H.: Method for estimating and modeling age and gender using facial image processing. In: Seventh International Conference on Virtual Systems and Multimedia, pp. 439–448 (2001)
6. Fukai, H., Takimoto, H., Mitsukura, Y., Fukumi, M.: Apparent age estimation system based on age perception. In: Proceedings of SICE, pp. 2808–2812 (2007)
7. Gao, F., Ai, H.: Face age classification on consumer images with gabor feature and fuzzy LDA method. In: Tistarelli, M., Nixon, M.S. (eds.) ICB 2009. LNCS, vol. 5558, pp. 132–141. Springer, Heidelberg (2009)
8. Mu, G., Guo, G., Fu, Y., Huang, T.S.: Human age estimation using bio-inspired features. In: Computer Vision and Pattern Recognition, pp. 112–119 (2009)
9. Choi, S.E., Lee, Y.J., Lee, S.J., Park, K.R., Kim, J.: Age estimation using a hierarchical classifier based on global and local facial features. Pattern Recogn. **44**, 1262–1281 (2011)
10. Lanitis, A., Taylor, C.J., Cootes, T.F.: Toward automatic simulation of aging effects on face images. IEEE Trans. Pattern Anal. Mach. Intell. **24**, 442–445 (2002)
11. Ueki, K., Hayashida, T., Kobayashi, T.: Subspace-based age-group classification using facial images under various lighting conditions. In: 7th International Conference on Automatic Face and Gesture Recognition, 6 p (2006)
12. Guo, G., Fu, Y., Huang, T.S., Dyer, C.R.: Locally adjusted robust regression for human age estimation. Urbana **51**, 61801 (2008)
13. Luu, K., Ricanek, K., Bui, T.D., Suen, C.Y.: Age estimation using active appearance models and support vector machine regression. In: IEEE 3rd International Conference on Biometrics: Theory, Applications, and Systems, pp. 1–5 (2009)
14. Kohli, S., Prakash, S., Gupta, P.: Hierarchical age estimation with dissimilarity-based classification. Neurocomputing **120**, 164–176 (2013)
15. Liu, J., Ma, Y., Duan, L., Wang, F., Liu, Y.: Hybrid constraint SVR for facial age estimation. Sig. Process. **94**, 576–582 (2014)
16. Minear, M., Park, D.C.: A lifespan database of adult facial stimuli. Behav. Res. Methods Instrum. Comput. **36**, 630–633 (2004)
17. Suo, J., Wu, T., Zhu, S., Shan, S., Chen, X., Gao, W.: Design sparse features for age estimation using hierarchical face model. In: 8th IEEE International Conference on Automatic Face & Gesture Recognition, pp. 1–6 (2008)
18. Guo, G., Mu, G., Fu, Y., Dyer, C., Huang, T.: A study on automatic age estimation using a large database. In: IEEE 12th International Conference on Computer Vision, pp. 1986–1991 (2009)
19. FGNET. http://www.fgnet.rsunit.com
20. Wang, J.-G., Sung, E., Yau, W.-Y.: Active learning with the furthest nearest neighbor criterion for facial age estimation. In: Kimmel, R., Klette, R., Sugimoto, A. (eds.) ACCV 2010, Part IV. LNCS, vol. 6495, pp. 11–24. Springer, Heidelberg (2011)
21. Kilinc, M., Akgul, Y.S.: Automatic human age estimation using overlapped age groups. In: Csurka, G., Kraus, M., Laramee, R.S., Richard, P., Braz, J. (eds.) VISIGRAPP 2012. CCIS, vol. 359, pp. 313–325. Springer, Heidelberg (2013)

22. Chen, K., Gong, S., Xiang, T., Loy, C.C.: Cumulative attribute space for age and crowd density estimation. In: Computer Vision and Pattern Recognition, pp. 2467–2474 (2013)
23. Guo, G., Wang, X.: A study on human age estimation under facial expression changes. In: Computer Vision and Pattern Recognition, pp. 2547–2553 (2012)
24. Ni, B., Song, Z., Yan, S.: Web image and video mining towards universal and robust age estimator. IEEE Trans. Multimedia **13**, 1217–1229 (2011)
25. Fu, Y., Guo, G., Huang, T.S.: Age synthesis and estimation via faces: a survey. IEEE Trans. Pattern Anal. Mach. Intell. **32**, 1955–1976 (2010)
26. Geng, X., Yin, C., Zhou, Z.-H.: Facial age estimation by learning from label distributions. IEEE Trans. Pattern Anal. Mach. Intell. **35**, 2401–2472 (2013)

Efficient On-the-fly Category Retrieval Using ConvNets and GPUs

Ken Chatfield[✉], Karen Simonyan, and Andrew Zisserman

Department of Engineering Science, University of Oxford, Oxford, UK
{ken,karen,az}@robots.ox.ac.uk

Abstract. We investigate the gains in precision and speed, that can be obtained by using Convolutional Networks (ConvNets) for on-the-fly retrieval – where classifiers are learnt at run time for a textual query from downloaded images, and used to rank large image or video datasets.

We make three contributions: (i) we present an evaluation of state-of-the-art image representations for object category retrieval over standard benchmark datasets containing 1M+ images; (ii) we show that ConvNets can be used to obtain features which are incredibly performant, and yet much lower dimensional than previous state-of-the-art image representations, and that their dimensionality can be reduced further without loss in performance by compression using product quantization or binarization. Consequently, features with the state-of-the-art performance on large-scale datasets of millions of images can fit in the memory of even a commodity GPU card; (iii) we show that an SVM classifier can be learnt within a ConvNet framework on a GPU *in parallel* with downloading the new training images, allowing for a continuous refinement of the model as more images become available, and simultaneous training and ranking. The outcome is an on-the-fly system that significantly outperforms its predecessors in terms of: precision of retrieval, memory requirements, and speed, facilitating accurate on-the-fly learning and ranking in under a second on a single GPU.

1 Introduction

On-the-fly learning offers a way to overcome the 'closed world' problem in computer vision, where object category recognition systems are restricted to only those pre-defined classes that occur in the carefully curated datasets available for training – for example ImageNet [1] for object categories or UCF-101 [2] for human actions in videos. What is more, it offers the tantalising prospect of developing large-scale general purpose object category retrieval systems which can operate over millions of images in a few seconds, as is possible in the specific instance retrieval systems [3–7] which have reached the point of commercialisation in products such as Google Goggles, Kooaba and Amazon's SnapTell.

Current on-the-fly systems typically proceed in three stages [8–11]: first, training data for the user query are compiled, commonly by bootstrapping the process via text-to-image search using *e.g.* Google Image Search as a source of

© Springer International Publishing Switzerland 2015
D. Cremers et al. (Eds.): ACCV 2014, Part I, LNCS 9003, pp. 129–145, 2015.
DOI: 10.1007/978-3-319-16865-4_9

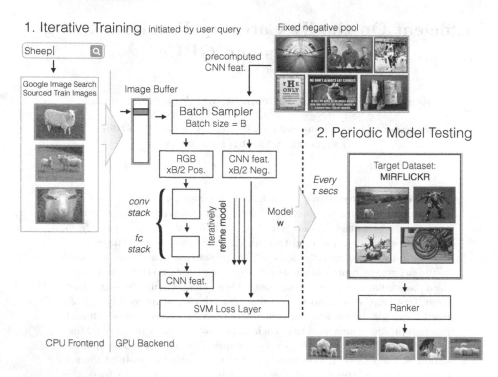

Fig. 1. Architecture of our on-the-fly object category retrieval system. The entire framework aside from the image downloader is resident on the GPU, with data stored in GPU memory outlined in green. Its operation is split into: (i) iterative training, as initiated by a user text query and (ii) periodic model testing to obtain a ranking over the target dataset (refer to text for further details) (Color figure online).

training images; second, a classifier or ranker is learnt for that category; third, all images/videos in a dataset are ranked in order to retrieve those containing the category. The aim is for these stages to happen on-line in a matter of seconds, rather than hours.

Previous methods for on-the-fly learning have been limited by the retrieval-performance/memory/speed trade off. In particular, very high-dimensional feature vectors were required for state-of-the-art classification performance [12–14], but this incurred both a severe memory penalty (as features for the dataset need to be in memory for fast retrieval) and also a severe speed penalty (as computing a scalar product for high-dimensional features is costly) both in training and ranking. Despite the excellent progress in compression methods for nearest neighbour search by using product quantization [15] or binary encoding [16,17], compromises still had to be made.

In this paper we show that in the context of on-the-fly category retrieval, Convolutional Networks (ConvNets) [18] with GPU training [19] can significantly improve on all three of: retrieval precision, memory requirements, and ranking speed. The whole pipeline, from computing the training image features and learning the model to scoring and ranking the dataset images is implemented on the GPU and runs in a highly-parallel, online manner. We thus demonstrate a system that is able to go from a cold-query to results in a matter of second(s) on a dataset of million(s) of images. The architecture of our proposed system, from input of text query to display of ranked results, is summarized in Fig. 1 (refer to Sect. 4 for details).

In terms of retrieval performance, we build on the recent research that shows that deep ConvNet features significantly outperform shallow features, such as Fisher Vectors [12,13], on the image classification task [19–21]. However, our contributions go further than simply using ConvNet features in an on-the-fly architecture: we take the full advantage of the GPU computation for all retrieval stages, in parallel with downloading the new training images on the CPU. This novel GPU-based architecture allows a time budget to be set, so that an SVM, trained on the available images within the time limit, can be used to (re-)rank the dataset images at any stage of the process (for instance, every 0.5 s). This architecture is in strong contrast to the standard on-the-fly architectures [8], where SVM training only begins once all training images have been downloaded and processed, and ranking follows after that.

We first perform a comprehensive evaluation of the performance of ConvNet-based image features for category-based image retrieval (Sect. 2). We start with a standard object category recognition benchmark (PASCAL VOC 2007 [22]), and then add a large number of distractor images to take the dataset size to 1M+ images (the datasets are described in Sect. 2). We assess retrieval performance over these two datasets (VOC and VOC + distractors) under variation in the training data – either using VOC training images (i.e. a curated dataset) or using images from Google Image search (i.e. the type of images, possibly with label noise, that will be available in the real-world on-the-fly system).

With our goal being ranking of millions of images on a conventional GPU-equipped PC, we then investigate, in Sect. 3, how retrieval performance is affected by using low-dimensional features (still originating from a ConvNet). Low-dimensional features (e.g. hundreds of components rather than thousands) have two advantages: they use less memory, and scalar products are faster, both in training and ranking. We cover a spectrum of methods for achieving a low-dimensional descriptor, namely: (i) reducing the dimensionality of the last ConvNet layer; (ii) product quantization of the ConvNet features and (iii) binarization of the ConvNet features. It is shown that a combination of a low-dimensional final ConvNet feature layer with product quantization produces features that are both highly-compact and incredibly performant.

Finally, based on these investigations, we propose a GPU architecture for on-the-fly object category retrieval in Sect. 4, highly scalable, capable of adapting to varying query complexity and all running on a single commodity GPU. An extended version of this paper is available on arXiv[1].

---

[1] http://arxiv.org/abs/1407.4764/.

2   Evaluating Large-Scale Object Category Retrieval

This section describes the evaluation protocol used to assess the performance of the image representations $\phi(I)$ described in Sect. 3 and of the on-the-fly training architecture introduced in Sect. 4. We begin by describing the datasets used for evaluation, and then describe the three different scenarios in which these datasets are used, with each subsequent scenario moving closer to modelling the conditions experienced by a real-world large-scale object category retrieval system.

One difficulty of evaluating a large-scale object category retrieval system is the lack of large-scale datasets with sufficient annotation to assess retrieval performance fully, in particular to measure recall. The PASCAL VOC dataset [22] provides full annotation for a set of twenty common object classes, facilitating evaluation using common ranking performance measures such as mean average precision (mAP), but is much too small (~10k images) to evaluate the performance of a real-world system. Conversely, the ILSVRC dataset [1], while being much larger (~1M+ images), does not have complete annotation of *all* object categories in each image. Therefore, ranking performance (*e.g.* recall or mAP) cannot be measured without further annotation, and only object category *classification* metrics (such as top-N classification error per image), which do not accurately reflect the performance of an object category *retrieval* scenario, can be used. Additionally, in this work we use the ImageNet ILSVRC-2012 dataset to pre-train the ConvNet, so can not also use that for assessing performance.

As a result, for evaluation in this paper, we use a custom combination of datasets, carefully tailored to be representative of the data that could be expected in a typical collection of web-based consumer photographs:

PASCAL VOC 2007 [22] is used as our base dataset, with assessment over seventeen of its twenty classes ('people', 'cats' and 'birds' are excluded for reasons explained below). We use the provided train, validation and test splits.

MIRFLICKR-1M [23, 24] is used to augment the data from the PASCAL VOC 2007 test set in our later experiments, and comprises 1M unannotated images (aside from quite noisy image tags). The dataset represents a snapshot of images taken by popularity from the image sharing site Flickr, and thus is more representative of typical web-based consumer photography than ImageNet, which although also sourced from Flickr was collected through queries for often very specific terms from WordNet. In addition, MIRFLICKR-1M has been confirmed to contain many images of the twenty PASCAL VOC classes.

2.1   Evaluation Protocol

A linear SVM is trained for all classes, and used to rank all images in the target dataset. For the object category retrieval setting the 'goodness' of the first few pages of retrieved results is critical, as the larger the proportion of true positives for a given object category at the top of a ranked list, the better the perceived performance. We therefore evaluate using precision @ K, where $K = 100$.

Adopting such an evaluation protocol also has the advantage that we are able to use the 1M images from the MIRFLICKR-1M dataset despite the fact that full annotations are not provided. Since we only need to consider the top K of the ranked list for each class during evaluation, we take can take a 'lazy' approach to annotating the MIRFLICKR-1M dataset, annotating class instaces only as far down the ranked list as necessary to generate a complete annotation for the top-K results (for more details of this procedure, refer to scenario 2 below). This avoids having to generate a full set of annotation for all 1M images.

2.2 Experimental Scenarios

Scenario 1: PASCAL VOC. We train models for seventeen of the twenty VOC object classes (excluding 'people', 'cats' and 'birds') using both the training and validation sets. Following this, a ranked list for each class is generated using images from the test set and precision @ K evaluated.

Scenario 2: Large-Scale Retrieval. Training is undertaken in the same manner as scenario 1, but during testing images are added from the MIRFLICKR-1M dataset. There are two sub-scenarios:

Scenario 2a – we test using images from the PASCAL VOC test set (as in scenario 1) with the addition of the entirety of the MIRFLICKR-1M dataset. For each class, we remove all (lazily annotated) positive class occurrences in the ranked list which are retrieved from MIRFLICKR-1M, as the purpose of this scenario is to test how our features perform when attempting to retrieve a small, known number of class occurrences from a very large number of non-class 'distractor' images.[2]

Scenario 2b – this time we exclude all images from the PASCAL VOC dataset, and instead evaluate precision @ K solely over the MIRFLICKR-1M dataset. The purpose of this scenario is to test how our features perform over a real-world dataset with unknown statistics. In practice, it is an easier scenario than scenario 2a, since the MIRFLICKR-1M dataset contains many instances of all of the PASCAL VOC classes.

Scenario 3: Google Training. Testing is the same as in scenario 2b, but instead of using PASCAL data for training, a query is issued to Google Image search for each of the PASCAL VOC classes, and the top $N \sim 250$ images are used in each case as training data. This scenario assesses the tolerance to training on images that differ from the VOC and MIRFLICKR-1M test images:

---

[2] The prevalence of the PASCAL VOC classes 'people', 'cats' and 'birds' in the MIRFLICKR-1M data explains why we exclude them, as restricting the annotation of these classes to reasonable levels proved to be impossible.

the Google images may be noisy and typically contain the object in the centre. It also mirrors most closely a real-world on-the-fly object category retrieval setting, as the queries in practice do not need to be limited to the PASCAL VOC classes. There are again two sub-scenarios, with different data used for the negative training samples in each case:

Scenario 3a – the images downloaded from Google Image Search for all other classes, except for the current class, are used as negative training data (this mirrors the PASCAL VOC setup).

Scenario 3b – a fixed pool of ~16,000 negative training images is used. These training images are sourced from the web by issuing queries for a set of fixed 'negative' query terms[3] to both Google and Bing image search, and attempting to download the first ~1,000 results in each case. This same pool of negative training data is also used in Sect. 4.

3   Retrieval Performance over Image Representations

In this section, we perform an evaluation of recent state-of-the-art image representations for the object category retrieval scenarios described in Sect. 2.2.

ConvNet-based features, which form the basis of our on-the-fly system described in Sect. 4, have been shown to perform excellently on standard image classification benchmarks such as PASCAL VOC and ImageNet ILSVRC [20, 21, 25, 26]. We therefore focus our evaluation on these features, employing 2048-dimensional 'CNN M 2048' image features of [21] as the baseline. We compare them to a more traditional shallow feature encoding in the form of the Improved Fisher Vector (IFV) [13]. Implementation details for ConvNets and IFV are given in Sect. 3.2. We explore the effects of reducing the dimensionality of our features on their retrieval performance using the following methods:

Lower-dimensional ConvNet output layer – One way of reducing the dimensionality of ConvNet features consists in retraining the network so that the last fully-connected (feature) layer has a lower dimensionality. Following [21], we consider the 'CNN M 128' network configuration with a 128-dimensional feature layer. Using such network in place of the baseline 'CNN M 2048' can be seen as discriminative dimensionality reduction by a factor of 16.

Product quantization (PQ) has been widely used as a compression method for image features [15, 27], and works by splitting the original feature into Q-dimensional sub-blocks, each of which is encoded using a separate vocabulary of cluster centres pre-learned from a training set. Here we explore compression using $Q = 4, 8$-dimensional sub-blocks.

---

[3] Miscellanea, random selection, photo random selection, random objects, random things, nothing in particular, photos of stuff, random photos, random stuff, things.

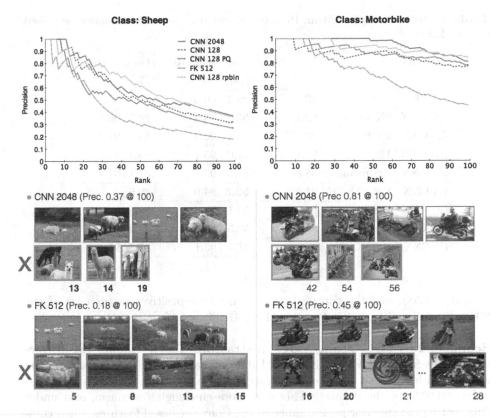

Fig. 2. Sample precision-rank curves and retrieved results for two queries over the combined VOC+MIRFLICKR data (Scenario 2a). In the bottom half of the figure, the top row in each case shows the first few results returned for each method and the second shows the top retrieved false positives with their rank.

Binarization is performed using the tight frame expansion method of [28], which has been recently successfully applied to local patch and face descriptors [29,30]. The binarization of zero-centred descriptors $\phi \in \mathbb{R}^m$ to binary codes $\beta \in \{0,1\}^n$, $n > m$ is performed as $\beta = \mathrm{sgn}(U\phi)$ where sgn is the sign function: $\mathrm{sgn}(a) = 1$ iff $a > 0$ and 0 otherwise, and the Parseval tight frame U is computed by keeping the first m columns of an orthogonal matrix, obtained from a QR-decomposition of a random $n \times n$ matrix.

3.1 Results and Analysis

Scenario 1 (VOC Train/VOC Test). The PASCAL VOC dataset does not pose any major challenges for any of our features, which is not surprising given the close to decade of research on representations which perform well on this dataset. Even for the most challenging classes (*e.g.* 'potted plant') IFV produces fairly good results, with the top 12 images being true positives (Prec

Table 1. Retrieval results (Mean Prec @ 100) for the evaluation scenarios described in Sect. 2.2.

Scenario		VOC Only	Large-scale Retr.		Google Training	
		[1]	[2a]	[2b]	[3a]	[3b]
(a) FK	512	82.3	29.3	80.5		
(b) CNN	2K	92.1	**55.4**	95.4	88.5	90.9
(c) CNN	2K PQ	90.7	55.1	96.4	88.2	91.9
(d) CNN	128	92.1	51.0	95.1	88.1	92.3
(e) CNN	128 noaug	88.8	45.4	93.1	87.1	91.1
(f) CNN	128 BIN 2K	91.5	**52.3**	94.0	89.6	
(g) CNN	128 BIN 1K	90.0	50.1	94.0	89.5	
(h) CNN	128 PQ	90.1	50.5	94.6	88.2	92.1
(i) CNN	128 PQ-8	88.8	47.4	93.1	87.7	91.1

@ 100 = 0.58), and the top 92 images being true positives in the case of our 2048-dimensional ConvNet features (Prec @ 100 = 0.83).

Scenario 2a (VOC Train/VOC+distractors Test). Adding 1M distractor images from the MIRFLICKR-1M dataset has a significant impact on the results, with the task now being to retrieve true positives that constitute less than ~0.02 % of the dataset. This is a more challenging scenario, and under this setting the superior performance of the ConvNet-based features, when compared to the state-of-the-art shallow representation (IFV), is much clearer to see. Some sample precision-rank curves for two queries, one particularly challenging ('sheep') and another less so ('motorbike') are shown in Fig. 2. We can make the following observations:

IFV Performance – It can be seen that IFV ([a] in Tables 1 and 2) performs the worst of all methods, despite being much higher dimensional (~1000×) and taking much longer to compute (~200×) compared to our CNN-128 method ([d]). Nonetheless, even for challenging classes such as 'sheep' IFV manages to pull out a few true positives at the top of the ranked list. However, the relative performance drop with rank is much sharper than with the ConvNet-based methods.

Bursty Images – Comparing the top-ranked negatives of the FK-512 method ([a] in Table 1) for 'sheep' to those of the CNN-2048 method ([b]), it can be seen that IFV appears to mistakenly rank highly 'bursty' images comprising repeating patterns or textures. This phenomenon is particularly evident for natural, outdoor scenes which explains why the performance drop of IFV is particularly severe in the 'sheep', 'cow' and 'horses' classes, as it appears that the ConvNet-based features are much more robust to such textured images.

Diversity – The diversity of the retrieved results is also much greater for ConvNet-based representations than for IFV, indicating that the classifier is able to make better generalisations using these features. For example, as seen in Fig. 2, whereas the top four retrieved results for the query 'motorbike' for the FK-512 method ([a]) all show a rider in a similar pose, on a racing bike on a race track, the top four retrieved results for the CNN-2048 method ([b]) depict a variety of different motorcycles (road, racing, off-road) from several different angles.

For the most part, compression of the ConvNet features does not appear to reduce their diversity appreciably, with the top-ranked results for all ConvNet methods, whether compressed or not, appearing to exhibit a similar diversity of results.

Compression – As mentioned above, the drop in performance in moving from ConvNet-based features to IFV is much greater than that incurred by any of the compression methods, and this seems to be strongly connected with the robustness of the ConvNet-based features, whether compressed or not, to the kind of 'bursty' textured images which IFV is susceptible to. This is remarkable given that comparing the size of the largest uncompressed ConvNet representation CNN-2048 ([b] in Table 2) to the smallest compressed one, CNN-128-PQ-8 ([i]), there is a $\sim$512$\times$ size difference. In the case of the CNN-128-BIN-2K method ([f]), the mPrec @ 100 actually increases marginally when compared to the non-compressed codes ([d]) which, when visually inspecting the rankings, again can be explained by the additional robustness brought by compression.

Table 2. Dimensionality, storage requirements and computation time. The rows in this table correspond to those in Table 1. Timings for compression methods are specified as additional time added to the total feature encoding time, and those in parenthesis indicate GPU timings where applicable.

	Dim	Compression (bytes)		New Dim	Storage/1M ims	Comp. Time/im (s)
(a)	83,968	–			312.8 GB	10.32
(b)	2048	–			7.63 GB	0.35 (0.061)
(c)	2048	PQ	4 dims/sq (16×)	512	488 MB	+0.061
(d)	128	–			488 MB	0.34 (0.061)
(e)	128	noaug			488 MB	0.083 (**0.024**)
(f)	128	BIN	2048 bytes (2×)	4096	244 MB	+0.38 ms
(g)	128	BIN	1024 bytes (4×)	2048	122 MB	+0.22 ms
(h)	128	PQ	4 dims/sq (16×)	32	30.5 MB	+3.9 ms
(i)	128	PQ	8 dims/sq (32×)	16	**15.3 MB**	+2.0 ms

VOC Training   Google Training

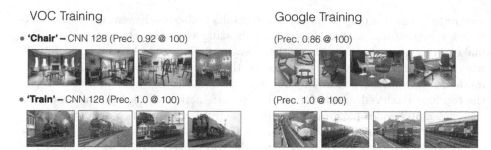

Fig. 3. Difference between retrieved results when training using VOC data and Google training data. Results are shown over the MIRFLICKR-1M dataset (Scenarios 2b and 3b).

The binary representations ([f] & [g]), combined with a linear SVM, also exhibit competitive performance despite the reduced memory footprint. The ranking of such features can be significantly sped-up using hardware-accelerated Hamming distance computation, which, however, requires a different ranking model, which is left for future work. For its superior compression ratios and negligible impact on performance, product quantization remains an obvious choice for the compression of ConvNet features. The fact that the ConvNet features are very sparse, with the CNN-128 representation typically being over 60 % zeros, is one reason why they are so amenable to compression, and it is possible that with compression methods geared specifically to capitalise on this sparsity even higher compression ratios could be achieved.

Scenario 2b (VOC Train/MIRFLICKR Test). Given that the MIRFLICKR-1M dataset contains many instances of all of the PASCAL VOC classes, moving to testing solely on MIRFLICKR leads to a jump in performance of the results across all methods. Nonetheless, this scenario provides a closer representation of the performance of a real-world on-the-fly object category retrieval system, given that the image statistics of the MIRFLICKR-1M dataset are not known in advance.

Scenario 3a (Google Train/MIRFLICKR Test). Switching to noisy training images from Google rather than the pre-curated PASCAL VOC training images as expected results in a small drop (∼6 %) across the board for all methods. However, the precision at the top of the ranking remains subjectively very good. Nonetheless, as shown in Fig. 3, the actual images returned from the dataset are very different, which reflects the differences in the training data sourced from Google Image search versus that from the curated dataset. For example, a query for 'chair' returns predominantly indoor scenes with regular dining-table chairs when using VOC training data, and more avant-garde, modern designs, generally centred in the frame when using Google training data.

Scenario 3b (Google Train + negative pool/MIRFLICKR Test). In this scenario, we switch to using a fixed pool of negative data sourced from a set of 'negative' queries, and it can be seen how this improves the results by up to ~5 %. This may be a result of the larger negative training pool size (~16,000 images *vs*. ~4,000 images when using queries for all other VOC classes to provide the negative data as we do in Scenario 3a). Given the assumed lack of coverage in the fixed negative image pool (as it is sourced by issuing queries for deliberately non-specific terms to facilitate its application to as broad a range of queries as possible), this suggests that to a certain extent lack of diversity can be made up for by using a larger number of negative training images.

3.2   Implementation Details

Our implementation of IFV and ConvNet image representations follows that of [21]. In more detail, for IFV computation we use their setting 'FK IN 512 (x,y)', which corresponds to: (i) dense rootSIFT [31] local features with spatial extension [32], extracted with 3 pixel step over 7 scales ($\sqrt{2}$ scaling factor); (ii) Improved Fisher vector encoding [13] using a GMM codebook with 512 Gaussians; (iii) intra normalisation [33] of the Fisher vector.

Our ConvNet training and computation framework is based on the publicly available Caffe toolbox [34]. The two ConvNet configurations, considered in this paper ('CNN M 2048' and 'CNN M 128') are pre-trained on the ImageNet ILSVRC-2012 dataset using the configurations described in [21][4]. Namely, they contain 5 convolutional and 2 fully-connected layers, interleaved with rectification non linearities and max pooling. The stack of layers is followed by a 1000-way soft-max classifier, which is removed after pre-training is finished (turning a ConvNet from an ImageNet classifier to a generic image descriptor). The only difference between the two ConvNets is the dimensionality of the second fully-connected layer, which is 2048 for 'CNN M 2048' and 128 for 'CNN M 128'.

In order to provide a similar setup to our on-the-fly architecture in Sect. 4, which uses a linear predictor $\langle \mathbf{w}, \phi(I) \rangle$ learnt using SVM hinge loss and a quadratic regulariser, as our learning stage we use a standard linear support vector machine implementation. The C parameter is determined using the VOC validation set for scenario 1, and fixed at 0.25 for all other experiments.

4   On-the-fly Architecture

Having evaluated various image representations in Sect. 3, we now describe the architecture of the object category retrieval system, which fully exploits the advantages of ConvNet image representations. From the user experience point of view, the main requirement to our system is instant response: the first ranking of the repository images should be obtained immediately (in under a second), with a potential improvement over time. This dictates the following design choice:

---

[4] http://www.robots.ox.ac.uk/~vgg/software/deep_eval/.

downloading the training images from the Internet should be carried out in parallel with training a model on the already downloaded images in the on-line fashion. As a result, at any point of time, the current model can be used to perform ranking of the dataset images.

For this approach to work, however, the chosen image representation should satisfy the following requirements: (i) highly discriminative, so that even a handful of training samples are sufficient to learn a linear ranking model; (ii) fast-to-compute, to maximise the amount of training data processed within the allocated time budget; (iii) low memory footprint, to allow for storing large-scale datasets in the main memory, and ranking them efficiently. As has been demonstrated in Sect. 3, a ConvNet image representation is a perfect match for these requirements. Indeed, pre-training on a large image collection (ImageNet) leads to highly discriminative representation, and even a few training samples are sufficient for training an accurate linear model; ConvNet features can be computed very quickly on the highly-parallel GPU hardware; they have low dimensionality (even without PQ compression) and can be instantly scored using a linear model on the GPU.

Our on-the-fly architecture is illustrated in Fig. 1. It is divided into the CPU-based front-end, which controls the graphical user interface and downloads the training images from the Internet, and the GPU-based back-end, which continually trains the ranking model on the downloaded images and periodically applies it to the repository. The category retrieval is carried out as follows:

Off-line (pre-processing). To allow for fast processing, the ConvNet features for the target dataset images are pre-computed off-line, using the CNN-128 architecture. We also prepare the fixed negative image pool for *all queries* by issuing our negative pool queries (see Sect. 2.2) to both Bing and Google image search, and downloading the returned URLs. The negative image feature features are also pre-computed. The memory requirements for storing the pre-computed features are as follows: 488 MB for the MIRFLICKR-1M dataset and 78 MB for the pool of 16K negative features. It is thus feasible to permanently store the features of both negative and dataset images in the high-speed GPU memory even without compression of any kind (a consumer-grade NVIDIA GTX Titan GPU, used in our experiments, is equipped with 6 GB RAM). As noted in Sect. 2, the ConvNet features can be compressed further by up to $16\times$ using product quantization without significant degradation in performance, making datasets of up to 160M images storable in GPU memory, setting 1 GB aside for storage of the model (compared to 10M images without compression), and more if multiple GPUs are used. Many recent laptops are fitted with a GPU containing similar amounts of memory, making our system theoretically runnable on a single laptop. Furthermore, whilst storing the target repository on the GPU is preferable in terms of the ranking time, in the case of datasets of 1B+ images it can be placed in the CPU memory, which typically has a larger capacity.

On-line (CPU front-end). Given a textual query, provided by a user (*e.g.* in a browser window), the front-end starts by downloading relevant images, which will be used as positive samples for the queried category and fed to the GPU

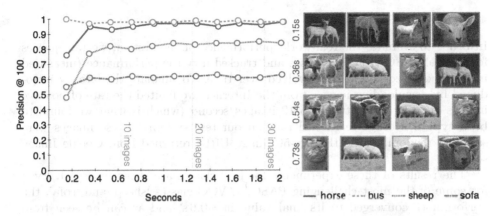

Fig. 4. Precision @ 100 against training time for four queries using our on-the-fly architecture. The number of images in the dynamically expanding positive image training pool over time is also marked on the plot. The top-4 returned images for the 'sheep' query at the first four time-steps (up to 0.73 s) is shown to the right. False positives are outlined in red, and new images in the top-4 at each time step are outlined in blue. Even for this moderately challenging query, the model settles in under a second (Color figure online).

back-end. At regular time intervals, the front-end receives a ranked list of dataset images from the back-end, and displays them in the user interface.

On-line (GPU back-end). The GPU back-end runs in parallel with the front-end, and is responsible for both training the ranking model and applying it to the dataset. *Training* an L_2-regularised linear SVM model is carried out using the mini-batch SGD with Pegasos updates [35]: at iteration t, the learning rate is $\frac{1}{\lambda t}$, where λ is the L_2-norm regularisation constant, set to 1 in our experiments. Each batch contains an equal amount of positive and negative samples; the total batch size was set to $B = 32$ in our experiments. The training commences as soon as the first positive image has been downloaded and is received from the front-end, after which B random crops are taken each iteration from the pool of positive training images downloaded so far. The front-end in the meantime will continue downloading new images from the Internet, constantly increasing the size of the positive image pool and the diversity of the extracted crops. We note that while the positive image features need to be computed on-the-fly, this is very quick in the case of ConvNets. *Ranking* takes place using the current SVM model every τ seconds (we used $\tau \sim 0.18$). As mentioned above, the pre-computed dataset features are pre-stored on a GPU, so the scores for 1M images are computed in ≈ 0.01 s. The 1M scores are then ranked (also on GPU, ≈ 0.002 s) and the list of the top-ranked images is passed to the front-end to be displayed to the user. All components of the GPU back-end are implemented within the same framework, derived from Caffe [34].

4.1   System Performance

In order to evaluate the real-world performance of the system, we ran queries for several PASCAL VOC classes and tracked how the performance (measured in terms of Precision @ 100) evolved over time. To simulate the latency introduced by downloading images from the Internet, we limited the rate of positive images entering the network to 12 images/second (which is what we found to be a typical average real-world rate on our test system). These images were sampled randomly from the top-50 image URLs returned from Google Image search.

The results of these experiments for four classes are shown in Fig. 4. Even for some of the most challenging PASCAL VOC classes 'sheep' and 'sofa', the performance converged to its final value in ~0.6 s, and as can be seen from the evolving ranking at each time-step the ordering at the top of the ranking generally stabilizes within a second, showing a good diversity of results. For easier classes such as 'aeroplane', convergence and stabilization occurs even faster.

In real terms, this results in a typical query time for our on-the-fly architecture, from entering the text query to viewing the ranked retrieved images, of **1–2 s and often less** to complete convergence and stabilization of results. However, one of the advantages of our proposed architecture is that it is adaptable to differing query complexity, and we can return good results early whilst still continuing to train in the background if necessary, exposing the classifier to an expanding pool of training data as it is downloaded from the web and updating the ranked list on-the-fly.

Novel On-the-fly Queries. Although experimental results have thusfar only been presented for the PASCAL VOC classes, the advantage of an on-the-fly architecture is that no limitation is imposed on the object categories which can be queried for, as a new classifier can be trained on demand (in our case using

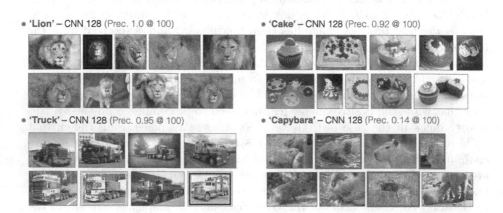

Fig. 5. Sample results for queries outside of the twenty PASCAL VOC classes. False positives are outlined in red (Color figure online).

Google Image search as a 'live' source of training data). We present some additional selected results of the on-the-fly system in Fig. 5, using the same setup as in *Scenario 3b* and query terms disjunct from the twenty PASCAL VOC classes. It can be seen that the architecture is very much generalisable to query terms outside of the PASCAL category hierarchy.

5   Conclusion

In this paper we have presented a system for on-the-fly object category retrieval, which builds upon the recent advances in deep convolutional image representations. We demonstrated how such representations can be efficiently compressed and used in a novel incremental learning architecture, capable of retrieval across datasets of 1M+ images within seconds and running entirely on a single GPU.

For larger datasets the CPU, or multiple GPU cards, could be employed for ranking once the classifier has been learnt on the GPU. Along with further investigation of how the diversity of the ranked results changes over time, this is the subject of future work.

Acknowledgements. This work was supported by the EPSRC and ERC grant Vis-Rec no. 228180. We gratefully acknowledge the support of NVIDIA Corporation with the donation of the GPUs used for this research.

References

1. Deng, J., Dong, W., Socher, R., Li, L.J., Li, K., Fei-Fei, L.: Imagenet: a large-scale hierarchical image database. In: Proceedings of CVPR (2009)
2. Soomro, K., Zamir, A.R., Shah, M.: UCF101: a dataset of 101 human actions classes from videos in the wild. CoRR abs/1212.0402 (2012)
3. Sivic, J., Zisserman, A.: Video Google: a text retrieval approach to object matching in videos. In: Proceedings of ICCV, vol. 2, pp. 1470–1477 (2003)
4. Nister, D., Stewenius, H.: Scalable recognition with a vocabulary tree. In: Proceedings of CVPR, pp. 2161–2168 (2006)
5. Philbin, J., Chum, O., Isard, M., Sivic, J., Zisserman, A.: Object retrieval with large vocabularies and fast spatial matching. In: Proceedings of CVPR (2007)
6. Jegou, H., Douze, M., Schmid, C.: Hamming embedding and weak geometric consistency for large scale image search. In: Forsyth, D., Torr, P., Zisserman, A. (eds.) ECCV 2008, Part I. LNCS, vol. 5302, pp. 304–317. Springer, Heidelberg (2008)
7. Jégou, H., Douze, M., Schmid, C., Pérez, P.: Aggregating local descriptors into a compact image representation. In: Proceedings of CVPR (2010)
8. Chatfield, K., Zisserman, A.: VISOR: towards on-the-fly large-scale object category retrieval. In: Lee, K.M., Matsushita, Y., Rehg, J.M., Hu, Z. (eds.) ACCV 2012, Part II. LNCS, vol. 7725, pp. 432–446. Springer, Heidelberg (2013)
9. Fernando, B., Tuytelaars, T.: Mining multiple queries for image retrieval: on-the-fly learning of an object-specific mid-level representation. In: Proceedings of ICCV (2013)

10. Liu, Y., Xu, D., Tsang, I.W., Luo, J.: Using large-scale web data to facilitate textual query based retrieval of consumer photos. In: Proceedings of the 17th ACM International Conference on Multimedia, MM 2009, pp. 55–64 (2009)
11. Parkhi, O.M., Vedaldi, A., Zisserman, A.: On-the-fly specific person retrieval. In: International Workshop on Image Analysis for Multimedia Interactive Services. IEEE (2012)
12. Chatfield, K., Lempitsky, V., Vedaldi, A., Zisserman, A.: The devil is in the details: an evaluation of recent feature encoding methods. In: Proceedings of BMVC (2011)
13. Perronnin, F., Sánchez, J., Mensink, T.: Improving the fisher kernel for large-scale image classification. In: Daniilidis, K., Maragos, P., Paragios, N. (eds.) ECCV 2010, Part IV. LNCS, vol. 6314, pp. 143–156. Springer, Heidelberg (2010)
14. Perronnin, F., Akata, Z., Harchaoui, Z., Schmid, C.: Towards good practice in large-scale learning for image classification. In: Proceedings of CVPR, pp. 3482–3489 (2012)
15. Jégou, H., Douze, M., Schmid, C.: Product quantization for nearest neighbor search. IEEE PAMI **33**(1), 117–128 (2011)
16. Torralba, A., Fergus, R., Freeman, W.T.: 80 million tiny images: a large dataset for non-parametric object and scene recognition. IEEE PAMI **30**, 1958–1970 (2008)
17. Raginsky, M., Lazebnik, S.: Locality sensitive binary codes from shift-invariant kernels. In: NIPS (2009)
18. LeCun, Y., Bottou, L., Bengio, Y., Haffner, P.: Gradient-based learning applied to document recognition. Proc. IEEE **86**, 2278–2324 (1998)
19. Krizhevsky, A., Sutskever, I., Hinton, G.E.: ImageNet classification with deep convolutional neural networks. In: NIPS, pp. 1106–1114 (2012)
20. Zeiler, M.D., Fergus, R.: Visualizing and understanding convolutional networks. CoRR abs/1311.2901 (2013)
21. Chatfield, K., Simonyan, K., Vedaldi, A., Zisserman, A.: Return of the devil in the details: delving deep into convolutional nets. In: Proceedings of BMVC (2014)
22. Everingham, M., Van Gool, L., Williams, C.K.I., Winn, J., Zisserman, A.: The PASCAL Visual Object Classes (VOC) challenge. IJCV **88**, 303–338 (2010)
23. Huiskes, M.J., Lew, M.S.: The MIR flickr retrieval evaluation. In: MIR 2008: Proceedings of the 2008 ACM International Conference on Multimedia Information Retrieval (2008)
24. Huiskes, M.J., Thomee, B., Lew, M.S.: New trends and ideas in visual concept detection: the MIR flickr retrieval evaluation initiative. In: MIR 2010: Proceedings of the 2010 ACM International Conference on Multimedia Information Retrieval, pp. 527–536 (2010)
25. Donahue, J., Jia, Y., Vinyals, O., Hoffman, J., Zhang, N., Tzeng, E., Darrell, T.: DeCAF: a deep convolutional activation feature for generic visual recognition. CoRR abs/1310.1531 (2013)
26. Razavian, A., Azizpour, H., Sullivan, J., Carlsson, S.: CNN Features off-the-shelf: an Astounding Baseline for Recognition. CoRR abs/1403.6382 (2014)
27. Sánchez, J., Perronnin, F.: High-dimensional signature compression for large-scale image classification. In: Proceedings of CVPR (2011)
28. Jégou, H., Furon, T., Fuchs, J.J.: Anti-sparse coding for approximate nearest neighbor search. In: Proceedings of ICASSP, pp. 2029–2032 (2012)
29. Simonyan, K., Vedaldi, A., Zisserman, A.: Learning local feature descriptors using convex optimisation. IEEE PAMI **36**, 1573–1585 (2014)
30. Parkhi, O.M., Simonyan, K., Vedaldi, A., Zisserman, A.: A compact and discriminative face track descriptor. In: Proceedings of CVPR. IEEE (2014)

31. Arandjelović, R., Zisserman, A.: Three things everyone should know to improve object retrieval. In: Proceedings of CVPR (2012)
32. Sánchez, J., Perronnin, F., Emídio de Campos, T.: Modeling the spatial layout of images beyond spatial pyramids. Pattern Recogn. Lett. **33**, 2216–2223 (2012)
33. Arandjelović, R., Zisserman, A.: All about VLAD. In: Proceedings of CVPR (2013)
34. Jia, Y.: Caffe: an open source convolutional architecture for fast feature embedding (2013). http://caffe.berkeleyvision.org/
35. Shalev-Shwartz, S., Singer, Y., Srebro, N.: Pegasos: primal estimated sub-gradient SOlver for SVM. In: Proceedings of ICML, vol. 227 (2007)

A Latent Clothing Attribute Approach for Human Pose Estimation

Weipeng Zhang[1]($\boxtimes$), Jie Shen[1], Guangcan Liu[2], and Yong Yu[1]

[1] Shanghai Jiao Tong University, Shanghai, China
weipengzhang@apex.sjtu.edu.cn
[2] Nanjing University of Information Science and Technology, Nanjing, China

Abstract. As a fundamental technique that concerns several vision tasks such as image parsing, action recognition and clothing retrieval, human pose estimation (HPE) has been extensively investigated in recent years. To achieve accurate and reliable estimation of the human pose, it is well-recognized that the clothing attributes are useful and should be utilized properly. Most previous approaches, however, require to manually annotate the clothing attributes and are therefore very costly. In this paper, we shall propose and explore a *latent* clothing attribute approach for HPE. Unlike previous approaches, our approach models the clothing attributes as latent variables and thus requires no explicit labeling for the clothing attributes. The inference of the latent variables are accomplished by utilizing the framework of latent structured support vector machines (LSSVM). We employ the strategy of *alternating direction* to train the LSSVM model: In each iteration, one kind of variables (e.g., human pose or clothing attribute) are fixed and the others are optimized. Our extensive experiments on two real-world benchmarks show the state-of-the-art performance of our proposed approach.

1 Introduction

Human oriented technology has a central role in computer vision and can greatly advance daily-life related applications. For example, face verification for surveillance [1] and clothing parsing for fashion search [2]. One of the most fundamental human oriented techniques is the well-known *human pose estimation* (HPE) in 2D images. In general, HPE could facilitate many applications, e.g., action recognition [3], image segmentation [4], etc. However, it is difficult to accurately estimate the human pose in unconstrained environments, especially in the presence of vision occlusions and background clutters.

To tackle the challenges, it is well-recognized that the contextual information (e.g., clothing attributes) is useful, as illustrated in Fig. 1. As a consequence, the so-called *context modeling*, which is to model properly the contextual information possibly existing in images, is widely regarded as a promising direction for HPE. A variety of approaches have been proposed and investigated in the literature over several years, e.g., [4–6]. In [5], it was proposed a model that encourages high contrast between background and foreground. Ladicky et al. [4] combined together pose estimation and image segmentation, aiming to take the advantages

© Springer International Publishing Switzerland 2015
D. Cremers et al. (Eds.): ACCV 2014, Part I, LNCS 9003, pp. 146–161, 2015.
DOI: 10.1007/978-3-319-16865-4_10

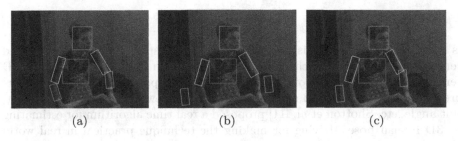

(a)   (b)   (c)

Fig. 1. Examples to demonstrate the benefit of integrating clothing attributes into HPE. In the three results of HPE, all human poses in (b) and (c) are correct except lower arms. we can assume that (c) is incorrect based on the great appearance difference between left and right lower arm, but there is slight appearance difference in (b). If we know the clothing attribute type, e.g. the sleeve type or color, we can remove (b) based on the inconsistent color between the upper and lower arms. Finally, we get the correct estimation (a).

of joint learning. In [6], a unified structured learning procedure was adopted to predict human pose and garment attribute simultaneously.

While effectual, the existing approaches require to label lots of contextual messages for training, and thus they are time-consuming and impractical. In this paper, we shall introduce a *latent* clothing attribute approach for HPE. Our approach formulates the HPE problem by extending the pictorial structure framework [7,8] and, in particular, models the clothing attributes as *latent variables*. Comparing to the previous approaches that rely on label information, our latent approach, in sharp contrast, requires no explicit labels of the clothing attributes and can therefore be executed in an efficient way. We define some clothing attributes and build their connections with human parts (e.g., sleeve with arms). Some domain specific features, including *pose-specific* features and *pose-attribute* features, are designed to describe the connections. We utilize the latent structured support vector machines (LSSVM) for the training procedure, where the attribute values are initialized by a simple K-Means clustering algorithm. Then the model parameters are learnt by employing a relabel strategy, which minimizes the objective function of LSSVM in an "alternating direction" manner. More precisely, we perform an iterative scheme to train the model: Given the (latent) clothing attributes, we perform a dynamic programming algorithm to find a suboptimal solution for human pose; Given the human pose, we seek the optimal attribute values by performing a greedy search on the attribute space. We empirically show that our approach can achieve the state-of-the-art performance on two benchmarks.

In summary, the contributions of this paper are three-folds: (1) We establish a latent clothing attribute approach that can implicitly utilize clothing attributes to enhance HPE. (2) We propose some domain specific features to describe the connections between human parts and clothing attributes. (3) We introduce an efficient algorithm to solve the optimization problem which is indeed challenging due to the presence of latent variables.

2   Related Work

As aforementioned, HPE is a difficult problem, especially in unconstrained scenes. Some of the researchers studied the problem under the context of 3D scenery [9,10]. In the work of [9], they extended the popular 2D pictorial structure [7,8] to 3D images and employed the new framework to model view point, joint angle, etc. Shotton et al. [11] proposed a real time algorithm for estimating the 3D human pose, striving for making the technique practical in real world applications.

Most studies (including this work) on HPE focus on 2D static images. In the early works, the human part was often modeled by oriented template. Although straightforward, the oriented templates may not properly handle the fore-shortening of the objects [12–14]. In [15], an advanced representation scheme was proposed to model the oriented human parts. The new model is formulated as a mixture of non-oriented components, each of which is attributed with a "type". Interestingly, the new model can approximate the fore-shortening by tuning the adjacent components in a spring structure.

Some work tried to incorporate "side" techniques, e.g., image segmentation, to enhance HPE. In [16], a variety of image features, e.g., boundary response and region segmentation, were utilized to produce more reliable HPE results. In [5], the background was modeled as a Gaussian distribution. In [17], the authors present a two-stage approximate scheme to improve the accuracy of estimating lower arms in videos. The algorithm was imposed to output the candidates with high contrast to the surroundings.

Besides of the shape feature which is very discriminative, the appearance feature (e.g. color, texture) is also important for HPE [18]. Generally, the appearance feature is actually a description of the clothing. As illustrated in Fig. 1, there is a strong correlation between human pose and clothing attribute. Some previous work such as [2,19–21] utilized the result of HPE to predict the clothing attribute or retrieve similar garments. Other methods (e.g., [6,22]) attempted to refine the clothing parsing by HPE and, in turn, refine HPE by clothing parsing. However, this requires a large annotation for clothing. In our work, it is not required to manually annotate the attributes as we take them as latent variables.

There is some work that has investigated clothing attributes in the tasks other than HPE. In [23], Liu et al. aimed to recommend garment for specific scenes. To bridge the gap between the low-level image evidence and the garment recommendation, they integrated an attribute-level representation that propagates semantic messages to the recommendation system. In [3], similar attribute techniques as ours were used for action recognition. However, there is a key difference: In [3], the attribute is used as a middle level prior and the high level task was facilitated by the knowledge of attribute; In our work, the attribute is modeled in a unified manner with human pose. Our model takes a relabel strategy to alternatively optimize the variables of the attribute and pose.

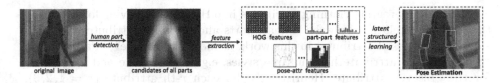

Fig. 2. Overview of our approach.

3   HPE with Latent Clothing Attributes

We summarize the pipeline of our approach in Fig. 2. First, we take a pre-processing step to detect potential human parts in the image. This step allows us to have a search space with manageable size. Then, we extract the domain specific features to characterize the human pose and clothing attributes. Finally, we utilize the LSSVM to actualize our attribute aware human pose model and present an efficient inference algorithm to find an approximate optimal solution to LSSVM. Note that our model can reveal the clothing attributes, and thus humans with similar attribute values will be grouped together (i.e., clustering human by their clothing attributes).

Table 1. The configuration of clothing attributes

Attribute	Human parts	Features	Number of values
Sleeve	All arms	Color Histogram	3
Neckline	Torso + Head	HOG	4
Pattern	Torso	LBP [24]	5

Before introducing the proposed approach in detail, we would like to introduce some notations. We write I for an image. A human part is represented as a bounding box (x, y, s, θ), where (x, y) is the coordinate, s is the size and θ is the rotation. To obtain an input space with manageable size, we use the existing HPE method [15] to produce 40 candidates for each human part. Thus, the input space $\mathcal{X}$ of our approach is defined as:

$$\mathcal{X} = \{\mathbf{x} | \mathbf{x} = (\mathbf{b}_1, \mathbf{b}_2, \cdots, \mathbf{b}_m)\}, \tag{1}$$

where m is the number of human upper-body parts ($m = 6$ in this work), and $\mathbf{b}_i$ denotes the candidate ensemble for the i-th human part (there are 40 candidates in each $\mathbf{b}_i$). The output space of human pose is defined as follows:

$$\mathcal{P} = \{\mathbf{p} | \mathbf{p} = (p_1, p_2, \cdots, p_m), \forall i, 1 \leq p_i \leq 40\}, \tag{2}$$

where p_i is a positive integer that indicates the index of the estimated candidate.

We aim to integrate clothing attributes into HPE task, striving for capturing the strong correlation between human parts and clothing attributes. We consider three types of attributes in this work, including "Neckline", "Pattern" and "Sleeve". Each attribute has multiple styles, e.g., short sleeve and long sleeve for the "Sleeve" attribute. Heuristically, for each r-th attribute ($r = 1, 2, 3$), the number of attribute values, T_r, are determined as in Table 1 (see the last column). Then the output space of the latent clothing attributes is as follows:

$$\mathcal{A} = \{\mathbf{a}|\mathbf{a} = (a_1, a_2, \cdots, a_n), \forall r, 1 \leq a_r \leq T_r\}. \tag{3}$$

where n is the number of clothing attributes ($n = 3$ in this work), and a_r is the label for the r-th attribute. Note here that it has no specific consideration to choose the value for a_r, e.g., $a_1 = 1$ may mean short sleeve or long sleeve. In this work it is an unsupervised clustering procedure that recognizes the clothing attributes.

Finally, the task of jointly estimating clothing attribute and human pose is formulated as follows:

$$f : \mathcal{X} \to \mathcal{Y}, \tag{4}$$

where $\mathcal{Y}$ is the output space given by

$$\mathcal{Y} = \{\mathbf{y}|\mathbf{y} = (\mathbf{p}, \mathbf{a}), \mathbf{p} \in \mathcal{P}, \mathbf{a} \in \mathcal{A}\}. \tag{5}$$

Regarding the prediction function f, we presume that there is a score function S which measures the fitness between any input-output pair $(\mathbf{x}, \mathbf{y})$ such that:

$$S(\mathbf{x}, \mathbf{y}; \beta) = \langle \beta, J(\mathbf{x}, \mathbf{y}) \rangle \tag{6}$$

where $\langle \cdot \rangle$ denotes the inner product between two vectors, $J(\cdot, \cdot)$ is the feature representation, and β is an unknown weight vector. In this way, the mapping function f in Eq. 4 can be written as:

$$f(\mathbf{x}; \beta) = \arg \max_{\mathbf{y} \in \mathcal{Y}} S(\mathbf{x}, \mathbf{y}; \beta) \tag{7}$$

This is a latent structured learning problem, where the latent variables are clothing attributes. Our learning procedure is motivated by [25], which employs a relabel strategy to increasingly improve the prediction of latent variables. Yet before proceeding to the training pipeline, we firstly introduce the design of the domain-specific features, as shown in the next section.

3.1   Feature Representation

The joint feature representation is an important component in structured learning [26]. We define the joint feature function $J(\mathbf{x}, \mathbf{y})$ by using two types of features, including *pose-specific* features denoted by $j_p(\mathbf{x}, \mathbf{p})$, and *pose-attribute* features denoted by $j_{pa}(\mathbf{x}, \mathbf{y})$; that is,

$$\langle \beta, J(\mathbf{x}, \mathbf{y}) \rangle = \langle \beta_p, j_p(\mathbf{x}, \mathbf{p}) \rangle + \langle \beta_{pa}, j_{pa}(\mathbf{x}, \mathbf{y}) \rangle \tag{8}$$

In the following, we present our techniques used to design each type of feature.

Pose-Specific Features. Given an input sample $\mathbf{x}$, we use the Histogram of Oriented Gradients (HOG) [27] to describe the shape of a candidate and consider the deformation constraint between two connected parts:

$$j_p(\mathbf{x}, \mathbf{p}) = \sum_{i=1}^{m} hog(\mathbf{x}, p_i) + \sum_{(i,j) \in E_p} d(\mathbf{x}, p_i, p_j), \tag{9}$$

where E_p is the set of connected limbs. The design of the deformation feature $d(\mathbf{x}, p_i, p_j)$ involves some basic geometry constraints between connected parts, including relative position, rotation and distance of part candidate p_i with respect to p_j, which is computed as $[x_j - x_i, y_j - y_i, (x_j - x_i)^2, (y_j - y_i)^2]$ [15].

Pose-Attribute Features. Now we try to integrate the clothing attributes into our model. Notice that an attribute is only associated with some of the human parts). For a given attribute r, we denote the human parts associated with it as r_p and the corresponding configuration as P_r. The detailed inter-dependency between human parts and clothing attributes is shown in the second column of Table 1. According to the work [2], for different attributes, different low-level features should be used to achieve good performance. The specific features used for each clothing attribute can be found in the third column in Table 1.

Formally, the pose-attribute features are defined as:

$$j_{pu}(\mathbf{x}, \mathbf{y}) = \sum_{r=1}^{n} \Psi(\mathbf{x}, P_r, a_r) \tag{10}$$

where $\Psi(\mathbf{x}, P_r, a_r)$ denotes the features extracted from the human part $\mathbf{x}$, with the configuration P_r and the attribute label a_r.

Algorithm 1. Structured Learning with Latent SVM

Input: Positive samples, negative samples, initial model β, number of relabel iteration t_1, number of hard negative mining iteration t_2.
Output: Final Model β^*.
1: Initialize the final model: $\beta^* = \beta$.
2: Let the negative sample set $F_n = \emptyset$.
3: **for** relabel $= 1$ to t_1 **do**
4:     Let the positive sample set $F_p = \emptyset$.
5:     Add positive samples to F_p.
6:     **for** iter $= 1$ to t_2 **do**
7:         Add negative samples to F_n.
8:         $\beta^* := \text{Pegasos}(\beta^*, F_p \bigcup F_n)$.
9:         Remove easy negative samples:
            Remove the samples whose feature vector v satisfying $\langle \beta^*, v \rangle < -1$ from F_n.
10:     **end for**
11: **end for**

Similar to [6], the pose-attribute feature is designed by an outer product of low-level features and an identity vector. We first convert the clothing attribute label a_r to a T_r-dimensional vector, denoted as $L(a_r)$, one element of which is assigned with valued "1" and all others are set to be "0". From Table 1, the low-level feature descriptors of the r-th clothing attribute depend on two aspects: (1) the corresponding human parts and (2) the feature type (denoted by F_r and has been specified in Table 1). We use $F_r(P_r)$ to denote features of the r-th clothing attribute associated with the part configuration P_r. Then our pose-attribute feature $\Psi(\mathbf{x}, P_r, a_r)$ is designed as follows:

$$\Psi_{pa}(\mathbf{x}, P_r, a_r) = F_r(P_r) \otimes L(a_r) \tag{11}$$

where the "$\otimes$" operator represents the (vectorized) outer product of two vectors.

3.2   Structured Learning with Latent SVM

Now we consider the problem of learning the prediction mapping f, given a collection of images labeled with human part locations. This is the type of data available in the all standard benchmark dataset for human pose estimation. Note that clothing attributes have no labels, and we treat them as latent variables.

We describe a framework for initializing the structure of a joint model and learning all parameters. Parameter learning is done by constructing a LSSVM training problem. We train the LSSVM using the relabel approach (details will be described later) together with the data-mining (hard negative mining), and we use Pegasos [28] for the online update to solve the problem of huge space for negative samples.

Algorithm 2. Inference for Clothing Attributes

Input: A sample $\mathbf{x}$, Model parameter β , Human parts label $\mathbf{p}$
Output: optimal clothing attributes value $\mathbf{a}^*$
 1: let T_r is the number of r-th clothing attribute type
 2: **for** r:= 1 **to** 3 **do**
 3:     select the attribute value which has highest score:
         $\mathbf{a}_r = \arg \max_{1 \leq r \leq T_r} \langle \beta_{pa}^r, j_{pa}(\mathbf{x}, P_r, a_r) \rangle$
 4: **end for**

Objective Function. We aim to learn the fitness function $S(\mathbf{x}, \mathbf{y}; \beta)$ defined in Eq. (6), which can later be used for joint estimation (see Eq. (7)). Given a positive training sample $(\mathbf{x}, \mathbf{y})$, we expect $S(\mathbf{x}, \mathbf{y}; \beta) \geq 1$. On the other hand, if a training sample $(\mathbf{x}, \mathbf{y})$ is negative, the output of the fitness function is required to be less than -1. In this way, given a training set $D = \{(\mathbf{x}_1, \mathbf{y}_1, z_1), \cdots, (\mathbf{x}_q, \mathbf{y}_q, z_q)\}$, where $z_k \in \{1, -1\}$ indicates the k-th sample is positive or not, we can optimize the following objective function to solve β:

$$\min_{\beta} \frac{1}{2}\|\beta\|^2 + C \sum_{k=1}^{q} \max(0, 1 - z_k S(\mathbf{x}_k, \mathbf{y}_k; \beta)). \tag{12}$$

Initialization. Since the clothing attributes are latent variables, we can only access the label of human pose. To start up, we take a relabel strategy to update the positive samples (more accurately, the clothing attribute labels) and the weight vector β in an alternative manner.

There are many ways to initialize the latent variables. One can randomly assign labels for training samples which may be unstable. In our work, we first use the groundtruth of human pose to extract low-level features (see Table 1) for each attribute. Then we perform a K-Means clustering algorithm to obtain the center of each attribute value, where K is exactly the number of attribute values we defined in Table 1. In this way, the initial label for the clothing attribute can be determined by the closest center.

Now all of the labels have been generated, we can solve Problem (12) to obtain the initial weight vector β (line 1 in Algorithm 1).

Relabel Strategy. As the initial clothing attribute labels are not accurate, we employ a relabel strategy to update the attribute labels. That is, given the model parameter β and human pose, we predict the clothing attribute by maximizing the fitness function $S(\mathbf{x}, \mathbf{y}; \beta)$, which is shown in Algorithm 2. Note that according to the design of our joint feature $J(\mathbf{x}, \mathbf{y})$, the pose-specific features are irrelevant for the inference of attributes. From Eq. (10), we know that there is no interaction between different attributes since J_{pa} is summation of n separate attributes associated features. Therefore, we can perform an efficient greedy search for each attribute to obtain a local optima (line 2–4 in Algorithm 2).

Algorithm 3. Approximate Inference for Clothing Attribute Aware HPE Task

Input: A sample $\mathbf{x}$, Model parameter β.
Output: Optimal estimation $\mathbf{y}^*$ and score $S*$.
1: Set $\mathbf{y}^* = \emptyset$.
2: Set the optimal score $S^* = -\infty$.
3: Initialize the parts estimation $\mathbf{p}_0$.
4: **repeat**
5:     Compute the local optimal clothing attributes $\mathbf{a}_t$.
6:     Compute the local optimal human pose $\mathbf{p}_t$.
7:     Compute the local score: $S = S(\mathbf{x}, \mathbf{y}_t; \beta)$.
8:     **if** $S > S^*$ **then**
9:         $S^* = S$, $\mathbf{y}^* = \mathbf{y}_t$
10:    **end if**
11: **until** S^* not change

Hard Negative Mining. For a recognition or detection task, one can obtain a positive sample set with manageable size. However, there is a huge space

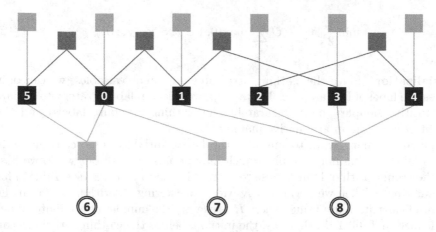

Fig. 3. Nodes with numbers from 0 to 5 are the human part variable and those 6 to 8 are clothing attributes. Colored nodes are the potentials (Color figure online).

for the negative samples. Actually, it is not possible for enumerate *all* negative samples. Thus, it is important to feed an algorithm with "hard" negative samples for efficiency and memory cost. In line 6–10 of Algorithm 1, we perform hard negative mining [25] to obtain valuable negative samples. This schema will call the inference algorithm 3 (see Sect. 3.3). More concretely, given an input sample $\mathbf{x}$ and weight vector β, we launch Algorithm 3 to find the optimal estimation $\mathbf{y}^*$. If $z \cdot S^*$ is less than -1 (a threshold we set), $\mathbf{x}$ is considered hard. The searching procedure on $\mathbf{x}$ will be stopped only when the S^* is greater than -1 (the $\mathbf{y}^*$ produced by the previous step is removed from the search space).

After collecting all the hard negative samples, we update β with Pegasos solver [28] (line 8 in Algorithm 1). Then we use the updated β to perform a shrinkage step to remove the easy negatives from the hard negative set F_n.

3.3 Inference

In Fig. 3, we represent our problem as a factor graph $\mathcal{G}$, where the rectangle node denotes a human part, the circle node with double boundaries denotes a clothing attribute. As our original problem is a cyclic graph, it cannot be optimized exactly and efficiently. Therefore, in Algorithm 3, we propose an iterative algorithm to search for an approximate solution. Our algorithm receives a sample x, the model parameter β as inputs and outputs a local optima for human parts and clothing attribute. In each iteration, by fixing the attributes, the inference can be performed on a tree structure, which can be optimized with a dynamic programming [8]. When the human parts are fixed, an efficient greedy search schema for clothing attribute is employed (see Algorithm 2).

Inference for Human Pose. We elaborate the inference procedure of human pose by extending the pictorial structure framework. In Fig. 3, we denote our

---

Algorithm 4. Inference for Human Pose

Input: A sample $\mathbf{x}$, Model parameter β , Clothing attributes value $\mathbf{a}$
Output: optimal human parts estimation $\mathbf{p}^*$
1: set the optimal human parts estimation $\mathbf{p}^* = \emptyset$
2: set the node 0 as the root node
3: **for** each candidate $\mathbf{p}_i$ of node i **do**
4:     set $m(\mathbf{p}_i) = \langle \beta_p^i, \phi_p(\mathbf{x}, p_i) \rangle + \langle \beta_{pa}^r, \Psi_{pa}(\mathbf{x}, P_r, a_r) \rangle$
5: **end for**
6: **for** each candidate $\mathbf{p}_j$ of parent node j and $\mathbf{p}_i$ of child node i **do**
7:     set $l(\mathbf{p}_i, \mathbf{p}_j) = \langle \beta_p^{ij}, \psi_p(\mathbf{x}, p_i, p_j) \rangle$
8:     **if** i is a leaf node **then**
9:         $B_i(\mathbf{p}_j) = \max_{\mathbf{p}_i}(m(\mathbf{p}_i) + l(\mathbf{p}_i, \mathbf{p}_j))$
10:    **else**
11:        $B_i(\mathbf{p}_j) = \max_{\mathbf{p}_i}(m(\mathbf{p}_i) + l(\mathbf{p}_i, \mathbf{p}_j) + \sum_{v \in C_i} B_v(\mathbf{p}_i))$
12:    **end if**
13: **end for**
14: select the best candidate for the root node:
    $\mathbf{p}_0^* = \arg\max_{\mathbf{p}_0}(m(\mathbf{p}_0) + \sum_{v \in C_0} B_v(\mathbf{p}_0))$
15: **for** each parent-child pair $(\mathbf{p}_j^*, \mathbf{p}_i)$ **do**
16:    $\mathbf{p}_i^* = \arg\max_{\mathbf{p}_i} B_i(\mathbf{p}_j^*)$
17: **end for**

---

score with colored nodes, with purple and red ones denoting the appearance and deformation scores. The main extension for the traditional PS model is the cyan nodes, which denoting the score to measure the fitness of human pose and clothing attribute (called pose-attribute score). Therefore, we propose the human pose inference procedure in Algorithm 4. We denote the children nodes as C_i for a node i. We compute the appearance and pose-attribute scores in line 3–5. In line 7, we compute the deformation score for each parent-child pair node i and j. In the line 8–12, we compute conventional message passing procedure by dynamic programming [7]. Then we perform a top-down process to find the best candidate for each human part in line 14–17.

4   Experiments

4.1   Datasets

We evaluate our approach using the Buffy dataset [29] and the DL (daily life) dataset. The Buffy Dataset contains 748 pose-annotated video frames from Buffy TV show. This dataset is presented as a benchmark for HPE task. The DL dataset contains 997 daily life photos collected from the Flickr website. We annotate the human pose for this dataset. Compared with Buffy, the DL dataset has more various clothing attribute values. In order to obtain quantitative evaluation results for attributes, we manually annotate the clothing attributes for Buffy and DL. There is a standard partition of Buffy for training and testing, where the training set consists of 472 images and the remaining are used for testing. For the

Table 2. Comparison with state-of-the-art algorithms on the Buffy dataset

Method	Torso	Upper arms	Lower arms	Head	Total
Andriluka et al. [30]	90.7	79.3	41.2	95.5	73.5
Sapp et al. [16]	**100**	95.3	63.0	96.2	85.5
Yang and Ramanan [15]	**100**	96.6	70.9	**99.6**	89.1
Our approach	**100**	**97.1**	**78.4**	99.1	**91.6**

Table 3. Comparison with state-of-the-art algorithms on the DL dataset

Method	Torso	Upper arms	Lower arms	Head	Total
Andriluka et al. [30]	97.0	91.7	84.5	94.0	90.6
Sapp et al. [16]	**100**	88.5	78.0	87.6	86.8
Yang and Ramanan [15]	99.8	95.7	87.5	95.6	93.6
Our approach	**100**	**97.2**	**91.3**	**99.1**	**95.7**

DL dataset, we select randomly 297 images for training and use the remaining 700 images for testing.

4.2 Baselines and Metric

We compare our approach with three state-of-the-art algorithms: Andriluka et al. [30], Sapp et al. [16], Yang and Ramanan [15]. For the HPE results, we evaluate them with a standardized evaluation protocol based on the probability of correct pose (PCP) [31], which measures the percentage of correctly localized human parts. For the clothing attributes results, we evaluate them with a standardized metric (F1 score) of clustering task. We use the K-Means clustering results as our baseline for clothing attributes. First we use the groundtruth of human pose to obtain the clustering center for each attribute value. Then we perform K-Means clustering under a given pose, which is produced by either the state-of-the-art HPE algorithms or the groundtruth (Fig. 4).

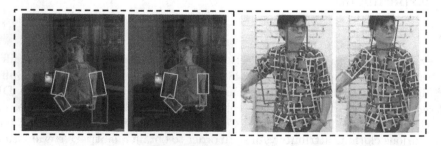

Fig. 4. Comparison of our approach with Yang and Ramanan [15] produces incorrect estimation (the 1st and 3rd) for upper and lower arms, while our latent clothing attribute approach produces correct.

Table 4. F1 scores for clothing attributes results on Buffy

HPE	Sleeve	Neckline	Pattern	Total
Andriluka et al. [30] + K-Means	24.1	26.6	34.2	28.3
Sapp et al. [16] + K-Means	22.9	27.9	40.5	30.4
Yang and Ramanan [15] + K-Means	38.3	25.7	22.6	28.9
Groundtruth + K-Means	34.7	36.1	39.5	36.8
Our approach	**55.6**	**68.8**	**80.8**	**68.4**

Table 5. F1 scores for clothing attributes results on DL

HPE	Sleeve	Neckline	Pattern	Total
Andriluka et al. [30] + K-Means	27.5	31.7	27.6	28.9
Sapp et al. [16] + K-Means	34.9	30.5	23.8	29.7
Yang and Ramanan [15] + K-Means	43.2	28.6	35.8	35.9
Groundtruth + K-Means	31	29.8	26.1	28.9
Our approach	**57.2**	**60.3**	**74.7**	**64.1**

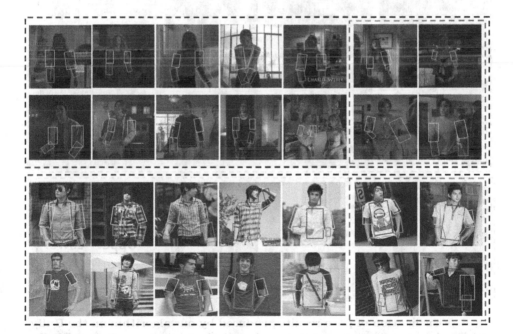

Fig. 5. Examples grouped on sleeve from Buffy and neckline from DL. The first row of the top panel (sleeve) shows the sleeveless type, the second is long type, while the first row of the bottom panel (neckline) shows the pointed type, the second is round type. The right two columns are the incorrect results.

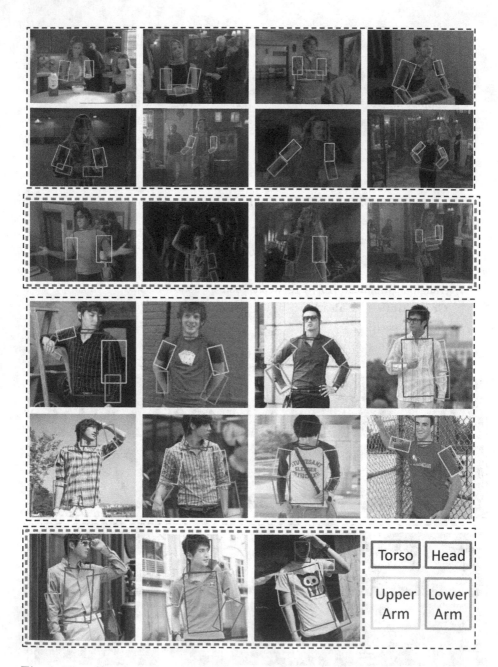

Fig. 6. Visualization of pose results produced by our algorithm on the Buffy and DL datasets. The top two panels are from Buffy and the others are from DL. We use the oriented bounding box to denote the pose estimation. The first panel of each dataset are correct results, while the second panel are incorrect results. The bounding box with red color denote the incorrect estimation (Color figure online).

4.3   Results

Figure 6 shows some exemplar HPE results produced by our approach. We provide the PCP evaluation results on Buffy and DL in Tables 2 and 3 respectively. For the Buffy dataset, Table 2 shows that our approach consistently outperforms Yang and Ramanan [15] which is a recently established algorithm. It is expected that the most difficult parts to estimate are the lower arms. Surprisingly, the improvement on the lower arms of our approach achieves 7.5 percent higher than Yang and Ramanan, possibly because of the integration of the sleeve attribute. For the DL dataset, our algorithm consistently outperforms all the competing baselines since the photos in DL are collected from daily life and have richer clothing attributes than Buffy.

As we also aim to reveal the clothing attribute, we show some results in Fig. 5 for Buffy and DL, where we arrange the images with same attribute value into one group (i.e. clustering humans by their clothing attributes). In the top pane of Fig. 5, we group humans by the sleeve attribute. The performance under the F1 score is demonstrated in Tables 4 and 5. Surprisingly, our approach enjoys a significant improvement on both datasets, mainly because of the relabel strategy and the iterative update role for our model parameter. Note that the result of "K-means + Groundtruth" provides the initial labels for the clothing attributes. In this way, we examine the effectiveness of our relabel strategy.

5   Conclusion

Inspired by the strong correlation between human pose and clothing attributes, we propose a latent clothing attribute approach for HPE, incorporating the clothing attributes into the traditional HPE model as latent variables. Compared with previous work [6], our formulation is more suitable for practical applications as we do not need to annotate the clothing attributes. We utilize the LSSVM to learn all the parameters by employing a relabel strategy. To start up, we take a simple K-Means step to initialize the latent variables and then update the model and the clothing attributes in an alternative manner. Finally, we propose an approximate inference schema to iteratively find an increasingly better solution. The experimental results justify the effectiveness of our relabel strategy and show the state-of-the-art performance for HPE.

References

1. Liu, L., Zhang, L., Liu, H., Yan, S.: Towards large-population face identification in unconstrained videos. In: IEEE Transactions on Circuits and Systems for Video Technology, p. 1 (2014)
2. Liu, S., Song, Z., Liu, G., Xu, C., Lu, H., Yan, S.: Street-to-shop: cross-scenario clothing retrieval via parts alignment and auxiliary set. In: IEEE Conference on Computer Vision and Pattern Recognition, pp. 3330–3337 (2012)

3. Liu, J., Kuipers, B., Savarese, S.: Recognizing human actions by attributes. In: IEEE Conference on Computer Vision and Pattern Recognition, pp. 3337–3344 (2011)
4. Ladicky, L., Torr, P.H.S., Zisserman, A.: Human pose estimation using a joint pixel-wise and part-wise formulation. In: IEEE Conference on Computer Vision and Pattern Recognition, pp. 3578–3585 (2013)
5. Rothrock, B., Park, S., Zhu, S.C.: Integrating grammar and segmentation for human pose estimation. In: IEEE Conference on Computer Vision and Pattern Recognition, pp. 3214–3221 (2013)
6. Shen, J., Liu, G., Chen, J., Fang, Y., Xie, J., Yu, Y., Yan, S.: Unified structured learning for simultaneous human pose estimation and garment attribute classification. arXiv preprint arXiv:1404.4923 (2014)
7. Fischler, M., Elschlager, R.: The representation and matching of pictorial structures. IEEE Trans. Comput. 22, 67–92 (1973)
8. Felzenszwalb, P., Huttenlocher, D.: Pictorial structures for object recognition. Int. J. Comput. Vision 61, 55–79 (2005)
9. Burenius, M., Sullivan, J., Carlsson, S.: 3D pictorial structures for multiple view articulated pose estimation. In: IEEE Conference on Computer Vision Pattern Recognition, pp. 3618–3625 (2013)
10. Ionescu, C., Carreira, J., Sminchisescu, C.: Iterated second-order label sensitive pooling for 3D human pose estimation. In: IEEE Conference on Computer Vision Pattern Recognition (2014)
11. Shotton, J., Sharp, T., Kipman, A., Fitzgibbon, A., Finocchio, M., Blake, A., Cook, M., Moore, R.: Real-time human pose recognition in parts from single depth images. Commun. ACM 56, 116–124 (2013)
12. Ramanan, D.: Learning to parse images of articulated bodies. In: Neural Information Processing Systems, pp. 1129–1136 (2006)
13. Sapp, B., Jordan, C., Taskar, B.: Adaptive pose priors for pictorial structures. In: IEEE Conference on Computer Vision and Pattern Recognition, pp. 422–429 (2010)
14. Morris, D.D., Rehg, J.M.: Singularity analysis for articulated object tracking. In: Conference on Computer Vision and Pattern Recognition (CVPR), pp. 289–296 (1998)
15. Yang, Y., Ramanan, D.: Articulated pose estimation with flexible mixture-of-parts. In: IEEE Conference on Computer Vision and Pattern Recognition, pp. 1385–1392 (2011)
16. Sapp, B., Toshev, A., Taskar, B.: Cascaded models for articulated pose estimation. In: Daniilidis, K., Maragos, P., Paragios, N. (eds.) ECCV 2010, Part II. LNCS, vol. 6312, pp. 406–420. Springer, Heidelberg (2010)
17. Cherian, A., Mairal, J., Alahari, K., Schmid, C.: Mixing body-part sequences for human pose estimation. In: IEEE Conference on Computer Vision Pattern Recognition (2014)
18. Eichner, M., Ferrari, V.: Better appearance models for pictorial structures. In: British Machine Vision Conference (2009)
19. Chen, H., Gallagher, A., Girod, B.: Describing clothing by semantic attributes. In: Fitzgibbon, A., Lazebnik, S., Perona, P., Sato, Y., Schmid, C. (eds.) ECCV 2012, Part III. LNCS, vol. 7574, pp. 609–623. Springer, Heidelberg (2012)
20. Bourdev, L., Maji, S., Malik, J.: Describing people: poselet-based attribute classification. In: International Conference on Computer Vision (ICCV) (2011)

21. Li, Y., Zhou, Y., Yan, J., Niu, Z., Yang, J.: Visual saliency based on conditional entropy. In: Zha, H., Taniguchi, R., Maybank, S. (eds.) ACCV 2009, Part I. LNCS, vol. 5994, pp. 246–257. Springer, Heidelberg (2010)
22. Yamaguchi, K., Kiapour, M.H., Ortiz, L.E., Berg, T.L.: You are what you wear: parsing clothing in fashion photos. In: IEEE Conference on Computer Vision and Pattern Recognition, pp. 3570–3577 (2012)
23. Liu, S., Feng, J., Song, Z., Zhang, T., Lu, H., Xu, C., Yan, S.: Hi, magic closet, tell me what to wear! In: ACM Multimedia Conference, pp. 619–628 (2012)
24. Ojala, T., Pietikainen, M., Harwood, D.: Performance evaluation of texture measures with classification based on kullback discrimination of distributions. In: International Conference on Pattern Recognition (1994)
25. Felzenszwalb, P., Girshick, R.B., McAllester, D., Ramanan, D.: Object detection with discriminatively trained part based models. IEEE Trans. Pattern Anal. Mach. Intell. 32, 1627–1645 (2010)
26. Tsochantaridis, I., Joachims, T., Hofmann, T., Altun, Y.: Large margin methods for structured and interdependent output variables. J. Mach. Learn. Res. 6, 1453–1484 (2005)
27. Dalal, N., Triggs, B.: Histograms of oriented gradients for human detection. In: IEEE Conference on Computer Vision and Pattern Recognition (2005)
28. Shalev-Shwartz, S., Singer, Y., Srebro, N.: Pegasos: primal estimated sub-Gradient SOlver for SVM. In: International Conference on Machine Learning, pp. 807–814 (2007)
29. Ferrari, V., Marin, M., Zisserman, A.: Progressive search space reduction for human pose estimation. In: IEEE Conference on Computer Vision and Pattern Recognition (2008)
30. Andriluka, M., Roth, S., Schiele, B.: Pictorial structures revisited: people detection and articulated pose estimation. In: IEEE Conference on Computer Vision and Pattern Recognition, pp. 1014–1021 (2009)
31. Ferrari, V., Marn-Jimnez, M.J., Zisserman, A.: Pose search: retrieving people using their pose. In: IEEE Conference on Computer Vision and Pattern Recognition, pp. 1–8 (2009)

NOKMeans: Non-Orthogonal K-means Hashing

Xiping Fu$^{(\boxtimes)}$, Brendan McCane, Steven Mills, and Michael Albert

Department of Computer Science, University of Otago, Dunedin, New Zealand
{xiping,mccane,steven,malbert}@cs.otago.ac.nz

Abstract. Finding nearest neighbor points in a large scale high dimensional data set is of wide interest in computer vision. One popular and efficient approach is to encode each data point as a binary code in Hamming space using separating hyperplanes. One condition which is often implicitly assumed is that the separating hyperplanes should be mutually orthogonal. With the aim of increasing the representation capability of the hyperplanes when used for indexing, we relax the orthogonality assumption without forsaking the alternate view of using cluster centers to represent the indexing partitions. This is achieved by viewing the data points in a space determined by their distances to the hyperplanes. We show that the proposed method is superior to existing state-of-the-art techniques on several large computer vision datasets.

1 Introduction

Finding nearest neighbor points is of wide interest in several areas of computer vision including feature matching [1], image retrieval [2] and object recognition [3]. For example, in content-based image retrieval (CBIR), the task is to retrieve similar images when given a query image. This is often done by representing all of the images as points in a specific space, and then retrieving the nearest neighbor points as similar images. Naive exhaustive searching is linear in the number of images in the collection and becomes infeasible for very large collections. Even specialised data structures such as KD-trees deteriorate to linear search complexity or worse if the dimensionality of the data is large [4]. Since computer vision problems often have very large collections and high dimensional data, approximation algorithms are of interest.

A popular approach for approximate nearest neighbor search is to represent each feature as a point (binary code/hash code) in Hamming space which enables fast retrieval and reduces storage space. As a case in point, one SIFT feature takes $128 \times 4 = 512$ bytes if it is stored as a 128 dimensional floating point vector, while it only occupies $128/8 = 16$ bytes if it is represented as a point in 128D Hamming space. Further, calculating the distance between two points in Hamming space is very quick since it only involves a bitwise XOR operation followed by a bit count.

Locality sensitive hashing (LSH) [5,6] pioneered the use of hashing for fast approximate nearest neighbor searching. In 1998, Indyk et al. introduced the concept of a locality sensitive function family. Each function in this family has

© Springer International Publishing Switzerland 2015
D. Cremers et al. (Eds.): ACCV 2014, Part I, LNCS 9003, pp. 162–177, 2015.
DOI: 10.1007/978-3-319-16865-4_11

the property that it can preserve the similarity between data points. Thus, by randomly choosing functions from this family, a binary code for each data point can be constructed. In order to preserve the similarity between data points when they are represented in Hamming space, however, a large number of bits are usually needed [7]. LSH has been generalized to Euclidean-LSH [8] for different similarity measures, and to shift kernel hashing [9] and Circulant Binary Embedding [10] by introducing different locality sensitive function families.

Machine learning techniques have also been used to design data dependent hashing algorithms. Borrowing ideas from manifold learning [11], Spectral Hashing [12] calculates the binary code by embedding the data points into Hamming space. The optimal embedding is determined by the following characteristics: neighbourhood relationships should be preserved, the code should be balanced (−1's and 1's should occur with roughly equal frequency), and bits should be pairwise independent. Spectral Hashing also leads to data dependent hashing algorithms. Various hashing algorithms have been proposed recently, including ones that use boosting based methods [13–16], exploit the spectral property [7,17,18], utilize the order of distance information [19,20], use supervised information [21–25], and so on.

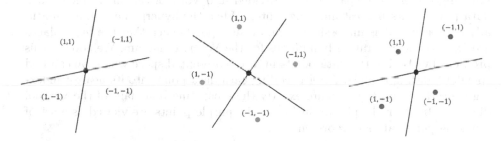

Fig. 1. Visualization of different encoding approaches. The left figure shows two hyperplanes in general position. The space is divided into four partitions. The binary code of a data point in this space can be determined by its relative positions to these hyperplanes. The middle figure shows that when the hyperplanes are mutually orthogonal, we can find a set of indexing centers (red points) whose binary codes have been predefined. The binary code of the points in this space can be determined by assigning the same code to its nearest indexing center. The right figure is a visualization of our proposed method. The purple points are the implicit indexing centers which are viewed in the re-represented space (Color figure online).

Since these algorithms use a binary encoding, the input space is divided into two pieces for each bit. Most of the hashing algorithms address this kind of partition problem by learning a set of hyperplanes which can be viewed either in the original space or in the Reproducing Kernel Hilbert space (RKHS). Each data point is encoded by its relative position to these hyperplanes, −1 for one side of the plane, 1 for the other. The left picture in Fig. 1 shows the space partitioned by two hyperplanes in 2D space. When the hyperplanes are mutually orthogonal, we can find a set of data points (indexing centers) such that the partition of the space (Voronoi diagram) according to this set coincides with the space partitioned by the hyperplanes. The hash code for the indexing centers can be predefined since these points are chosen from the vertices of a hyper-cube [26] or hyper-cuboid [27]. The middle picture in Fig. 1 shows such a set of indexing centers (red points). Thus the encoding process for each data point can also be viewed as assigning the same binary code to its nearest indexing center. Both ITQ [26] and Orthogonal K-means (OKmeans) [27] aim to learn the mutually orthogonal hyperplanes such that the total quantization error between the data point and its indexing center is minimized.

The focus of this paper is to design a compact binary code based on minimizing quantization error. We propose a novel hashing algorithm: Non-Orthogonal K-means (NOKMeans). The essential idea of this algorithm is that increasing the freedom of the separating hyperplanes can lead to a better binary code in the sense of the recall of retrieval performance. We achieve this by relaxing the orthogonality constraints in [26,27] to a near orthogonal assumption. One problem introduced by this relaxation is that the explicit indexing centers cannot be found in the original feature space any more. This is because for any given indexing centers, the space will be divided into Voronoi cells if we index each data point by its nearest indexing center. When the hyperplanes are not mutually orthogonal, it is impossible to find center points such that the hyperplanes are exactly the separating boundaries for the Voronoi diagram. We address this problem by viewing the data points in a re-represented space where we can find specific indexing centers. After encoding each data point into its nearest indexing center, the hyperplanes are exactly the separating boundary of the Voronoi diagram. In the right picture in Fig. 1, the purple points are viewed as a set of indexing points after re-representation.

2   Background

2.1   Notation

Here are the common notations we use throughout the paper. Suppose we want to build a binary code index for the data set $\{x_1, x_2, \cdots, x_N\}, x_i \in \mathcal{R}^D$. Denote $X \in \mathcal{R}^{N \times D}$ as the data matrix where each row is a data point. The binary code for this data set is denoted as $B \in \{-1, 1\}^{N \times d}$ where each row corresponds to a d bit binary code in Hamming space. sign(X) is a function returning a Hamming matrix of equal size to X, with -1 or 1 as entries depending on the sign of the input entries. Assuming the data set is already centered and the hyperplanes pass through the origin, each hyperplane can be fixed by its normal direction. Therefore, the d hyperplanes, which are used to determine the binary code, can be specified by a hyperplane matrix (projection matrix) $A \in \mathcal{R}^{D \times d}$ where each column corresponds to one normal direction. Another view of the space which is partitioned by the hyperplanes is that the space is divided into regions (partitions) where the data points in the same region have the same binary code. We use **1** to represent an all ones column vector and I is the identity matrix.

2.2 Related Work

When given a set of indexing centers, the encoding process shares some similarity with the K-mean clustering algorithm. Each data point is encoded into a binary code according to its nearest indexing center which behaves as a cluster center in the K-means algorithm. ITQ [26] aims to find an optimal binary code in the sense of minimal quantization error. Specifically, the data points are preprocessed by centering and then projecting to a low dimensional space by PCA, and then solving an optimization problem. The main idea of the optimization problem is to find a rotation $R \in \mathcal{R}^{d \times d}$ in order to minimize the quantization error between the rotated data points and their corresponding indexing centers. Suppose $V \in R^{N \times d}$ is the preprocessed data, and $B \in \{-1, 1\}^{N \times d}$ is the encoding binary matrix. The optimization problem of ITQ is:

$$\min \quad J(R, B) = ||B - VR||_F^2 \tag{1}$$
$$s.t. \qquad R'R = I$$
$$B \in \{-1, 1\}^{N \times d}$$

If we combine the PCA projection matrix P and the final orthogonal matrix R together, we can see that ITQ aims to find a set of mutually orthogonal hyperplanes, and its optimization model is to find minimum quantization error in the subspace obtained from PCA, and its index centers are from the vertices of a rotated d-dimensional hyper-cube in the PCA subspace. The left picture in Fig. 2 shows a visualization of ITQ. Two hyperplanes are used to partition the data points. The red points are the corresponding indexing centers. The data points in the space can be encoded by either its relative position to the hyperplanes or its nearest indexing center.

OKmeans [27] generalizes ITQ by embedding the vertices of a d dimensional hyper-cube in $\mathcal{R}^D$, then the vertices are rotated by $R \in \mathcal{R}^{d \times D}$, scaled by $S \in \mathcal{R}^{d \times d}$ (S is a diagonal matrix) in the corresponding directions and translated by $\mu \in \mathcal{R}^D$. Thus the indexing centers can be viewed as points chosen from the vertices of a rectangular hyper-cuboid. Finally, the optimization objective is modelled as minimizing the quantization error which is formulated as:

$$\min \quad J(R, \mu, B, S) = ||X - 1\mu - BSR||_F^2 \tag{2}$$
$$s.t. \qquad R'R = I$$
$$\mu \in \mathcal{R}^D$$
$$B \in \{-1, 1\}^{N \times d}$$
$$S \in \mathcal{R}^{d \times d}, \qquad S_{i,j} = 0 \text{ if } i \neq j \in \{1, 2, \cdots, d\}$$

If we view $\mu \in \mathcal{R}^D$ as the 'origin' of the data points, the columns of the rotation matrix behave as the normal directions of the corresponding hyperplanes, the regions of the data points which have the same index are separated by these hyperplanes. A visualization of OKmeans is shown in the right picture of Fig. 2. From the visualization of both ITQ and OKmeans, we can see that both of the partitions from ITQ and OKmeans are divided by mutually orthogonal hyperplanes, and the indexing centers of ITQ and OKmeans are chosen from a unit hyper-cube and a rectangular hyper-cuboid respectively.

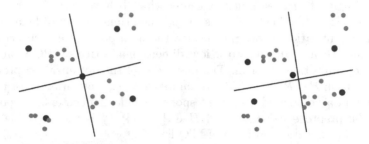

Fig. 2. Visualization of data points encoded by ITQ and OKmeans. The black point is the center of the data points. The red points are the indexing centers. The indexing centers are chosen from the vertices of a square (ITQ) and rectangle (OKMeans) respectively (Color figure online).

3   Proposed Algorithm

As discussed above, the main idea of ITQ and OKmeans is to find a set of mutually orthogonal hyperplanes. The hyperplanes are used to divide the data points into partitions, thus we can index each data point as a point in $\{-1,1\}^d$ according to its relative position to the hyperplanes. In this work, we investigate the situation when the orthogonality assumption used in ITQ and OKmeans is relaxed. Specifically, we adopt the 'near' mutually orthogonal property which is also used in [24]. One advantage of the relaxation is that it will increase the representation capability of the hyperplanes. The quality of the hash code is closely related to the position of the hyperplanes since the hyperplanes behave as the separating boundary of different index regions. Thus the flexibility of the position of the hyperplanes can lead to smaller overall quantization error. Furthermore, as discussed in [24], the 'near' mutually orthogonal condition is favored since the mutually orthogonal condition has some practical problems even though it is an approximation to the bit independent property. Therefore, to some degree, the near orthogonal constraint is a trade off between independence [12] and representation capability.

When the separating hyperplanes are orthogonal to each other, we can find appropriate indexing centers in the original space. For example, if we view the red points in Fig. 2 as indexing centers, and then index each data point according to its nearest indexing center, we will find that the region of different index partitions is exactly the same as the space partitioned by hyperplanes. When the hyperplanes are not orthogonal, it is impossible to find indexing centers in the original space; when given a set of data points as indexing centers, the resulting segmented space will have a general Voronoi diagram structure and the hyperplanes will not coincide with the boundary diagram when the corresponding hyperplanes are not orthogonal. The left picture of Fig. 3 shows the resulting Voronoi cells for the indexing centers (purple points) in the original space. We can see that it is impossible to find two hyperplanes to separate these cells.

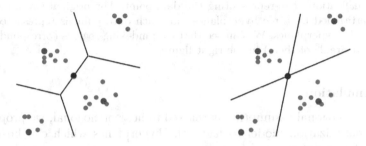

Fig. 3. Visualization of the Voronoi diagrams under different views. The purple points in the left picture are viewed as the indexing centers in the original space. The resulting Voronoi cells can never be separated by two hyperplanes since the indexing centers are in general position rather than from the vertices of a square or a rectangular. The right picture shows the resulting Voronoi cells when the purple points are viewed as the indexing centers in the re-represented space (Color figure online).

In this work, we view the indexing centers in a transformed space used to re-represent the data points. In this way, if we index each data point by its nearest center, the hyperplanes coincide with the boundaries of different index regions. The intuitive idea is as follows: suppose the hyperplanes are fixed, we can re-represent each data point by its relative distance to the hyperplanes. Figure 4 shows one way to re-represent the data points. There are three hyperplanes in the original space. After re-representation, the data point is represented as a point in 3D space. In the new representation space, the vertices $\{-1, 1\}^d$ can be viewed as the indexing centers. If we encode every data point as the binary code of its nearest indexing center, we can see that the hyperplanes are exactly the boundary of the different indexing regions. An example of partitioning with non-orthogonal hyperplanes is shown in Fig. 3, the purple points can be viewed as the indexing centers in the new representation space. One advantage of this view is that the hyperplanes can be viewed as the boundary of the different indexing regions. This re-representation trick allows us to formulate the problem by minimising the quantisation error between data points and indexing centers.

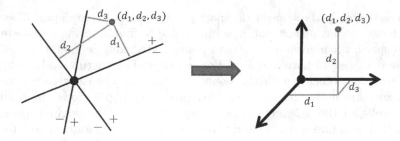

Fig. 4. Visualization of re-representing the data point. The original two dimensional space is partitioned by three hyperplanes, and each data point is represented by its distance to the hyperplanes. We can see that each indexing regions corresponds to one octant (there are 2^3 of them) in the right figure.

3.1 Formulation

When the orthogonal assumption is relaxed to near orthogonal, we propose the following optimization model to learn the hyperplanes which can be used to index the data points:

$$\min \quad J(A, B) = \frac{1}{2N}||XA - B||_F^2 + \frac{\lambda}{4}||A'A - I||_F^2 \tag{3}$$

$$s.t. \qquad A \in \mathcal{R}^{D \times d}$$

$$B \in \{-1, 1\}^{N \times d}$$

In above optimization model, the columns of A behave as the normal directions of the hyperplanes, and $B \in \{-1, 1\}^{N \times d}$ is the encoding matrix. When each column of A has a unit norm, the resulting re-represented data points are represented using the distance information of the data point to each hyperplane, i.e. each data point is represented by a vector where each element is corresponding to the signed distance between the data point and one specific hyperplane. When the columns do not satisfy the unit norm property, the new representation can be viewed as a scaling effect on the data points represented by distance information. The first part in the objective function is used to minimize the average quantization error, the second part is used as a regularizer in order to maintain the near orthogonal property, λ is the regularization parameter and the fraction is kept for convenience in further calculation. The constraint on hyperplanes has an effect on the final binary matrix indirectly since it guarantees the balance condition on B to some degree.

For solving the above optimization problem, we use alternating descent to find a locally optimal solution:

Fix. A it is easy to see that $B = \text{sign}(XA)$ is the optimal solution.
Fix. B we use first order gradient descent to update the projection matrix A:

$$\frac{\partial J(A, B)}{\partial A} = \frac{1}{N}X'(XA - B) + \lambda(AA' - I)A \tag{4}$$

Therefore, A can be updated by $A - \gamma \frac{\partial J(A,B)}{\partial A}$. For the step length γ, we use a simple line search strategy, i.e. start with $\gamma = 1$, if the updated A does not improve the cost function, update the step length γ with $s\gamma$. The process is continued until the total cost is reduced.

Algorithm 1. Non-Orthogonal K-means

Input: N training data points $x_1, x_2, \cdots, x_N$, I_{max} is the maximum iteration for the overall optimization problem and I_{step} is the maximum iteration for finding the step length.

Output: The hyperplane matrix A

1: Center the training data points, denote the centered data points as $X \subset \mathcal{R}^{D \times N}$, and initializing the hyperplane matrix A.

2: **for** $i = 1$ to I_{max} **do**

3:     Update B:
$$B \leftarrow \text{sign}(XA)$$

4:     Calculate the gradient direction by (4)

5:     Search the step length γ by backtracking line search with at most I_{step} iterations. If the maximum number of step length search iterations is reached, stop training stage.

6:     Update A by:
$$A \leftarrow A - \gamma \frac{\partial J(A,B)}{\partial A}$$

7: **end for**

In all of the following experiments, the initialization of A is obtained by the PCA projection times a random rotation matrix which is a common approach used in hashing algorithms, and the s is set to be 0.125. The backtracking line search process takes 10 to 20 iterations to find the appropriate step length. Thus, in order to make the computational complexity of the proposed algorithm measurable, we set the maximum iteration for the line search step as $I_{step} = 50$. When the maximum number of iterations is reached, we stop the training stage since the projection is almost unchanged if we continue to update A by a very small step length. Finally, the maximum iteration I_{max} for the alternative descent method is set to 50 which is the same value used in ITQ and OKmeans.

3.2 Computational Complexity

In each iteration, updating B takes $\Theta(NDd)$. For updating the projection matrix A, it takes two steps. The first step is to calculate the gradient which takes $\Theta(ND^2 + NDd)$. Here $\Theta(ND^2)$ is used for calculating $X'X$. For establishing the step length, in each iteration, we have to check the appropriateness of the current γ, this involves calculating the objective function which takes $\Theta(NDd)$. Suppose the maximum iteration for the overall optimization problem is I and the maximum iteration for finding the step length is I_{step}, thus the overall computational complexity is $\Theta(I_{max}(NDd + ND^2 + NDd + I_{step}(NDd))) = \Theta(I_{max}ND^2 + I_{max}I_{step}NDd)$. $\Theta(ND^2)$ is used for calculating the $X'X$ which can be precalculated, therefore the overall computational complexity of the training stage is $\Theta(ND^2 + I_{max}I_{step}NDd)$ which takes more computation than ITQ and OKmeans ($\Theta(I_{max}(Nd^2 + d^3))$ and $(\Theta(I_{max}(NDd + D^3)))$ respectively). During the training stage on our machine (implemented in MATLAB with single core), NOKMeans takes about 2.820 s per iteration when N, D and d are set to 10^5, 128 and 64 respectively, while for the same setting, the ITQ and OKmeans take 0.259 and 0.419 respectively. Since the line search step requires the most computation in the current implementation, the training stage can be sped up by choosing an appropriate initial step length γ and backtracking parameter s or a faster line search algorithm.

Finally, for encoding data and query points, it takes the same computational complexity as most hashing based algorithms, i.e. each data point takes $\Theta(Dd)$ time to compute the binary code. For retrieving the K nearest neighbor points in Hamming distance, we use exhaustive search in all of our experiments since the distance calculation is efficient in Hamming space and it is easy to find the nearest neighbor points due to the distance property which only take values from $\{0, 1, 2, \cdots, d\}$. To speed up this process, one can build a hash table or use fast nearest neighbor searching designed for Hamming space [28].

3.3   Discussion

The proposed method shares some similarity with ITQ. For ITQ, the final projection matrix is the PCA projection matrix P multiplied by the learned rotation matrix R, and, for the proposed algorithm, the projection matrix is learned during the optimization process directly. When the parameter λ is infinite, the projection matrix A in NOKMeans shares the orthogonal property, i.e. $A'A = I$. Nevertheless there are still some differences between these two algorithms even as λ tends to infinity. For example, the quantization error in ITQ is calculated in the PCA subspace, while the quantization error in the proposed method is calculated in the space determined by A which is learned during the optimization process.

Compared to OKmeans, the proposed algorithm also utilizes a rectangular hyper-cuboid to some degree. When the parameter λ is positive, the learned projection matrix can be decomposed into $A = QS$ where each column in $Q \in \mathcal{R}^{D \times d}$ has a unit norm, and S is a diagonal matrix which has a scaling effect in each direction. Notice that the overall quantization error $||XA - B||_F^2 = |S|^2||XQ - BS^{-1}||_F^2$, thus our proposed method can be viewed as re-representing each data point by its distance information to each hyperplane, and then encoding the data point according to the indexing centers from the vertices of a hyper-cuboid. This hyper-cuboid is obtained by scaling the unit hyper-cube by S^{-1} in the corresponding directions. On the other hand, the S in the optimization objective in OKmeans is viewed as an independent variable. One advantage of modeling the scale effect is that the resulting indexing centers will fit better to the data points in the sense of the quantization error, but it also introduces a distortion problem. For example, the Hamming distance between neighboring vertices is always 1, but their Euclidean distance is not fixed due to the scale effect of the hyper-cuboid in different directions. With the regularization parameter λ in our method, the scale value will be constrained to around 1, and therefore the scale distortion is minimal.

4 Experiments

We evaluate the proposed hashing algorithm on four real data sets: SIFT1M [29], SIFT10M, SIFT1B [30], GIST1M [29], and compare the performance of related algorithms: LSH [5], Spectral Hashing [12], ITQ [26], OKmeans [27], on these data sets. SIFT1M, SIFT1B, and GIST1M are three benchmark data sets which are used for testing the performance of different nearest neighbor searching algorithms. In SIFT1M and SIFT1B, each data point is a 128D SIFT feature [31] extracted from Flickr images and INRIA Holidays images [32]. In GIST1M, each data point is a 960D GIST feature which is extracted from the tiny image set of [33], Holidays image set and Flickr1M [34].

SIFT10M is our own dataset. Each data point in this set is a SIFT feature which is extracted from Caltech-256 [35] by the open source VLFeat library [36]. Caltech-256 is a benchmark image data set in computer vision, that features a large number of classes (256) and high intra-class variations in each category. For SIFT10M, the base data points, training data points, and the query points are randomly chosen from all SIFT features extracted from the image set. The true nearest neighbor points are provided by exhaustive nearest neighbor search in 128D Euclidean space. For the other three benchmark data sets, we use the publicly available base points, training points, and query points, and true nearest neighbor information for the query points directly. Detailed information about these data sets including the number of training points, query points and base data points used in our experiments are summarized in Table 1.

Table 1. Datasets which are used for evaluating different approximate nearest search algorithms

Data set	Data type	Dimension	Base points	Training points	Query points
SIFT1M	SIFT feature	128	1,000,000	100,000	10,000
SIFT10M	SIFT feature	128	10,000,000	1,000,000	10,000
SIFT1B	SIFT feature	128	1,000,000,000	1,000,000	10,000
GIST1M	GIST feature	960	1,000,0000	500,000	1,000

4.1 Performance Measurements

We adopt recall as an indicator of retrieval performance since this is an important indicator of retrieval performance and it also has internal relationships with other common measurements. For instance, higher recall often corresponds to higher precision. For each query data point, we retrieve its nearest N data points in the sense of the Hamming distance. Recall@N is the percentage of true nearest neighbor points in the retrieved data set, i.e.:

$$\text{Recall@}N = \frac{\#\text{retrieved true nearest neighbor points}}{\#\text{true nearest neighbor points}}$$

We have varied N from 1 to $N_{max} = 10,000$ to give a better overall picture of performance. In order to evaluate the overall retrieval performance of the hashing algorithm, we introduce the m-Recall (mean recall) measure. m-Recall is calculated as:

$$\text{m-Recall}(\lambda) = \frac{\sum_{i=1}^{N_{max}} Recall_\lambda(i)}{N_{max}}$$

here N_{max} is the maximum retrieved nearest points in Hamming space and $Recall_\lambda(i)$ is the average recall of retrieving i nearest neighbor points for the regularization parameter λ.

m-Recall shares some similarity with mean average precision which is often used to measure the overall performance of retrieval algorithms. The main difference between these two measurements is that N_{max} is set to the total number of data points in mean average precision, while here, N_{max} is relatively small compared to the whole data base. For evaluating the performance of hashing algorithms, the data sets often contain millions or billions of points and retrieving part of the data set is of interest in practice. m-Recall is introduced to evaluate the overall performance when only part of the data set is retrieved.

4.2   Parameter Selection

When using this model to learn the hyperplanes, we have to decide the value of the parameter λ. In order to test the sensitivity of the parameter λ in the optimization, we choose λ from $\{10^1, 10^2, 10^3, 10^4, 10^5, 10^6, 10^7\}$. The m-Recall for different λ is shown in the right image in Fig. 5. From Fig. 5, we can see that, at beginning, the m-Recall increases as λ increases. After reaching the peak, the m-Recall dips moderately as λ keeps increasing. This motivates us to have a strategy to learn the index for different data sets. For each data set, λ is fixed by choosing from $\{10^1, 10^2, 10^3, 10^4, 10^5, 10^6, 10^7\}$ for one specific task, and choosing the parameter such that it reaches peak performance, then use this parameter for the whole data set. In the following experiments, the parameter is fixed as $10^4, 10^5, 10^6, 10^5$ for SIFT1M, SIFT10M, SIFT1B and GIST1M respectively. However it is worth noting that performance is similar for values of λ in the range 10^4–10^6 on all four data sets.

4.3   Results

We have evaluated the proposed algorithm, ITQ, OKmeans, Spectral Hashing and LSH on the four data sets. Figure 6 shows the recall curves of different algorithms for searching nearest neighbor points. For each SIFT feature data set,

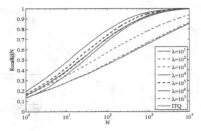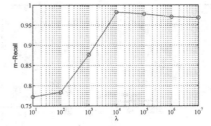

Fig. 5. Retrieval performance on SIFT1M data set with different λ. Each data point is encoded into 128 bits, and the task is to retrieve the nearest neighbor point for each query. The performance of ITQ (red line) is also reported as a baseline (Color figure online).

we report the recall performance when the data points are encoded by 64, 96 and 128 bits respectively. The experimental results enable us to view the performance of different algorithms from two dimensions, i.e. increase the number of bits to encode the SIFT feature and the scale of the data sets. From these two dimensions, we can see that, generally speaking, the more bits used to encode the feature points, the higher the recall. On the other hand, the nearest neighbor point searching problem becomes more difficult for bigger data sets. When each data point is indexed to a 64 bit binary code, the proposed algorithm has a comparable recall performance to the state of art result (OKmeans), and has a much better recall performance than the remaining algorithms. When we use more bits to encode the data set, we find that the proposed algorithm has the highest performance among these algorithms. For the GIST1M data set (Fig. 7), which has the highest number of dimensions among our test scenarios, a similar pattern is observed. From the plot, we can see that the performance gain of our proposed algorithm is larger when the number of encoding bits is increased.

The performance of the proposed algorithm coincides with our model assumption. This is because when few bits are used, the independence property, which leads to the mutually orthogonal condition, plays the main role when designing the hash code. When more bits are used to index the feature points, the mutual orthogonality condition leads to the loss of representation capability. Take the following toy example. Suppose the data points are distributed in a 2D subspace in 3 dimensional space, and we use three bits to encode the data points. If the three hyperplanes are mutually orthogonal, the data points are effectively encoded with two bits since the 2D subspace is partitioned into 4 different index regions. When the orthogonality condition is relaxed, the 2D space can be partitioned into 6 different indexing regions. So when the mutual orthogonality condition is relaxed, the separating capability of the hyperplanes will increase.

As discussed in [18,37], retrieving different numbers of nearest neighbor points affects the performance of searching algorithms. Figure 8 shows the performance of retrieving different K neighbors. Here the K ranges from $\{1, 5, 10, 20, 50, 100\}$, and each data point is encoded as a 256 bit binary code. The top left figure presents the performances of different algorithms for retrieving 1 nearest

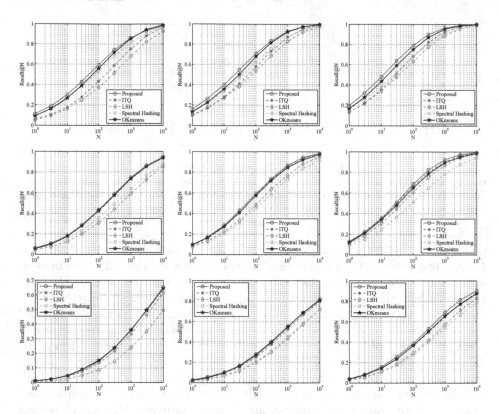

Fig. 6. Retrieval performance on SIFT feature data sets. Different data sets are reported in different rows (SIFT1M, SIFT10M, SIFT1B respectively). For each SIFT feature data set, we show the *Recall@N* when each data point is encoded with 64, 96, 128 bits for columns 1, 2 and 3 respectively.

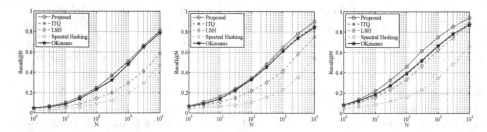

Fig. 7. Retrieval performance on GIST1M data set. The left figure shows the retrieval performance of different algorithms when each data points are encoded into 64 bit binary code. The following two figures show the retrieval performance when using 128 or 256 bits to encode.

neighbor point. The top middle shows the performances of retrieving 5 nearest neighbor points, followed by retrieving 10, 20, 50, and 100 nearest neighbor points. As the trend shows, we can see that the overall recall value keeps going

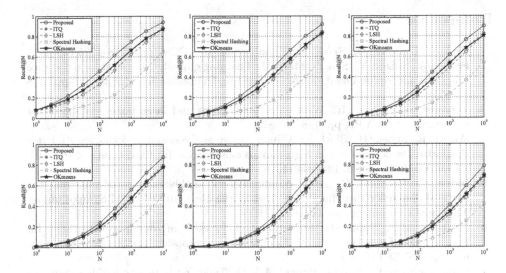

Fig. 8. Retrieval results on GIST1M data set for retrieving different K nearest neighbor points. Here, the K ranges from $\{1, 5, 10, 20, 50, 100\}$, and each GIST feature is encoded by 256 bits.

down. This means that retrieving the K-th nearest neighbor point is more difficult as K increases. Another phenomenon we can see from the plot is that, in order to retrieve more true nearest neighbor points, it is better to retrieve a relatively large number of points in the Hamming distance. For example, if we retrieve 1000 nearest neighbor points in Hamming space, the recall of finding 100 nearest neighbor points is much lower than the recall of searching 1 nearest neighbor point, while for retrieving 10,000 points in Hamming space, the recall gap between different nearest neighbor points is relatively small.

5   Conclusion

In this paper, we have investigated a minimum quantization error based hashing algorithm. Specifically, our focus is on the quantization error of the re-represented data points. In this way, the Voronoi diagram in the original space is the same as the space which is separated by hyperplanes. Compared to the previous quantization based algorithms, the hyperplanes learned in our algorithm are without the constraint that they are mutually orthogonal. We believe this relaxation leads to a better binary code index for large scale high dimensional data. We have tested the proposed algorithm on three benchmark data sets as well as a new SIFT data set. The experimental results shows that our method performs better than current state of the art methods especially when encoding high dimensional data points.

References

1. Brown, M., Lowe, D.: Recognising panoramas. In: ICCV, pp. 1218–1225 (2003)
2. Frome, A., Singer, Y., Sha, F., Malik, J.: Learning globally-consistent local distance functions for shape-based image retrieval and classification. In: ICCV, pp. 1–8 (2007)
3. Torralba, A., Fergus, R., Weiss, Y.: Small codes and large image databases for recognition. In: CVPR pp. 1–8 (2008)
4. Weber, R., Schek, H., Blott, S.: A quantitative analysis and performance study for similarity-search methods in high-dimensional spaces. In: Proceedings of the 24th VLDB Conference, pp. 194–205 (1998)
5. Indyk, P., Motwani, R.: Approximate nearest neighbors: towards removing the curse of dimensionality. In: Proceedings of the 30th Annual ACM Symposium on Theory of Computing, pp. 604–613 (1998)
6. Charikar, M.S.: Similarity estimation techniques from rounding algorithms. In: Proceedings of the Thiry-Fourth Annual ACM Symposium on Theory of Computing, pp. 380–388 (2002)
7. Shen, F., Shen, C., Shi, Q., Hengel, A.V.D., Tang, Z.: Inductive hashing on manifolds. In: CVPR, pp. 1562–1569 (2013)
8. Datar, M., Immorlica, N., Indyk, P., Mirrokni, V.S.: Locality-sensitive hashing scheme based on p-stable distributions. In: Symposium on Computational Geometry, pp. 252–262 (2004)
9. Raginsky, M., Lazebnik, S.: Locality-sensitive binary codes from shift-invariant kernels. In: NIPS (2009)
10. Yu, F.X., Sanjiv, K., Gong, Y., Chang, S.F.: Circulant binary embedding. In: ICML (2014)
11. Belkin, M., Niyogi, P.: Laplacian eigenmaps and spectral techniques for embedding and clustering. In: NIPS (2001)
12. Weiss, Y., Antonio, T., Robert, F.: Spectral hashing. In: NIPS, pp. 1753–1760 (2008)
13. Jin, Z.M., Hu, Y., Lin, Y., Zhang, D.B., Lin, S.D., Cai, D., Li, X.: Complementary projection hashing. In: ICCV, pp. 257–264 (2013)
14. Kim, S., Kang, Y., Choi, S.: Sequential spectral learning to hash with multiple representations. In: Fitzgibbon, A., Lazebnik, S., Perona, P., Sato, Y., Schmid, C. (eds.) ECCV 2012, Part V. LNCS, vol. 7576, pp. 538–551. Springer, Heidelberg (2012)
15. Xu, H., Wang, J., Li, Z., Zeng, G., Li, S., Yu, N.: Complementary hashing for approximate nearest neighbor search. In: ICCV, pp. 1631–1638 (2011)
16. Wang, J., Kumar, S., Chang, S.F.: Sequential projection learning for hashing with compact codes. In: ICML, pp. 1127–1134 (2010)
17. Liu, W., Wang, J., Kumar, S., Chang, S.F.: Hashing with graphs. In: ICML, pp. 1–8 (2011)
18. Weiss, Y., Fergus, R., Torralba, A.: Multidimensional spectral hashing. In: Fitzgibbon, A., Lazebnik, S., Perona, P., Sato, Y., Schmid, C. (eds.) ECCV 2012, Part V. LNCS, vol. 7576, pp. 340–353. Springer, Heidelberg (2012)
19. Wang, J., Liu, W., Sun, A., Jiang, Y.: Learning hash codes with listwise supervision. In: ICCV, pp. 3032–3039 (2013)
20. Wang, J., Wang, J., Yu, N., Li, S.: Order preserving hashing for approximate nearest neighbor search. In: Proceedings of the 21st ACM International Conference on Multimedia, pp. 133–142 (2013)

21. Norouzi, M., Fleet, D., Salakhutdinov, R.: Hamming distance metric learning. In: NIPS, pp. 1070–1078 (2012)
22. Norouzi, M., Fleet, D.: Minimal loss hashing for compact binary codes. In: ICML, pp. 353–360 (2011)
23. Kulis, B., Darrell, T.: Learning to hash with binary reconstructive embeddings. In: NIPS, pp. 1042–1050 (2009)
24. Wang, J., Kumar, S., Chang, S.F.: Semi-supervised hashing for scalable image retrieval. In: CVPR, pp. 3424–3431 (2010)
25. Liu, W., Wang, J., Ji, R., Jiang, Y., Chang, S.F.: Supervised hashing with kernels. In: CVPR, pp. 2074–2081 (2012)
26. Gong, Y., Lazebnik, S.: Iterative quantization: a procrustean approach to learning binary codes. In: CVPR, pp. 817–824 (2011)
27. Norouzi, M., Fleet, D.: Cartesian k-means. In: CVPR, pp. 3017–3024 (2013)
28. Norouzi, M., Punjani, A., Fleet, D.: Fast search in hamming space with multi-index hashing. In: CVPR, pp. 3108–3115 (2012)
29. Jegou, H., Douze, M., Schmid, C.: Product quantization for nearest neighbor search. IEEE Trans. Pattern Anal. Mach. Intell. **33**, 117–128 (2011)
30. Jegou, H., Tavenard, R., Douze, M., Amsaleg, L.: Searching in one billion vectors: re-rank with source coding. In: ICASSP, pp. 861–864 (2011)
31. Lowe, D.G.: Distinctive image features from scale-invariant keypoints. Int. J. Comput. Vision **60**, 91–110 (2004)
32. Jegou, H., Douze, M., Schmid, C.: Improving bag-of-features for large scale image search. Int. J. Comput. Vision **14**, 316–336 (2010)
33. Torralba, A., Fergus, R., Freeman, W.T.: 80 million tiny images: a large database for non-parametric object and scene recognition. IEEE Trans. Pattern Anal. Mach. Intell. **30**, 1958–1970 (2008)
34. Jegou, H., Douze, M., Schmid, C.: Hamming embedding and weak geometric consistency for large scale image search. In: Forsyth, D., Torr, P., Zisserman, A. (eds.) ECCV 2008, Part I. LNCS, vol. 5302, pp. 304–317. Springer, Heidelberg (2008)
35. Griffin, G., Holub, A., Perona, P.: Caltech-256 object category dataset. Technical report, pp. 1–20 (2007)
36. Vedaldi, A., Fulkerson, B.: VLFeat: an open and portable library of computer vision algorithms. In: Proceedings of the International Conference on Multimedia, pp. 1469–1472 (2008)
37. He, K., Wen, F., Sun, J.: K-means hashing: an affinity-preserving quantization method for learning binary compact codes. In: CVPR, pp. 2938–2945 (2013)

Visual Vocabulary with a Semantic Twist

Relja Arandjelović[✉] and Andrew Zisserman

Department of Engineering Science, University of Oxford, Oxford, UK
relja@robots.ox.ac.uk

Abstract. Successful large scale object instance retrieval systems are typically based on accurate matching of local descriptors, such as SIFT. However, these local descriptors are often not sufficiently distinctive to prevent false correspondences, as they only consider the gradient appearance of the local patch, without being able to "see the big picture".

We describe a method, SemanticSIFT, which takes account of local image semantic content (such as grass and sky) in matching, and thereby eliminates many false matches. We show that this enhanced descriptor can be employed in standard large scale inverted file systems with the following benefits: improved precision (as false retrievals are suppressed); an almost two-fold speedup in retrieval speed (as posting lists are shorter on average); and, depending on the target application, a 20 % decrease in memory requirements (since unrequired 'semantic' words can be removed). Furthermore, we also introduce a fast, and near state of the art, semantic segmentation algorithm.

Quantitative and qualitative results on standard benchmark datasets (Oxford Buildings 5 k and 105 k) demonstrate the effectiveness of our approach.

1 Introduction

Large scale specific object retrieval is a well studied topic due to its usefulness in a range of applications, amongst others: geolocalization [1–4], personal photo search and automatic tagging [5,6], product and logo recognition [7–10], video search [11] and 3-D reconstruction [12].

All successful systems rely on matching local image patches using their appearance, usually via matching of local descriptors such as SIFT [13]. The bag-of-visual-words (BoW) framework [11] accomplishes this by quantizing descriptors into visual words and performing efficient retrieval for large scale datasets by using an inverted index. Many improvements to this seminal work have been made by increasing the quality of descriptor matches. These include: higher precision by using large visual vocabularies [7,14]; storing compact versions of descriptors inside the inverted index [15–17]; spatial reranking and query expansion [18–22]; and learning better descriptors (than SIFT) [23,24].

However, all these methods are built around the core system based on matching local patches/descriptors. In this paper we aim at improving the core system

---

Electronic supplementary material The online version of this chapter (doi:10.1007/978-3-319-16865-4_12) contains supplementary material, which is available to authorized users.

© Springer International Publishing Switzerland 2015
D. Cremers et al. (Eds.): ACCV 2014, Part I, LNCS 9003, pp. 178–195, 2015.
DOI: 10.1007/978-3-319-16865-4_12

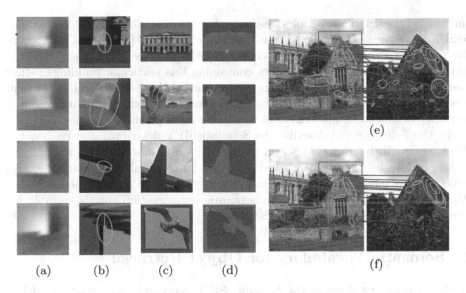

(a)   (b)   (c)   (d)   (f)

Fig. 1. Patch matching with semantic reasoning. (a) Four normalized image patches extracted from the images in (c); (b) zoom-in around the patches (with standard size and rotation normalization). The four patches are very similar, their descriptors match and it is therefore impossible to filter these false matches using the patches alone. (d) Automatic segmentation of the image into {sky,grass/trees,other} shown as blue, green and red, respectively. The local patches' semantic content provides sufficient information to discard most of these false matches. The four patches (from top to bottom) contain {grass,other}, {sky,other}, {other}, {sky,other}, and consequently only the {sky,other} patches can match in this case. (e, f) Matched patches without and with semantic reasoning, respectively. The number of matches falls from 25 to 12 due to correctly removing correspondences which were falsely established based on patches alone. Note that no spatial consistency check is performed.

and going beyond blind matching of local patches by also taking account of the semantic content of the query and database images. This addresses one of the principal problems of local descriptor matching: that often the patches are not sufficiently discriminative to avoid false matches – see Fig. 1. The key idea in this work is to use semantic information to filter out such false matches. We term the augmented SIFT descriptor, 'SemanticSIFT'.

The proposed approach can be seen as belonging to an emerging theme in recent computer vision papers of using semantic information to aid classical computer vision tasks, e.g. in stereo correspondence [25], 3D reconstruction [26] and Semantic SLAM [27,28]. For example, Haene et al. [26] show that 3D reconstruction can be improved by simultaneously reasoning about the classes of objects present in the image, since the objects provide geometric cues about surface normals.

Despite the obvious benefits of using semantic information in various areas of computer vision, semantic segmentation has not yet been applied to large scale object retrieval. Rather, erroneous SIFT matches have been removed using the context of other descriptors and spatial matching [1,3,29–31]. These methods, and the others listed above, are complementary to SemanticSIFT. Note, SemanticSIFT should be distinguished from "semantic retrieval" [32–34] in CBIR where the goal is to retrieve visual concepts. Here our focus is on *specific* object retrieval, so queries are "find images containing this particular building" rather than "find images of cars in urban environments". However, as will be seen, in specific object search knowing that a set of pixels represents a building or not is certainly beneficial as false matches to non-building pixels can be discarded.

In the following, we describe the SemanticSIFT descriptor and its benefits (Sect. 2). It will be seen that it can reduce the size of posting lists, which leads to a speed up in retrieval times, with no loss in retrieval performance. It also removes many erroneous retrievals, and thereby improves retrieval performance. We also describe a method for fast semantic segmentation that is suitable for large scale and real time systems (Sect. 3).

2   Semantic Vocabulary for Object Retrieval

In this section we develop the SemanticSIFT representation, starting with a semantic vocabulary based on a semantic segmentation of the image into multiple classes. We then describe how this semantic vocabulary is used to match local patches, and its combination with a standard BoW visual vocabulary, to form the hybrid SemanticSIFT vocabulary.

2.1   Semantic Vocabulary

Suppose we have a semantic segmentation method that provides a pixel-wise labelling into C semantic classes. High accuracy segmentations are desired and therefore for this work we only focus on the following relatively "easy" classes: sky, flora (i.e. grass, trees and bushes), and "other" (containing everything else, including building, road, human, car, table, sea, etc.); therefore $C = 3$. However, the choice of classes is free and the retrieval method is capable of handling any choice given that the semantic segmentation quality is high.

A local image patch is assigned a "semantic word" based on the semantic class/classes it contains: if the patch contains at least one pixel of a particular semantic class c, then it is deemed to contain class c. There are $K_s = 2^C - 1$ possible semantic words representing all possible combinations of a class appearing or not appearing in the patch (note the "-1" is because a patch has to contain at least one semantic class). For our choice of semantic classes ({sky,flora,other}, $C = 3$), there are $K_s = 7$ semantic words formed from all possible non-empty sub-sets: {sky}, {flora}, {other}, {sky,flora}, {sky,other}, {flora,other} and {sky,flora,other}.

2.2   Matching Patches: SemanticSIFT

As with the standard bag-of-visual-words retrieval methods, two local patches are deemed to match each other if they are assigned to the same word. For visual words this typically means that the relevant local descriptors have been assigned to the same cluster obtained by (approximate) k-means. For the semantic word case, words are naturally defined as the combination of classes appearing in the local patch, and no clustering is required. Figure 1 demonstrates the effectiveness of this approach, where several local patches are assigned to the same visual word as they have almost identical appearance and therefore very similar SIFT descriptors (in fact their Hamming signatures also match – see Sect. 4.1). However, looking at the corresponding images it is clear that the matches are invalid due to the difference in their semantic content. Most of the false matches obtained by using visual words can be eliminated by requiring that the semantic words have to match as well. The procedure therefore increases precision, as will be demonstrated in Sect. 4.2.

2.3   Product Vocabulary and Speedup

In order to deem two patches to be matching, both their visual words and semantic words have to be the same. This behaviour is identical to defining a hybrid, SemanticSIFT, vocabulary and demanding that the hybrid words match. The SemanticSIFT vocabulary is effectively a product vocabulary of the visual and the semantic one – its size is $K = K_v \times K_s$, where K_v and K_s are the sizes of the visual and semantic vocabularies, respectively. In other words, the Semantic-SIFT vocabulary has all combinations of visual and semantic words. If the visual words are v_1, v_2, .., v_{K_v} and semantic words are s_1, s_2, ..., s_{K_s}, then Semantic-SIFT words are (v_1, s_1), (v_1, s_2), ..., (v_1, s_{K_s}), (v_2, s_1), (v_2, s_2), ..., (v_2, s_{K_s}), ..., (v_{K_v}, s_{K_s}).

Standard large scale retrieval systems based around the bag-of-words concept use very large visual vocabularies, ranging between 100 k to 16 M words, making the bag-of-word image representation very sparse. Fast ranking is performed using an inverted index which exploits the BoW sparsity, where images containing a particular visual word are arranged in a posting list. Larger vocabularies cause BoWs to be sparser, which makes average posting list length smaller, and therefore improves the retrieval speed as a smaller number of entries in the inverted index are visited during the scoring. Since the SemanticSIFT vocabulary size is $K_v \times K_s$, i.e. K_s times larger than the baseline vocabulary (where our $K_s = 7$), the average posting list length decreases K_s times making retrieval significantly faster. However, ranking is not actually K_s faster as some semantic words are much rarer than others (e.g. patches which contain all three semantic classes are rarer than patches which contain only "other"). Nevertheless, we experimentally obtain an almost two-fold speedup (see Sect. 4.2).

2.4   Reduction in Memory Requirements

As discussed earlier, SemanticSIFT increases precision by removing some false matches, while simultaneously improving retrieval speed by visiting shorter posting lists. Both of these improvements come at no storage cost at all as the number of entries in the inverted index doesn't change (the average posting list length decreases as the vocabulary size increases, but the total number of entries remains the same). It is possible to reduce storage requirements, and therefore reduce the RAM consumption of the retrieval system if it is known *a priori* that a particular class of objects is not interesting to the user. For example, it is reasonable to assume that pure sky features are of no use in most retrieval applications as it is unlikely that a user will search for a particular detail in the sky or a particular cloud. It is also likely that features which only contain flora are also not useful or even detrimental as they are often not distinctive enough. Note that we are not proposing to remove all features that contain flora, just the ones that contain only flora or only {flora,sky}, because {flora,other} can indeed be distinctive. For example, a feature from an interface between a building and grass is potentially useful. Note that, apart from reducing storage requirements, removal of features also decreases computational cost as there is a further reduction in the number of visited items in the inverted index.

2.5   Accounting for Segmentation Uncertainty

In an ideal case when perfect semantic segmentation of all images is available, SemanticSIFT is guaranteed to improve precision. However, in a real-world scenario the "hard" nature of the matching procedure, i.e. requiring that semantic words have to be identical, could potentially hurt recall. This is particularly evident near the borders between two different semantic classes, where uncertainty in the exact position of the border can lead to noisy semantic word assignments, resulting in false rejection of matching patches.

Here we describe a simple extension to SemanticSIFT, called SoftSemanticSIFT, which can take these uncertainties into account. It only assumes that the underlying semantic segmentation method can output an extra special label, *unknown*, without placing any constraints on the way this information is obtained. For example, one could use the method in Sect. 3 which compares costs across classes, or have an *ad hoc* post-processing step which simply marks pixels close to estimated semantic discontinuities as "unknown".

SemanticSIFT matching, as before, enforces that the underlying patch semantic content has to be identical, but the special "unknown" label is allowed to match any other label(s). For example, {sky,other} are allowed to match {unknown} because the "unknown" pixels could potentially contain "sky" and "other". Note that a patch which contains "unknown" cannot simply match any other patch, as for example {flora,unknown} cannot match {other} as "unknown" can match "other" but the latter patch does not contain "flora".

Impact on Speed and Memory Requirements. The SoftSemanticSIFT is slower than SemanticSIFT because of its smaller rejection rate of visual word matched features, but is also faster than the BoW matching as many patches will remain rejected. The number of semantic words increases to $K_s = 1 + 2 \times 7 = 15$, because an extra {unknown} word is added, and all of the original 7 semantic words can appear in two variants (with or without "unknown"). However, unlike SemanticSIFT, multiple posting lists are visited for a single query feature; for example, for a query {flora} posting lists for {flora}, {flora, unknown} and {unknown} need to be visited (obviously, the search is restricted to the same visual word, as before). Likewise, storage savings with respect to the baseline visual retrieval system are smaller than SemanticSIFT, but still exist.

2.6   Challenges

Some images are very challenging for automatic semantic segmentation, even for the seemingly simple task of finding sky, flora and other. Therefore, it is expected that failures occur. However, not all miss-classifications are catastrophic for the task considered in this paper. As illustrated in Fig. 2, provided that mistakes are consistent matches will not be lost.

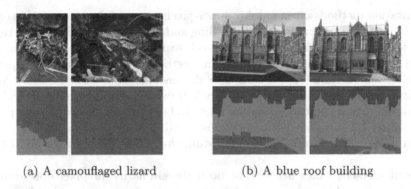

(a) A camouflaged lizard   (b) A blue roof building

Fig. 2. Hard cases for semantic segmentation. Two pairs of challenging images are shown in the top row, and the corresponding semantic segmentation is shown in the bottom row. The left pair shows a green lizard which due to camouflage looks like grass, the right pair shows an Oxford college with a sky-colour roof. Even though semantic segmentation fails in these two challenging cases, the retrieval system is not hampered because the miss-segmentation is systematic and repeatable, e.g. the green lizard is always classified as grass and therefore correctly matched features will not be removed.

3   Fast Semantic Segmentation

For the proposed SemanticSIFT method we have two principal requirements for the semantic segmentation: first, *speed*, as we envisage large scale deployment (millions to billions of images) and real time processing of uploaded query images; and second, *accuracy*, as incorrect segmentations may reduce recall. Of course, these two requirements often conflict: currently the methods of [35–37] produce state of the art semantic segmentations (e.g. on the Stanford background dataset [38]) but take several minutes per image; conversely, existing fast approaches either produce results of insufficient quality, such as Semantic Texton Forest [39] (see supplementary material for examples), or make assumptions which are often violated in real world images, such as the "Tiered Scene" assumption [40] where sky is, if present in the image, forced to be above any other label (this assumption is often invalid in real images, see bottom row of Fig. 1 or supplementary material).

For this reason we introduce our own semantic segmentation method, dubbed Fast Semantic Segmentation via Soft Segments (FSSS), which is described next. It proceeds in two stages: first, a number of soft segments are defined across the image centred on a regular grid; second, these soft segments are used to provide context when labelling pixels with their semantic class. Note, however, that any available fast and accurate semantic segmentation method could be employed for SemanticSIFT.

3.1 Soft Segments

Segmentation methods often employ super-pixels or multiple-segmentations [35, 36, 41] to provide context for pixel labelling and/or to reduce complexity. Here, rather than making a hard decision on such segments, we obtain soft-segments (or soft super-pixels) using the embedding method of [42] together with spatial proximity. The method [42] provides an 8 dimensional embedding for every pixel in an image, such that a small L2 distance between a pair of pixels in this feature space signifies that the two pixels are likely to be a part of the same superpixel. The squared L2 distance between pixels i and j is denoted as $D_s(i,j)$. The method is very fast, producing an embedding for a 500×500 image in 1.7 s on a CPU.

A soft-segment takes account of both the similarity in pixel appearances (from $D_s(i,j)$) and also their spatial distance (e.g. a blue car shouldn't be in the same soft-segment as blue sky because they are not close in the image space). Suppose a soft-segment is centred on pixel i (pixel i is the seed), then we define the association of pixel j to this soft-segment by the weight

$$w_{i,j} = \exp(-\alpha D_s(i,j) - \beta D_p(i,j)) \tag{1}$$

where $D_p(i,j)$ is the squared L2 distance between normalized pixel locations, and α and β are parameters (to be learnt). Figure 3b shows several examples of soft-segments. A set of soft-segments is obtained for an image by seeding segments on a regular grid (i.e. the i pixels above are chosen on a regular grid).

3.2 Labelling

A labelling of the pixels of the image (into the semantic classes) *and* of the set of soft-segments (into the same semantic classes) is obtained by minimizing an energy function. As usual, there are two terms, but in this case the unary is over soft-segments and is low when the label is consistent with the appearance; and the second term is between soft-segments and pixels, and is low when the labelling of the soft-segment is consistent with the labelling of pixels (softly) associated with it. More formally, the energy $E(l, L)$ of a labelling l is defined as follows.

$$E\left(l,L\right) = \sum_i \left(\lambda\phi_i\left(L_i\right) - \sum_j w_{i,j}\delta\left(L_i = l_j\right) \right) \qquad (2)$$

where l_j is the label of pixel j, L_i is a latent variable signifying the label of the soft superpixel defined at the grid point i, $\phi_i(L_i)$ is the penalty for superpixel i having the label L_i (i.e. the "unary potential"), $w_{i,j}$ is the reward obtained when soft-segment i and pixel j have the same label, $\delta(L_i = l_j)$ is an indicator function which yields 1 if L_i equals l_j and 0 otherwise, and λ is the relative weighting of the unary and pairwise terms. The graphical model corresponding to this energy is shown in Fig. 3a. The unary term is described in more detail below.

Efficient Inference. From Eq. (2) and the corresponding graphical model in Fig. 3a, it is clear that, by design, the pixel labels l are conditionally independent from each other given the soft segment labels L, and vice versa. The energy function is optimized by initializing the segment labels L according to the unary potentials, followed by iterating between fixing L and optimizing for pixel labels l, and fixing l and optimizing for L. The procedure can be interpreted as message passing, where the first set of messages are sent top-down from soft superpixels to the underlying pixels, and the second set of messages are sent bottom-up from pixels to soft superpixels.

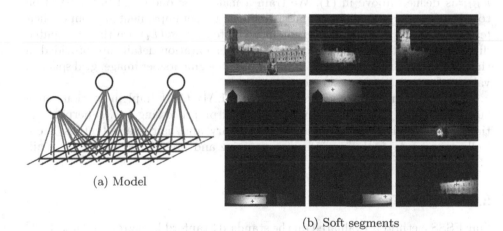

(a) Model

(b) Soft segments

Fig. 3. Graphical model and soft-segments. (a) The graphical model corresponding to the energy (2). Pixels (rectangular grid) are connected to multiple soft-segments (shown as circles), where (b) illustrates the support of the soft-segments. (b) Top left: the original image, all other images show soft-segments as defined in Eq. (1). Each image shows the "seed" for the soft-segment as a red cross, and the brightness depicts the weight $w_{i,j}$ between the seed pixel i and all pixels j. Note, (i) that the soft-segments are localized and do not cross semantic boundaries, and (ii) the varying effective sizes, e.g. soft-segments containing sky and buildings are large while the one centred on a person is small.

The iterations finish when a step does not change any label; in practice the algorithm converges quickly, in 1 to 7 iterations depending on the complexity of the scene. Several examples of the produced semantic segmentations are shown in Fig. 4 and more are available in the supplementary material.

Segmentation Uncertainty. It is sometimes beneficial for a semantic segmentation algorithm to be able to provide an extra "unknown" label when it is uncertain about the true labelling, instead of making a hard and potentially wrong decision; such functionality is exploited by the SoftSemanticSIFT method (Sect. 2.5). A pixel is assigned the "unknown" label if perturbing its optimal label does not change its contribution to the energy (Eq. (2)) more than a threshold value. The uncertainty estimation does not impact computational efficiency as it is obtained directly during the optimization of the energy function; the supplementary material contains more details.

Implementation Details. The features used are a histogram of colours in HSV space, a bag-of-words of dense RootSIFT [18], and a histogram of normalized y pixel locations. These are concatenated into a single feature vector. Each pixel generates one very sparse feature vector (e.g. the histogram of colours component has exactly one non-zero element). The feature vector for a soft-segment L_i is a weighted sum of pixel-wise feature vectors, where the weight for pixel j is $w_{i,j}$, as defined above in (1). We train a multi-class one-vs-all linear SVM on top of soft-segment features, using a Hellinger kernel implemented as an explicit feature map [43]. The soft-segment unary potentials $\phi_i(L_i)$ are then computed directly as negative classifier scores. All implementation details are provided in the supplementary material, i.e. number of soft-segments per image, grid spacing, values of α and β parameters, etc.

The run time is 7 s, with a pure MATLAB CPU implementation, on a 500×500 pixel image, including all required preprocessing (i.e. superpixelization, feature extraction, computation of unary and pairwise potentials, etc.). Full source code, including inference, training and pre-trained models, is available at [44].

3.3   Segmentation Results

Our FSSS method is evaluated on the standard Stanford background dataset [38] which contains 715 320×240 images and 8 semantic categories. This is the most suitable standard benchmark for our task, as others, such as PASCAL VOC, concentrate on objects rather than 'stuff'. As is standard procedure [36–38], segmentation quality is assessed as the average pixel accuracy across five random splits of the data. Our method achieves competitive performance, 78.0 %, while only taking 3.7 s end-to-end (i.e. including all feature extraction, soft-segment computation and pixel labelling). The results compare favourably to existing methods which generally use far more complicated features and take longer to compute. For example [38] achieves 76.5 % (and uses additional features

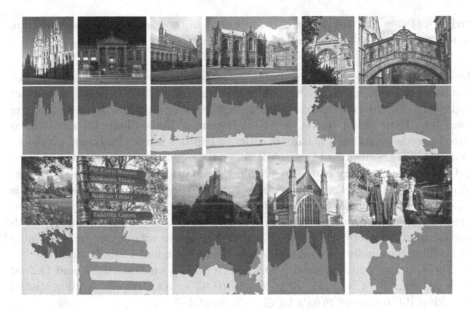

Fig. 4. Example semantic segmentations. Pairs of rows show the original image on the top, and the automatic semantic segmentation on the bottom. The three classes {sky,flora,other} are shown in blue, green and red, respectively. Best viewed in colour. See the supplementary material for more examples.

including the horizon location information and segment shape), and reports that inference takes up to 10 min; Tighe and Lazebnik [45] achieve 77.5 % with a large collection of features: superpixel shape, GIST, location, texton histograms, SIFT histogram, SIFT histogram on superpixel boundary, colour, context, etc. The best reported accuracy is 81.9 % [36], but this method takes minutes per image as it relies on gPb contour detector [46] and superpixelization [47].

We have demonstrated that FSSS is 'fit for purpose': it has been designed for fast and accurate semantic segmentation, and achieves this whilst being comparable to the state of the art in terms of multi-class semantic segmentation performance.

4 Experimental Setup and Retrieval Results

4.1 Evaluation, Datasets and Baseline

Retrieval performance is assessed using the standard and publicly available Oxford Buildings benchmark [14]. The basic dataset, Oxford 5 k, contains 5062 high-resolution images downloaded from Flickr. Retrieval quality is measured in terms of mean average precision (mAP) over the 55 pre-defined test queries. In order to test larger scale retrieval, the dataset is often expanded with 100 k Flickr images acting as distractors, thus forming the Oxford 105 k dataset. We follow the common practice [15,20,48,49] of using an independent dataset,

Paris 6 k [48], for all training (e.g. computation of the visual vocabulary, training for semantic segmentation, etc.).

Baseline. We have implemented a baseline retrieval system based on the Hamming Embedding [15] with burstiness normalization [50]. In detail, we extract RootSIFT [18] descriptors from Hessian-Affine interest points [51], and quantize them into 100 k visual words. A 64-bit Hamming Embedding [15] signature is stored together with each feature in order to improve feature matching precision. Two features are deemed to match if they are assigned to the same visual word and their Hamming signatures are within a standard threshold of 24 on the Hamming distance [15,52]. For a given query, a similarity score for a database image is obtained by summing all the Gaussian weighted votes of the image's matching features (a standard parameter value of $\sigma = 16$ is used, as in [50,52]). Finally, burstiness normalization of [50] is applied as well. The visual vocabulary and Hamming Embedding parameters are all trained on the independent Paris 6k dataset.

The baseline achieves good performance (mAP) on Oxford 5 k and Oxford 105 k benchmarks (Table 1): 70.70 % and 61.63 %, respectively. Adding spatial reranking [14] improves mAPs to 71.95 % and 64.38 %.

Semantic Segmentation. We have found that the Stanford background dataset [38], commonly used for semantic segmentation benchmarks, is inappropriate for training a segmentation method working on real-world unconstrained Flickr images. It contains 715 relatively small (320×240) images, with, for example, less than 8 million sky pixels. Furthermore, the set only contains outdoor images shot in daytime. Other datasets, e.g. MSRC [53], suffer from similar drawbacks. We have therefore annotated [54] 360 high resolution images (1024×768), randomly sampled from the Paris 6 k [48] and Sculptures 6 k [55] datasets, both of which have no images in common with Oxford 5 k and 105 k datasets. The set (named ParisSculpt360) contains many more labelled pixels: 122, 30 and 43 million for sky, flora and other, respectively, compared to the Stanford background dataset which contains only 55 M pixels in total. The images are unconstrained, i.e. there are indoors and outdoors photos, taken at day or night, colour and grayscale, and are not necessarily vertically aligned. The 5-fold average accuracy of FSSS on this dataset is 91.6 %.

All SemanticSIFT results and qualitative examples are generated using models trained on this ParisSculpt360 training data.

4.2 Retrieval Results

In this section we evaluate the three benefits of using SemanticSIFT versus the baseline, namely: improved retrieval quality, speedup and reduced storage/memory requirements.

Retrieval Quality. Table 1 shows the retrieval performance of the baseline, SemanticSIFT and SoftSemanticSIFT. The baseline achieves the mAP of 70.70 %

Table 1. Retrieval performance (mAP). All methods use exactly the same features, 100 k visual vocabulary and Hamming signatures with all training performed on the Paris6k dataset (Sect. 4.1). "+Spat." denotes spatial reranking [14]. SoftSemanticSIFT clearly outperforms the baseline and SemanticSIFT methods

Method	Oxford 5 k	+spat	Oxford 105 k	+spat
Baseline	0.7070	0.7195	0.6163	0.6438
SemanticSIFT	0.7082	0.7196	0.6228	0.6434
SoftSemanticSIFT	**0.7117**	**0.7238**	**0.6234**	**0.6487**

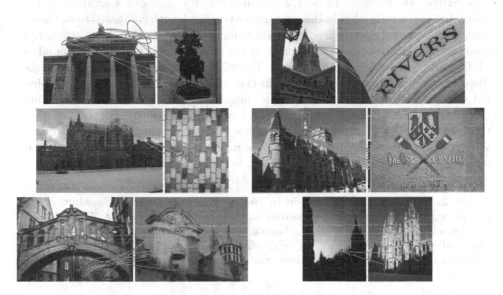

Fig. 5. Filtered false matches. Six pairs of images showing patch correspondences based on baseline descriptor-only based matching (i.e. matching visual word and Hamming signatures). Patches are shown as red ellipses, matching patches are connected with green lines. All displayed matches are correctly filtered out using SemanticSIFT because of the semantic content mismatch. Note, for example, the very challenging pair in the bottom-right, where patches corresponding to spires match patches showing shadows of spires; SemanticSIFT correctly discards these as the former contain {sky,other} while the latter only contain {other}.

and 61.63 % on the Oxford 5 k and 105 k benchmarks, respectively. Our SemanticSIFT method improves precision increasing the mAP to 70.82 % and 62.28 %. However, it struggles to bring an improvement after spatial reranking, because segmentation errors reduce recall. SoftSemanticSIFT, which is robust to some uncertainties in the automatic semantic segmentation, gives better results, 71.17 % and 62.34 %, and does outperform both the baseline and SemanticSIFT after spatial reranking as well. We further evaluate the statistical significance of the obtained improvements by employing five different visual vocabularies (corresponding to different random initializations of the approximate k-means algorithm). In all five cases SoftSemanticSIFT outperforms the baseline, for Ox105 k the relative improvement is +1.2 % on average, the minimal being +1 %.

Thus, even a small number of semantic classes leads to an improvement in retrieval mAP performance. It is to be expected that as more classes are introduced this improvement will increase. Figure 5 shows a selection of examples where the use of SemanticSIFT removes false matches (arising from the visual words and Hamming signatures alone).

Speedup. As discussed in Sect. 2.3, SemanticSIFT provides a significant speedup due to the reduction in the average posting list length compared to the baseline. The retrieval speed directly depends on the number of posting list entries that are traversed during the ranking stage, which is also equal to the number of Hamming distance computations. Therefore, the appropriate and accurate measure of speedup is the reduction in the average number of traversed posting list entries when using SemanticSIFT compared to the baseline. The speedup (Table 2), is 31.6 % and 41.1 % for the Oxford 5 k and Oxford 105 k tests, respectively. For the SoftSemanticSIFT case, where more posting list entries are traversed due to handling uncertainty of semantic segmentation, the speedup is smaller but still large: 23.1 % and 30.7 % for the two tests, respectively.

Table 2. Speedup and reduction in memory requirements. "Speedup" shows the reduction in the number of posting list entries traversed for the 55 pre-defined queries in the Oxford Buildings benchmark, achieved due to using a semantic vocabulary. Relative reduction in memory requirements (index size) is achieved by removing {flora} and {sky,flora} features, while "total speedup" denotes the speedup achieved after the index reduction

Method	Oxford 5 k			Oxford 105 k		
	Speedup	Memory savings	Total speedup	Speedup	Memory savings	Total speedup
SemanticSIFT	31.6 %	13.2 %	31.9 %	41.1 %	19.6 %	41.5 %
SoftSemanticSIFT	23.1 %	9.4 %	23.3 %	30.7 %	14.5 %	31.0 %

The above speedup measurements are based on the predefined 55 queries in the Oxford Buildings benchmarks. Another way of assessing retrieval speed across inverted indexes with varying properties is to compare the expected number of inverted index entries the system has to process for an average query [56]. In the supplementary material we give the details of the computation for the case of SemanticSIFT. The result is that the expected speedup over the baseline for an average query is 40.7 % and 50.4 %, for the Oxford 5 k and Oxford 105 k tests, respectively.

One alternate way of improving retrieval speed is to increase the visual vocabulary (as this also reduces the length of posting lists on average). However, this leads to increased quantization errors and the retrieval performance suffers: with a 700 k visual vocabulary, equal to the size of SemanticSIFT's product vocabulary, the baseline only achieves mAP of 54.9 % on Oxford 5 k, compared to 70.7 % obtained with a 100 k vocabulary. In contrast, SoftSemanticSIFT gets 71.2 % while preserving the same speedup.

Memory Savings. As discussed in Sect. 2.4, features can be removed from the inverted index based on their semantic content if it is known *a priori* that they are not useful for the application in question. When searching for buildings (which belong to the "other" class), as in the Oxford Buildings tests, it is clear that flora features are not useful. Therefore, the database features assigned to semantic words {flora} or {flora,sky} are removed, whilst the semantic word {flora,other} is kept as it can still be useful. With these changes the retrieval quality (mAP) remains virtually unchanged for both Oxford 5 k and Oxford 105 k tests. The memory/storage saving on the other hand is significant (Table 2): 13.2 % and 19.6 % of features are removed from the SemanticSIFT index for Oxford 5 k and 105 k, respectively. Furthermore, there is an additional slight improvement in speed due to the decreased number of posting lists that have to be traversed for query images which contain the removed features. The total speedup for the two datasets with respect to the baseline is 31.9 % and 41.5 %, compared to the 31.6 % and 41.1 % achieved without feature removal. The speedup is minor because the 55 predefined queries for the Oxford Buildings benchmarks don't contain many flora features.

Colour. One might argue that the SemanticSIFT's increase in retrieval performance is purely due to the use of colour (used indirectly for semantic segmentation), which the baseline method does not use. However, OpponentSIFT [57], the state-of-the-art colour SIFT variant, actually performs slightly worse than SIFT (the mAP decreases by 0.7 %) on Oxford 5 k. This proves that the improvement from SemanticSIFT is not due to the use of colour, but to taking proper account of the semantic classes when matching.

5   Conclusions and Future Work

We have presented a method, SemanticSIFT, which improves the standard large scale specific object retrieval by leveraging semantic information to efficiently filter out some falsely matched descriptors, thereby increasing precision and improving retrieval performance. Furthermore, there is a "win-win-win" situation: the gain in recognition accuracy is obtained simultaneously with a nearly two-fold speedup, due to visiting shorter posting lists, and a 20 % decrease in storage (RAM) requirements. The method can be used as an improvement to any standard retrieval systems based on matching local patches – a 'plug in' to boost speed and retrieval performance.

Semantic reasoning for object retrieval is a very promising idea that opens many directions for future work, which are out of scope and length limitations of this paper. With future improvements of semantic segmentation methods (which will surely happen over time), one can hope to take more classes into consideration, e.g. people/faces (successful face detection already exists), buildings, cars, roads, flowers, etc. A finer scale reasoning can be used too – for the "buildings" class example one could remove falsely matched features between a window and a door. Successful fine-grained distinctions within a class would be very useful as well.

Another interesting direction is to employ the semantic labels as a form of automatic supervision which could be used in descriptor learning. Automatic generation of training data for descriptor learning in the form of matching and non-matching image patches using object retrieval has been done in [58,59], but unsupervised discovery of hard negatives has always been a problem. Semantic-SIFT can provide the needed automatic supervision.

Acknowledgement. We are grateful for financial support from ERC grant VisRec no. 228180 and a Royal Society Wolfson Research Merit Award.

References

1. Cummins, M., Newman, P.: Highly scalable appearance-only SLAM - FAB-MAP 2.0. In: RSS (2009)
2. Schindler, G., Brown, M., Szeliski, R.: City-scale location recognition. In: Proceedings of the CVPR (2007)
3. Knopp, J., Sivic, J., Pajdla, T.: Avoiding confusing features in place recognition. In: Daniilidis, K., Maragos, P., Paragios, N. (eds.) ECCV 2010, Part I. LNCS, vol. 6311, pp. 748–761. Springer, Heidelberg (2010)
4. Torii, A., Sivic, J., Pajdla, T., Okutomi, M.: Visual place recognition with repetitive structures. In: Proceedings of the CVPR (2013)
5. Quack, T., Leibe, B., Van Gool, L.: World-scale mining of objects and events from community photo collections. In: Proceedings of the CIVR (2008)
6. Gammeter, S., Bossard, L., Quack, T., Van Gool, L.: I know what you did last summer: object-level auto-annotation of holiday snaps. In: Proceedings of the ICCV (2009)
7. Nister, D., Stewenius, H.: Scalable recognition with a vocabulary tree. In: Proceedings of the CVPR, pp. 2161–2168 (2006)
8. Shen, X., Lin, Z., Brandt, J., Wu, Y.: Mobile product image search by automatic query object extraction. In: Proceedings of the CVPR (2012)
9. Romberg, S., Lienhart, R.: Bundle min-hashing for logo recognition. In: ACM ICMR (2013)
10. Google Goggles. http://www.google.com/mobile/goggles
11. Sivic, J., Zisserman, A.: Efficient visual search of videos cast as text retrieval. IEEE PAMI **31**, 591–606 (2009)
12. Agarwal, S., Snavely, N., Simon, I., Seitz, S.M., Szeliski, R.: Building Rome in a day. In: Proceedings of the ICCV (2009)
13. Lowe, D.: Distinctive image features from scale-invariant keypoints. IJCV **60**, 91–110 (2004)
14. Philbin, J., Chum, O., Isard, M., Sivic, J., Zisserman, A.: Object retrieval with large vocabularies and fast spatial matching. In: Proceedings of the CVPR (2007)

15. Jégou, H., Douze, M., Schmid, C.: Hamming embedding and weak geometric consistency for large scale image search. In: Forsyth, D., Torr, P., Zisserman, A. (eds.) ECCV 2008, Part I. LNCS, vol. 5302, pp. 304–317. Springer, Heidelberg (2008)

16. Jégou, H., Douze, M., Schmid, C.: Exploiting descriptor distances for precise image search. Technical report, INRIA (2011)

17. Aly, M., Munich, M., Perona, P.: Compactkdt: compact signatures for accurate large scale object recognition. In: IEEE Workshop on Applications of Computer Vision (2012)

18. Arandjelović, R., Zisserman, A.: Three things everyone should know to improve object retrieval. In: Proceedings of the CVPR (2012)

19. Chum, O., Philbin, J., Sivic, J., Isard, M., Zisserman, A.: Total recall: automatic query expansion with a generative feature model for object retrieval. In: Proceedings of the ICCV (2007)

20. Chum, O., Mikulik, A., Perďoch, M., Matas, J.: Total recall II: query expansion revisited. In: Proceedings of the CVPR (2011)

21. Shen, X., Lin, Z., Brandt, J., Avidan, S., Wu, Y.: Object retrieval and localization with spatially-constrained similarity measure and k-NN reranking. In: Proceedings of the CVPR (2012)

22. Qin, D., Gammeter, S., Bossard, L., Quack, T., Van Gool, L.: Hello neighbor: accurate object retrieval with k-reciprocal nearest neighbors. In: Proceedings of the CVPR (2011)

23. Simonyan, K., Vedaldi, A., Zisserman, A.: Descriptor learning using convex optimisation. In: Fitzgibbon, A., Lazebnik, S., Perona, P., Sato, Y., Schmid, C. (eds.) ECCV 2012, Part I. LNCS, vol. 7572, pp. 243–256. Springer, Heidelberg (2012)

24. Winder, S., Hua, G., Brown, M.: Picking the best daisy. In: Proceedings of the CVPR, pp. 178–185 (2009)

25. Ladicky, L., Sturgess, P., Russell, C., Sengupta, S., Bastanlar, Y., Clocksin, W., Torr, P.H.S.: Joint optimisation for object class segmentation and dense stereo reconstruction. IJCV 100(2), 122–133 (2012)

26. Haene, C., Zach, C., Cohen, A., Angst, R., Pollefeys, M.: Joint 3D scene reconstruction and class segmentation. In: Proceedings of the CVPR (2013)

27. Castle, R.O., Klein, G., Murray, D.W.: Combining monoSLAM with object recognition for scene augmentation using a wearable camera. Image Vis. Comput. 28(11), 1548–1556 (2010)

28. Civera, J., Gálvez-López, D., Riazuelo, L., Tardós, J.D., Montiel, J.M.M.: Towards semantic SLAM using a monocular camera. In: IEEE Intelligent Robots and Systems (IROS) (2011)

29. Turcot, T., Lowe, D.G.: Better matching with fewer features: the selection of useful features in large database recognition problems. In: ICCV Workshop on Emergent Issues in Large Amounts of Visual Data (WS-LAVD) (2009)

30. Wu, Z., Ke, Q., Isard, M., Sun, J.: Bundling features for large scale partial-duplicate web image search. In: Proceedings of the CVPR (2009)

31. Fernando, B., Tuytelaars, T.: Mining multiple queries for image retrieval: on-the-fly learning of an object-specific mid-level representation. In: Proceedings of the ICCV (2013)

32. Wang, J.Z., Li, J., Wiederhold, G.: SIMPLIcity: semantics-sensitive integrated matching for picture libraries. IEEE PAMI 23, 947–964 (2001)

33. Duygulu, P., Barnard, K., de Freitas, J.F.G., Forsyth, D.: Object recognition as machine translation: learning a lexicon for a fixed image vocabulary. In: Heyden, A., Sparr, G., Nielsen, M., Johansen, P. (eds.) ECCV 2002, Part IV. LNCS, vol. 2353, pp. 97–112. Springer, Heidelberg (2002)

34. Li, J., Wang, J.Z.: Automatic linguistic indexing of pictures by a statistical modeling approach. IEEE PAMI **25**(9), 1075–1088 (2003)
35. Munoz, D., Bagnell, J.A., Hebert, M.: Stacked hierarchical labeling. In: Daniilidis, K., Maragos, P., Paragios, N. (eds.) ECCV 2010, Part VI. LNCS, vol. 6316, pp. 57–70. Springer, Heidelberg (2010)
36. Lempitsky, V., Vedaldi, A., Zisserman, A.: A pylon model for semantic segmentation. In: NIPS (2011)
37. Ladicky, L., Russell, C., Kohli, P., Torr, P.H.S.: Associative hierarchical random fields. IEEE PAMI **36**(6), 1056–1077 (2014)
38. Gould, S., Fulton, R., Koller, D.: Decomposing a scene into geometric and semantically consistent regions. In: Proceedings of the ICCV (2009)
39. Shotton, J., Johnson, M., Cipolla, R.: Semantic texton forests for image categorization and segmentation. In: Proceedings of the CVPR (2008)
40. Felzenszwalb, P.F., Veksler, O.: Tiered scene labelling with dynamic programming. In: Proceedings of the CVPR (2010)
41. Russell, B.C., Efros, A.A., Sivic, J., Freeman, W.T., Zisserman, A.: Using multiple segmentations to discover objects and their extent in image collections. In: Proceedings of the CVPR (2006)
42. Leordeanu, M., Sukthankar, R., Sminchisescu, C.: Efficient closed-form solution to generalized boundary detection. In: Fitzgibbon, A., Lazebnik, S., Perona, P., Sato, Y., Schmid, C. (eds.) ECCV 2012, Part IV. LNCS, vol. 7575, pp. 516–529. Springer, Heidelberg (2012)
43. Vedaldi, A., Zisserman, A.: Efficient additive kernels via explicit feature maps. In: Proceedings of the CVPR (2010)
44. Arandjelović, R., Zisserman, A.: Fast semantic segmentation code (2014). http://www.robots.ox.ac.uk/~vgg/software/fast_semantic_segmentation
45. Tighe, J., Lazebnik, S.: Superparsing: scalable nonparametric image parsing with superpixels. In: Daniilidis, K., Maragos, P., Paragios, N. (eds.) ECCV 2010, Part V. LNCS, vol. 6315, pp. 352–365. Springer, Heidelberg (2010)
46. Maire, M., Arbelaez, P., Fowlkes, C., Malik, J.: Using contours to detect and localize junctions in natural images. In: Proceedings of the CVPR (2008)
47. Arbelaez, P., Maire, M., Fowlkes, C., Malik, J.: From contours to regions: an empirical evaluation. In: Proceedings of the CVPR (2009)
48. Philbin, J., Chum, O., Isard, M., Sivic, J., Zisserman, A.: Lost in quantization: improving particular object retrieval in large scale image databases. In: Proceedings of the CVPR (2008)
49. Jégou, H., Chum, O.: Negative evidences and co-occurences in image retrieval: the benefit of pca and whitening. In: Fitzgibbon, A., Lazebnik, S., Perona, P., Sato, Y., Schmid, C. (eds.) ECCV 2012, Part II. LNCS, vol. 7573, pp. 774–787. Springer, Heidelberg (2012)
50. Jégou, H., Douze, M., Schmid, C.: On the burstiness of visual elements. In: Proceedings of the CVPR (2009)
51. Mikolajczyk, K., Schmid, C.: Scale & affine invariant interest point detectors. IJCV **1**, 63–86 (2004)
52. Tolias, G., Jégou, H.: Local visual query expansion: exploiting an image collection to refine local descriptors. Technical report RR-8325, INRIA (2013)
53. Shotton, J., Winn, J.M., Rother, C., Criminisi, A.: *TextonBoost*: joint appearance, shape and context modeling for multi-class object recognition and segmentation. In: Leonardis, A., Bischof, H., Pinz, A. (eds.) ECCV 2006, Part I. LNCS, vol. 3951, pp. 1–15. Springer, Heidelberg (2006)

54. Arandjelović, R., Zisserman, A.: Parissculpt360 annotations (2014). http://www.robots.ox.ac.uk/~vgg/data/data-various.html
55. Arandjelović, R., Zisserman, A.: Smooth object retrieval using a bag of boundaries. In: Proceedings of the ICCV (2011)
56. Stewénius, H., Gunderson, S.H., Pilet, J.: Size matters: exhaustive geometric verification for image retrieval accepted for ECCV 2012. In: Fitzgibbon, A., Lazebnik, S., Perona, P., Sato, Y., Schmid, C. (eds.) ECCV 2012, Part II. LNCS, vol. 7573, pp. 674–687. Springer, Heidelberg (2012)
57. van de Sande, K.E.A., Gevers, T., Snoek, C.G.M.: Evaluating color descriptors for object and scene recognition. IEEE PAMI **32**, 1582–1596 (2010)
58. Philbin, J., Isard, M., Sivic, J., Zisserman, A.: Descriptor learning for efficient retrieval. In: Daniilidis, K., Maragos, P., Paragios, N. (eds.) ECCV 2010, Part III. LNCS, vol. 6313, pp. 677–691. Springer, Heidelberg (2010)
59. Simonyan, K., Vedaldi, A., Zisserman, A.: Learning local feature descriptors using convex optimisation. IEEE PAMI **36**(8), 1573–1585 (2014)

Context Based Re-ranking for Object Retrieval

Yanzhi Chen[1,2]([✉]), Anthony Dick[2], Xi Li[2,3], and Rhys Hill[2]

[1] United Technologies Research Center (China) Ltd, Room 3502, 35/F,
Kerry Parkside Office, Shanghai, China
chenyz@utrc.utc.com

[2] Australian Centre for Visual Technologies, The University of Adelaide,
Adelaide, SA 5005, Australia

[3] College of Computer Science and Technologies, Zhejiang University,
Hangzhou, China

Abstract. We propose a simple but effective re-ranking method for improving the results of object retrieval. Our method considers the contextual information embedded in a dataset. This is based on the observation that if there are multiple images containing the same object in a dataset, then these images can often be grouped into clusters. We make the following two contributions. Firstly, we gain this contextual information by a *random dimension partition* of the dataset. This enables online query model expansion if needed. Secondly, we use the collected contextual information to refine the initial retrieval results by taking into account the context in which each retrieved image occurs. Experimental results on several datasets demonstrate the effectiveness of our method in both accuracy and computation cost: our method refines retrieval results without relying on low-level feature matching or re-issuing the query.

1 Introduction

The goal of object retrieval is to find other images in a dataset containing a target object given in a query image. The target object may appear under varying image conditions, including scale, viewpoint, lighting changes, or partial occlusion of the objects [1]. Therefore, many successful object retrieval systems are based on local invariant descriptors [1–5], that are robust to scale, affine transformations and partial occlusion [6].

In order to scale to large datasets, an image is reduced into a compressed "Bag-of-Words" (BoW) format [2] instead of using thousands of local invariant descriptors. In the BoW model, each "word" is a quantised image feature, typically weighted according to its frequency in the image (term frequency, tf) and rarity in the dataset (inverse document frequency, idf). However, the compressed format decreases the retrieval accuracy because of the quantisation process [7].

Over the past decade, there has been considerable improvement on the BoW based retrieval system, focusing on better exploiting low-level feature information [1,7–12]. It has also been noticed [10,11,13] that an image dataset usually contains multiple images showing the same object. Nevertheless, little attention has been paid to the fact that these images containing the same object will

© Springer International Publishing Switzerland 2015
D. Cremers et al. (Eds.): ACCV 2014, Part I, LNCS 9003, pp. 196–210, 2015.
DOI: 10.1007/978-3-319-16865-4_13

appear as clusters in the dataset as opposed to background noise (see Fig. 1 for example). These clustered images can be treated as contextually associated. To this end, we define a "**context**" as a group of images having common visual properties and show its benefits in improving the retrieval performance.

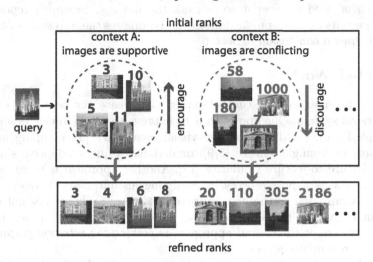

Fig. 1. Illustration of context based re-ranking. The initial retrieval results (sorted by similarity Ψ) contain both true and false positives. The numbers above images are rankings. The accuracy is increased after re-ranking by contextual information. Best viewed in color (Color figure online).

Unlike many previous methods that require an expensive offline training stage, the first contribution of this paper is a simple, efficient clustering method for online context generation. Traditional methods, *e.g.* k-means, are unable to cluster the BoW vectors efficiently, because the vectors are very sparse and high dimensional. Instead, we propose a *random space partition* method, by which the dataset is clustered into groups of images by partitions along randomly selected dimensions. This is effective because of the sparsity of the BoW vectors, and efficient despite their high dimensionality because only a small number of dimensions are selected. The scheme of this simplified clustering method is similar to [14], in which a random projection of high dimensional data is conducted for multiple runs as well.

Our second contribution is to improve the initial retrieval results once the contexts are available, by the analysis of image ranks in each context. The idea is that the similarity between a query and a dataset image should not be determined solely by those two images (as in the standard dot-product similarity [2]), but also influenced by their association with other contextually related images. As illustrated in Fig. 1, images in a context are promoted if they support each other, *i.e.* high retrieval ranks dominate, and therefore ranked highly (context A). Otherwise, images are demoted if there are low or conflicting ranks in their context (context B). Our context based re-ranking method refines the retrieval results by improving the standard one-to-one comparison (dot-product similarity) with the contextual information at query time.

The rest of the paper is organised as follows: Sect. 2 discusses the related work to our method. Section 3 presents the method to extract the contextual information, which is used in Sect. 4 to re-rank the dataset. Section 5 reports the re-ranking results on some public datasets and compares them to state-of-the-art. Finally we draw a conclusion in Sect. 6.

2 Related Work

There have been extensive studies aiming to increase the accuracy of BoW based retrieval system. One approach is to improve the BoW image descriptors, for example forming a discriminative visual vocabulary [8], mapping multiple visual words to a single feature [7,9], or deriving a query adaptive similarity based on feature-to-feature similarity [12]. Another approach is to re-rank the retrieval results as a post-process by analysing an initial set of query results [1,4,15,16]. Compared to the first approach, online re-ranking does not require re-construction of the visual vocabulary, nor does it require training data. In this paper, we adopt the second approach: *improving the retrieval performance by an online re-ranking process*.

A popular approach to online re-ranking is to utilise low-level spatial information to promote dataset images whose features are spatially consistent with those in the query. Spatial verification [1] examines a truncated list of retrieved results by computing a geometric transformation between features in both query and dataset images. However, the computation of geometric transformation is expensive, so that only a short-list of images can be examined. To speed it up, weak geometric consistency (WGC) [4] filters mismatching descriptors without applying geometric transformation. Instead, the method assumes that matching descriptors are related by a fixed orientation and scale. Re-ranking can also be achieved by testing reciprocal similarity of query and dataset images [13]—that is, whether the images retrieve each other when both used as queries. Reciprocal similarity is discovered by a k-reciprocal nearest neighbour structure that is built offline. In addition, features from verified top ranked results can be added to the query which is then re-issued, in order to improve recall [15,16]. These methods succeed in finding more query relevant images, but at the cost of online feature matching or query re-issuing, which is computationally expensive.

Rather than examining individual features, the ranking information embedded in a set of top ranked results can be used to further refine the results [17,18]. In [17], a distance matrix is defined by the similarity of the ranks to take into account the contextual information, while the method proposed in [18] measures the similarity between the query and dataset images based on the idea that images are visually similar if they have intersections among top ranked results when using them as queries. However, these methods need to re-query the dataset in order to re-define the distance between query and dataset images.

In this paper, we present a novel re-ranking method for BoW based object retrieval, which achieves both efficiency and effectiveness. Our work is also inspired by [10] in terms of adjusting the similarity scores of images. Their method applies an offline image graph creation step in which each node represents an image and an edge indicates the connection of same objects in a pair of images, such that neighbouring images are grouped. Our work is different from [10] in two aspects: (i) our method softly adjusts the similarity scores of dataset images at runtime with the help of the contextual information (although the offline step is optional); (ii) the adjustments of similarity scores are based on query-specific rank analysis performed at runtime.

3   Context Generation

A key ingredient of our method is to generate "contexts" from the dataset. This section describes how to derive such information efficiently from the BoW vectors. The usage of contextual information for re-ranking is discussed in the following Section.

3.1   Random Space Partition

Let T be a set of dataset images. The goal of our method is to cluster T into D groups: $C := \{c_k\}_{k=1}^{D}$, where each group c_k is a context that contains a small number (n_k) of dataset images. The clustering of T involves two issues: (i) scalability: the clustering is conducted on high-dimensional BoW vectors, for which standard k-means methods or graph cut of the image dataset [19] are not feasible; and (ii) efficiency: as it runs at query time, the partition should have low computation and memory requirements.

In order to address these two issues, we use a *random space partition* method which utilises the specific properties of the BoW model. A visual vocabulary is composed of N visual words: $\mathbf{W} := \{w_i\}_{i=1}^{N}$, where N is typically large ($N = 10^6$ in our implementation). The dataset images are represented as a collection of visual word vectors $T := \{\mathbf{d}_j\}_{j=1}^{V}$, in which V is number of images and $\mathbf{d}_j$ is the corresponding tf-idf image vector.

The dataset vectors T are very sparse: on average, there are only 2200 non-zero entries in a 10^6 dimensional vector (in our implementation). The high sparsity simplifies the partitioning of T. As illustrated in Fig. 2(a), the dataset vectors T are separated into two groups by a random dimension of the image vectors, according to whether each vector contains a non-zero entry in a specific dimension. Note that each dimension of $\mathbf{d}_j$ corresponds to one visual word w_i, so the images can be quickly accessed by an inverted file [2], which maps each visual word to images it appears in. Thus, each "column" of the file, as is shown in Fig. 2(b), corresponds to a visual word w_i and forms an image group c_k:

$$\mathbf{c}_k = \{\mathbf{d}_j\}_{j=1}^{n_k} \text{ if } F_j(w_i) > 0 \tag{1}$$

where $F_j(w_i)$ is the frequency of w_i in image j. Scalable clustering of T is achieved by repeated random partitions. As the inverted file is already used for

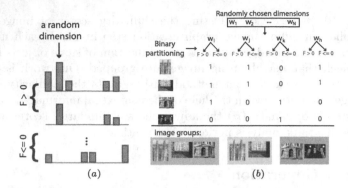

Fig. 2. (*a*): Image vector separation by a random dimension into two parts. (*b*): Illustration of random space partition method by using the inverted file. Best viewed in color (Color figure online).

the calculation of tf-idf weights, this involves almost no extra computation or storage beyond the standard BoW pipeline.

The efficiency of our method is achieved by performing only D ($D \ll N$) data partitions to generate groups $\mathcal{C}$. Intuitively, it is inefficient to use all dimensions (visual words) because only a small number of them are informative. These words are usually the query words $\mathbf{Q}$, thus the random dimension partition is conducted on $\mathbf{Q}$ by default. In addition, an extra set of words $\mathbf{S}$ ($\mathbf{Q}, \mathbf{S} \subset \mathbf{W}$), which are relevant to the query, can also be considered.

Query-relevant words $\mathbf{S}$ can be generated either offline or online as follows: (*i*) **offline**: obtain $\mathbf{S}$ by a thesaurus structure built offline [20], which includes the frequently co-occurring visual words in fixed spatial regions. (*ii*) **online**: obtain $\mathbf{S}$ by query expansion [15], in which the visual words included in the spatially verified regions are appended.

3.2   Expansion of Contexts

In order to promote the query-relevant words $\mathbf{S}$ (as well as keep the query words $\mathbf{Q}$), we propose an expansion method during context generation which adopts a weighted random selection scheme to select the dimensions. Because each dimension in the BoW vector is also associated to a visual word, this method can be seen as an expansion of the original query words $\mathbf{Q}$ obtained without re-issuing the query. The expansion proceeds as follows.

Firstly, we randomly choose a subset of words in which $\mathbf{Q}$ and $\mathbf{S}$ are given a higher probability of selection than those words that are non relevant. This is done by associating visual words to random keys under a mapping function f:

$$f(w_i) = \begin{cases} a \cdot x \text{ if } w_i \in \mathbf{Q} \\ b \cdot x \text{ if } w_i \in \mathbf{S} \backslash (\mathbf{Q} \cap \mathbf{S}) \\ x \quad \text{ otherwise} \end{cases} \tag{2}$$

where $w_i \in \mathbf{W}$, x is a uniformly distributed random variable $x \in U(0,1)$ and the parameters a, b are the weights. The D dimensions used for partition are selected in decreasing order of $f(w_i)$. This scheme of random dimension selection is similar to [21].

Secondly, we define three cases based on the values of a and b, such that the query information can be incrementally appended by adjusting the parameters: (i) **Random selection:** $a = 1$, $b = 1$: each visual word has uniform probability of being selected. (ii) **Query-dependent selection:** $a > 1$, $b = 1$: words in the given query $\mathbf{Q}$ are more likely to be selected. (iii) **Query-expansion selection:** $a > 1$, $b > 1$: words in the query and the query-relevant set $\mathbf{S}$ are more likely to be selected than others. After obtaining D dimensions, image groups $\mathcal{C} := \{\mathbf{c}_k\}_{k=1}^{D}$ are used to estimate the context scores for re-ranking.

4   Context Based Re-ranking

This section describes our context based re-ranking scheme. We start with the baseline method that sorts the dataset images according to their dot-product similarity [2] between the tf-idf vectors $\mathbf{q}$ and $\mathbf{d}$, corresponding to query image q and a dataset image d:

$$\Psi(q,d) = \frac{\mathbf{q} \cdot \mathbf{d}}{\| \mathbf{q} \| \| \mathbf{d} \|} \tag{3}$$

Each dataset image d then obtains a rank order r_d under $\Psi(q,d)$, for which top ranks are probably relevant to query while low ranks are likely irrelevant to the query. The ranking is efficient, but neglects contextual information linking the returned results as it only measures similarity between the query and each dataset image in isolation.

As illustrated in Fig. 1, the ranks of all dataset images in a given context can be informative. If many images in a context are relevant to a query, then this supports ranking all images in that context more highly. Conversely, if many images in a context have low rank, then a high ranked exception is likely to be a false positive. Therefore, our method aims to improve one-to-one matching by embedding this information in the similarity measure Ψ (Eq. 3), such that contextually similar images boost each other up. To this end, we use the contextual ranking information to adjust the dot-product similarity Ψ:

$$\Phi(q,d) = \Psi(q,d) \cdot \exp(\Theta(q,d)) \tag{4}$$

where $\Phi(q,d)$ is the improved ranking score. The context factor $\Theta(q,d)$ in Eq. (4) is calculated according to the ranks of result images belonging to each context, and is discussed below. Images are re-ranked by sorting $\Phi(q,d)$ (Eq. (4)). Our method is outlined in Algorithm 1.

4.1   Computing the Context Factor for Re-ranking

Our context based re-ranking method introduces the contextual information to the similarity measure by a pair of contextual measures: a context factor and a

---
Algorithm 1. Context based re-ranking

Input: Query image q, number of random dimensions D.
Output: Retrieval results.
1. Rank dataset images by sorting the dot-product similarity Ψ (Eq. (3)).
2. Obtain initial ranks of dataset images.
3. Select D dimensions (Eq. (2)).
4. Generate image groups $\mathcal{C} := \{c_k\}_{k=1}^{D}$ from inverted file (Eq. (1)).
5. Compute the context score $W(q, c_k)$ for each image group (Eq. (5)).
6. Compute the context factor $\Theta(q, d)$ for each dataset image d (Eq. (6)).
7. Adjust image similarity and re-rank (Eq. (4)).
Return: Re-ranked results.

---

context score. A query-specific context score $W(q, c_k)$ describes the association of each image group c_k, while the context factor $\Theta(q, d)$ of a dataset image d is formed by context scores learnt from n_d image groups it has been assigned to. The dataset image d is then re-ranked by the similarity score refined by the context factor (Eq. (4)). Specifically, our method proceeds in two steps.

Firstly, each image group is assigned a context score $W(q, c_k)$, which summarises the ranks of images in the group. This is composed of two parts:

- The coherence of image ranks in c_k: $\frac{1}{n_k^2}\sum_{j=1}^{n_k}\sum_{s=1}^{n_k}K(\frac{r_j-r_s}{\rho})$, where r_j and r_s are the image ranks in c_k, n_k is the group size, K is a Gaussian kernel and ρ is its bandwidth. In this way, the coherence of a context is measured by the association of image ranks in c_k. The parameter ρ is automatically tuned, based on estimating the standard deviation of the input image ranks [22]. Thus, image groups which are distributed widely in the ranking list have less coherence, and will not be weighted strongly in the refined similarity.
- The number of top and bottom image ranks: $\frac{t_q(c_k,H)-b_q(c_k,H)}{n_k}$, where functions $t_q(c_k, H)$ and $b_q(c_k, H)$ count the number of members c_k in the top-H and bottom-H places, respectively. This indicates whether the contexts are close to query q or not. The context score of group c_k is the product of both:

$$W(q, c_k) = \left[\frac{1}{n_k^2}\sum_{j=1}^{n_k}\sum_{s=1}^{n_k}K(\frac{r_j - r_s}{\rho})\right] \cdot \frac{t_q(c_k, H) - b_q(c_k, H)}{n_k} \quad (5)$$

Secondly, the re-ranking process utilises these context scores to improve the similarity score of a dataset image d. We index each dataset image d by a set of D indicators $\{\mathbb{I}_k^d\}_{k=1}^{D}$, where $\mathbb{I}_k^d$ indicates whether d appears in c_k or not. As each image is assigned to several groups, the re-ranking then makes use of the average context score. The context factor is obtained from these context scores, and is defined for a response image d to query image q as:

$$\Theta(q, d) = \frac{1}{\sum_{k=1}^{D}\mathbb{I}_k^d} \cdot \sum_{k=1}^{D}\mathbb{I}_k^d W(q, c_k) \quad (6)$$

According to Eq. (4), the initial similarity of images having negative context factor ($\Theta(q, d) < 0$) is decreased, while those having positive context factor ($\Theta(q, d) > 0$) is increased.

5   Experimental Results

5.1   Experimental Setup

We investigate the performance of our context based re-ranking method in the following aspects: (i) varying the key parameters applied to context generation (random space partition and context expansion). (ii) varying the context re-ranking parameters, which include the number of iterations as well as the top (bottom) truncation. (iii) comparison to state-of-the-art. The details of our experimental settings are as follows.

Datasets: The retrieval experiments are conducted on three public object retrieval datasets: two small scale datasets (Oxford 5K and Paris 6K [23]) and a large scale dataset Oxford 105K consisting of Oxford 5K images and 100K images from MIRFLICKR-1M [24]. Both the Oxford 5K and Paris 6K datasets [23] contain 11 building landmarks for evaluation. Each image within these datasets is represented as a histogram of SIFT words after tf-idf weighting.

Implementation details: The visual words are obtained by quantising the SIFT feature descriptors using approximate k-means [1,25]. The vocabulary size is 1 million. After that, images are stored in an inverted file structure such that the online process only needs to access those containing query words (or query related words as discussed in Sect. 3.2). We run our experiments on 2×8-Core Xeon E5-2680 at 2.70 GHz with 10 G memory.

Evaluation: In order to quantify the retrieval performance, we evaluate the retrieval accuracy by the widely used mean average precision (mAP), as defined in [2]. The mAP scores reported in the following are from our implementation, excepts those cited from other sources.

5.2   Evaluation of Random Space Partition

Initially, we evaluate the effects of various parameter settings in the random space partition. As discussed in Sect. 3.1, the random space partition involves two key parameters:

(1) Query-dependent set Q selection weight, achieved by adjusting the weight a in the random mapping function (Eq. 2). We illustrate the effects of query-dependent set **Q** by varying a while fixing the other weighting parameter ($b = 1$). In this way, the weight a ($a > 1$) gives more priority to the query words than those not in the query ($a = 1$). Table 1 assesses these effects as follows: (i) (f_1): $a = 1$, random selection of visual words (dimensions). (ii) (f_2): $a = 10$, query words 10× more likely to be selected. (iii) (f_3): $a = tf$, similar to f_2 but weight a is proportional to the term frequency of the query word, rather than constant as in f_2. As reported in Table 1, the retrieval results of f_1 are as good as spatial verification on the Oxford 5K dataset, while achieving slightly higher accuracy on the Paris 6K dataset. Note that f_1 can be completed offline, so our random selection method is able to re-rank the dataset effectively and efficiently but with less information required than the standard spatial verification method. In contrast, the mapping functions f_2 and f_3 are query-specific, namely the dimensions are decided according to the given query online. They result in more accurate retrieval accuracy than the offline version (f_1), as well as outperform the spatial verification results on both datasets. The difference between f_2 and f_3 is negligible when a is large. As a result, we set weight $a = 10$ whenever query words require priority in random space partition.

Table 1. Retrieval performance with varying weighting functions in ordering the query words. See text for details. Total number of visual words selected: 3×10^4.

Methods		Oxford 5K	Paris 6K
Baseline (without re-ranking)		0.612	0.639
Spatial Re-ranking		0.645	0.653
$a = 1, b = 1$	f_1	0.644	0.674
$a > 1, b = 1$	f_2	0.670	0.690
	f_3	0.674	0.690
$a > 1, b > 1$	f_4	0.676	0.691
	f_5	0.684	0.697
	f_6	**0.701**	**0.700**
	f_7	0.692	**0.700**

(2) Number of randomly chosen dimensions D. Figure 3(a) reports the retrieval accuracy for increasing D dimensions selected. Note that the context generation utilises these dimensions to collect contextual information during re-ranking. As illustrated in Fig. 3(a), the accuracy improves as D increases, and then plateaus above a threshold, e.g. $D = 7 \times 10^4$ on both Oxford 5K and Paris 6K datasets. Figure 3(a) also validates that the re-ranking performance improves by diminishing amounts as D increases. In addition, Table 2 shows the average CPU time as D increases, in which the CPU time rises consistently with increasing dimension number D. Considering both accuracy and runtime, we set $D = 3 \times 10^4$.

5.3 Effects of Context Expansion

In this section we illustrate the effects of context expansion in improving the re-ranking performance in two aspects:

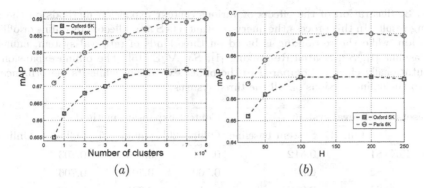

(a)   (b)

Fig. 3. (*a*): Retrieval result comparison with increasing dimension D. (*b*): Retrieval result comparison with increasing top/bottom-H.

Table 2. Computational cost comparison of spatial verification and our method, where D is the selected dimension (context) number. The results are measured by CPU second.

Methods		Oxford 5K	Paris 6K	Oxford 105K
Spatial Re-ranking		2.10	4.71	4.34
f_2	$D = 1 \times 10^4$	0.030	0.034	0.44
	$D = 3 \times 10^4$	0.039	0.043	0.48
	$D = 5 \times 10^4$	0.045	0.052	0.51
	$D = 7 \times 10^4$	0.054	0.060	0.54

(1) Query-relevant set (S) collection. This can be done offline [20] or online [15], as discussed in Sect. 3.2. We investigate the effects of various query-relevant set **S** collection methods by applying them to re-rank three retrieval systems: the baseline system (S1), spatial verification (S2), and average query expansion (AQE) (S3). Initially, we investigate the effects of various ways to collect **S** based on re-ranking the baseline system (S1). As seen in Table 3, the retrieval accuracy is 14.5 % (9.5 %) higher than S1 on the Oxford 5K (Paris 6K) dataset, when **S** is formed by offline expansion. In addition, online expansion is performed by including **S** as all words included in the spatially verified regions **S** (as done by AQE in [15]). The difference between the retrieval results is minor, *e.g.* 0.701 *v.s.* 0.696 on the Oxford 5K dataset. Moreover, combining offline and online expansion leads to a small rise in mAP scores for S1. Similar to S1, offline expansion also enables an increase in retrieval accuracy when re-ranking the results returned by S2 and S3, while the online expansion methods lead to mAP scores close to the offline version but with more expensive computational cost during runtime. Therefore, we use the computationally cheaper offline expansion in the experiments.

(2) Query-relevant (S) selection weight. We investigate the effects of query-relevant set (**S**) on the re-ranking results. This is done by enlarging weight b in

Table 3. Illustration of the effects of various context expansion methods on the re-ranking results. In this process,the query-relevant sets **S** are collected by online or offline expansion, while the re-ranking is based on three kinds of retrieval system, namely: $S1$, Baseline [1]; $S2$, Spatial Re-ranking [1]; $S3$, AQE [15]. The offline expansion is computationally cheaper compared to the online expansion, while its performance is close to the online versions on all the three systems.

Datasets	Retrieval system		Context expansion method		
	System ID	System baseline	Offline [20]	Online [15]	Offline + Online
Oxford5K	S1	0.612	0.701	0.696	0.703
	S2	0.645	0.700	0.703	0.706
	S3	0.806	0.814	0.825	0.830
Paris6K	S1	0.639	0.700	0.705	0.705
	S2	0.653	0.704	0.709	0.709
	S3	0.769	0.770	0.777	0.773

the random mapping function (Eq. 2) while fixing weight $a = 10$ in Table 1: (i) f_4: $b = \frac{a}{8}$; (ii) f_5: $b = \frac{a}{4}$; (iii) f_6: $b = \frac{a}{2}$; (iv) f_7: $b = a$. The query-relevant words are collected by offline query expansion. Note that the parameters $a > 1$, $b > 1$ in Eq. 2 indicate that both the query and query-relevant words have priority to be selected. We set $b = \frac{a}{2}$ by default in the following experiments as it achieves the best performance on both datasets.

5.4   Evaluation of Context Re-ranking

In the previous sections, we evaluate various parameters when generating contexts. As expected, the context re-ranking parameters, also affect the re-ranking results, which are discussed as follows:

(1) The range of top/bottom ranks. This is set by parameter H in Eq. 5. Figure 3(b) reports the retrieval accuracy with the increasing top/bottom-H. Intuitively, the range of top (bottom) ranks need to be relatively small compared to the dataset size so that it indicates whether a context is close to the query. As shown in Fig. 3(b), we obtain stable retrieval accuracy when H exceeds a threshold, where $H = 200$. Thus, we set $H = 200$ as default.

(2) The number of re-ranking iterations. Note that the re-ranking process is an updating scheme: the similarity score of each dataset image is refined according to the contextual information extracted from the ranking list. This process can be repeated such that each iteration generates re-ordered ranks, leading to updated contextual information. Figure 4 reports the re-ranking accuracy as the iteration number grows, on the Oxford 5K and Paris 6K datasets. As seen in Fig. 4, retrieval accuracy is increased when the iteration number raises from 0 (baseline) to 3. During this process, the highest performance gain occurs at the first iteration. However, the accuracy begins to drop after several iterations.

This is because random space partition usually includes noise due to the simplified clustering method. The noisy contextual information is accumulated within several iterations, thus decreasing the accuracy. Based on the above, we perform context based re-ranking once only in order to balance the efficiency and effectiveness.

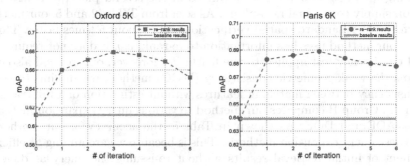

Fig. 4. Illustration of the effects of re-ranking iterations on the Oxford 5K and Paris 6K datasets. The iteration number raises from 0 (baseline) to 6, gradually. Best viewed in color (Color figure online).

Table 4. Comparison of the effectiveness and efficiency of various re-ranking methods on three datasets, measured by CPU second. Note that the runtime of AQE includes spatial verification and re-issuing query of the dataset. We only calculate the runtime of re-ranking, while do not include the CPU time spent on the initial baseline retrieval.

Method	Oxford 5K		Paris 6K		Oxford 105K	
	Runtime	mAP	Runtime	mAP	Runtime	mAP
Spatial verification	2.10	0.645	4.71	0.653	4.34	0.571
Our method	0.039	0.701	0.043	0.700	0.48	0.585
AQE	2.21	0.796	4.85	0.769	6.01	0.767

5.5   Comparison to State-of-the-Art

This section compares the accuracy and computation cost of our method to state-of-the-art.

1. Computational cost: As our method makes use of the inverted file structure, it requires no extra memory usage compared to the baseline tf-idf matching. Moreover, the runtime of our method consistently increases with D in terms of CPU time (Table 2) and accuracy (Fig. 3(a)). By truanting the dimension number, our method balances effectiveness and efficiency. In addition, Table 4 compares our method to the spatial verification and AQE methods in terms of both accuracy and runtime. As seen in Table 4, our method outperforms the spatial verification method, while it is not as accurate as AQE. However, as AQE requires re-issuing the query from spatial verified results, our method is able to reduce the computational cost while still increasing the accuracy over the baseline and spatial verification methods.

2. Accuracy: Table 5 compares the accuracy of our method to state-of-the-art in three groups. Group A compares our method to some widely used spatial re-ranking methods. Our method is ranked in the second place, although it is based on simply contextual re-ranking. As seen from Tables 2 and 5, our method outperforms the standard spatial verification and is about 5 times faster. This is because our method uses less information to re-rank, *e.g.* it does not require the spatial consistency test applied to the features. Moreover, our method also outperforms the weak geometric consistency (WGC) method, which aims to verify the consistency between matching features without estimation of a full transformation [4]. Group B compares our method to various query expansion methods, such as AQE and DQE. As shown in Table 5, the accuracy of our method is below these query expansion methods. This is because we are aiming at efficient refinement of initial retrieval results without re-issuing the query as done by these query expansion methods. Compared to the query expansion methods, our method does not need online collection of query relevant visual words. The final group investigates the effect when our context re-ranking method is combined with other re-ranking methods, for example AQE and DQE. The results illustrate that our method can be combined with various query expansion methods, which leads to further improvement of retrieval performance.

Table 5. Retrieval performance comparison with state-of-the-art. Our method in this table is based on tf-idf similarity (S1). The results are all obtained from our implementation except those are taken from literatures. Note that our results are slightly different from the results reported in the original paper due to the repetition in implementation.

Method		Oxford 5K	Paris 6K	Oxford 105K
Group A	Baseline	0.612	0.639	0.515
	WGC [4] (no prior)	0.621	0.644	0.574
	Spatial Re-ranking [1]	0.645	0.653	0.571
	Our method	0.701	0.700	0.585
	iSP [16]	0.741 [16]	0.769 [16]	0.649 [16]
Group B	QE baseline [15]	0.708	0.736	0.679
	AQE [15]	0.796	0.769	0.767
	DQE [11]	0.798	0.783	0.802
	Hello neighbor [13]	0.814 [13]	0.803 [13]	0.767 [13]
Group C	**Our method + AQE** [15]	0.814	0.770	0.757
	Our method + DQE [11]	0.832	0.793	0.790

6 Conclusion

In this paper, we proposed a simple yet effective re-ranking method for improving the BoW based object retrieval system. In contrast to the standard re-ranking methods, our method analyses the image ranks in terms of shared contextual information rather than expensive spatial consistency examination. We exploit contextual information in two steps. Firstly, we use a random space partition method to cluster the dataset into a large number of image groups. Secondly, the image groups, namely contexts, are used to refine the similarity scores of dataset images by considering their context factors. The experimental results show that our method can provide a significant accuracy boost with minimal computational cost. In future, we plan to test our method on non-rigid object retrieval, since unlike other re-ranking methods we do not rely on spatial rigidity.

References

1. Philbin, J., Chum, O., Isard, M., Sivic, J., Zisserman, A.: Object retrieval with large vocabularies and fast spatial matching. In: Proceedings of the IEEE Conference on Computer Vision and Pattern Recognition, pp. 1–8 (2007)
2. Sivic, J., Zisserman, A.: Video Google: A text retrieval approach to object matching in videos. In: Proceedings of International Conference on Computer Vision, pp. 1470–1477 (2003)
3. Nister, D., Stewenius, H.: Scalable recognition with a vocabulary tree. In: Proceedings of the IEEE Conference on Computer Vision and Pattern Recognition, pp. 2161–2168 (2006)
4. Jegou, H., Douze, M., Schmid, C.: Hamming embedding and weak geometric consistency for large scale image search. In: Forsyth, D., Torr, P., Zisserman, A. (eds.) ECCV 2008, Part I. LNCS, vol. 5302, pp. 304–317. Springer, Heidelberg (2008)
5. Jégou, H., Douze, M., Schmid, C.: Improving bag-of-features for large scale image search. Int. J. Comp. Vis. **87**, 316–336 (2010)
6. Mikolajczyk, K., Tuytelaars, T., Schmid, C., Zisserman, A., Matas, J., Schaffalitzky, F., Kadir, T., Van Gool, L.: A comparison of affine region detectors. Int. J. Comp. Vis. **65**, 43–72 (2005)
7. Philbin, J., Chum, O., Isard, M., Sivic, J., Zisserman, A.: Lost in quantization: Improving particular object retrieval in large scale image databases. In: Proceedings of IEEE Conference on Computer Vision and Pattern Recognition (2008)
8. Mikulík, A., Perdoch, M., Chum, O., Matas, J.: Learning a fine vocabulary. In: Daniilidis, K., Maragos, P., Paragios, N. (eds.) ECCV 2010, Part III. LNCS, vol. 6313, pp. 1–14. Springer, Heidelberg (2010)
9. Jegou, H., Harzallah, H., Schmid, C.: A contextual dissimilarity measure for accurate and efficient image search. In: Proceedings of IEEE Conference on Computer Vision and Pattern Recognition, pp. 1–8 (2007)
10. Turcot, P., Lowe, D.: Better matching with fewer features: The selection of useful features in large database recognition problems. In: ICCV Workshop on Emergent Issues in Large Amounts of Visual Data, pp. 2109–2116 (2009)
11. Arandjelović, R., Zisserman, A.: Three things everyone should know to improve object retrieval. In: Proceedings of IEEE Conference on Computer Vision and Pattern Recognition (2012)

12. Qin, D., Wengert, C., Van Gool, L.: Query adaptive similarity for large scale object retrieval. In: Proceedings of IEEE Conference on Computer Vision and Pattern Recognition. IEEE (2013)
13. Qin, D., Gammeter, S., Bossard, L., Quack, T., van Gool, L.: Hello neighbor: accurate object retrieval with k-reciprocal nearest neighbors. In: Proceedings of IEEE Conference on Computer Vision and Pattern Recognition (2011)
14. Fern, X.Z., Brodley, C.E.: Random projection for high dimensional data clustering: A cluster ensemble approach. In: Proceedings of International Conference on Machine Learning, vol. 3, pp. 186–193 (2003)
15. Chum, O., Philbin, J., Sivic, J., Isard, M., Zisserman, A.: Total recall: Automatic query expansion with a generative feature model for object retrieval. In: Proceedings of IEEE Conference on Computer Vision and Pattern Recognition, pp. 1–8 (2007)
16. Chum, O., Mikulik, A., Perdoch, M., Matas, J.: Total recall ii: Query expansion revisited. In: Proceedings of IEEE Conference on Computer Vision and Pattern Recognition (2011)
17. Guimarães Pedronette, D.C., da S. Torres, R.: Image re-ranking and rank aggregation based on similarity of ranked lists. In: Real, P., Diaz-Pernil, D., Molina-Abril, H., Berciano, A., Kropatsch, W. (eds.) CAIP 2011, Part I. LNCS, vol. 6854, pp. 369–376. Springer, Heidelberg (2011)
18. Chen, Y., Li, X., Dick, A., Hill, R.: Ranking consistency for image matching and object retrieval. Pattern Recogn. **47**, 1349–1360 (2014)
19. Philbin, J., Sivic, J., Zisserman, A.: Geometric latent dirichlet allocation on a matching graph for large-scale image datasets. Int. J. Comp. Vis. **95**, 138–153 (2011)
20. Chen, Y., Dick, A., van den Hengel, A.: Image retrieval with a visual thesaurus. In: 2010 International Conference on Digital Image Computing: Techniques and Applications, pp. 8–14 (2010)
21. Chum, O., Philbin, J., Zisserman, A.: Near duplicate image detection: min-hash and tf-idf weighting. In: Proceedings of the British Machine Vision Conference, vol. 3, p. 4 (2008)
22. Bowman, A.W., Azzalini, A.: Applied Smoothing Techniques for Data Analysis. Oxford University Press, Oxford (1997)
23. http://www.robots.ox.ac.uk/~vgg/data/
24. http://press.liacs.nl/mirflickr/dlform.php
25. http://www.robots.ox.ac.uk/~vgg/software/fastcluster/

Adaptive Structural Model for Video Based Pedestrian Detection

Junjie Yan, Bin Yang, Zhen Lei$^{(\boxtimes)}$, and Stan Z. Li

Center for Biometrics and Security Research and National Laboratory of Pattern Recognition, Institute of Automation, Chinese Academy of Sciences, Beijing, China
{jjyan,bin.yang,zlei,szli}@nlpr.ia.ac.cn

Abstract. The performance of generic pedestrian detector usually declines seriously for videos in novel scenes, which is one of the major bottlenecks for current pedestrian detection techniques. The conventional works improve pedestrian detection in video by mining new instances from detections and adapting the detector according to the collected instances. However, when treating the two tasks separately, the detector adaptation suffers from the defective output of instance mining. In this paper, we propose to jointly handle the instance mining and detector adaption using an adaptive structural model. The regularization function of the model is applied on detector to prevent overfitting in adaption, and the loss function is designed to evaluate the combination of mined instances set and detector. Particularly, we extend the Deformable Part Model (DPM) to adaptive DPM, where an adaptive feature transformation defined on low-level HOG cell is learned to reduce the domain shift, and the regularization function for the detector is conducted on the transformation. The loss of the instance set and detector is measured by a cost-flow network structure which incorporates both the appearance of frame-wise detections and their spatio-temporal continuity. We demonstrate an alternating minimization procedure to optimize the model. The proposed method is evaluated on ETHZ, PETS2009 and Caltech datasets, and outperforms baseline DPM by 7 % in terms of mean miss rate.

1 Introduction

Pedestrian detection has been a hot research topic for decades. Benefitting from the advances in low-level feature and high-level model, static image based pedestrian detection has achieved impressive progresses in both effectiveness [1–8] and efficiency [9–13]. With well-designed feature and model, current detectors trained on a large set can handle some occlusions, pose and viewpoint variations. However, the performance on novel scenes may drop disastrously due to the domain shift. For example, according to the evaluation in [14], the state-of-the-art pedestrian detector Crosstalk [12] achieves 19 % mean miss rate on INRIA test set, while increases to 54 % on Caltech Pedestrian Benchmark.

To handle the domain shift, one promising solution is the automatic adaption of the generic detector to the target scenes, as recently explored in [15–22]. Most of the works followed an unsupervised paradigm since the annotations in novel scenes are often unavailable. These works usually considered two tasks in

© Springer International Publishing Switzerland 2015
D. Cremers et al. (Eds.): ACCV 2014, Part I, LNCS 9003, pp. 211–226, 2015.
DOI: 10.1007/978-3-319-16865-4_14

detector adaptation. The first is to mine new positive and negative instances of the target video in an unsupervised manner, and the second is to adapt the generic detector when the training instances of the target video are collected. The standard paradigm in these works is as follows (Fig. 1(a)), (1) conduct frame-wise detection on video; (2) use various information (e.g., tracking, background substraction and optical flow) to mine instances from the detection result; (3) take the mined instances as online training samples to update the detector.

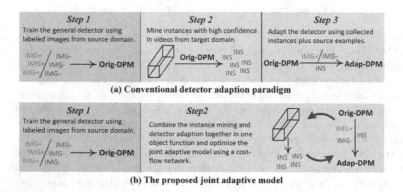

(a) Conventional detector adaption paradigm

(b) The proposed joint adaptive model

Fig. 1. Different paradigms of detector adaptation for video based pedestrian detection. The conventional methods take the training instance mining and detector adaptation as two separate tasks. In this paper, to explore the benefit from each other, we propose to optimize the instance mining and detector adaptation jointly in a structural model.

The motivation of our approach is that the instance mining and detector adaptation procedures should be explored jointly. For example, the detector can benefit from the confidently mined clear instances in adaptation, and the well adapted detector can further improve the quality of mined instances. Given the frame-wise detection result, we build a joint structural model to find an optimal combination of adapted detector and new instances from the video (Fig. 1(b)). Particularly, we build a frame-wise detector with DPM. To avoid the complexity in shifting the high dimensional DPM parameters directly, we propose to use a linear transformation to capture the domain shift on low-level HOG cell, which can effectively capture the variations in different conditions with much less parameters. The loss function in the structural model is built on a cost-flow network to capture the structure in video, where both the frame-wise appearance and the video continuity among frames are encoded. We show that when the instance set is fixed, the optimal detector can be solved by standard quadratic programming, and when the detector is fixed, the model can be solved by efficient successive shortest-path algorithm. In optimizing the structural model, we conduct an alternating scheme to conduct frame-wise detection and structural model adaptation iteratively.

We validate the detection performance following the protocol provided in [14] on challenging videos from ETHZ, Caltech, and PETS2009. Our structural model decreases mean miss rate by more than 7% compared to the baseline DPM (version 5), and outperforms the best published results by a 2% margin.

The rest of the paper is organized as follows. We discuss the related work in Sect. 2 and provide the background of DPM and cost-flow network based data association in Sect. 3. The joint structural model and the corresponding optimization method are described in Sect. 4. We demonstrate the experimental results in Sect. 5 and finally conclude the paper in Sect. 6.

2   Related Work

There are numerous works on pedestrian detection, and we refer readers to [14,23,24] for the detailed survey. Our work is most related to the work on adapting the generic pedestrian detector to videos, which is recently explored in [16–22,25,26]. These works differ in the training instances mining and detector adaptation methods. Methods presented in [16,18,19] mined new instances from detections according to a pre-defined threshold. To reduce the noise in the detected results, context cues were applied to refine the detections. References [19,20,25] explored context cues on background to remove the detections with high scores. Reference [16] used multiple target tracking to associate detections with trajectories, and took the non-associated detections as negative instances. Reference [18] conducted KLT tracking to collect positive instances with low detection scores. Reference [17] proposed an unsupervised tree coding method to cluster the detections. Reference [20] proposed a confidence score SVM to encode the confidence scores in the model updating. The learning algorithms largely depend on the models used in the generic detector. For example, [16,21,25,26] were built on boosting detectors, [17–20] were built on SVM detectors, [22] was built on the deep neural network. To the best of our knowledge, this is the first work to jointly consider the instance mining and detector adaptation in one objective function.

The problem setting is also related to the domain adaptation, which has been studied extensively in computer vision. We learn a feature transformation between the source and the target domain, as explored in [27–29] in an unsupervised manner. The most similar models as ours are the unsupervised approaches proposed in [30,31]. However, these unsupervised approaches were based on generative models, making themselves unsuitable for real world detection tasks where discriminative models are always adopted. In addition, these work are designed for images instead of videos.

Our detector is built on DPM (Deformable Part Model) [6], which is one of the state-of-the-art detectors for generic detection tasks on static images. However, as evaluated in [14], its performance is unsatisfying for videos in real applications (e.g., Caltech benchmark [14]). Our method can be seen as an extension of DPM to adaptive-DPM for videos, where the detector is adapted automatically and the spatio-temporal continuity in videos is explored. Since the feature dimension in DPM is very high (more than 20 K), it's infeasible to adapt it directly. Instead we introduce a feature transform on the cell level of HOG features, which can effectively capture the holistic low-level appearance change caused by domain shift. In the description of the model, we use a bilinear form of DPM used in [32] to simplify our notation.

We employ cost-flow network as part of our structural model, which is related to detection based multiple-target tracking [33–39]. Previous detection based multiple-target tracking methods rely on a fixed detector, while we adapt the detector automatically. The tracker outputs the trajectories of detections of multiple targets, while we focus on improving the detection performance. Due to the noticeable improvement of object detection in videos, our work can serve as a more reliable initialization for detection based tracking.

3   Preliminaries

In this section, we briefly introduce the bilinear form of DPM [6] and the cost-flow based data association [33]. The former model is the basis of our pedestrian detector, and the latter one is the structure on which we define the objective function with both appearance and spatio-temporal constraints.

3.1   Bilinear DPM

The popular DPM provides a hierarchical representation for pedestrians (as well as other objects). It contains a root filter and a set of deformable part filters. Without loss of generalization, we take the root as a special part here. Given an image I and a configuration of parts $\zeta = \{l_0, l_1, \cdots, l_m\}$ in the detection window, we define the detection score of the configuration with respect to the DPM detector $\mathcal{F}$ as

$$score(\mathcal{F}, I, \zeta) = \sum_{i=0}^{m} w_i^T \phi_a(I, l_i) + w_s^T \phi_s(\zeta), \tag{1}$$

where w_i is the filter of the ith part, and $\phi_a(I, l_i)$ is the HOG [1] feature vector extracted at l_i. w_s is the shape prior which prefers a particular configuration, and $\phi_s(\zeta)$ is the spatial feature vector of the configuration ζ. Here l_0 is the location of the root, and l_i is the location of the ith part. It is straightforward to introduce the mixture components in Eq. 1, so we leave them out to simplify the exposition.

In this paper, we use the bilinear form of DPM originally introduced in [32]. It equals to the standard DPM, but can simplify the notation of our adaptive DPM introduced in the next section. Similar formulation is also proposed in [8]. The HOG feature of the ith part is denoted as a $n_f \times n_k$ dimensional matrix $\phi_a(I, l_i)$, where n_k is the number of cells in the part, and n_f is the dimension of gradient histogram feature vector for a cell. Each column in $\phi_a(I, l_i)$ is a feature vector of a cell. $\phi_a(I, l_i)$ are further concatenated to be a large matrix $\Phi_a(I, \zeta) = [\phi_a(I, l_0), \phi_a(I, l_1), \cdots \phi_a(I, l_m)]$. The appearance filters in the detector are concatenated to be a matrix W_a in the same way. With these notations, the detection score of DPM [6] equals

$$score(\mathcal{F}, I, \zeta) = Tr(W_a^T \Phi_a(I, \zeta)) + w_s^T \phi_s(\zeta), \tag{2}$$

where $Tr(\cdot)$ is the trace operation which is defined as summation of the elements on the main diagonal of a matrix. The bilinear form DPM detector is parameterized by the appearance parameter matrix W_a and spatial parameter matrix w_s. For a scanning window in detection, only the root location l_0 is given, and all the part locations are taken as latent variables which are optimized at runtime. The detection score of the sliding window is denoted as $score(I, \zeta^*)$, where ζ^* is the best possible part configuration when the root location is fixed to be l_0. Using quadratic function to model the spatial deformation of each part, the problem can be effectively solved with linear complexity [6].

3.2   Cost-Flow Based Data Association

Cost-flow based data association is proposed in [33] to associate detections in a video to be long trajectories. Finding the globally optimal trajectories for detections in video is reformulated as finding the min-cost flow in a network. Let us define the detection set in a video as $\mathcal{D} = \{d_1, \cdots, d_n\}$, where $d_i = \{\zeta_i, \sigma_i, t_i\}$ and n is the number of detections. ζ_i, σ_i, and t_i stand for the location, scale, and frame index respectively. The detection d_i corresponds to an edge from node u_i to v_i in the network. The c_i is the weight to represent the cost for d_i to be a pedestrian activation. For detections between different frames that have the possibility to belong to the same trajectory, an edge (v_i, u_j) is created and $c_{i,j}$ is used to represent the cost for the transition between v_i and u_j in one trajectory. To start the flow, source node s and sink node t are added to the network, where s links to all the u_i with cost $c_{s,i}$ and all the v_i are linked to the sink node t with cost $c_{t,i}$. The cost $c_{s,i}$ and $c_{t,i}$ are used to punish the number of trajectories. For each edge in the flow, there is an indicator to represent whether the edge is included in one trajectory, which is denoted as y_i, $y_{i,j}$, $y_{s,i}$ and $y_{t,i}$ for the edge $(u_i, v_i), (v_i, u_j), (s, u_i)$ and (v_i, t), respectively. To interpret the network flow as no overlap trajectory, the model uses the following constraints

$$y_{s,i} + \sum_{j=1}^{n} y_{j,i} = y_i = y_{t,i} + \sum_{j=1}^{n} y_{i,j}, \forall i \tag{3}$$

$$y_i, y_{s,i}, y_{t,i}, y_{i,j} \in \{0, 1\},$$

where y_i is 1 when the detection d_i is included in current trajectory, and otherwise 0. The above constraints guarantee that no paths share a common edge. The flow in the network is specified by $\mathcal{Y} = \{y_i, y_{i,j}, y_{s,i}, y_{t,i}\}$. Given the network and a configuration of $\mathcal{Y}$, the total cost is

$$L(\mathcal{D}, \mathcal{Y}) = \sum_{i=1}^{n} c_i y_i + \sum_{i=1}^{n} c_{s,i} y_{s,i} + \sum_{i=1}^{n} c_{t,i} y_{t,i} + \sum_{i=1}^{n} \sum_{j=1}^{n} c_{i,j} y_{i,j}, \tag{4}$$

where costs of all activated edges are summarized. When the cost terms are properly defined, finding the globally optimal trajectories is equivalent to solving the min-cost flow problem, where the cost is defined in Eq. 4 with constrains in Eq. 3. The optimization problem has been well explored. For example, [34] has shown an efficient successive shortest-paths algorithm with the complexity of $O(knlogn)$, where k is the number of trajectories and n is the number of detections. It is efficient enough in real applications (e.g., fewer than 10 s for a 10^3-frame video with 10^6 detections).

4   Adaptive Structural Model

Conventional methods consider the instance mining and detector adaptation as two separate tasks. In this way, the errors in instance mining could result in the drift of the detector, and the drift in detector adaptation could further harm the instance mining. To avoid the vicious circle, in this work, we propose to capture instance mining and detector adaptation jointly, where the instance mining and detector adaptation are handled in one objective function, and the joint optimization procedure outputs a combination of new instances and adapted detector.

Given the target video, we first conduct frame-wise detection and denote the detection result as $\mathcal{D}$. Due to the noise in detection, the detections in $\mathcal{D}$ cannot be taken as ground truth, instead we take them as latent variables, and label $\mathcal{D}$ by $\mathcal{Y}$ via an instance mining module. Here the indicator set $\mathcal{Y} = \{y_1, \cdots, y_n\}$ and $y_i \in \{0, 1\}$, where $y_i = 1$ indicates that the detection d_i is taken as the true positive, otherwise $y_i = 0$. Given the original detector $\mathcal{F}^0$ and the detection set $\mathcal{D}$, we propose to find the optimal adapted detector $\mathcal{F}^*$, and the new indicator set $\mathcal{Y}^*$ with our designed objective function as

$$(\mathcal{F}^*, \mathcal{Y}^*) = \arg\min_{\mathcal{F}, \mathcal{Y}} R(\mathcal{F}, \mathcal{F}^0) + \eta L(\mathcal{D}, \mathcal{F}, \mathcal{Y}), \tag{5}$$

where $R(\mathcal{F}, \mathcal{F}^0)$ is used to regularize the new detector $\mathcal{F}$ by the original detector $\mathcal{F}^0$, and $L(\mathcal{F}, \mathcal{D}, \mathcal{Y})$ is the loss term to measure the fitness between the adapted model $\mathcal{F}$ and the final detection result, which is specified by $\mathcal{D}$ and its indicator set $\mathcal{Y}$. The loss function is designed to encode the structural information in the target video. Two kinds of information can be encoded, the first is the appearance in detections, and the second is the spatio-temporal continuity in the video. The objective function in Eq. 5 naturally combines the instances mining and detector adaptation in a unified framework, and enables two tasks to benefit from each other. In the following parts, we define the regularization and loss function, and show how to optimize the objective function.

4.1   Adaptive DPM and Regularization

We use the generic DPM detector [6] as the initial detector $\mathcal{F}^0$ and aim to find an optimized DPM detector $\mathcal{F}$ on the target video. To avoid the direct adaptation of parameters of high dimensionality in DPM, we introduce a simple but effective adaptive DPM and show how to regularize it in the structural model defined below.

In DPM based representation, pedestrian consists of a number of local parts, and each part is represented by HOG cells. In applying the generic pedestrian detector to a novel scene, we only consider the domain shift in appearance (e.g., illumination, imaging condition) and ignore the variations in viewpoint, since the viewpoint variations could be naturally handled by the DPM mixture model. Under this assumption, we argue that the structure of parts and HOG spatial relationship between different parts should remain unchanged in detector adaptation process, while domain shift can be captured at feature level. Particularly, we use a linear transformation P to model the mapping between the source and target domain in HOG cell level, which is a $n_f \times n_f$ dimensional matrix. When the transformation matrix P is given, the detection score in the *adaptive DPM* for a part configuration ζ is defined as

$$score(\mathcal{F}, I, \zeta) = Tr(W_a^T P \Phi_a(I, \zeta)) + w_s^T \phi_s(\zeta), \tag{6}$$

where an additional feature transformation P is conducted before the feature $\Phi_a(I, \zeta)$, which is then fed into the appearance filter W_a. Here the model $\mathcal{F}$ is specified by W_a, w_s and P. The Eq. 2 can be taken as a special case of Eq. 6 when the transformation matrix P is the identity matrix. To avoid the overfitting in model adaptation, we use the identity matrix I to regularize P by

$$R(\mathcal{F}, \mathcal{F}^0) = \|P - I\|_F^2, \tag{7}$$

where the Frobenius norm $\| \cdot \|_F$ is defined as the square root of the sum of the absolute squares of the elements in a matrix. It is of particular importance for video based detection since the feature vector is high dimensional while the number of mined instances is usually about a few hundred. The number of variables needed for adaptation is $n_f \times n_c$ in the original DPM, where n_c is the number of HOG cells in all parts. In adaptive DPM, we only need to adapt $n_f \times n_f$ parameters, which brings about more efficiency (in typical DPM models, n_c is one order larger than n_f).

4.2   Loss Function

The loss function is used to measure the detector $\mathcal{F}$ and indicator set $\mathcal{Y}$ on the target video. In this paper, two kinds of information are considered. The first is the frame-wise detection information, which means that detections activated in $\mathcal{Y}$ should have low appearance loss (i.e. high detection score). The second is that the activated detections should satisfy the video continuity, for example a stand alone detection in video is very likely to be a false positive and should be indicated as a false detection in $\mathcal{Y}$. To capture the above two types of information, we borrow the idea from cost-flow based data association, and measure the loss of indicator set $\mathcal{Y}$ and detector $\mathcal{F}$ jointly with the following function

$$L(\mathcal{F}, \mathcal{D}, \mathcal{Y}) = \sum_{i=1}^{n} (c_{t,i} y_{t,i} + c_{s,i} y_{s,i} + c_i y_i) \tag{8}$$

$$where \quad c_i = \max(\xi_1, \xi_2 - score(\mathcal{F}, I, \zeta_i))$$

$$s.t. \quad y_{s,i} + \sum_{j=1}^{n} y_{j,i} = y_i = y_{t,i} + \sum_{j=1}^{n} y_{i,j}, \forall i$$

$$and \quad y_i, y_{i,j}, y_{s,i}, y_{t,i} \in \{0, 1\},$$

where the indicator $\mathcal{Y}$ now includes auxiliary variables. The $score(\mathcal{F}, I, \zeta_i)$ is defined in adaptive DPM as Eq. 6. The above problem can be seen as an instantiation of the general cost-flow based data association problem introduced in Eq. 4. The appearance cost c_i is defined as a generalized hinge loss of adaptive DPM detection score. The intuition inside the definition is that detections with high appearance scores should be activated with a negative loss value, while the detections with low appearance scores should be suppressed with a positive value. The parameter ξ_1 and ξ_2 can be tuned according to the range of detection scores. The costs $c_{s,i}$ and $c_{t,i}$ which involve the source and sink nodes are fixed to be positive constraint. They can be considered as a punishment to the number of trajectory, which can help to remove the discontinuous false positives.

4.3 Adaptive Optimization

In video based detection, we need to determine the new detector $\mathcal{F}$ specified by P, the frame-wise detection set $\mathcal{D}$, and the indicator set $\mathcal{Y}$ of the detection set. Advocated by recent latent structural learning works, we adopt the alternating minimization procedure to optimize them.

Algorithm 1. Adaptive Structural Optimization for Video based Pedestrian Detection.

1: **Input:**
   The video V, and the generic detector $\mathcal{F}_0$.
2: Set $\mathcal{F} = \mathcal{F}_0$, i.e. $P = I$.
3: **for** i=1 **to** T_1 **do**
4:    Conduct the frame-wise adaptive DPM detection procedure with detector $\mathcal{F}$ by Eq. 6, and get the detection set $\mathcal{D}$ of the video.
5:    **for** j=1 **to** T_2 **do**
6:       Fix the P, and solve the optimal indicator set $\mathcal{Y}$ by minimizing $L(P, \mathcal{D}, \mathcal{Y})$ with the successive shortest-paths algorithm.
7:       Fix the $\mathcal{Y}$, and solve the optimal P in Eq. 11 with standard quadratic programming procedure.
8:    **end for**
9: **end for**
10: **return** $(\mathcal{F}, \mathcal{D}, \mathcal{Y})$.

The whole optimization procedure is shown in Algorithm 1. In the outer loop, we conduct the adaptive DPM detector for frame-wise detection to get the detection set D. When $\mathcal{D}$ is fixed, the detection indicator $\mathcal{Y}$ and the adapted detector $\mathcal{F}$ are jointly optimized by the following problem

$$(\mathcal{Y}^*, P^*) = \arg\min_{\mathcal{Y}, P} \|P - I\|_F^2 + \eta L(P, \mathcal{D}, \mathcal{Y}) \tag{9}$$

$$s.t. \quad y_{s,i} + \sum_{j=1}^{n} y_{j,i} = y_i = y_{t,i} + \sum_{j=1}^{n} y_{i,j}, \forall i$$

$$and \quad y_i, y_{s,i}, y_{t,i}, y_{i,j} \in \{0,1\},$$

where the $L(P, \mathcal{D}, \mathcal{Y})$ is exactly the $L(\mathcal{F}, \mathcal{D}, \mathcal{Y})$, since F can be specified by P. The filters W_a and w_s in $\mathcal{F}$ are from the generic detector and fixed in the whole procedure. It is a difficult mixed programming non-convex problem when both $\mathcal{Y}$ and P are free. We therefore resort to an iterative algorithm based on the fact that solving $\mathcal{Y}$ given P, and solving P given $\mathcal{Y}$ are convex problems, and there exists off-the-shelf solvers. In detail, we solve the following two problems.

Fix $\mathcal{Y}$ to solve P When $\mathcal{Y}$ is given, the constrains in Eq. 9 can be removed, and the problem becomes to be

$$\arg\min_{P} \|P - I\|_F^2 \tag{10}$$

$$+ \eta \sum_{i=1}^{n} y_i \cdot max(\zeta_1, \zeta_2 - (Tr(W_a^T P \Phi_a(I, \zeta_i)) + w_s^T \phi_s(\zeta_i))),$$

Since $Tr(W_a^T P \Phi_a(I, \zeta_i))$ is equal to $Tr(P \Phi_a(I, \zeta_i) W_a^T)$, the above problem equals

$$\arg\min_{P} \|vec(P) - vec(I)\|^2 \tag{11}$$

$$+ \eta \sum_{i=1}^{n} y_i \cdot max(\xi_1, \xi_2 - (vec(P)^T vec(\Phi_a(I, \zeta_i) W_a^T) + w_s^T \phi_s(\zeta))),$$

where $vec(\cdot)$ is the operator to reshape the matrix to be a vector in a column-wise manner. The above problem can be solved effectively by standard quadratic programming solvers [40].

Fix P to solve $\mathcal{Y}$ When the transformation matrix P is given, Eq. 5 becomes $\arg\min_{\mathcal{Y}} L(P, \mathcal{D}, \mathcal{Y})$ under the cost-flow constraint, which can be effectively solved by successive shortest-paths algorithm described in [34]. In the algorithm, we iteratively find the minimum-cost parts γ from the source to the sink in the residual graph, and update the flow by pushing the unit-flow along γ if the total cost of the path is negative.

Since the objective value is reduced in both of the two subproblems of the inner loop, it can be easily proved that the inner loop will converge to a local minima. We set the loop number T_1 to be 5, the loop number T_2 to be 8 and validate the convergence of the whole optimization procedure in experiments.

5 Experiment

Experiments are conducted on challenging videos from ETHZ [41], Caltech [10] and PETS2009[1] pedestrian datasets. The ETHZ and Caltech are captured from moving camera, while the PETS2009 is captured from stationary camera. Particularly, the Bahnhof sequences from ETHZ, S2-L2 from PETS2009, and 8 sequences from Caltech with most people are selected for evaluation. The ETHZ-Bahnhof sequences contain 999 frames and 8467 pedestrians; the PETS2009-S2-L2 sequences contain 436 frames and 8927 pedestrians; the 8 sequences from Caltech testset are with the length of about 1800 frames. These videos are challenging for cluttered background, large illumination variations, and heavy occlusion. The DPM detector (Version 5) trained on the INRIA dataset [1] is taken as the baseline. Since the detector can only detect pedestrians of above 120 pixels in height, we resize every video frame with a scale of 2.5, and only measure pedestrians of above 50 pixels in height as suggested in [14]. For all the experiments, ξ_1, ξ_2, $c_{s,i}$ and $c_{t,i}$ used in Eq. 8 are fixed to be -1, 0.2, 10 and 10, respectively.

We follow the publicly available evaluation protocol in [14], except that the evaluations are conducted for each video separately. Full ROC curve and mean miss rate[2] are used to compare different algorithms. In the following parts, we compare different detector adaptation methods and examine the convergence of the outer loop in Algorithm 1, and finally compare the detection performance with other state-of-the-art detectors.

5.1 Different Methods for Video Based Detection

In this part, we compare four different approaches for video based pedestrian detection on PETS2009-S2-L2, which is challenging for appearance variations in illumination and occlusion. These approaches include: (1) Generic DPM, the baseline DPM detector (version 5) learned on INRIA; (2) DPM + Adaptation, which iteratively adds new training instances according to the frame-wise detection score, and then adapts the DPM detector using the collected instances; (3) DPM + Tracking + Adaptation, which uses the tracked detections as the new instances to adapt the DPM detector, where the tracking is solved by cost-flow network; (4) The proposed method that jointly considers instance mining and detector adaptation.

ROC curves and mean miss rates of the four methods are demonstrated in Fig. 2. Due to the noise in training instances used, direct adaptation could cause the drift problem, and in this experiment it only improves a small margin over the original generic detector. Since a lot of false positives can be removed by optimizing the cost-flow network, the instances used in adapting the detector are

---

[1] http://www.cvg.rdg.ac.uk/PETS2009/.

[2] The mean miss rate defined in P. Dollár's toolbox is used here, which is the average miss rate at 0.0100, 0.0178, 0.0316, 0.0562, 0.1000, 0.1778, 0.3162, 0.5623 and 1.0000 false-positive-per-image.

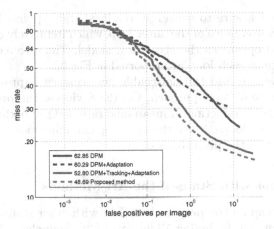

Fig. 2. Pedestrian detection results of different methods on PETS2009-S2-L2.

clear enough in the DPM + Tracking + Adaptation procedure, and it improves the performance with quite a large margin. Benefiting from the joint model, our approach achieves the best performance and outperforms the baseline generic DPM with 14 % reduction in mean miss rate. Compared with the sequential instance mining and detector adaptation approach, the proposed joint learning method further reduces the mean miss rate by 4 %.

5.2 The Convergence

In this part, we validate the convergence of the proposed method. 8 videos from Caltech testset with most pedestrians are selected for evaluation. Since the inner

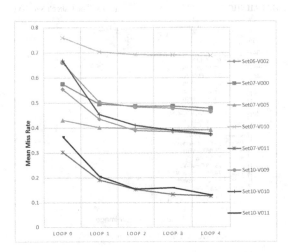

Fig. 3. The convergence illustration of the proposed optimization method in video based pedestrian detection.

loop in Algorithm 1 is sure to converge to a local stable point, in this part, we only validate the convergence of the outer loop, which iteratively conducts framewise detection and optimizes the structural model. The selected video ID and the mean miss rate at each loop are reported in Fig. 3.

From Fig. 3, we can find the noticeable performance improvement and the fast convergence rate of our approach. On the 8 videos, the proposed method has an average of 16 % reduction in mean miss rate and the performance is close to convergence after 3 loops. Since the first loop can mine most of the instances, it contributes most to the performance.

5.3   Comparisons with State-of-the-Art Methods

In this part, we compare the proposed method with other state-of-the-art algorithms, collected in [14], including Viola-Jones [42], Shapelet [43], LatSVM-V1,

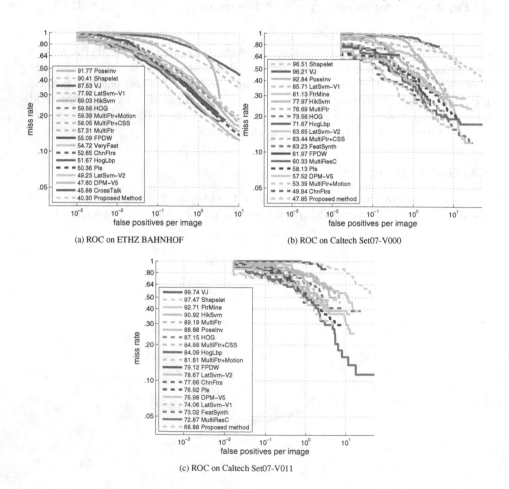

(a) ROC on ETHZ BAHNHOF

(b) ROC on Caltech Set07-V000

(c) ROC on Caltech Set07-V011

Fig. 4. Quantitative evaluations on ETHZ and Caltech.

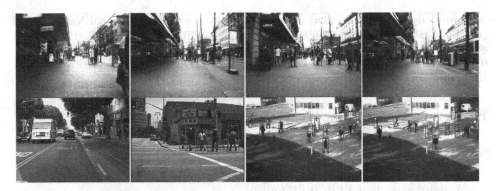

Fig. 5. Qualitative results of the proposed video base pedestrian detection on the ETHZ, Caltech and PETS2009.

LatSVM-V2 [6], PoseInv [44], HOGLbp [4], HikSVM [3], HOG [1], FtrMine [45], MultFtr [43], MultiFtr+CSS [43], Pls [46], MultiFtr+Motion [43], FPDW [10], FeatSynth [47], ChnFtrs [48], MultiResC [7], Veryfast [11], and CrossTalk [12]. We show the results of the video Bahnhof in ETHZ, the set07-V000 and set07-V011 in Caltech[3].

Figure 4 illustrates the quantitative results of different methods. On all the three videos, the proposed method outperforms the baseline DPM (version 5) by more than 7 %, and outperforms the published state-of-the-art results. It improves about 5 % on the ETHZ Bahnhof, 2 % on Caltech Set07-V000, and 4 % on Caltech Set07-V011 than the best published results. Some qualitative examples are shown in Fig. 5.

While the structural model optimization step is very efficient, most of the calculation is spent on frame-wise detection. In our implementation, we modify the code of the FFT based implementation [49] for fast convolution computation. Some techniques can be used to further accelerate the loop, such as the cascade detection or only detecting a subset in the early steps of the outer loop in Algorithm 1, and we leave it in future work.

6 Conclusion

In this paper, we propose a joint structural model to adapt the generic pedestrian detector for video based pedestrian detection. The instance mining and detector adaptation are formulated in one objective function, and an alternating minimization procedure is adopted to optimize it. The DPM is extended to be adaptive-DPM, where a feature transformation defined on low-level HOG cell is used to reduce the domain shift. We demonstrate noticeable improvement over the methods that treat the two tasks independently, and other state-of-the-art detectors on challenging videos from Caltech, ETHZ and PETS2009.

---

[3] The two videos are selected as they contain more people than other videos.

Acknowledgement. This work was supported by the Chinese National Natural Science Foundation Projects #61105023, #61103156, #61105037, #61203267, #61375037, #61473291, National Science and Technology Support Program Project #2013BAK 02B01, Chinese Academy of Sciences Project No. KGZD-EW-102-2, and AuthenMetric R&D Funds.

References

1. Dalal, N., Triggs, B.: Histograms of oriented gradients for human detection. In: CVPR. IEEE (2005)
2. Yan, J., Lei, Z., Yi, D., Li, S.Z.: Multi-pedestrian detection in crowded scenes: A global view. In: CVPR. IEEE (2012)
3. Maji, S., Berg, A., Malik, J.: Classification using intersection kernel support vector machines is efficient. In: CVPR. IEEE (2008)
4. Wang, X., Han, T., Yan, S.: An hog-lbp human detector with partial occlusion handling. In: ICCV. IEEE (2009)
5. Walk, S., Majer, N., Schindler, K., Schiele, B.: New features and insights for pedestrian detection. In: CVPR. IEEE (2010)
6. Felzenszwalb, P., Girshick, R., McAllester, D., Ramanan, D.: Object detection with discriminatively trained part-based models. TPAMI (2010)
7. Park, D., Ramanan, D., Fowlkes, C.: Multiresolution models for object detection. In: Daniilidis, K., Maragos, P., Paragios, N. (eds.) ECCV 2010, Part IV. LNCS, vol. 6314, pp. 241–254. Springer, Heidelberg (2010)
8. Yan, J., Zhang, X., Lei, Z., Liao, S., Li, S.Z.: Robust multi-resolution pedestrian detection in traffic scenes. In: CVPR. IEEE (2013)
9. Huang, C., Nevatia, R.: High performance object detection by collaborative learning of joint ranking of granules features. In: CVPR. IEEE (2010)
10. Dollár, P., Belongie, S., Perona, P.: The fastest pedestrian detector in the west. In: BMVC 2010 (2010)
11. Benenson, R., Mathias, M., Timofte, R., Van Gool, L.: Pedestrian detection at 100 frames per second. In: CVPR. IEEE (2012)
12. Dollár, P., Appel, R., Kienzle, W.: Crosstalk cascades for frame-rate pedestrian detection. In: Fitzgibbon, A., Lazebnik, S., Perona, P., Sato, Y., Schmid, C. (eds.) ECCV 2012, Part II. LNCS, vol. 7573, pp. 645–659. Springer, Heidelberg (2012)
13. Yan, J., Lei, Z., Wen, L., Li, S.Z.: The fastest deformable part model for object detection. In: CVPR (2014)
14. Dollár, P., Wojek, C., Schiele, B., Perona, P.: Pedestrian detection: An evaluation of the state of the art. TPAMI (2012)
15. Yang, M., Zhu, S., Lv, F., Yu, K.: Correspondence driven adaptation for human profile recognition. In: CVPR. IEEE (2011)
16. Sharma, P., Huang, C., Nevatia, R.: Unsupervised incremental learning for improved object detection in a video. In: CVPR. IEEE (2012)
17. Wang, X., Hua, G., Han, T.X.: Detection by detections: Non-parametric detector adaptation for a video. In: CVPR. IEEE (2012)
18. Tang, K., Ramanathan, V., Fei-Fei, L., Koller, D.: Shifting weights: Adapting object detectors from image to video. In: NIPS (2012)
19. Wang, M., Wang, X.: Automatic adaptation of a generic pedestrian detector to a specific traffic scene. In: CVPR. IEEE (2011)
20. Wang, M., Li, W., Wang, X.: Transferring a generic pedestrian detector towards specific scenes. In: CVPR. IEEE (2012)

21. Sharma, P., Nevatia, R.: Efficient detector adaptation for improved object detection in a video. In: CVPR. IEEE (2013)
22. Yang, Y., Shu, G., Shah, M.: Semi-supervised learning of feature hierarchies for object detection in a video. In: CVPR. IEEE (2013)
23. Enzweiler, M., Gavrila, D.: Monocular pedestrian detection: Survey and experiments. TPAMI (2009)
24. Geronimo, D., Lopez, A., Sappa, A., Graf, T.: Survey of pedestrian detection for advanced driver assistance systems. PAMI (2010)
25. Roth, P.M., Sternig, S., Grabner, H., Bischof, H.: Classifier grids for robust adaptive object detection. In: CVPR. IEEE (2009)
26. Pang, J., Huang, Q., Yan, S., Jiang, S., Qin, L.: Transferring boosted detectors towards viewpoint and scene adaptiveness. TIP (2011)
27. Saenko, K., Kulis, B., Fritz, M., Darrell, T.: Adapting visual category models to new domains. In: Daniilidis, K., Maragos, P., Paragios, N. (eds.) ECCV 2010, Part IV. LNCS, vol. 6314, pp. 213–226. Springer, Heidelberg (2010)
28. Kulis, B., Saenko, K., Darrell, T.: What you saw is not what you get: Domain adaptation using asymmetric kernel transforms. In: CVPR. IEEE (2011)
29. Gao, T., Stark, M., Koller, D.: What makes a good detector? – Structured priors for learning from few examples. In: Fitzgibbon, A., Lazebnik, S., Perona, P., Sato, Y., Schmid, C. (eds.) ECCV 2012, Part V. LNCS, vol. 7576, pp. 354–367. Springer, Heidelberg (2012)
30. Gopalan, R., Li, R., Chellappa, R.: Domain adaptation for object recognition: An unsupervised approach. In: ICCV. IEEE (2011)
31. Gong, B., Shi, Y., Sha, F., Grauman, K.: Geodesic flow kernel for unsupervised domain adaptation. In: CVPR. IEEE (2012)
32. Pirsiavash, H., Ramanan, D.: Steerable part models. In: CVPR. IEEE (2012)
33. Zhang, L., Li, Y., Nevatia, R.: Global data association for multi-object tracking using network flows. In: CVPR. IEEE (2008)
34. Pirsiavash, H., Ramanan, D., Fowlkes, C.C.: Globally-optimal greedy algorithms for tracking a variable number of objects. In: CVPR. IEEE (2011)
35. Berclaz, J., Fleuret, F., Fua, P.: Multiple object tracking using flow linear programming. In: PETS-Winter. IEEE (2009)
36. Jiang, H., Fels, S., Little, J.J.: A linear programming approach for multiple object tracking. In: CVPR. IEEE (2007)
37. Yang, B., Huang, C., Nevatia, R.: Learning affinities and dependencies for multi-target tracking using a crf model. In: CVPR. IEEE (2011)
38. Andriyenko, A., Schindler, K.: Globally optimal multi-target tracking on a hexagonal lattice. In: Daniilidis, K., Maragos, P., Paragios, N. (eds.) ECCV 2010, Part I. LNCS, vol. 6311, pp. 466–479. Springer, Heidelberg (2010)
39. Wen, L., Li, W., Yan, J., Lei, Z., Yi, D., Li, S.Z.: Multiple target tracking based on undirected hierarchical relation hypergraph (2014)
40. Boyd, S., Vandenberghe, L.: Convex Optimization. Cambridge University Press, Cambridge (2009)
41. Ess, A., Leibe, B., Schindler, K., van Gool, L.: A mobile vision system for robust multi-person tracking. In: CVPR. IEEE (2008)
42. Viola, P., Jones, M., Snow, D.: Detecting pedestrians using patterns of motion and appearance. IJCV 63(2), 153–161 (2005)
43. Wojek, C., Schiele, B.: A performance evaluation of single and multi-feature people detection. In: Rigoll, G. (ed.) DAGM 2008. LNCS, vol. 5096, pp. 82–91. Springer, Heidelberg (2008)

44. Lin, Z., Davis, L.S.: A pose-invariant descriptor for human detection and segmentation. In: Forsyth, D., Torr, P., Zisserman, A. (eds.) ECCV 2008, Part IV. LNCS, vol. 5305, pp. 423–436. Springer, Heidelberg (2008)
45. Dollár, P., Tu, Z., Tao, H., Belongie, S.: Feature mining for image classification. In: CVPR. IEEE (2007)
46. Schwartz, W., Kembhavi, A., Harwood, D., Davis, L.: Human detection using partial least squares analysis. In: ICCV. IEEE (2009)
47. Bar-Hillel, A., Levi, D., Krupka, E., Goldberg, C.: Part-based feature synthesis for human detection. In: Daniilidis, K., Maragos, P., Paragios, N. (eds.) ECCV 2010, Part IV. LNCS, vol. 6314, pp. 127–142. Springer, Heidelberg (2010)
48. Dollár, P., Tu, Z., Perona, P., Belongie, S.: Integral channel features. In: BMVC (2009)
49. Dubout, C., Fleuret, F.: Exact acceleration of linear object detectors. In: Fitzgibbon, A., Lazebnik, S., Perona, P., Sato, Y., Schmid, C. (eds.) ECCV 2012, Part III. LNCS, vol. 7574, pp. 301–311. Springer, Heidelberg (2012)

Fusion of Auxiliary Imaging Information for Robust, Scalable and Fast 3D Reconstruction

Hainan Cui[✉], Shuhan Shen, Wei Gao, and Zhanyi Hu

National Laboratory of Pattern Recognition,
Institute of Automation, Chinese Academy of Sciences, Beijing, China
{hncui,shshen,wgao,huzy}@nlpr.ia.ac.cn

Abstract. One of the potentially effective means for 3D reconstruction is to reconstruct the scene in a global manner, rather than incrementally, by fully exploiting available auxiliary information on imaging condition, such as camera location by GPS, orientation by IMU(or Compass), focal length from EXIF etc. However these auxiliary information, though informative and valuable, is usually too noisy to be directly usable. In this paper, we present a global method by taking advantage of such noisy auxiliary information to improve SfM solving. More specifically, we introduce two effective iterative optimization algorithms directly initiated with such noisy auxiliary information. One is a robust iterative rotation estimation algorithm to deal with contaminated EG(epipolar graph), the other is a robust iterative scene reconstruction algorithm to deal with noisy GPS data for camera centers initialization. We found that by exclusively focusing on the inliers estimated at the current iteration, called potential inliers in this work, the optimization process initialized by such noisy auxiliary information could converge well and efficiently. Our proposed method is evaluated on real images captured by UAV(unmanned aerial vehicle), StreetView car and conventional digital cameras. Extensive experimental results show that our method performs similarly or better than many of the state-of-art reconstruction approaches, in terms of reconstruction accuracy and scene completeness, but more efficient and scalable for large-scale image datasets.

1 Introduction

With the progress of modern technology, many imaging devices come with built-in sensors, such as GPS, compass and inclinometer. In addition, UAV (unmanned aerial vehicle), which is usually equipped with GPS and IMU (inertial measurement unit), has become widely available to generate high resolution DSM (digital surface model). Fortunately, sensor data are recorded simultaneously during image acquisition phase and from which approximate camera poses, though too noisy to be directly useful for 3D reconstruction [1,2], can be obtained.

SfM approaches have been widely used to build 3D scene from images in the past few years. The state-of-art IBA(incremental bundle adjustment) approaches [3–5] start by selecting a few seed images for initial reconstruction, then repeatedly add new images to incrementally reconstruct the scene and refine the result

© Springer International Publishing Switzerland 2015
D. Cremers et al. (Eds.): ACCV 2014, Part I, LNCS 9003, pp. 227–242, 2015.
DOI: 10.1007/978-3-319-16865-4_15

by bundle adjustment. Although such an incremental mode finds its success in a variety of applications, it suffers from drift, large error accumulation, and heavy computational load. Contrary to IBA, many global algorithms [1,2,7–10] which simultaneously operate on all images are reported recently, in which the bundle adjustment, a time consuming module, is activated once rather than repeatedly. However, sometimes such global methods do not work well because the estimated parameters are not accurate enough for the bundle adjustment.

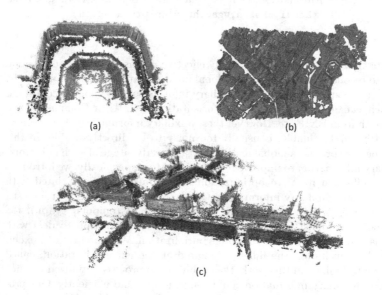

Fig. 1. 3D reconstruction results: (a) reconstruction by a conventional moving digital camera (MP; 144 images); (b) reconstruction by UAV (TK2; 501 images); (c) reconstruction by StreetView car (SV1; 2468 images). In order to better reflect the scene structure, here the results are further reconstructed by dense reconstruction method PMVS2 [6], which is a follow-up step of our method.

In this paper, we present a novel global strategy to solve SfM problem by fully exploiting available noisy auxiliary imaging information, such as GPS, IMU info, and compass angle. One key advantage of our method is its versatility, applicable to both ordered images (Fig. 1b and c) and unordered images (Fig. 1a). Another advantage of our method is its computational efficiency, and it works well for large scene reconstruction as shown in our experiments. For example, our SV2 image dataset contains 16600 images. Our proposed method has three steps. The first one is to build an EG (epipolar graph). The second one is a robust iterative rotation estimation. Since even under RANSAC paradigm, pairwise geometry estimates may still contain gross errors, global camera rotations are iteratively estimated by rotation consistency in this step. The last step is to iteratively perform triangulation and bundle adjustment. In order to tackle the problem of gross errors in pairwise geometry estimates as well as the inaccuracy of initializing camera centers with noisy GPS data, we introduce a concept called "potential inlier" for the iterative optimization process, which constitutes one of our major novelties.

We think although auxiliary imaging information is not accurate enough, it still contains some degree of truthfulness on the imaging condition, and can be used as a good initializer for our potential inliers selection. In our work, a constraint is considered as a *potential inlier* if its residual at the current iteration is less than an adaptive threshold. Note that by such a setting, a potential inlier is not necessarily meant a real inlier, it is merely meant that the probability of a potential inlier to be a real inlier is much larger than a potential outlier. In addition, potential inlier is meaningful only at the current iteration this is because a potential inlier is changeable at its status from iteration to iteration. It is possible a potential inlier at the current iteration changes to a potential outlier at the next iteration, and vice versus. But with a good initialization of potential inliers with auxiliary imaging information and iteratively filtering out the potential outliers, our proposed iterative method can rapidly converge with a few iterations, as demonstrated in our later experiments. To some degree, our proposed iterative method possesses some analogy with the well-known Boosting scheme. In Boosting, by iteratively combining weak classifiers, a strong classifier is obtained. In our method, by iteratively filtering potential outliers, potential inliers converge to real inliers, and the parameters, such as camera poses and 3D scene points, become more and more precise. Unlike Boosting where the convergence is slow due to the less impact of later weak classifiers, our method is quite computationally efficient as demonstrated in our later experiments. This computational efficiency is mainly due to the following two interleaved factors: Firstly, only potential inliers are used, which is a subset of the total constraints. Second, with iteration going on, the set of the selected potential inliers contains less and less real outliers, and the estimated parameters become closer and closer to the correct ones, then less number of iterations is needed.

Our proposed method is validated on various datasets, including images captured by UAV, StreetView car and a moving conventional digital camera. The reconstruction results are compared with those by state–of–art methods, such as Bundler [3], MRF-based [1], VSFM [8], OpenMVG [9] and Linear Method [10].

2   Related Work

Many reported approaches [3–5,11] to solve SfM problem are based on incremental mode which repeatedly uses bundle adjustment to refine the scene and camera poses. The state-of-art representative is Bundler [3], which may suffer from drift due to the accumulation of errors in addition to its heavy computational load when handling large image dataset. Besides, Bundler's reconstruction result largely depends on the selection rule of the seed images and the order of subsequent image addition. Haner et al. [11] presented a new selection and addition rule which makes use of covariance propagation, and they pointed out that a well-determined camera should have both small estimated covariance and low reprojection error for next view planning. For Bundler, the worst-case running time of image matching part and bundle adjustment part is $O(n^2)$ and $O(n^4)$ in the number of images respectively, which becomes prohibitive when the number of images is large, many attempts are proposed to tackle this problem recently.

For the image matching part, graph-based algorithm [12,13] are proposed to improve the efficiency by pruning original image set. However, the graph construction is always time consuming, and sometimes the completeness of scene cannot be guaranteed. The other typical solution is to employ image retrieval method to explore candidate matching image pairs [14,15]. Nister et al. [14] proposed a vocabulary tree based approach to find out potential matching image pairs. Besides, based on the rank of Hamming distance, Cheng et al. [16] proposed a Cascade Hashing strategy to speed up the image matching. For bundle adjustment part, global methods [1,2,7–10], which only optimize the reconstruction result once, are considered of great potentiality. These approaches usually take three steps to solve the SfM problem. The first step is to compute camera rotations by rotation consistency, the second is to calculate camera translations, and the third one is to refine camera poses and 3D points by performing a final bundle adjustment. In particular, Jiang et al. [10] proposed a linear method for global camera pose registration from pairwise relative poses. This method requires a large set of precise pairwise geometries to perform the SVD decomposition. However, for many real applications, for example for StreetView images, pairwise geometry estimates are always noisy. As a result, many images may be discarded by [10] because their weak visual connections with other images.

Other works fuse auxiliary imaging information during the SfM solving [17,18]. Carceroni et al. [17] computed camera rotations by using GPS. Pollefeys et al. [18] reported a real-time SfM in urban scene reconstruction with the support of GPS/IMU sensors. However, these two methods rely on high-precision GPS sensors which are not available in common devices. Several methods [1,19] are proposed to reconstruct 3D scene by exploiting noisy auxiliary imaging information. Crandall et al. [1] proposed a discrete-continuous optimization method, in which noisy auxiliary info (GPS and vertical vanishing point) is incorporated into the SfM process. Note that VPs (Vertical vanishing points) are used to estimate the tilt angle. They used BP (belief propagation) on a discretized space of camera orientations and 2D camera positions to find a good parameter initialization, then run non-linear least squares and bundle adjustment to refine these estimates. Sinha et al. [19] also proposed a linear SfM method in which vanishing points are incorporated. However, these two methods are not applicable to the SfM problem on UAV images because the VPs cannot be estimated when the UAV faces a large tract of land where evident lines is not available. Although the tilt angle is available in IMU, it is usually unusable because of the influence of gravity. Besides, the extent of scene should be predetermined in [1], and discrete position labels take up a huge storage when the scene covers a large area.

In this paper, we present an efficient and versatile global approach, which is fully exploiting noisy auxiliary imaging information, to improve the SfM solving. Our proposed method is applicable to various kinds of images, including common digital images, UAV images and StreetView images.

3   A Global Approach by Iteratively Optimizing Potential Inliers

Our SfM method, shown in Fig. 2, consists of three main steps. Step1 is a pre-processing step, its main aim is to build an EG (epipolar graph). In this step, an image retrieval technique is used to speed up the image matching. In Step2, global camera rotations are iteratively estimated through rotation consistency. At each iteration, in order to increase the percentage of real edge inliers, gross edge outliers are filtered out. In Step3, camera poses and 3D scene points are iteratively estimated. In this step, we focus on tackling inevitable track outliers and the resulting inaccuracy problem by initializing camera centers with noisy GPS data. Next we elaborate on these three steps.

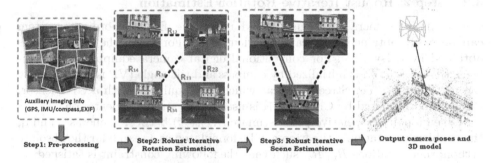

Fig. 2. The flowchart of our method. Step1: features are detected and then matched across images. Step2: rotation estimation by iteratively optimizing potential pairwise geometry inliers(showed by red solid lines) and discarding gross pairwise geometries (showed by black dotted lines). Step3: scene estimation by iteratively optimizing potential track inliers(showed by red solid lines) and discarding gross tracks (showed by black dotted lines). Finally, camera poses showed by cyan cones and 3D scene points are obtained (Color figure online).

3.1   Step 1: Pre-processing

At first, SIFT points are extracted from images. Note that raw GPS data is in the form of longitude, latitude and altitude defined in the WGS84 coordinate system. For the convenience of further processing, these data are converted into the ECEF (Earth Centered, Earth Fixed) coordinate system, which is usually called the local east-north-up. Here ECEF is used as the global coordinate system.

In order to accelerate the matching process, a vocabulary tree [14] is used to detect candidate matching image pairs. Furthermore, based on GPS, too distant image pairs are discarded. For each candidate pair, we compute SIFT matches using Cascade Hashing strategy [16]. Each 3D scene point is identified by finding their corresponding track-interest points across multiple images which have similar SIFT descriptors. However, sometimes a feature point may be contained by different tracks. Since such tracks are ambiguous when used for subsequent triangulation and bundle adjustment, they are considered unstable and discarded. After matching relevant images, geometric verification based on 5-point algorithm [20] is performed. Two images are considered as a matched pair if the number of their matched SIFT points is more than a threshold (in our work, it is set to 20). Moreover, pairwise relative rotations and translation directions are computed from every matched pair of images.

The final matching result is represented by a graph called EG (epipolar graph), whose vertices $V = \{I_1, I_2 \cdots I_N\}$ correspond to images and edges $E = \{e_{ij} | i, j \in V\}$ link matched image pairs, then the LCC (largest connected component) of EG is extracted and used in the subsequent reconstruction.

3.2 Step 2: Robust Iterative Rotation Estimation

Coarse initial camera rotations defined under the ECEF coordinate system can be easily obtained from camera orientations. For UAV, the orientation is obtained by noisy IMU. For conventional digital camera equipped with compass, the orientation is initialized by compass and tilt angle (VP is calculated by the method [21]). For StreetView car which only equipped with a GPS sensor, the method proposed by Crandall [1] is used to get a rough orientation.

Given a pairwise relative pose estimate (R_{pq}, t_{pq}) between cameras p and q, the problem of rotation estimation can be formulated as a search for the absolute orthonormal rotations R_p, R_q, such that the following constraint is satisfied:

$$R_{pq} = R_p R_q^T \tag{1}$$

Every edge in EG forms such a constraint. Thus, an overdetermined equation system is obtained since EG always consists of redundant edges. Note that the residual of an edge between cameras p and q is measured by the Frobenius norm of $\|R_{pq} - R_p R_q^T\|$. As proposed by Martinec [22], the solution of this overdetermined equation system can be initially computed without considering the orthonormality constraint and then enforced by subsequently projecting the approximate rotation to the closest rotation under Frobenius norm using SVD decomposition. However there always exist outliers, whose relative pose estimates are either incorrect or the epipolar constraints are actually non-existent, in EG.

In order to tackle the inevitable edge outliers in EG and increase the percentage of real edge inliers in the optimization process, we propose a robust rotation estimation algorithm by iteratively and exclusively optimizing the so-called potential edge inliers. An edge in EG is regarded as a potential edge inlier in the ith iteration if its corresponding residual ($\|R_{pq} - R_p R_q^T\|_F$) is less than a threshold $T^{(i)}$. Given a threshold α, $T^{(i)}$ in the ith iteration is computed as follows:

$$T^{(i)} = \min\{T : \frac{\sum_{j=1}^M \eta_j^{(i)}}{M} \geq \alpha\} \tag{2}$$

$$s.t. \qquad \eta_j^{(i)} = \begin{cases} 0, & \text{if } r_j^{(i)} > T; \\ 1, & \text{if } r_j^{(i)} \leq T; \end{cases} \qquad (3)$$

where $r_j^{(i)}$ is the residual of the jth edge in the ith iteration; $j = 1...M$; M is the number of edges in the LCC of EG. Moreover, the following covering condition should be satisfied: the current potential edge inliers should cover all the vertices in the LCC of EG. If this condition is not satisfied, the threshold α in Eq. (2) should be increased. In our work, initial α is set to 0.9. With this threshold, the goal of Eq. (2) is to calculate a minimal threshold $T^{(i)}$ such that the percentage of potential edge inliers over the total edges is equal or larger than 90 %. By ordering edge residuals from small to large, we consider that the last 10 % of EGs are erroneous or potential outliers, then discarded in the current iteration. Discarding such EGs will increase the percentage of real edge inliers over used EGs in the optimization.

Note that some real edge inliers may be labelled as potential edge outliers due to the inaccurate camera rotations as well as the empirical threshold α. In order to tackle such inaccuracy problem and make more real edge inliers be used in the optimization, we estimate the absolute camera rotations $\mathbf{R} = \{R_1, ..., R_N\}$ iteratively by minimizing the sum of the residuals of the potential edge inliers, where N is the number of images. In the ith iteration:

$$\mathbf{R}^{(i+1)} = \min\{\mathbf{R} : \sum_{p=1}^{N} \sum_{q=1}^{N} E_{pq}^{(i)} \|R_{pq} - R_p^{(i)} R_q^{(i)T}\|_F\} \qquad (4)$$

subject to that each matrix in $\mathbf{R}$ is orthonormal. $E_{pq}^{(i)}$ is set to 1 if the edge between image p and image q is a potential edge inlier in the ith iteration, otherwise set to 0. With the camera rotations become more and more accurate with iteration, more and more real edge inliers will be included in the optimization process. For the sake of efficiency, the iteration is usually stopped when the number of the changes of the potential edge inliers between two consecutive iterations is less than a threshold (in our work, it is set to 20).

3.3   Step 3: Robust Iterative Scene Reconstruction

The camera projection matrix set $\mathbf{P} = \{P_i; i = 1...N\}$, can be approximately initialized as:

$$P_i = K_i R_i[\mathbf{I} - C_i] = \begin{bmatrix} f_{exif\_i} & 0 & 0 \\ 0 & f_{exif\_i} & 0 \\ 0 & 0 & 1 \end{bmatrix} R_i[\mathbf{I} - C_i] \qquad (5)$$

where f_{exif_i} denotes the focal length from the ith image EXIF tag; R_i denotes the estimated absolute rotation of image i in Step 2; $\mathbf{I}$ denotes the identity matrix; C_i denotes the converted GPS of image i. Given the camera projection matrices and a track set of corresponding images, 3D scene points can be initially reconstructed by triangulation and bundle adjustment. However, due to the inaccuracy of the current initialization, mostly one-time bundle adjustment is not sufficient to produce satisfactory reconstruction result, and additional alternated triangulation and bundle adjustment process need to be carried out.

For each track, we pick the image pair which has the maximal baseline among all possible visible image pairs to perform the triangulation. For the robustness concern, a 3D point will not be triangulated if the maximal baseline of its corresponding track is too small, and a 3D point is saved as a candidate for further processing when its current average reprojection error across all visible images is less than 20 pixels and maximal reprojection error across all visible images is less than 100 pixels.

Given the camera projection matrix set $\mathbf{P}$ and the set of currently reliable reconstructed 3D points $\mathbf{X}$, the discrepancy between the measured 2D image point locations and predicted 3D scene points is minimized subsequently. For N images and K tracks, the cost function $\mathcal{G}$ is formulated as the weighted geometric projection errors:

$$\mathcal{G}\left(\mathbf{P}, \mathbf{X}\right) = \sum_{i=1}^{N} \sum_{j=1}^{K} v_{ij} \|x_{ij} - \gamma(P_i, X_j)\|^2 \tag{6}$$

where 2D image point locations x_{ij} are the observation of the 3D point X_j in the ith image; v_{ij} is set to 1 if X_j is visible in the ith image, otherwise set to 0. $\gamma(P_i, X_j)$ denotes the projection of X_j in the ith image. Note that in our work only the first two camera radial distortion parameters are used. The nonlinear least square problem defined in Eq. (6) always needs a good parameter initialization. However, converted GPS locations are not precise enough to be used as the camera positions initialization. Besides, there always exist outliers, which are caused by mismatching, in tracks set. Thus, direct optimization on Eq. (6) is not a sensible choice, and an iterative approach is here proposed by only performing optimization on potential track inliers to tackle this problem.

A track is regarded as a potential track inlier in the lth iteration if its average reprojection error across visible images is less than $H^{(l)}$. Given a threshold β, $H^{(l)}$ in the lth iteration is calculated as:

$$H^{(l)} = \min\{H : \frac{\sum_{j=1}^{K} \delta_j^{(l)}}{K} \geq \beta\} \tag{7}$$

$$s.t. \quad \delta_j^{(l)} = \begin{cases} 0, & \text{if } r_j^{(l)} > H; \\ 1, & \text{if } r_j^{(l)} \leq H; \end{cases} \tag{8}$$

where $r_j^{(l)}$ denotes the averaged reprojection error across all visible images of the jth track in the lth iteration; $j = 1...K$; K denotes the number of tracks. In addition, these potential track inliers should also satisfy the following covering condition: the visible images of the current potential track inliers should cover all vertices in the LCC of EG. If this condition is not satisfied, the potential track inliers should be recomputed by increasing β. Since there are still outliers present in the obtained potential tracks inliers, we use a robust Huber norm by setting its parameter as 25 pixels on the reprojection error. In our work, β is set to 0.9. Similarly as that in Sect. 3.2, by ordering average reprojection errors from small to large, the last 10 % of the tracks are considered as potential outliers, and they are not used in the optimization of current iteration.

Considering that the focal lengths obtained from image EXIF tags are relatively reliable, an enforcement term is added to the cost function (Eq. (6)). As a result, at the lth iteration, our cost function on potential track inliers is formulated as:

$$\mathcal{F}\left(\mathbf{P}^{(l)}, \mathbf{X}^{(l)}\right) = \mathcal{G}_{huber}\left(\mathbf{P}^{(l)}, \mathbf{X}^{(l)}\right) e_j^{(l)} + \sum_{i=1}^{N} \lambda \left(f_i^{(l)} - f_{exif\_i}\right)^2 \tag{9}$$

where $f_i^{(l)}$ is the focal length of the ith image in the lth iteration; $e_j^{(l)}$ is set to 1 if the jth track is considered as a potential track inlier in the lth iteration, otherwise set to 0. Conventionally, repeated bundle adjustment is regarded as the most time-consuming part in 3D reconstruction. However, as our following experimental part shows, the time-cost of repeated bundle adjustment in this step is acceptable. The reason is two-fold: on the one hand, only a part of tracks are optimized in each iteration, and the iteration number is always less than 5; on the other hand, the sparse structure of SfM problem is taken into account. In our work, the weighting factor λ in Eq. (9) is set to 10^{-4}, and the version(1.8.0) of ceres-solver [23] is adopted to perform the bundle adjustment.

4 Experiments

The experiments are carried out on a PC with an Intel Core2 i5-2400 3.10 GHz CPU(4 cores) and 16 G RAM. Our method is evaluated on real images captured by different devices, including (1) an UAV with integrated GPS and IMU sensors; (2) a conventional digital camera with a GPS receiver and compass inside; (3) a StreetView car equipped with a GPS sensor. The specifications of five image datasets are listed in Table 1. Due to the limited space, only the first 4 datasets are compared in detail.

4.1 Comparison Methods and Comparison Criteria

Our method is compared with Bundler [3], MRF-based method [1], OpenMVG [9], VSFM [8] and the Linear Method [10]. Note that since OpenMVG in [24] requires images to have the same initial focal length, OpenMVG cannot be run on MP. In addition, MRF-based approach [1] stresses the importance of tilt. Due to the lack of straight lines in UAV images, MRF-based method cannot be performed on TK1 and TK2.

Both qualitative and quantitative comparisons are carried out. In the qualitative comparison, not only the scene structures are assessed, but the camera trajectories are also compared for the UAV and StreetView images. Gross calibration errors or evident artifacts are the direct indicators of the algorithm's

Table 1. Specifications of image datasets

Name	# of images # in LCC	Capturing device	GPS precision	IMU/Compass precision	Same initial focal length?
MP	144	Canon 5D Mark III	$5 \sim 10\,\mathrm{m}$	$5 \sim 10°$	No
TK1	145	UAV	$5 \sim 10\,\mathrm{m}$	$5 \sim 10°$	Yes
TK2	501	UAV	$5 \sim 10\,\mathrm{m}$	$5 \sim 10°$	Yes
SV1	2468	StreetView car	$3 \sim 5\,\mathrm{m}$	–	Yes
SV2	16600	StreetView car	$3 \sim 5\,\mathrm{m}$	–	Yes

inadequacy. In the quantitative comparison, we evaluate the accuracy of the reconstructed cameras by comparing their positions to the ground truth locations. For the Arts Quad dataset, the truth GPS locations are publicly available in [1]. The running-time of the evaluated algorithms after image matching part is recorded to compare the computational load.

4.2 Results and Analysis

Results of Step 3. Since Step3 described in Sect. 3.3 is the key step in our algorithm, we show its results in Figs. 3 and 4. It can be clearly seen from Fig. 3 that our method almost converges after four iterations. Since initial parameters are not good enough, only a subset of tracks are regarded as potential track inliers at the first iteration. With iterations going on, more potential track inliers appear in the subsequent iterations, which indicates that the camera poses become more and more precise. Some results with respect to the iteration time are shown in Fig. 4. From the results in the first iteration, it can be seen that one-off bundle adjustment is obviously not enough when camera centers are directly initialized with GPS. Specifically, in the result of MP(Iter_1), both camera positions and scene structure are bad and unreasonable. With the iterations going on, the scene structure becomes more and more precise and reasonable.

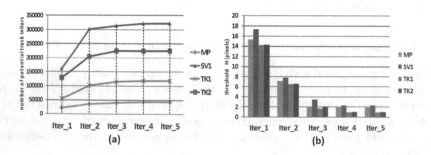

Fig. 3. (a) Number of potential track inliers with respect to the iteration number; (b) the threshold $H^{(l)}$ with respect to the iteration number.

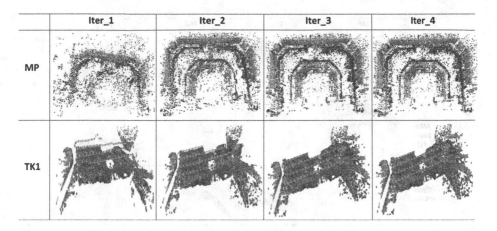

Fig. 4. Sparse reconstruction results with respect to the iteration number. Red and green points denote the camera positions (Color figure online).

Moreover, tracks are always clean in UAV images as no occlusions exist in the view. However, tracks are always contaminated in images captured by free shooting or StreetView car because of the large changes of view angles or the existence of numerous self-symmetric features. In our experiment, relative to the respective whole tracks, the percentage of final potential track inliers on MP, TK1, TK2 and SV1 is 54.07 %, 89.73 %, 89.71 %, 59.03 %, which shows our proposed method is robust to both cluttered and clean scenes.

Qualitative Comparison. For OpenMVG and Linear Method, accurate camera poses estimation are mainly dependent on the existence of many accurate triplets. However, triplets are not many in UAV and StreetView images because the speed of UAV or street view car is usually fast. Especially for StreetView images, many pairwise geometry estimates are usually not accurate enough. As shown in Fig. 5, these two methods generate obvious error results on TK1, TK2 and SV1. Note that the results on MP are comparable among five methods (Bundler, MRF-based approach, VSFM, Linear Method and our method), which indicates that most existing SfM methods are more suited for this scenario.

For TK1, the results produced by openMVG and Linear Method are obviously incomplete. For the camera trajectory of TK1, one obvious calibration error (a camera is under the scene), which is highlighted by a blue circle, appears in Bundler's result. Compared with VSFM's result on TK1, the camera trajectory of our result is more reasonable (unreasonable jitters appear in VSFM's result highlighted by a blue circle). In addition, for TK2, the result produced by openMVG is appearantly wrong. The reason is that OpenMVG does not account the image distortion. More elaborate reasons are reported by Wu [25]. Furthermore, results on TK2 produced by Bundler and Linear Method are obviously wrong, and there are some obvious calibration errors (sudden leap on camera centers) in VSFM's result, while our result on TK2 is more reasonable than others.

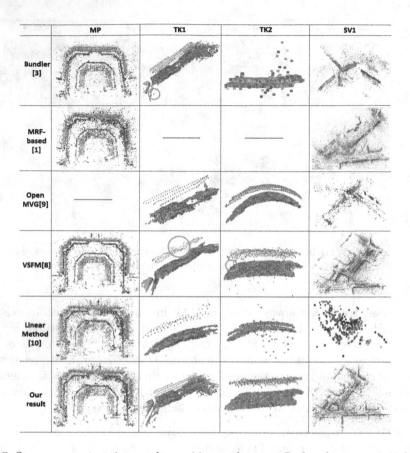

Fig. 5. Sparse reconstruction results on 4 image datasets. Red and green points denote the camera positions. Blue ellipses mark the sampled unreasonable areas in the results (Color figure online).

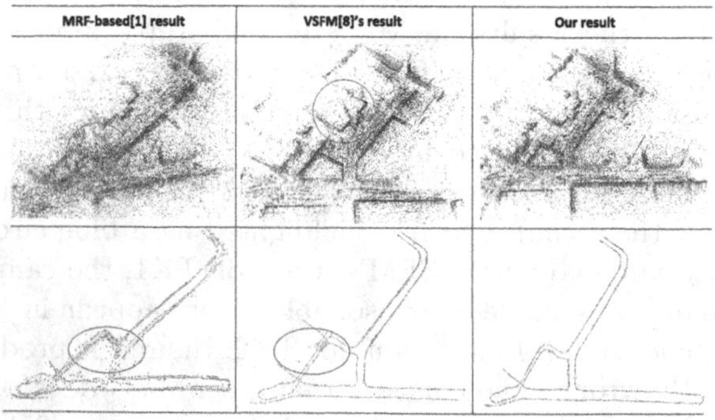

Fig. 6. The first row shows the reconstruction results on SV1 and the second shows the corresponding camera centers. Red circles and blue ellipses mark the unreasonable areas in the reconstructed results (Color figure online).

For SV1, the results produced by Bundler, openMVG and Linear Method are obviously incomplete or wrong. In order to make the comparison more evident, the scene structure and camera trajectory of other results are respectively shown in Fig. 6. For the scene structure, some obvious errors, which are highlighted by red circles, appear in the results produced by MRF-based approach and VSFM. For the camera trajectory, our result is more convincing as no obvious jitters appear on the route of car. Two blue ellipses mark the unreasonable parts on the results of VSFM and MRF-based method.

The reason of why our results are better than those produced by MRF-based method is mainly due to the following two factors. Firstly, the 2D camera positions in MRF-based method may be not dense enough (in our experiments, a label corresponds a 4 m*4 m square). As a result, parameter initializations may be not good enough for the bundle adjustment. Secondly, the accuracy of initial translations in MRF-based method largely depend on the initial selected tracks, so it is sensitive to track outliers. In sum, in term of qualitative comparison, our method outperforms the other five ones. Furthermore, our reconstruction result on SV2 is shown in Fig. 7b where the area marked by red dotted line is the reconstruction on SV1. Since the other five methods could not work well on SV1, they are not run on SV2. From our results, many dense reconstruction methods can be used. As shown in Fig. 1, dense reconstruction is performed by PMVS2 [6].

Quantitative evaluation. The accuracy of the calibrated cameras is evaluated by comparing their positions with ground truth locations. For the dataset Arts Quad which is publicly available in [1], there are 6514 images in total while 4255 images have geotags, and 348 images with high accurate differential GPS positions are used as ground truth. Since we need GPS to initialize camera centers, our method is only performed on geotaged images. The reconstruction results generated by our method is shown in Fig. 7a, in which 251 out of the 348 ground truth images are found. Then RANSAC is used to estimate a 3D similarity transformation between the 251 camera locations and their ground truth coordinates. The registration result shows that our camera positions have a median error of 1.13 m, which is comparable with 1.16 m reported by [1].

Time Efficiency and Scalability. The running-time of OpenMVG [9] is not compared here because its reconstruction results on our four datasets are either incomplete or obviously wrong. As a result, the time-cost of our method are compared with those of other four methods. Neither parallel computation nor GPU acceleration is used here to ensure the fairness of comparison. Note that if the cameras is partly calibrated, only the number of calibrated images of the corresponding method is showed in Table 2. It can be seen from Table 2 that our method performs better than other approaches on TK1, TK2 and SV1.

Our method is about 6 times faster than MRF-based approach on SV1. The detailed comparison of these two global reconstruction methods is shown in Table 3. Obviously, MRF-based approach spends a lot of time in estimating translations, while our main time-cost is spent on bundle adjustment. In the third row of Table 3, 4.0 min*5 is meant that each triangulation spends 4.0 min

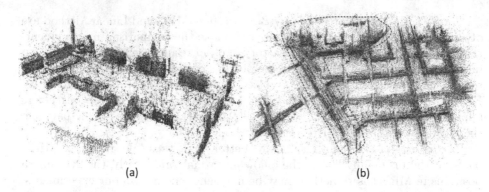

(a)   (b)

Fig. 7. Sampled reconstructions on Arts Quad (a) and SV2 (b). The area marked by red dotted line in (b) is the reconstruction results on SV1 (Color figure online).

Table 2. Running time of our method compared to other methods. (#) denotes the number of calibrated images by the corresponding method.

	Bundler	MRF-based	VSFM	Linear method	Our method
MP	20.1 min(144)	13.2 min(144)	1.6 min(144)	**1.1 min**(144)	1.8 min(144)
TK1	(142)	–	9.0 min(145)	(79)	**7.5 min**(145)
TK2	12.1 h(501)	–	(499)	(360)	**25.5 min**(501)
SV1	(90)	31.2 h(2468)	(1910)	(179)	**5.0 h**(2468)

Table 3. Time-cost comparison between MRF-based method and our method on SV1

	Rotations estimation	Translations estimation	Triangulation	Bundle adjustment	Total time-cost
MRF-based [1]	9.0 min	30.0 h	4.0 min	1.0 h	31.2 h
Our method	9.0 min	0 min	4.0 min * 5	4.5 h	**5.0 h**

and 5 iterations are carried out. The results show that our method has a better scalability than the MRF-based approach.

5   Conclusion

In this paper, we propose an efficient and accurate reconstruction method by fully exploiting auxiliary imaging information. The main novelty of our work is the exclusive use of the so-called potential inliers at each iterative optimization step to effectively deal with the inevitable constraint outliers, which is made possible in turn by employing auxiliary imaging information. Experimental results show that our approach outperforms the state-of-art reconstruction approaches, especially for UAV and StreetView images. In the future work, the iterative convergence of potential inliers to true inliers will be further investigated.

Acknowledgement. This work was supported by National High Technology *R&D* Program of China(863 program) under the grant No 2013*AA*12*A*202 and NSFC under the grant No (61333015, 61273280).

References

1. Crandall, D., Owens, A., Snavely, N., Huttenlocher, D.: SfM with MRFs: discrete-continuous optimization for large-scale structure from motion. PAMI **35**, 2841–2853 (2013)
2. Irschara, A., Hoppe, C., Bischof, H., Kluckner, S.: Efficient structure from motion with weak position and orientation priors. In: CVPRW, pp. 21–28. IEEE (2011)
3. Snavely, N., Seitz, S.M., Szeliski, R.: Modeling the world from internet photo collections. IJCV **80**, 189–210 (2008)
4. Agarwal, S., Furukawa, Y., Snavely, N., Simon, I., Curless, B., Seitz, S.M., Szeliski, R.: Building rome in a day. ACM **54**, 105–112 (2011)
5. Moulon, P., Monasse, P., Marlet, R.: Adaptive structure from motion with *a contrario* model estimation. In: Lee, K.M., Matsushita, Y., Rehg, J.M., Hu, Z. (eds.) ACCV 2012, Part IV. LNCS, vol. 7727, pp. 257–270. Springer, Heidelberg (2013)
6. Furukawa, Y., Ponce, J.: Accurate, dense, and robust multiview stereopsis. PAMI **32**, 1362–1376 (2010)
7. Strecha, C., Pylvanainen, T., Fua, P.: Dynamic and scalable large scale image reconstruction. In: CVPR, pp. 406–413. IEEE (2010)
8. Wu, C.: Towards linear-time incremental structure from motion. In: International Conference on 3D Vision, pp. 127–134 (2013)
9. Moulon, P., Monasse, P., Marlet, R.: Global fusion of relative motionsfor robust, accurate and scalable structure from motion. In: ICCV (2013)
10. Nianjuan Jiang, Zhaopeng Cui, P.T.: A global linear method for camera pose registration. In: ICCV (2013)
11. Haner, S., Heyden, A.: Covariance propagation and next best view planning for 3D reconstruction. In: Fitzgibbon, A., Lazebnik, S., Perona, P., Sato, Y., Schmid, C. (eds.) ECCV 2012, Part II. LNCS, vol. 7573, pp. 545–556. Springer, Heidelberg (2012)
12. Snavely, N., Seitz, S.M., Szeliski, R.: Skeletal graphs for efficient structure from motion. In: CVPR (2008)
13. Lou, Y., Snavely, N., Gehrke, J.: MatchMiner: efficient spanning structure mining in large image collections. In: Fitzgibbon, A., Lazebnik, S., Perona, P., Sato, Y., Schmid, C. (eds.) ECCV 2012, Part II. LNCS, vol. 7573, pp. 45–58. Springer, Heidelberg (2012)
14. Nister, D., Stewenius, H.: Scalable recognition with a vocabulary tree. In: CVPR (2006)
15. Chum, O., Mikulik, A., Perdoch, M., Matas, J.: Total recall ii: query expansion revisited. In: CVPR (2011)
16. Jian, C., Cong, L., Jiaxiang, W., Hainan, C., Hanqing, L.: Fast and accurate image matching with cascade hashing for 3d reconstruction. In: CVPR (2014)
17. Carceroni, R., Kumar, A., Daniilidis, K.: Structure from motion with known camera positions. In: CVPR (2006)
18. Pollefeys, M., Nistér, D., Frahm, J.M., Akbarzadeh, A., Mordohai, P., et al.: Detailed real-time urban 3d reconstruction from video. IJCV **78**, 143–167 (2008)

19. Sinha, S.N., Steedly, D., Szeliski, R.: A multi-stage linear approach to structure from motion. In: Kutulakos, K.N. (ed.) ECCV 2010 Workshops, Part II. LNCS, vol. 6554, pp. 267–281. Springer, Heidelberg (2012)
20. Nistér, D.: An efficient solution to the five-point relative pose problem. PAMI **26**, 756–770 (2004)
21. Tardif, J.P.: Non-iterative approach for fast and accurate vanishing point detection. In: ICCV (2009)
22. Martinec, D., Pajdla, T.: Robust rotation and translation estimation in multiview reconstruction. In: CVPR (2007)
23. Agarwal, S., Mierle, K., Others: Ceres solver. http://ceres-solver.org/
24. Moulon, P.: openMVG. https://github.com/openMVG/openMVG/tree/master
25. Wu, C.: Critical configurations for radial distortion self-calibration. In: CVPR (2014)

What Visual Attributes Characterize an Object Class?

Jianlong Fu[1](✉), Jinqiao Wang[1], Xin-Jing Wang[2],
Yong Rui[2], and Hanqing Lu[1]

[1] National Laboratory of Pattern Recognition, Institute of Automation,
Chinese Academy of Sciences, No. 95, Zhongguancun East Road,
Beijing 100190, China
{jlfu,jqwang,luhq}@nlpr.ia.ac.cn
[2] Microsoft Research, No. 5, Dan Ling Street, Haidian District,
Beijing 10080, China
{xjwang,yongrui}@microsoft.com

Abstract. Visual attribute-based learning has shown a big impact on many computer vision problems in recent years. Albeit its usefulness, most of works only focus on predicting either the presence or the strength of pre-defined attributes. In this paper, we discuss how to automatically learn visual attributes that characterize an object class. Starting from the images of an object class that are collected from the Web, we first mine visual prototypes of attributes (i.e., a clean intermediate representation for learning attributes) by clustering with Gaussian mixtures from multi-scale salient areas in noisy Web images. Second, a joint optimization model is proposed to fulfill the attribute learning with feature selection. As sparse approximation is adopted for feature selection during the joint optimization, the learned attributes tend to present a more representative visual property, e.g., stripe pattern (when texture features are selected), yellow-color (when color features are selected). Finally, to quantify the confidence of attributes and restrain the noisy attributes learned from the Web, a ranking-based method is proposed to refine the learned attributes. Our approach ensures the learned visual attributes to be visually recognizable and representative, in contrast to manually constructed attributes [1] that contain properties difficult to be visualized, e.g., "smelly," "smart." We evaluated our approach on two benchmark datasets, and compared with state-of-the-art approaches in two aspects: the quality of the learned visual attributes and their effectiveness in object categorization.

1 Introduction

A visual attribute presents a certain type of property (e.g., striped, yellow, long-neck) that can describe an object class [2]. Recent research on visual attributes

---

Jianlong Fu—This work was conducted when Jianlong Fu was a research intern at Microsoft Research.

© Springer International Publishing Switzerland 2015
D. Cremers et al. (Eds.): ACCV 2014, Part I, LNCS 9003, pp. 243–259, 2015.
DOI: 10.1007/978-3-319-16865-4_16

has shown a big impact on both research achievements and practical applications, e.g., face verification [3], image retrieval [4,5], object recognition [6,7], and adopting attributes such as size, color to refine search results by commercial search engines.

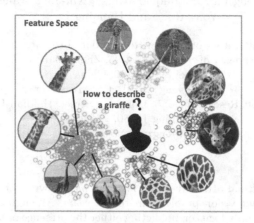

Fig. 1. An illustration of the attribute learning of "giraffe." We start with a large collection of Flickr images (small circles) and produce attributes with example images (large circles) indicating that a giraffe has a long neck, deer-like face, stripes and four legs.

However, existing approaches on attribute learning and attribute-based object recognition generally work on the pre-defined vocabulary of attributes, and the task is to predict the presence or relative strength of an attribute in an image or an object class [8,9]. Few works were done to automatically generate or discover attributes so that images of this class can be discriminated from images of other object classes when projected into a more specific and representative attribute space. Moreover, few works were done which considered the "visualness" of an attribute[1], and generated only *visual attributes* that could be effectively modeled with low-level visual features. Osherson and Wilkie collected 85 attributes of 48 animal classes via manual judgments [1], but not all of the attributes are visual, e.g., "smelly."

In this paper, we propose an unsupervised approach to learn the visual attributes that characterize an object class. That is, given an object class with its associated Web images (e.g., Flickr images), our approach outputs a ranked list of visual attributes that capture the key properties of the object class, where a rank score suggests the confidence for each attribute. Figure 1 shows a few attributes our approach learned from 5,000 Flickr images of "giraffe." It is clear that some attributes are visually recognizable and can present the property of long-neck, skin patterns, deer-like face and four legs, though we don't focus on assigning semantics in this work.

---

[1] Visualness [10] is a quantitative measure of how likely a concept can be visualized with example images.

Learning from the Web has demonstrated great success due to the huge quantities of images and unlimited vocabulary [11]. However, the challenge for learning attributes from noisy Web images can derive from two aspects. First, Web images often consist of both main objects and complex background. Second, the text to image association is far less controlled. For example, an image may be irrelevant to its user-contributed tag in Flickr. To solve the two problems, we propose an approach with three steps: (1) A Gaussian mixture model (GMM) [12] is first applied onto the multi-scale salient areas of a certain class images from Flickr, which generates visual prototypes of attributes, with each Gaussian one prototype. The intuition of building the visual prototypes is to reduce the background noises from Flickr images, which ensures a good intermediate representation for the attribute learning of a targeted object class. (2) Visual prototypes with specific properties are further learned and represented as attributes, where each attribute is an ensemble of Gaussian mixtures on the selected features. (3) Each attribute is ranked according to a confidence score by accumulating the rank scores from its contained visual prototypes. Thus, noisy attributes learned from irrelevant images can be restrained by low scoring.

We conducted comprehensive evaluations of the approach on two standard datasets, Animal with Attributes [13] and PASCAL VOC 2007. The evaluations show the effectiveness of our approach, which not only learned clean and intuitive attributes of object classes (e.g., the attribute of "long neck" is ranked at the top for giraffe and "stripe" is ranked at the top for zebra), but also achieved higher accuracy in object categorization, compared to state-of-the-art approaches.

The **main contribution** of this work is the unsupervised data-driven approach which automatically learns visual attributes from noisy Web images. Specifically, (1) the proposed visual prototype and attribute ranking scheme can effectively reduce the impact of noises from Web images. (2) The design of spectral analysis with feature selection ensures that the learned attribute can reflect a more representative visual property against previous approaches. (3) This approach is highly efficient and scalable as the training data is directly collected from the Web without any human cleanup.

2   Related Work

In this section, we review some works related to ours in two categories, i.e., pre-defined attributes and data-driven attributes.

Learning pre-defined attributes: A large body of works on attribute learning are based on pre-defined attributes. The list of pre-defined attributes can be generally formed by human [13,14] or mining online text [15]. Li et al. [16] and Torresani et al. [17] both consider the output of many object class classifiers of pre-defined categories as attributes for high-level visual recognition. To utilize the rich data on the Web, Ferrari et al. [18] learn visual models of a list of given attributes by Web image search results. A similar work is done by Tamara et al. [15] who automatically mine both texts and images on the Web to recognize attributes, thus it can dramatically alleviate human efforts. However, the pre-defined attribute lists crawled from the Web or collected from existing classifiers are limited and cannot be discriminative to a new specific categorization task. Besides, some are even not predictable by visual features, e.g., "smell."

Learning data-driven attributes: As the pre-defined attributes cannot fully discover specific properties for an object class, data-driven attributes have been proposed to learn attributes from data itself. Yang *et al.* [19] propose an automatic event detection approach from a large collection of unconstrained videos using data-driven approaches. Jingen *et al.* [20] automatically infer data-driven attributes from training data using an information theoretic approach. Yu *et al.* [2] and Wang *et al.* [6] design discriminative attribute learning approaches to improve object recognition, where the large-margin framework and latent models are adopted, respectively.

Compared to previous data-driven approaches where the attributes are considered as bag-of-words representation in [19], latent variables in [6] or linear model in [2], our learned attributes are visually recognizable and tend to present a more representative visual property with an importance rank score since features are selected in optimization processes. Meanwhile, we specially design the generating of visual prototypes and the scheme of attribute ranking to reduce the impact of noises from Web images, instead of using them directly as in [17,18].

3   Unsupervised Visual Attributes Learning

In this section, we present the details of the proposed unsupervised attributes learning approach for an object class. The framework is shown in Fig. 2. As we can observe from this figure, our approach takes as input a set of noisy Flickr images associated with an object class (shown in (a)) and returns as output a series of ranked attributes (shown in (e)). To achieve this goal, we first generate the visual prototypes from multi-scale salient areas (shown in (b) and (c)). Second, a joint optimization model is conducted to do the attribute learning

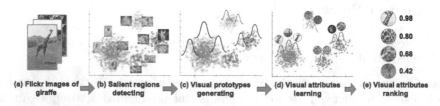

Fig. 2. The proposed unsupervised visual attributes learning approach. In (b), the detected regions are projected into the low-level feature space. In (c), visual prototypes are first learned from multi-scale salient regions in the original feature space. In (d), the attributes are further discovered from visual prototypes in the selected feature space which guarantees to present a certain property, e.g., long-neck (when shape features are selected), striped (when texture features are selected).

with feature selection (shown in (d)). Finally, we compute a confident score for each attribute by accumulating the scores from its contained visual prototypes in the selected feature space.

3.1 Visual Prototypes Generating

To reduce the background interference and ensure that the object-located region of an image can be selected for attribute learning, we propose a method of generating visual prototypes. A visual prototype is defined as a clean intermediate representation for attribute learning. First, we adopt a saliency detection approach [21] with multiple parameters, which generates a series of salient regions with different scales in an image. As it is hard to determine which scale the object can locate in, we cluster multi-scale salient areas by Gaussian mixture models and use the Gaussian mean with covariance matrix as the visual prototypes. This idea has an intuitive explanation that the object-located region can be determined by a soft voting from the multi-scale salient areas. Considering there can be similar images in the set of Flickr images associated with an object class, this clustering is conducted on the salient regions of all training images. The learning model is given in Eq. 1:

$$G(x|\omega) = \sum_{i-1}^{K} \pi_i G_i(x|\omega_i)$$

$$= \sum_{i=1}^{K} \pi_i \frac{1}{(2\pi)^{D/2}|\Sigma_i|^{1/2}} exp\{-\frac{1}{2}(x - \mu_i)^T \Sigma_i^{-1}(x - \mu_i)\} \tag{1}$$

where x is the visual feature of a salient region and $G_i(x|\omega_i)$ is a visual prototype. $\omega = \{\omega_1, ..., \omega_K\} = \{(\pi_1, \mu_1, \Sigma_1), ..., (\pi_K, \mu_K, \Sigma_K)\}$ denotes the parameter set of G. D is the dimension of x. π_i is the weight of each component, $\pi_i >= 0$ and $\sum_{i=1}^{K} \pi_i = 1$. $\mu = \{\mu_1, ..., \mu_K\}$ and $\Sigma = \{\Sigma_1, ..., \Sigma_K\}$. μ_i is the mean vector and Σ_i is the covariance matrix of the ith component.

The two parameters in Eq. 1, ω and K, need to be optimized. First, we use the Expectation Maximization (EM) algorithm [22] to estimate ω. The EM algorithm is a general method of finding the maximum-likelihood estimate of the parameters of an underlying distribution from a given data set. Second, as K affects the descriptive ability of visual prototypes, we apply an n-fold cross-validation approach to determine the best K, rather than setting it empirically. We separate training data into n pieces and pick $n - 1$ pieces of data to estimate ω. Then we calculate the loglikelihood on the rest one piece of data. The procedure is performed n times and produces an average loglikelihood. Previous work [12] has demonstrated that with the increasing number of K, the average loglikelihood increases but seems to be converging to some upper bound. It also shows that a small number of K is indeed insufficient to achieve good performance. Therefore, we increase K starting from 50 to $+\infty$ and stop when the difference of loglikelihoods between two successive calculations is smaller than a threshold (denoted as T_1).

3.2   Visual Attributes Learning

Once we have obtained the reliable intermediate representations, i.e., visual prototypes, we further learn visual attributes by a joint optimization with feature selection. The visual attributes are learned from a set of similar prototypes in a selected feature space, which ensures that the learned attributes can describe a certain visual property for an object class, e.g., round (when shape features are selected), striped (when texture features are selected). Note that whether presenting a specific property is the key difference between attributes and prototypes, while prototypes just represent the appearances of main objects in images.

For a set of visual prototypes $G = \{G_1, G_2, ..., G_K\}$, each prototype G_i is represented by (μ_i, Σ_i). A full-connected graph is constructed between any two prototypes to reflect a global structure on Gaussian space. Specifically, a label matrix $Y \in R^{K \times C}$ is defined as $y_{i,j} = 1$ if the ith prototype can be grouped into the jth attribute, otherwise 0, where C denotes the number of attributes. Furthermore, to find the specific visual property in attribute representations, a feature selection matrix $W \in R^{D \times C}$ is leveraged.

A Joint Objective Function. Given a spectral clustering term $\mathcal{F}(Y)$ and a feature selection term $\mathcal{L}(Y, W)$, the joint objective function is proposed as:

$$\min_{Y,W} \mathcal{F}(Y) + \mathcal{L}(Y, W)$$

$$= \min_{Y,W} \mathrm{Tr}[Y^T L Y] + \alpha(||\boldsymbol{\mu}^T W - Y||_F^2 + \beta||W||_{2,1}) \qquad (2)$$

$$s.t. \quad Y^T Y = I_C, Y \geq 0$$

where α and β are two nonnegative parameters.

In the spectral clustering term, an effective affinity matrix is obviously beneficial to reflect the relationship among different visual prototypes. As each prototype is a Gaussian, we use KL divergence to depict this relationship. To construct the affinity matrix $S \in R^{K \times K}$, we define:

$$S_{i,j} = exp\{-\frac{KL(i,j)^2}{\sigma^2}\} \qquad (3)$$

where σ is a free parameter to control the decay rate and KL divergence between two prototypes has a closed formed expression:

$$KL(i,j) = \frac{1}{2}[\log \frac{|\Sigma_j|}{|\Sigma_i|} + \mathrm{Tr}[\Sigma_j^{-1} \Sigma_i] - D + (\mu_i - \mu_j)^T \Sigma_j^{-1}(\mu_i - \mu_j)] \qquad (4)$$

Then the spectral clustering term is defined as minimizing the following formula:

$$\mathcal{F}(Y) = \frac{1}{2} \sum_{i,j=1}^{K} S_{ij} ||\frac{y_i}{\sqrt{A_{ii}}} - \frac{y_j}{\sqrt{A_{jj}}}||_2^2 = \mathrm{Tr}[Y^T L Y] \qquad (5)$$

where A is a degree matrix defined as the diagonal matrix with the degrees $a_1, ..., a_K$ on the diagonal. $a_i = \sum_{j=1}^{K} S_{i,j}$ and $L = I - A^{-1/2} S A^{-1/2}$.

In the feature selection term, mean vector μ_i is used to describe the visual appearance of the ith prototype. The l_{21}-norm is defined as $||W||_{2,1} = \sum_{i=1}^{D} \sqrt{\sum_{j=1}^{C} W_{i,j}^2}$, which is viewed as a regularization term to ensure the sparsity of W in row. We constrain one prototype can be grouped to one visual attribute, therefore an orthogonal constraint is imposed. Besides, to make Y more accurate and discriminative, a nonnegative constraint is also introduced. Both the orthogonal and nonnegative constraints guarantee that there is only one element in each row of Y that is much larger than zero and the others tend to be zeroes.

In the optimization process, on one hand, the spectral clustering learns the pseudo cluster labels. On the other, to minimize the overall loss, the algorithm automatically searches the most discriminative features to pseudo cluster labels and learns feature selection matrix W.

Optimization. Note that the l_{21}-norm is non-smooth and the objective function is not convex for W and Y simultaneously, then an efficient iterative optimization strategy is applied. First, we relax the orthogonal term and rewrite the optimization problem as:

$$
\begin{aligned}
&\min_{Y,W} \mathcal{F}(Y) + \mathcal{L}(Y,W) \\
&= \min_{Y,W} \mathrm{Tr}[Y^T L Y] + \alpha(||\mu^T W - Y||_F^2 + \beta||W||_{2,1}) \\
&\quad + \frac{\gamma}{2}||Y^T Y - I_C||_F^2 \\
&s.t. \quad Y \geq 0
\end{aligned}
\tag{6}
$$

where $\gamma \geq 0$ is a parameter to control the orthogonal constraint. It can be set large enough to ensure the constraint satisfied as in [23]. Following [23, 24], we define $\mathscr{F}(Y,W) = \mathcal{F}(Y) + \mathcal{L}(Y,W)$. Setting $\frac{\partial \mathscr{F}(Y,W)}{\partial W} = 0$, we have:

$$
\begin{aligned}
\frac{\partial \mathscr{F}(Y,W)}{\partial W} &= 2\alpha(\mu(\mu^T W - Y) + \beta B W) = 0 \\
&\Rightarrow W = (\mu\mu^T + \beta B)^{-1}\mu Y
\end{aligned}
\tag{7}
$$

Here B is a diagonal matrix with $B_{ii} = \frac{1}{2||w_i||_2}$. Representing W by Eqs. 6, and 7 is induced as:

$$
\min_{Y} \mathrm{Tr}[Y^T Z Y] + \frac{\gamma}{2}||Y^T Y - I_C||_F^2 \quad s.t. \quad Y \geq 0
\tag{8}
$$

where $Z = L + \alpha[I_K - \mu^T(\mu\mu^T + \beta B)^{-1}\mu]$ and $I_K \in R^{K \times K}$ is an identity matrix. Then we introduce multiplicative updating rules. Letting $\phi_{i,j}$ be the Lagrange multiplier for constraint $Y_{ij} \geq 0$ and $\Phi = [\phi_{ij}]$, the lagrange function is:

$$
\mathrm{Tr}[Y^T Z Y] + \frac{\gamma}{2}||Y^T Y - I_C||_F^2 + \mathrm{Tr}(\Phi Y^T)
\tag{9}
$$

Setting its derivative of Y to zero and using the KKT condition where $\phi_{ij}Y_{ij} = 0$, Y can be updated according to the following rules:

$$Y_{ij} \leftarrow Y_{ij} \frac{(\gamma Y)_{ij}}{(ZY + \gamma YY^T Y)_{ij}} \tag{10}$$

Then Y is normalized by $(Y^T Y)_{ii} = 1, i = 1, ..., K$. Convergence of the iterative algorithm can be proven in [23].

3.3 Visual Attributes Ranking

The resultant visual attribute models are the clusters of visual prototypes with selected features. Each cluster represents one attribute representation. We first describe the visual prototypes in the selected feature space, then the generating of visual attributes with ranking scheme is further proposed.

After the above optimization, the position of zero rows in W indicates the position of the feature dimensions which are not discriminative and can be abandoned. Therefore, we delete the related rows and columns of μ_i and Σ_i in G_i to obtain the new prototype G'_i on the selected features, where these related rows and columns correspond to the abandoned feature dimensions. Then we recalculate the KL divergence as $KL(i,j)'$ and the affinity matrix as S'.

Let the columns of S' be a standard simplex [25], then S' has the largest eigenvalue equal to one and a real eigenvector r^*. The ranking process can be achieved according to spectral analysis by solving the following objective function:

$$r^* = \arg_r \min \|S'r - r\|_2^2 \tag{11}$$

here r^* contains all the rank scores for each new prototype G'_j with selected features and the optimization can be solved by iterative method [26]. Then the rank score for each attribute is defined as:

$$R(M_i) = \sum_{j=1}^{|N_i|} r_j^* \tag{12}$$

where M_i denotes the ith attribute and r_j^* denotes the rank score of G'_j which is selected from r^*. This sum runs over the scores of all the prototypes grouped to M_i. $|N_i|$ measures the size of M_i by its contained prototypes. Attributes are ranked by $R(M_i)$ with decreasing order. Each produced attribute is a Gaussian mixture, which is presented as the ensemble of visual prototypes with their ranks:

$$M_i = \sum_{j=1}^{|N_i|} r_j^* * G'_j \tag{13}$$

where $i = 1, ..., C$. The complete unsupervised attributes learning algorithm is summarized in Algorithm 1.

Algorithm 1. Unsupervised Visual Attributes Learning

Input: Noisy Flickr images given an object class
        parameters $K, \omega, \alpha, \beta, \gamma$
1. Saliency detection and feature extraction
2. Visual prototypes generating by Eq. 1
   ω is determined by EM algorithm
   K is determined by cross-validation
3. Visual attributes learning by solving Eq. 2
   The iteration step $t = 1$
   Initialize $Y \in R^{K \times C}$ and $W \in R^{D \times C}$
   Set $B^{(t)} \in R^{D \times D}$ as an identity matrix
   Repeat:
   $$Z^{(t)} = L + \alpha[I_K - \mu^T(\mu\mu^T + \beta B^{(t)})^{-1}\mu]$$
   $$Y_{ij}^{(t+1)} = Y_{ij}^{(t)} \frac{(\gamma Y^{(t)})_{ij}}{(Z^{(t)}Y^{(t)} + \gamma Y^{(t)}(Y^{(t)})^T Y^{(t)})_{ij}}$$
   $$W^{(t+1)} = (\mu\mu^T + \beta B^{(t)})^{-1}\mu Y^{(t+1)}$$
   update $B^{(t+1)}$ with $B_{ii}^{(t+1)} = \frac{1}{2||w_i^{t+1}||_2}$
   $t = t + 1$
   Until Convergence or $t = 500$
4. Visual attributes ranking
   calculate S'
   $r^* = \arg_r \min ||S'r - r||_2^2$
   $R(M_i) = \sum_{j=1}^{|N_i|} r_j^*$
   $M_i = \sum_{j=1}^{|N_i|} r_j^* * G_j'$
Output: Attributes for the object class

---

4   Experiments

In this section, we evaluated the proposed approach on two aspects: the quality of the learned visual attributes for each object class and their effectiveness for object categorization tasks.

4.1   Datasets

For attribute learning, we collected $5,000$ images from Flickr for each object class by searching user-contributed tags. We extracted features of color (RGB color histogram), texture [27], shape (PHOG [28] and self-similarity histograms [29]). Different features were normalized and concatenated into a feature vector with the dimension of 1073.

For object categorization, we trained classification models and evaluated them on two datasets. One is Animal with Attributes (AwA) [13] which contains $30,475$ images of 50 animal object classes. The other is PASCAL VOC 2007 which consists of $9,963$ images of 20 different object classes.

4.2 Experiment Settings

Parameter Settings for Attribute Learning. There are two key parameters in saliency detection [21], i.e., "sigma" and "level." The former one controls the spatial spread of weights between different image locations. The latter one controls the resolution of the feature map. To produce multi-scale salient regions, the range of "sigma" is set from 0.1 to 1.0 with the step of 0.1, and the "level" is set as [2, 3, 4] and [5, 6, 7]. Hence, there are totally 20 groups of parameters that can generate 20 salient regions with different scales for an image in attribute learning.

In the visual prototype generating, we set the threshold T_1 as 0.01 and our experiments showed that K varied from 1,000 to 2,000 for most object classes. In the visual attribute learning, σ in Eq. 3 is set to 2 empirically. The three parameters α, β, γ should be determined in Eq. 6. γ is set to be 10^8 to ensure the orthogonal constraint as used in [23]. To evaluate the effect of α and β, a ratio is defined between intra-attribute similarity and inter-attribute similarity as:

$$Ratio = \frac{S(intra\_attribute)}{S(inter\_attribute)} \tag{14}$$

where $S(intra\_attribute)$, $S(inter\_attribute)$ can be obtained by calculating the sum of similarity of any two prototypes within any attribute (i.e., KL distance between Gaussians) and the sum of the similarity of any two attributes (i.e., KL distance between Gaussian mixtures), respectively. α and β are set to $\{1, 10, 10^2, 10^3, 10^4, 10^5, 10^6\}$. The results on the classes of AwA are shown in Fig. 3. $\alpha = 10^2$ and $\beta = 10^4$ were chosen when the ratio reached the highest value.

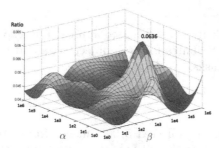

Fig. 3. Parameters setting for α and β for 50 object classes in AwA.

Compared Approaches for Object Categorization. The following approaches are compared for performance evaluation of object categorization tasks.

1. low-level feature: a typical image representation approach with the low-level features described in Sect. 4.1.
2. Classemes [17]: an approach using the output of existing object class classifiers of pre-defined categories as attributes.

3. category-level attribute designing approach (CLA) [2]: an automatic attribute learning approach with large-margin framework.
4. LDA-based [30] attribute learning approach: an automatic attribute learning approach using latent dirichlet allocation to generate attributes for each object class.

Note that attribute-based approaches leverage the outputs on different attributes as features, e.g., the output of classifiers in Classemes [17] and CLA [2], the response of topics in LDA [30] and the response of attributes (i.e., Gaussian mixtures) in our approach. Classemes was implemented using the author-released code. We implemented CLA as in [2]. The LDA-based attribute learning approach was trained on noisy Flickr images as ours, with each topic one attribute. We used a non-linear SVM (χ^2 kernel) as the classification model. The training, testing and validation images were selected according to [2, 31] for AwA dataset and PASCAL VOC 2007 dataset, respectively.

4.3 Attribute Learning Results

We first showed the attribute learning results of our unsupervised approach by fixing the number of attributes (i.e., C in Eq. 13) to 30, as the performance cannot increase with larger numbers examined in the following sections. For different object classes, we visualized the attributes ranked in No. 1, No. 5 and No. 30 by showing the top five salient regions from Flickr images with the highest responses to each attribute. The results are shown in Figs. 4 and 5. For an attribute, the higher the score, the more representative it is. As we can observe from Fig. 4, the most representative attribute for "Deer" is the salient "antler," which can discriminate deer from other animals such as sheep or horse. And their body postures are ranked in the fifth place. As we expected, "long neck" and "stripe texture" are the two most representative attributes for "giraffe" and "zebra," respectively. As an interesting discovery, the last image of the top attribute of

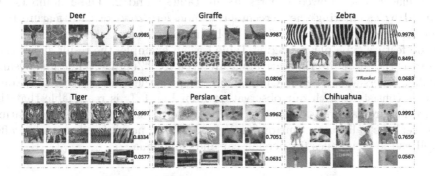

Fig. 4. Attribute learning results for six object classes of AwA dataset. For each object class, we visualize attributes ranked in No. 1, No. 5, No. 30 within the 30 attributes by showing the top five salient regions from Flickr images with their rank scores.

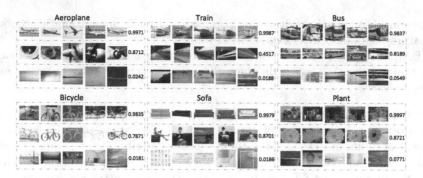

Fig. 5. Attribute learning results for six object classes of PASCAL VOC 2007 dataset (The illustration is same as Fig. 4).

zebra is actually a pedestrian crossing due to its similar visual appearance to the skin of zebras. For "Tiger," "Persian cat" and "Chihuahua," the results indicate that their facial cues are the most representative attributes, followed by body postures or textures. It is reasonable because it is often difficult for humans to separate cat and dog only by their furry body, but we can easily recognize them by their faces.

From Fig. 5, we can observe some implicit or even social attributes. For example, the learned attribute located in the second row of "Train" can be interpreted as "fast." For "Sofa," the second-row attribute reveals that the sofa is a kind of furniture with its specific function that human can comfortably sit on it. In addition, our approach can greatly weaken the noisy attributes which correspond to irrelevant images for an object class. For instance, the third-row attributes ranked in No. 30 for all classes have the lowest rank scores, which reflect those appearances of irrelevant images. The role of these attributes can be neglected as the responses on them can approach to zero.

Moreover, we examined the most discriminative visual features for different object classes and showed the results in Tables 1 and 2. These numbers are obtained by calculating the percentage of non-zero rows of each feature type in the feature selection matrix W. The higher percentages, the more important role the feature type plays. Taking Table 1 as an example, the result shows that texture is the most discriminative feature type for "Zebra." While for "Dear," "Giraffe," "Persian cat" and "Chihuahua," shape is the most discriminative one, which is consistent with our observation from Fig. 4. It is reasonable that the texture feature can well reflect the "stripe pattern" of zebra, the shape feature can reveal the salient contour of "antler" and "long neck" for dear and giraffe, as well as the facial cues for persian cat and chihuahua.

4.4 Object Categorization on AwA

In this part, we showed the superiority of the learned attributes by applying them to the task of object categorization on AwA dataset. We first conducted an

Table 1. The analysis of feature selection for six object classes in AwA.

	Color	Texture	Shape
Deer	0.55	0.47	**0.97**
Giraffe	0.6	0.47	**0.97**
Zebra	0.55	**0.98**	0.33
Tiger	**0.65**	0.44	0.12
Persian_cat	0.45	0.14	**0.93**
Chihuahua	0.55	0.12	**0.96**

Table 2. The analysis of feature selection for six object classes in PASCAL VOC 2007.

	Color	Texture	Shape
Aeroplane	0.52	0.44	**0.85**
Train	0.45	0.16	**0.81**
Bus	0.49	0.42	**0.82**
Bicycle	0.45	0.34	**0.87**
Sofa	**0.81**	0.47	0.75
Plant	**0.83**	0.45	0.73

experiment on 40 known classes. Each object class produced attributes with the number of C, and thus there were totally attribute features of $40*C$ dimensions. We examined the influence of the number of attributes C of an object class. We can observe from Fig. 6(b), C increases from 10 to 40. There is no significant accuracy improvement when the C reaches 30, compared to the performance of $C = 40$. Therefore, we consider 30 attributes can effectively cover the properties of an object class and we keep this number for all object classes in the following experiments.

To compare the performance for object categorization, different compared approaches were constrained to produce the attribute features of the same dimensions. For example, Classemes can generate attribute features of $2,659$ dimensions. We used PCA to reduce this feature representation to the dimension of $1,200$. For LDA-based attribute learning approach, we produced 30 attributes for each object class and generated $1,200$ attributes for the 40 classes as ours.

Figure 6(a) shows the comparison result with different attribute learning approaches. We can observe the following conclusions. First, attribute-based approaches can achieve higher accuracy against the low-level-feature-based approach when we have enough training samples, e.g., 30 or 50. Second, our approach surpasses Classemes with pre-defined attributes, which demonstrates the superiority of the data-driven attribute learning approach that can detect specific attributes from data itself. Third, compared to CLA and LDA, the proposed approach consistently achieves better performance. The reason can be concluded in two folds. On one hand, the feature selection scheme ensures to present a certain type of properties, which enhance the discrimination ability in object categorization against the CLA approach. On the other, our approach can effectively weaken the noisy attributes learned from irrelevant images and provide a cleaner attribute representations against the LDA-based approach, which directly learns the attribute from noisy Web images.

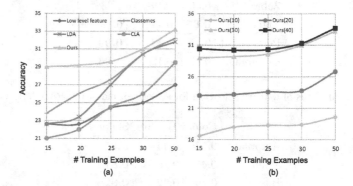

Fig. 6. Multi-class classification on 40 known object classes. (a) shows the accuracy of various approaches with the increasing of training examples. (b) shows the influence of different numbers of attributes in an object class to the classification results (the numbers are in brackets).

To show the performance for 10 novel classes defined in [13], we conducted an interesting experiment which projected images of a novel object class onto the learned attributes of known classes. As we can observe from Fig. 7, our approach achieves the best performance compared with both the low-level-feature-based and the attribute-based approaches. We achieve the accuracy gain of 4.5 % against the second-best approach (Classemes) when using half training samples. We also find that the accuracy seems to reach an upper bound with the increasing of training samples, which reveals the limitation of the shared attributes between different object classes.

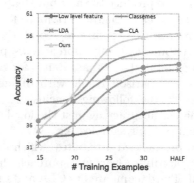

Fig. 7. Multi-class classification on 10 novel object classes.

4.5   Object Categorization on PASCAL VOC 2007

We conducted another object categorization comparison on PASCAL VOC 2007 dataset. We kept 30 attributes for each object class. As there were 20 classes in the dataset, we obtained an attribute space of 30 * 20 dimensions. The images of training, testing and validation were projected into the attribute space, with each response of an attribute as one attribute feature. Table 3 shows the comparison with the four baselines and the best result reported in [31]. Our proposed attribute-based approach improves the best result on 8 out of the 20 classes and boosts the mean average precision (mAP) with 2.8 %.

Table 3. Classification result on PASCAL VOC 2007

	aeroplane	bicycle	bird	boat	bottle	bus	car	cat	chair	cow	table
Low level feature	43.1	36.5	42.6	48.7	27.5	40.6	43.9	38.3	42.5	45.1	46.3
BestResult [31]	**77.5**	63.6	56.1	**71.9**	33.1	60.6	**78.0**	58.8	53.5	42.6	54.9
Classemes(600)	70.5	48.5	**66.7**	68.3	44.7	**66.8**	64.4	**68.0**	**65.6**	60.7	71.7
CLA(600)	65.8	49.0	47.8	57.2	40.0	56.3	60.0	62.4	61.2	46.3	52.6
LDA(600)	61.2	62.8	53.6	56.3	37.5	45.3	46.5	61.3	53.9	60.2	64.8
Ours(600)	67.5	**74.6**	64.8	62.4	**44.8**	59.0	50.2	60.0	63.2	**70.9**	**73.4**

	dog	horse	mbike	person	plant	sheep	sofa	train	tv	mAP
Low level feature	39.4	47.5	40.2	35.3	21.4	31.4	41.6	40.3	18.5	38.5
BestResult [31]	45.8	**77.5**	64.0	**85.9**	36.3	44.7	50.6	**79.2**	**53.2**	59.4
Classemes(600)	58.3	59.3	52.2	46.1	25.4	68.1	**67.5**	69.1	35.5	58.9
CLA(600)	47.8	56.2	62.4	44.1	27.9	41.4	45.3	53.9	25.7	50.1
LDA(600)	52.6	64.5	63.6	67.3	34.0	67.7	48.7	68.5	28.3	54.9
Ours(600)	**61.2**	66.0	**69.7**	74.9	**40.0**	**73.4**	59.5	73.7	35.5	**62.2**

5   Conclusion

In this paper, we have studied the problem of automatic visual attributes learning. To achieve this goal, we proposed an approach with three steps, i.e., prototypes generating, attributes learning and attributes ranking, which can effectively reduce the impact of noises in Web images and ensure that the learned attributes can present a certain property. Extensive experiments showed the good quality of the learned visual attributes and their effectiveness in object categorization. Note that this paper focuses only on visual attribute learning rather than assigning semantic meanings to each learned attribute. We will study the semantic association in our future work.

Acknowledgement. This work was supported by 863 Program (2014AA015104), and National Natural Science Foundation of China (61273034, and 61332016).

References

1. Osherson, D.N., Stern, J., Wilkie, O., Stob, M., Smith, E.E.: Default probability. Cogn. Sci. **15**, 251–269 (1991)
2. Yu, F.X., Cao, L.L., Feris, R.S., Smith, J.R., Chang, S.F.: Designing category-level attributes for discriminative visual recognition. In: CVPR (2013)
3. Kumar, N., Berg, A.C., Belhumeur, P.N., Nayar, S.K.: Attribute and simile classifiers for face verification. In: ICCV (2009)
4. Siddiquie, B., Feris, R.S., Davis, L.S.: Image ranking and retrieval based on multi-attribute queries. In: CVPR, pp. 801–808 (2011)
5. Yu, F.X., Ji, R., Tsai, M.H., Ye, G., Chang, S.F.: Weak attributes for large-scale image retrieval. In: CVPR, pp. 2949–2956 (2012)
6. Wang, Y., Mori, G.: A discriminative latent model of object classes and attributes. In: Daniilidis, K., Maragos, P., Paragios, N. (eds.) ECCV 2010, Part V. LNCS, vol. 6315, pp. 155–168. Springer, Heidelberg (2010)
7. Branson, S., Wah, C., Schroff, F., Babenko, B., Welinder, P., Perona, P., Belongie, S.: Visual recognition with humans in the loop. In: Daniilidis, K., Maragos, P., Paragios, N. (eds.) ECCV 2010, Part IV. LNCS, vol. 6314, pp. 438–451. Springer, Heidelberg (2010)
8. Wang, G., Forsyth, D.A.: Joint learning of visual attributes, object classes and visual saliency. In: ICCV, pp. 537–544 (2009)
9. Parikh, D., Grauman, K.: Relative attributes. In: ICCV, pp. 503–510 (2011)
10. Xu, Z., Wang, X.J., Chen, C.W.: Mining visualness. In: ICME, pp. 1–6 (2013)
11. Wang, X.J., Zhang, L., Ma, W.Y.: Duplicate-search-based image annotation using web-scale data. Proc. IEEE **100**, 2705–2721 (2012)
12. Zoran, D., Weiss, Y.: Natural images, gaussian mixtures and dead leaves. In: NIPS, pp. 1745–1753 (2012)
13. Lampert, C.H., Nickisch, H., Harmeling, S.: Learning to detect unseen object classes by between-class attribute transfer. In: CVPR, pp. 951–958 (2009)
14. Farhadi, A., Endres, I., Hoiem, D., Forsyth, D.: Describing objects by their attributes. In: CVPR (2009)
15. Berg, T.L., Berg, A.C., Shih, J.: Automatic attribute discovery and characterization from noisy web data. In: Daniilidis, K., Maragos, P., Paragios, N. (eds.) ECCV 2010, Part I. LNCS, vol. 6311, pp. 663–676. Springer, Heidelberg (2010)
16. Li, L.-J., Su, H., Xing, E.P., Fei-Fei, L.: Object bank: a high-level image representation for scene classification and semantic feature sparsification. In: NIPS (2010)
17. Torresani, L., Szummer, M., Fitzgibbon, A.: Efficient object category recognition using classemes. In: Daniilidis, K., Maragos, P., Paragios, N. (eds.) ECCV 2010, Part I. LNCS, vol. 6311, pp. 776–789. Springer, Heidelberg (2010)
18. Ferrari, V., Zisserman, A.: Learning visual attributes. In: NIPS (2007)
19. Yang, Y., Shah, M.: Complex events detection using data-driven concepts. In: Fitzgibbon, A., Lazebnik, S., Perona, P., Sato, Y., Schmid, C. (eds.) ECCV 2012, Part III. LNCS, vol. 7574, pp. 722–735. Springer, Heidelberg (2012)
20. Liu, J., Kuipers, B., Savarese, S.: Recognizing human actions by attributes. In: CVPR, pp. 3337–3344 (2011)
21. Harel, J., Koch, C., Perona, P.: Graph-based visual saliency. In: NIPS, pp. 545–552 (2006)
22. Dempster, A.P., Laird, N.M., Rubin, D.B.: Maximum likelihood from incomplete data via the EM algorithm. J. Roy. Stat. Soc. Ser. B **39**, 1–38 (1977)

23. Yang, Y., Shen, H.T., Ma, Z., Huang, Z., Zhou, X.: $l_{2,1}$-norm regularized discriminative feature selection for unsupervised learning. In: IJCAI, pp. 1589–1594 (2011)
24. Nie, F., Huang, H., Cai, X., Ding, C.H.Q.: Efficient and robust feature selection via joint; 2, 1-norms minimization. In: NIPS, pp. 1813–1821 (2010)
25. Luxburg, U.: A tutorial on spectral clustering. Stat. Comput. **17**, 395–416 (2007)
26. Golub, G.H., van der Vorst, H.A.: Eigenvalue computation in the 20th century. J. Comput. Appl. Math. **123**, 35–65 (2000)
27. Lazebnik, S., Schmid, C., Ponce, J.: A discriminative framework for texture and object recognition using local image features. In: Ponce, J., Hebert, M., Schmid, C., Zisserman, A. (eds.) Toward Category-Level Object Recognition. LNCS, vol. 4170, pp. 423–442. Springer, Heidelberg (2006)
28. Bosch, A., Zisserman, A., Munoz, X.: Representing shape with a spatial pyramid kernel. In: CIVR, pp. 401–408 (2007)
29. Shechtman, E., Irani, M.: Matching local self-similarities across images and videos. In: CVPR (2007)
30. Blei, D.M., Ng, A.Y., Jordan, M.I.: Latent dirichlet allocation. J. Mach. Learn. Res. **3**, 993–1022 (2003)
31. Everingham, M., Van Gool, L., Williams, C.K.I., Winn, J., Zisserman, A.: The PASCAL Visual Object Classes Challenge 2007 (VOC2007) Results (2007). http://www.pascal-network.org/challenges/VOC/voc2007/workshop/index.html

Accurate Object Detection with Location Relaxation and Regionlets Re-localization

Chengjiang Long[1], Xiaoyu Wang[2](✉), Gang Hua[1], Ming Yang[3], and Yuanqing Lin[2]

[1] Stevens Institute of Technology, Hoboken, NJ 07030, USA
[2] NEC Laboratories America, Cupertino, CA 95014, USA
fanghuaxue@gmail.com
[3] Facebook, Menlo Park, CA 94026, USA

Abstract. Standard sliding window based object detection requires dense classifier evaluation on densely sampled locations in scale space in order to achieve an accurate localization. To avoid such dense evaluation, selective search based algorithms only evaluate the classifier on a small subset of object proposals. Notwithstanding the demonstrated success, object proposals do not guarantee perfect overlap with the object, leading to a suboptimal detection accuracy. To address this issue, we propose to first relax the dense sampling of the scale space with coarse object proposals generated from bottom-up segmentations. Based on detection results on these proposals, we then conduct a top-down search to more precisely localize the object using supervised descent. This two-stage detection strategy, dubbed *location relaxation*, is able to localize the object in the continuous parameter space. Furthermore, there is a conflict between accurate object detection and robust object detection. That is because the achievement of the later requires the accommodation of inaccurate and perturbed object locations in the training phase. To address this conflict, we leverage the rich spatial information learned from the Regionlets detection framework to determine where the object is precisely localized. Our proposed approaches are extensively validated on the PASCAL VOC 2007 dataset and a self-collected large scale car dataset. Our method boosts the mean average precision of the current state-of-the-art (41.7 %) to 44.1 % on PASCAL VOC 2007 dataset. To our best knowledge, it is the best performance reported without using outside data (Convolutional neural network based approaches are commonly pre-trained on a large scale *outside* dataset and fine-tuned on the VOC dataset.).

1 Introduction

An object may appear in any locations and scales in an image defined by the continuous parameter space spanned by (x, y, s, a), where (x, y) is the object center point, and s and a are the scale and aspect ratio of the object. In particular, different aspect ratios generally correspond to different viewpoints, leaving a difficult open question for robust object detection.

© Springer International Publishing Switzerland 2015
D. Cremers et al. (Eds.): ACCV 2014, Part I, LNCS 9003, pp. 260–275, 2015.
DOI: 10.1007/978-3-319-16865-4_17

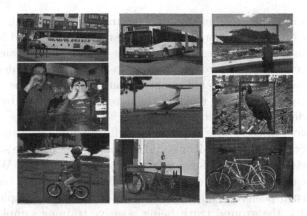

Fig. 1. Sample detection results applying our detection framework to the PASCAL VOC 2007 dataset. First row: bus and boat detection. Second row: bottle, aeroplane and bird detection. Third row: bicycle detection.

In order to accurately localize the object in the image, sliding window based detector [1–5] requires densely sampling a fixed size candidate object window (*i.e.*, a base window) from the continuous parameter space at each scale of a scale-space image pyramid. Then, a binary decision is made for each specific window to predict whether it contains the object or not. To deal with different viewpoints of the object, one often discretizes the space of aspect ratio to define different base windows, and one classifier needs to be trained for each base window to detect the same object with different viewpoints.

Obviously, sliding window based approaches could be computationally prohibitive to obtain precise localization of the object, as it may potentially involve evaluating the classifier on millions or even billions of candidate windows. To reduce the computational cost, as suggested by the seminal Viola-Jones detector [6], a cascade classifier allows to early reject obvious non-object window, and hence achieves real-time performance. This strategy has been widely adopted in the literature. However, unless the weak classifier in the cascade can be efficiently evaluated, *e.g.*, by leveraging Haar features with integral images, the computational cost even with early rejection may still be very high.

Beyond cascade classifiers, the computational cost could be further reduced either from top-down or bottom-up approaches. Top-down methods, such as branch-and-bound [7], divide and conquer [8], and crosstalk [9] *etc.*, take advantage of observations from already evaluated windows to prune the windows which are not likely to have the object. While bottom-up methods guide their search by firstly identifying category independent candidate object locations before applying category specific detectors. This can be achieved either through low-level segmentations [10,11] or through some "objectness" [12] measurement of a candidate window. Since the number of classifier evaluation is drastically pruned in such bottom-up methods, even computational intensive spatial pyramid matching [13], which is very successful in image classification, can be adopted for object detection.

Notwithstanding the great success of these methods for reducing the computational cost for object detection, none of these methods searched for the object in the full continuous parameter space, *i.e.*, the center point, scale, and aspect ratio of the object. In other words, for top-down approaches, the detection accuracy is still bounded by the level of quantization these algorithms operating on. For bottom-up approaches, the recall of the detector is bounded by the recall of the category independent object proposal.

Moreover, most of the above approaches still rely on classification models to localize the object. While a classifier could be robust due to large scale training, it is not necessarily optimized for accurate object localization. What worsens the situation is that many detectors such as DPM [4] are not trained on the exact ground truth positive samples. These detectors allow samples with sufficient overlap with the ground truth being positive training samples, for either data augmentation purpose or a more comprehensive modeling of visual appearance among different positive samples. Thus in contrast to aiming at precise localization as much as possible, the visual classification models are learned to accommodate inaccurate localizations.

These observations motivate us to develop a detection framework which is capable of precisely searching for the object in a full parameter space with favorable efficiency. To achieve this goal, we first relax dense sampling of the object location and scale, dubbed the name *location relaxation*, and only evaluate the detector at a much coarser set of locations and scales. For coarse detection windows which have relatively high response, we apply supervised descent search [14] to find potential object hypothesis by simultaneously optimizing their center point, scale, and aspect ratio. The resulting detections are much more improved with supervised descent search but still not sufficient in terms of accurate localization. Thus we introduce Regionlets Re-localization, which is naturally built based on the quantized Regionlets features, to directly predict the true object location based on results from supervised descent search.

Figure 2 takes person detection as an example to illustrate our object detection framework. By applying an object detector to bottom-up object proposals, we obtain coarse detections, *i.e.*, the bounding boxes shown in Fig. 2(b). Among them, the red box is relatively confident detection compared to others. Through the supervised descent search starting from the red bounding box, a better detection is obtained as the dash box in Fig. 2(c). Finally we apply Regionlets Re-localization to determine the object location as shown in Fig. 2(d). We show some sample detection results on the PASCAL VOC 2007 dataset in Fig. 1.

The contribution of this paper lies on three aspects. Firstly, it proposed coarse detection plus supervised descent search in a fully parameterized location space for generic object detection which shows promising performance. Secondly, it proposed a novel Regionlets Re-localization method which complements the suboptimal object localization performance given by object detectors. Finally, our detection framework achieves the best performance on the PASCAL VOC 2007 dataset without using any outside data. It also demonstrates superior performance on our self-collected car dataset.

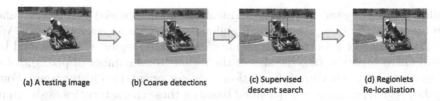

(a) A testing image   (b) Coarse detections   (c) Supervised descent search   (d) Regionlets Re-localization

Fig. 2. Illustration of the proposed object detection framework. (a) A testing image on which we want to detect all persons. (b) Coarse detection results obtained from object detectors applied to bottom-up proposals. The red bounding box indicates a relatively confident detection. (c) More confident detections obtained through supervised descent search. (d) The Regionlets Re-localization is employed to produce better localization. A non-max suppression procedure is followed to generate the final detection result (Color figure online).

2 Our Approach

Our object detection framework is composed of three key components: bottom-up object hypotheses generation, top-down object search with supervised descent and object re-localization with a localization model.

There are several alternatives to obtain object hypotheses. For example, through the objectness measurement [12], the saliency analysis or their combinations [15], or using segmentation cues [10]. Because our top-down search algorithm is applied locally, we expect the bottom-up object hypotheses to split the object location space evenly, to avoid the search algorithm converging to the same local minimum. To this end, we employ low-level segmentation to propose the object hypotheses. The superpixel segmentation merges similar pixels locally into disjoint sets which perfectly matches our need. However, over-segments only provide small object candidates. To obtain object hypotheses for large objects, the over segmented superpixels are gradually merged to produce larger candidates.

The detection with location relaxation takes coarse detection results from a detector applied on the bottom up object proposals. Then it searches the object location guided by discriminatively learned descent model inspired by Xiong and De la Torre [14]. The learned supervised descent model is used to predict the next more accurate object location to explore based on observations from the current location. Although our method is applicable with any black box object detector, we use the Regionlets detector [16] due to its outstanding performance and flexibility to detect objects in any viewpoints.

All the detection results, including the original coarse detections as well as detections generated by supervised descent search, are fed to our Regionlets Re-localization process to more accurately locate the target objects.

2.1 Bottom-Up Object Proposal

To complement our top-down searching strategy, we employ a segmentation based bottom-up scheme to generate our initial set of candidate searching locations.

Similar to [10], we start with over-segments (*i.e.*, superpixels) of an image and then hierarchically group these small regions to generate object hypotheses. We use [17] to generate superpixel segments. A segmented region r_i is described by several characteristics, *i.e.*, the size of the region (total number of pixels), color histograms, and the texture information (gradient orientation histograms). Four neighbor region similarities are defined based on these characteristics as shown in the following equations:

$$S_c(r_i, r_j) = \sum_{k=1}^{n} \min(c_i^k, c_j^k), \tag{1}$$

$$S_s(r_i, r_j) = 1 - \frac{sz(r_i) + sz(r_j)}{sz(im)}, \tag{2}$$

$$S_t(r_i, r_j) = \sum_{k=1}^{n} \min(t_i^k, t_j^k), \tag{3}$$

$$S_f(r_i, r_j) = 1 - \frac{sz(bb_{ij}) - sz(r_i) - sz(r_j)}{sz(im)}. \tag{4}$$

where c_i^k is the kth dimension of the color histogram, $sz(r_i)$ is the number of pixels in image region r_i, im stands for the whole image, t_i^k is the kth dimension of the texture histogram, bb_{ij} is the rectangular region which tightly bound region r_i and r_j. S_c, S_s and S_t are the color similarity, size similarity, texture similarities, respectively. S_f measures how the combined two regions will occupy the rectangular bounding box which tightly bounds them. The similarity of two adjacent regions can be determined by any combination of the four similarities.

The two regions with the highest similarity *w.r.t* the similarity measurement are merged first and this greedy process is repeated following an agglomerative style clustering scheme. Each merging step produces a bounding box which bounds the merged two regions. In principle, we want regions from the same object to be merged together. Each low level cue contributes from its aspect. For example, the color similarity measures the color intensity correlation between neighbor regions which encourage regions similar in color to be merged together. The size similarity encourages small regions to merge first. The fill similarity encourages the bounding box to tightly bound the merged region. The texture similarity measures the similarity of appearance in gradient, which is complementary to color similarity. The usage of similarity measures and segmentation parameters are detailed in the experiment section.

2.2   Top-Down Supervised Object Search

Once the coarse object hypotheses are obtained, we apply an object detector to determine relatively confident detections. The top-down supervised descent search is only applied to these confident detections.

Supervised descent is a general approach to optimize an objective function which is neither analytically differentiable nor practical to be numerically approximated. It is very suitable for vision problems when visual feature is involved in optimizing the objective function, because most visual features such as SIFT, HOG, and LBP histogram are not differentiable with respect to locations. Instead of computing the descent direction from the gradient, supervised descent uses a large number of examples to train a regression model to predict the descent direction. The training process requires features, which serves as the regressor, to be a fixed length vector, while bottom up segmentations naturally produces arbitrary size proposals. To deal with this issue, we normalize the bounding boxes to a fixed size. In the following, we explain how the supervised descent is adopted to find objects in a full parameter space.

Given an initial object hypothesis location $\mathbf{o}_0 = [x_0, y_0, s_0, a_0]^T$, which may not accurately bound the object, our objective is to use supervised descent to greedily adjust the bounding box by a local movement $\Delta\mathbf{o} = [\Delta x, \Delta y, \Delta s, \Delta a]^T$, leading to a more accurate localization of the object. The goal of the supervised descent training process is hence to learn a sequence of K models to predict the optimal descent direction of the bounding box for each step of the supervised descent, where the needed supervised descent step K is also automatically identified from the training process.

More specifically, denote $\Phi(\mathbf{o}_{k-1})$ to be the n dimensional feature vector extracted from the bounding box defined by $\mathbf{o}_{k-1}$ in the $k-1$ step of the supervised descent process, we learn an $n \times 4$ linear projection matrix $\mathbf{R}_{k-1} = [\mathbf{r}_{k-1}^x, \mathbf{r}_{k-1}^y, \mathbf{r}_{k-1}^s, \mathbf{r}_{k-1}^a]^T$ and a four dimensional bias vector $\mathbf{b}_{k-1} = [b_{k-1}^x, b_{k-1}^y, b_{k-1}^s, b_{k-1}^a]^T$ so that the bounding box movement can be predicted as $\Delta\mathbf{o}_k = \mathbf{R}_{k-1}^T \Phi(\mathbf{o}_{k-1}) + \mathbf{b}_{k-1}$ based on the location from the $k-1$ step. $\Phi(\cdot)$ indicates the feature extracted which is HOG and LBP histogram in our experiments.

We first explain the training process for the first supervised descent model, followed by details to train models sequentially after. Given a set of labeled ground truth object locations $\{\mathbf{o}_*^i = (x_*^i, y_*^i, s_*^i, a_*^i)\}$, we construct the starting locations $\{\mathbf{o}_0^i = (x_0^i, y_0^i, s_0^i, a_0^i)\}$ of the object by applying a random perturbation from the ground truth but assure that they are overlapped. The training of the projection matrix $\mathbf{R}_0$ and the bias $\mathbf{b}_0$ is to solve the following optimization problem:

$$\arg\min_{\mathbf{R}_0, \mathbf{b}_0} \sum_i ||\Delta\mathbf{o}_{0*}^i - \Delta\mathbf{o}_0^i||^2, \tag{5}$$

where $\Delta\mathbf{o}_{0*}^i = \mathbf{o}_*^i - \mathbf{o}_0^i$ is the true movement and $\Delta\mathbf{o}_0^i = \mathbf{R}_0^T \Phi(\mathbf{o}_0^i) + \mathbf{b}_0$ is the predicted displacements of the state vector. The optimal $\mathbf{R}_0$ and $\mathbf{b}_0$ are computed in a closed-form by a linear least square method.

The subsequent $\mathbf{R}_k$ and $\mathbf{b}_k$ for $k = 1, 2, \ldots,$ can be learned iteratively. At each iteration, we update the new locations determined by the previous model $\mathbf{R}_{k-1}$ and $\mathbf{b}_{k-1}$,

$$\mathbf{o}_k^i = \mathbf{o}_{k-1}^i + \mathbf{R}_{k-1}^T \Phi(\mathbf{o}_{k-1}^i) + \mathbf{b}_{k-1}. \tag{6}$$

By updating $\Delta\mathbf{o}_{k*}^i = \mathbf{o}_*^i - \mathbf{o}_k^i$ and $\Delta\mathbf{o}_k^i = \mathbf{R}_k^T \Phi(\mathbf{o}_{k-1}^i) + \mathbf{b}_{k-1}$ the optimal $\mathbf{R}_k$ and $\mathbf{b}_k$ can be learned from a new linear regression problem by minimizing

$$\arg\min_{\mathbf{R}_k, \mathbf{b}_k} \sum_i ||\Delta\mathbf{o}_{k*}^i - \Delta\mathbf{o}_k^i||^2. \tag{7}$$

The error empirically decreases as more iterations are added [14]. In our experiments, this training of supervised descent models often converged in 20–30 steps.

Given a testing image, we firstly apply the cascade regionlets detector [16] to the coarse bottom-up object candidates. Object hypotheses which produces high detection scores are fed to the iterative supervised descent search process to perform local search. New locations output by supervised descent search are re-evaluated by the object detector to obtain the detection score. By ranking all the detection scores from searched locations, we keep the most confident detections.

2.3 Regionlets Object Re-localization

The supervised descent search introduced in the previous subsection significantly improve the detection rate by scanning more predicted object candidates. In this section, we assume the object has already been detected, but with non-perfect localization. To further improve the object detection system, we train a model specific for object localization taking advantage of features extracted from the Regionlets detection model.

The Regionlets detector [16] is composed of thousands of weak classifiers learned with RealBoost. These weak classifiers are formed as several cascades for early rejection, yielding fast object detection. The cascade structure is not related to our re-localization approach and would not be included in the following presentation without any misunderstanding. The input of each weak classifier in the Regionlets model is a 1-D feature extracted from a rectangular region in the detection window. In the training process, these 1-D features are greedily chosen to minimize the logistic loss over all training samples, which is based on classification errors. More details about the Regionlets learning and testing are beyond the scope of this paper and can be found from [16].

Not only does the Regionlets training process greedily select discriminative visual appearances, but also it determines the spatial regions to extract the 1-D feature. Thus the resulting weak features extracted from regionlets implicitly encode thousands of spatial locations, which could be used to further predict the precise location of an object. It is worth noting that the detector learning only targets on minimizing the classification error which does not necessarily guarantee that the localization error is also minimized at the same time.

To leverage the rich spatial information encoded in the Regionlets model, we let each Regionlet vote the object's position. Given the object location (l, t, r, b) detected by the object detector $((l, t, r, b)$ represents the object's left, top, right and bottom coordinates, respectively), the problem is equivalent to predict the localization error $(\Delta l_n, \Delta l_t, \Delta l_r, \Delta l_b)$ of the current detection so that the true object location is computed as:

$$
\begin{aligned}
l^* &= l + w\Delta l_n, & t^* &= t + h\Delta t_n, \\
r^* &= r + w\Delta r_n, & b^* &= b + h\Delta b_n.
\end{aligned}
\tag{8}
$$

Here (l^*, t^*, r^*, b^*) is the ground truth object location. (l, t, r, b) is the bounding box detected with the Regionlets model. $w = r - l + 1$, $h = b - t + 1$ are the detected bounding box width and height respectively. $(\Delta l_n, \Delta t_n, \Delta r_n, \Delta b_n)$ are the relative localization error between the ground truth and the current detection. It is normalized by the width and height of the detected objects[1]. Detections from Regionlets model have various sizes, we observe that normalizing displacement errors is critical to stabilize the training and prediction.

Training the localization model is to learn a vector V, so that we can predict the localization error : $\Delta L = V^T R$, where ΔL is either Δl_n, Δt_n, Δr_n, or Δb_n, R is the feature extracted for from regionlets. We minimize the squared localization error in the model training phase. More specifically, we solve a support vector regression problem for each of the four coordinates respectively:

$$\min_V \left\{ \frac{\|V\|}{2} + C \sum_{m=1}^{M} \max(0, |\Delta L_m - V^T R_m| - \epsilon)^2 \right\}, \tag{9}$$

where V is the coefficient vector to be learned, ΔL_m is the normalized localization error of training sample m, R_m is the feature extracted from all the Regionlets in the object detection model for the mth sample as explained in the following, M is the total number of training examples. The first term in the Eq. (9) is the regularization term, while C is a trade-off factor between the regularization and the sum of squared error, ϵ is the tolerance factor. The problem can be effectively solved using the publicly available liblinear package [18].

The feature R is extracted from the discriminatively learned Regionlets detection model. However, directly applying Regionlets features produces poor performance. Based on the weak classifier learned on each Regionlets feature, we transfer the 1-D Regionlet feature into a sparse binary vector. Each Regionlets weak classifier is a piece-wise linear function implemented using a lookup table:

$$h_i = \sum_{j=1}^{8} w_{i,j} \delta(Q(f_i) - j), \tag{10}$$

where f_i is the 1-D feature extracted from a group of regionlets, $Q(f_i)$ quantize the feature f_i into an integer from 1 to 8. $\delta(x) = 1$ when $x = 0$ otherwise 0. $\{w_{i,j}\}_{j=1}^{8}$ is the classifier weights learned in the boosting training process. We transfer $Q(f_i)$ into an 8-dimensional binary vector r, where the jth dimension is computed as $r(j) = \mathbb{1}(Q(f_i) = j)$, and $\mathbb{1}(\cdot)$ is the indicator function. Apparently, there is one and only one nonzero dimension in r. Note that the Regionlets object detector is a combination of N weak classifiers:

$$H = \sum_{i=1}^{N} h_i. \tag{11}$$

Thus by concatenating these binary vectors from all weak classifiers, the detection model naturally produces $8N$ dimensional sparse vectors, denoted as

---

[1] We empirically found that using the four coordinates for our localization model produces better performance than using (x, y, s, a). Thus we choose (l, t, r, b) in our Regionlets Re-localization approach.

$R = (r_1^T, r_2^T, \ldots, r_N^T)^T$. It serves as the feature vector R_m in Eq. (9). Intuitively, each Regionlets feature f_i has 8 options to vote for the actual object location depending on the binarized feature vector r_i. Learning the weight vector V in Eq. (9) is to jointly determine the votes (regression coefficients) in 8 different scenarios for all Regionlets features.

The sparse binary features extracted from regionlets are very high dimensional. We observed significant over-fitting problem if there are not enough training samples. To avoid over-fitting during training, we randomly sample 80k bounding boxes around ground truth objects to train the localization model.

Discussion. The supervised descent search is designed to search more object candidates in a principled way to increase the detection rate, and a following discriminative visual model (Regionlets detector) is mandatory to determine the detection scores of new locations. Regionlets Re-localization is only used to predict the accurate object location. There is no detector followed to evaluate the new location as in the supervised search. Thus it adjusts the detection to a more precise location without changing the detection score. In contrast, using the object detector to re-evaluate the detection score decreases the performance. Because the newly predicted location usually gives lower detection score which causes the predicted location being eliminated in the post non-max suppression process. To summarize, the role of supervised descent search is to find objects based on detections with coarse locations. Regionlets Re-localization is conducted on fine detections from supervised descent search. It aims at further improvement in accurate localization based on reasonable good localizations from supervised descent search. Leaving out any of these two schemes would significantly hurt the detection performance according to our observation.

3   Experiments

We evaluate the proposed detection framework with the Regionlets detector [16] on the PASCAL VOC2007 dataset and a self-collected car dataset. Our collected car dataset contains 5559 images (17501 cars) for training and 3893 images (12546 cars) for testing. We use the average precision (AP) and mean average precision (mAP) as performance measurement. We first analyze the performance of location relaxation search detection, followed with quantitative results of Regionlets Re-localization.

3.1   Location Relaxation Search

In the training phase of supervised descent, our starting points include the one from the Regionlets [16] confident detection and a set of random perturbations from the ground-truth. We found adding such starting points with perturbation samples to be necessary for a stable training. In testing phase, it always starts from Regionlets coarse detections. In this subsection, Regionlets [16] is used as a baseline for performance comparison to better understand the location relaxation

Table 1. Cues used to generate object hypotheses. The last column shows average number of object hypotheses generated per image based on these cues.

#cues	Color space	Segmentation	Similarity	#object hypotheses
1	RGB	F-g (k=50)	(S_c, S_t, S_s, S_f)	955
2	RGB	F-g (k=50)	$(S_c, S_t, S_s, S_f), (S_t, S_s, S_f)$	1454
4	RGB	F-g (k=50, k=100)	$(S_c, S_t, S_s, S_f), (S_t, S_s, S_f)$	2045
8	RGB, Lab	F-g (k=50, k=100)	$(S_c, S_t, S_s, S_f), (S_t, S_s, S_f)$	3367

search. We first study the performance of the location relaxation search with different bottom-up object proposals. Then we choose the best bottom-up setting for a thorough performance evaluation.

Effects of Bottom-Up Object Proposal. The top-down search strategy is evaluated on bottom-up object hypotheses using several different settings based on (1) the color space used for over-segmentation. (2) the algorithm parameter used for over-segmentation, (3) the similarity functions (defined in Sect. 2.1) used for generating object proposals.

We use the graph-based image segmentation proposed by Felzenszwalb *et al.* [17] (denoted as F-g) with the scale parameter k = 50 or k=100 to capture both small and large regions. Two color space are investigated in our experiments, *i.e.*, the RGB color space and the Lab color space. Following Sect. 2.1, the four different similarity measures used are color similarity S_c, size similarity S_s, texture similarity S_t, and fill similarity S_f. There are two levels of combination of these four similarity measurements. (1) Similarity level: combining these similarities as the final similarity measurement for merging neighbor regions. For example, (S_t, S_f) means the final similarity is the weighted summation of texture similarity and fill similarity. (2) Object hypotheses level: object proposals generated using different similarity combinations are collected together for coarse detection. The first combination does not increase the number of object proposals but it affects the neighbor merging activity. The second combination increases the total number of object proposals.

We call one bottom-up object hypotheses generation setup as one cue. The number of object hypotheses is increased by applying different cues independently and collecting all the resulting object hypotheses. Obviously, employing more cues increases the chance of covering the target object. Figure 3 shows the detection performance of our top-down supervised search. We evaluated four detection settings which gradually increase the number of cues to get object hypotheses. The configurations are summarized in Table 1. Figure 3 presents the result including the performance of the original coarse Regiolets detection, the performance of our top-down search without optimizing object aspect ratio (a setup close to branch-and-bound, cross-talk, divide and conquer search) and the performance of our top-down search with optimizing the object aspect ratio. Although achieving promising improvement by searching only for the correct object center and scale, ignoring the aspect ratio during supervised descent

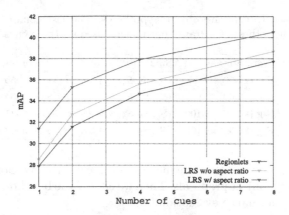

Fig. 3. The detection mean average precision vs number of cues used on the PASCAL VOC 2007 dataset. **Regionlets:** the performance of regionlets without local search. **LRS w/o aspect ratio:** Location relaxation search without searching optimal object aspect ratio. **LRS w/ aspect ratio:** Location relaxation search with aspect ratio optimization.

search substantially suppresses the best detection accuracy we can obtain. Augmented with aspect ratio search, our top-down supervised search consistently improve the detection performance with a large margin. The more cues we used, the better performance we have. That is because our supervised descent search is targeted to find a local maximum which cannot save missing objects which are far away from the coarse detection.

Overall Performance. Table 2 shows the detailed performance for each object category using 8 cues for coarse detection. Without aspect ratio search, our method only improves the detection mean average precision by 1%. Adding aspect ratio to the supervised descent procedure significantly boost the performance by 3%. Note that the detection results of the Regionlets [16] detector reported here is the average precision without conducting the exhaustive local

Table 2. Performance comparison with the baselines on the PASCAL VOC 2007 dataset (average precision %). LRS w/o aspect ratio: location relaxation search without optimizing aspect ratio. LRS w/ aspect ratio: location relaxation search with optimizing aspect ratio. **mAP** is the mean average precision over all the 20 categories.

AP %	aero	bike	bird	boat	bottle	bus	car	cat	chair	cow	table
Regionlets [16]	53.1	49.5	16.7	25.9	16.3	49.8	64.2	37.9	16.7	39.3	44.7
LRS w/o aspect ratio	53.3	49.1	17.0	25.9	17.9	50.6	64.5	41.5	17.2	40.1	**46.8**
LRS w/ aspect ratio	**54.2**	**52.4**	**18.0**	**27.3**	**22.5**	**53.8**	**68.6**	**43.1**	**20.6**	**42.8**	45.6
	dog	horse	mbike	person	plant	sheep	sofa	train	tv	mAP	
Regionlets [16]	23.2	50.4	52.7	35.6	11.7	29.5	31.3	56.1	50.0	37.7	
LRS w/o aspect ratio	25.0	51.6	53.3	36.6	13.0	29.6	34.4	55.6	50.5	38.7	
LRS w/ aspect ratio	**26.2**	**56.2**	**57.2**	**42.7**	**16.0**	**37.0**	**38.7**	**57.1**	**51.7**	**41.6**	

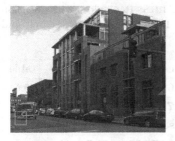

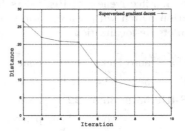

Fig. 4. The trace of the searched bounding box center in supervised descent.

Fig. 5. The distance between the searched bounding box center and the true object center in supervised descent.

grid search (*i.e.*, only a coarse detection is applied in order to validate the effectiveness of our supervised descent search). If such exhaustive local grid search is conducted, it bumps the mAP to be 41.7 % as reported in [16]. Table 2 suggests that our principled supervised descent search achieves comparable results with exhaustive dense local search.

Understanding Supervised Descent. As aforementioned, training the supervised descent models in our experiments takes about 20 to 30 iterations to converge. Hence in testing, the supervised descent would run up to 20 to 30 steps. To better understand the supervised descent steps, we use an example to visualize how the bounding box would be evolving with the progress of the supervised descent, as illustrated in Figs. 4 and 5. In Fig. 4, it shows the trace of the object center (the pink curve) when supervised descent is gradually applied. The blue box is the initial coarse detection based on the bottom-up segmentation and the red box is where the search converged. We plot the distance between the searched bounding box center and the ground truth object center in Fig. 5. The distance is gradually reduced in the search process. Note that this is just an illustration for understanding the process. In practice, the algorithm does not necessarily always converge to a true detection. An initialization with a false detection which is far away from any ground truth objects may result in a higher false positive during the local search. We rely on the object detector to eliminate false positives.

3.2 Regionlets Re-localization

Table 3 shows the performance of our Regionlets Re-localization approach built upon the location relaxation search on the PASCAL VOC 2007 dataset. Our localization model improves 19 out of 20 object categories. For the person category which usually has many articulated poses, our approach dramatically boosts the average precision by 6.3 %. It suggests that even a dense search with the classification model does not solve the precise localization problem. This can be explained by the fact that the classification model is targeted for robust detection which

Table 3. Effectiveness of Regionlets Re-localization. LRS: Regionlets with location relaxation search with aspect ratio search. LRS-RR: Location relaxation search and Regionlets Re-localization

AP %	aero	bike	bird	boat	bottle	bus	car	cat	chair	cow	table
LRS	54.2	52.4	18.0	27.3	22.5	53.8	68.6	43.1	20.6	42.8	45.6
LRS-RR	**55.8**	**53.5**	**22.1**	**28.8**	**25.1**	**54.1**	**71.5**	**45.9**	**22.3**	**45.7**	**50.6**
	dog	horse	mbike	person	plant	sheep	sofa	train	tv	**mAP**	
LRS	26.2	56.2	**57.2**	42.7	16.0	37.0	38.7	57.1	51.7	41.6	
LRS-RR	**29.6**	**58.4**	55.6	**49.0**	**17.6**	**41.1**	**42.4**	**59.5**	**54.2**	**44.1**	

Table 4. Performance comparison between our Regionlets Re-localization and the bounding box prediction used in deformable part base model. DPM base: base DPM performance in [19]; DPM with BB: DPM with bounding box prediction in [19]. LRS base: our base location relaxation search with aspect ratio search. LRS with RR: LRS with Regionlets Re-localization.

DPM base	DPM with BB	Improvement
26.3 %	26.8 %	0.5 %
LRS base	LRS with RR	Improvement
41.6 %	44.1 %	2.5 %

Table 5. Comparison with state of the arts using mAP over 20 classes. "WC" means the method utilizes context cues. We do not use any context information in our method.

	VOC 2007	Results year
DPM(WC) [4]	35.4	2008
UCI_2009 [20]	27.1	2009
INRIA_2009 [21]	28.9	2009
MIT_2010 [2]	29.6	2010
Song *et al.* (WC) [22]	37.7	2011
Li *et al.* (WC) [23]	35.2	2011
SS_SPM [10]	33.8	2011
Cinbis *et al.* (WC) [24]	35.0	2012
Regionlets [16]	41.7	2013
Ours(LRS + RR)	**44.1**	2014

accommodates inaccurate object locations, while a localization model largely complements the effort for accurate object localization.

Table 4 shows the comparison between our Regionlets Re-localization and the location prediction approach used in DPM (DPM-BB). In contrast to DPM-BB for which the improvements are within 0.5 % for most of the object categories, our

Table 6. Performance of Regionlets Re-localization on the car dataset. **0.5 ov:** A true detection must have more than 50 % overlap with the ground truth. **0.7 ov:** A true detection much have more than 70 % overlap with ground the truth.

	0.5 ov	0.7 ov
LRS	62.7 %	34.8 %
LRS-RR	65.3 %	43.9 %
Improvement	2.6 %	9.1 %

method yields a larger improvement, in average 2.5 %. Combined with location relaxation search, our detection approach produces 44.1 % mean average precision on the PASCAL VOC 2007 dataset, which to our best knowledge, is the best performance reported on this dataset without using outside data. Table 5 presents the performance comparison of our detector with recent state-of-the-art detection systems.

The detection performance of Regionlets Re-localization on the car dataset is evaluated with two different criteria. The first criterion treats a detection as true detection if it has more than 50 % overlap (intersection/union) with the ground truth. The second criterion set the threshold to be 70 %, which requires much better localization. As shown in Table 6, with the 0.5 overlap criterion, our Regionlets Re-localization improves the performance by 2.6 %. With the 0.7 overlap criterion, it largely improves the average precision by 9.1 %. This experiment strongly demonstrates that the detections are much more accurate after Regionlets Re-localization.

3.3 Run-Time Speed

Our detection system runs at 4 frames per second if the over-segments are ready. The over segmentation took 1 seconds per image. However, recent approaches [25] show it is possible to obtain real-time over segmentation.

4 Conclusions

In this paper, we proposed an object detection strategy which is a combination of bottom-up object hypotheses generation and top-down local object search for generic object detection. Our framework optimizes the object location in a full parameter space which can also search the aspect ratio of the object. The Regionlets Re-localization model complement existing classification models and can produce more precise localization, pushing even more accurate object detection.

Acknowledgements. The main part of the work was carried out when the first author was a summer intern at NEC Laboratories America in Cupertino, CA. Research reported in this publication was also partly supported by the National Institute Of

Nursing Research of the National Institutes of Health under Award Number R01NR015371. The content is solely the responsibility of the authors and does not necessarily represent the official views of the National Institutes of Health. This work is also partly supported by US National Science Foundation Grant IIS 1350763, China National Natural Science Foundation Grant 61228303, GH's start-up funds form Stevens Institute of Technology, a Google Research Faculty Award, a gift grant from Microsoft Research, and a gift grant from NEC Labs America.

References

1. Chen, G., Ding, Y., Xiao, J., Han, T.X.: Detection evolution with multi-order contextual co-occurrence. In: CVPR (2013)
2. Zhu, L., Chen, Y., Yuille, A., Freeman, W.: Latent hierarchical structural learning for object detection. In: CVPR (2010)
3. Wang, X., Han, T.X., Yan, S.: An HOG-LBP human detector with partial occlusion handling. In: ICCV (2009)
4. Felzenszwalb, P., McAllester, D., Ramanan, D.: A discriminatively trained, multi-scale, deformable part model. In: CVPR (2008)
5. Dalal, N., Triggs, B.: Histograms of oriented gradients for human detection. In: CVPR (2005)
6. Viola, P., Jones, M.: Robust real-time object detection. IJCV (2001)
7. Lampert, C.H., Blaschko, M.B., Hofmann, T.: Beyond sliding windows: object localization by efficient subwindow search. In: CVPR (2008)
8. Lampert, C.H.: An efficient divide-and-conquer cascade for nonlinear object detection. In: CVPR (2010)
9. Dollár, P., Appel, R., Kienzle, W.: Crosstalk cascades for frame-rate pedestrian detection. In: Fitzgibbon, A., Lazebnik, S., Perona, P., Sato, Y., Schmid, C. (eds.) ECCV 2012, Part II. LNCS, vol. 7573, pp. 645–659. Springer, Heidelberg (2012)
10. Van de Sande, K.E.A., Uijlings, J.R.R., Gevers, T., Smeulders, A.W.M.: Segmentation as selective search for object recognition. In: ICCV (2011)
11. Cinbis, R.G., Verbeek, J., Schmid, C.: Segmentation driven object detection with fisher vectors. In: ICCV (2013)
12. Alexe, B., Deselaers, T., Ferrari, V.: Measuring the objectness of image windows. IEEE T-PAMI **34**, 2189–2202 (2012)
13. Lazebnik, S., Schmid, C., Ponce, J.: Beyond bags of features: spatial pyramid matching for recognizing natural scene categories. In: CVPR (2006)
14. Xiong, X., De la Torre, F.: Supervised descent method and its applications to face alignment. In: CVPR (2013)
15. Chang, K.Y., Liu, T.L., Chen, H.T., Lai, S.H.: Fusing generic objectness and visual saliency for salient object detection. In: ICCV (2011)
16. Wang, X., Yang, M., Zhu, S., Lin, Y.: Regionlets for generic object detection. In: ICCV (2013)
17. Felzenszwalb, P.F., Huttenlocher, D.P.: Efficient graph-based image segmentation. IJCV **59**, 167–181 (2004)
18. Fan, R., Chang, K., Hsieh, C., Wang, X., Jin, C.: Liblinear: a library for large linear classification. JMLR **9**, 1871–1874 (2008)
19. Felzenszwalb, P., Girshick, R., McAllester, D., Ramanan, D.: bject detection with discriminatively trained part-based models. IEEE T-PAMI **32**, 1627–1645 (2010)
20. Desai, C., Ramanan, D., Fowlkes, C.: Discriminative models for multi-class object layout. In: ICCV (2009)

21. Harzallah, H., Jurie, F., Schmid, C.: Combining efficient object localization and image classification. In: ICCV (2009)
22. Song, Z., Chen, Q., Huang, Z., Hua, Y., Yan, S.: Contextualizing object detection and classification. In: CVPR (2011)
23. Li, C., Parikh, D., Chen, T.: Extracting adaptive contextual cues from unlabeled regions. In: ICCV (2011)
24. Cinbis, R.G., Sclaroff, S.: Contextual object detection using set-based classification. In: Fitzgibbon, A., Lazebnik, S., Perona, P., Sato, Y., Schmid, C. (eds.) ECCV 2012, Part VI. LNCS, vol. 7577, pp. 43–57. Springer, Heidelberg (2012)
25. Van den Bergh, M., Boix, X., Roig, G., de Capitani, B., Van Gool, L.: SEEDS: superpixels extracted via energy-driven sampling. In: Fitzgibbon, A., Lazebnik, S., Perona, P., Sato, Y., Schmid, C. (eds.) ECCV 2012, Part VII. LNCS, vol. 7578, pp. 13–26. Springer, Heidelberg (2012)

Unsupervised Feature Learning for RGB-D Image Classification

I-Hong Jhuo[1]([✉]), Shenghua Gao[2], Liansheng Zhuang[3],
D.T. Lee[1,4], and Yi Ma[2,5]

[1] Institute of Information Science, Academia Sinca, Taipei, Taiwan
ihjhuo@gmail.com
[2] School of Information Science and Technology, ShanghaiTech University,
Shanghai, China
gaoshh@shanghaitech.edu.cn
[3] CAS Key Laboratory of Electromagnetic Space Information, USTC, Hefei, China
lszhuang@ustc.edu.cn
[4] Department of Computer Science, National Chung Hsing University,
Taichung, Taiwan
dtlee@ieee.org
[5] Department of ECE, University of Illinois at Urbana-Champaign, Champaign, USA
mayi@shanghaitech.edu.cn

Abstract. Motivated by the success of Deep Neural Networks in computer vision, we propose a deep Regularized Reconstruction Independent Component Analysis network (R^2ICA) for RGB-D image classification. In each layer of this network, we include a R^2ICA as the basic building block to determine the relationship between the gray-scale and depth images corresponding to the same object or scene. Implementing commonly used local contrast normalization and spatial pooling, we gradually enhance our network to be resilient to local variance resulting in a robust image representation for RGB-D image classification. Moreover, compared with conventional handcrafted feature-based RGB-D image representation, the proposed deep R^2ICA is a feedforward network. Hence, it is more efficient for image representation. Experimental results on three publicly available RGB-D datasets demonstrate that the proposed method consistently outperforms the state-of-the-art conventional, manually designed RGB-D image representation confirming its effectiveness for RGB-D image classification.

1 Introduction

Image classification is a fundamental problem in computer vision. It has many potential applications for both robotic vision and social networking applications. With recent advances and the popularity of sensing hardware in ranging devices, e.g., RGB-D Kinect cameras, the acquisition of depth information has become easier and provides effective support for the inference of objects or scenes beyond

© Springer International Publishing Switzerland 2015
D. Cremers et al. (Eds.): ACCV 2014, Part I, LNCS 9003, pp. 276–289, 2015.
DOI: 10.1007/978-3-319-16865-4_18

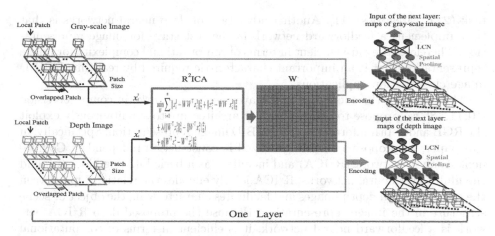

Fig. 1. Illustration of the proposed method for image representation based on feature extraction of basic building block with one layer deep neural network. We first randomly sample some gray-scale patches and their corresponding depth patches to learn the R^2ICA filters. After learning the filters, we apply them on the gray-scale image and depth image respectively. Then we apply the commonly used spatial pooling and local contrast normalization (LCN) to enhance the robustness of the image representation. The outputs is then used as the inputs to the next layer. Repeating these operations for several layers, a deep R^2ICA network can be built for the RGB-D image representation. This figure is best viewed in color (Color figure online).

traditional RGB information. Therefore, a method to effectively and efficiently combine RGB information with depth information for robust image representation has become a core issue in RGB-D based image classification.

Significant research [3,4,6] has been undertaken and promising results have been achieved in this field. However, almost all the previous work [2,4,5,8] focus on handcrafted feature-based image representation for RGB-D image representation, such as 3-dimensional (3D), Local Binary Patterns (3D-LBP) and RGB-D kernel descriptor-based image representation [1,3]. Although these features boost the image classification accuracy on RGB-D images compared with that based only on the RGB image, their design and application require strong domain-specific knowledge. More importantly, the feature extraction stage of these methods is extremely time consuming, limiting their application in real-time robotic image classification [3,4].

Recently, with the development of machine learning techniques, Deep neural networks (DNNs) have demonstrated success in many computer vision tasks [18,22,28–30]. Compared to manually designing the features, deep neural networks automatically extract the features from the raw pixels. Using layer-wise stacking of the basic building blocks, for example, Restricted Boltzmann Machine (RBM) and Convolutional Neural Nets (CNN), deep neural networks gradually extract additional semantic meaningful features in the higher layers, including object parts [18,19]. It is worth noting that deep neural network-based methods significant outperform the traditional manually designed features in terms of classification accuracy on the extremely challenging ImageNet classification task (22 K categories) [11]. Another advantage of deep neural networks is that they implement a feedforward network in the test stage for image representation. Therefore, they are efficient in terms of computational complexity for image representation that is an important characteristic required by real-time RGB-D image classification applications.

Motivated by the success of multi-layer neural networks in computer vision [10,11,18], we propose to utilize the deep architecture to simultaneously exploit the RGB and depth information for RGB-D image representation. Specifically, in this paper, we propose a deep Regularized Reconstruction Independent Component Analysis network (R^2ICA) and include it as a basic building block to build the multi-layer neural networks. R^2ICA jointly encodes the relationship between the gray-scale and depth images and facilitates characterizing the object or scene structure in the image representation. Because the proposed deep R^2ICA network is a feedforward neural network, it is efficient in terms of computational complexity in the test phase for image classification. Figure 1 illustrates the proposed architecture model and an overview of the framework in one layer.

The contribution of the proposed work can be summarized as follows: (1) To our knowledge, this is the first attempt in the direction of discovering the relationship between the gray-scale and depth images in building a deep neural network for RGB-D image classification.[1] The resultant deep neural network boosts both the accuracy and efficiency for RGB-D image classification; (2) we propose the R^2ICA algorithm and implement it as a new building block to create the deep neural network. R^2ICA encodes the relationships between the gray-scale and depth images for building the deep neural networks; (3) the proposed image representation outperforms manually designed feature-based image representations in both accuracy and efficiency.

We organize the rest of the paper as follows: work related to deep neural networks based image classification and RGB-D image classification will be discussed in Sect. 2. In Sect. 3, our R^2ICA based deep neural networks structure will be explained in details, and it would be evaluated in Sect. 4. We conclude our work in Sect. 5.

2 Related Work

2.1 Work Related to Deep Neural Networks for Image Classification

Many building blocks have been proposed to develop deep neural networks for image representation. These building blocks can generally be categorized as global image representation-based and local image patch-based building blocks. Global image representation-based building blocks include the Restricted Boltzmann Machine (RBM) [10], Auto-Encoder (AE), and other building blocks that are extensions of RBM and AE, such as Deep Belief Machine (DBM), Denoising Auto-Encoder [29], and Contractive Auto-encoder [24]. These global

---

[1] [25] applies the DNNs on RGB and depth image representation separately, and simply concatenates the resultant representations for the RGB-D image presentation.

image representation-based building blocks are trained on the entire image. Therefore, they typically require more training samples for training the robust neural networks. This seriously restricts the advantage of automatically learned features from the raw data [18,19]. On the other hand, local patch-based building blocks such as Convolutional Neural Nets (CNN) [20] and Deconvolutional Networks (DN) [32] usually operate on image patch levels to train a stable network. Compared with global image representation-based building blocks, these local image patch-based building blocks are more flexible to address cases where the intra-class variance is more significant. Therefore, they frequently achieve better performance on challenging image classification datasets, such as CIFAR-10, CIFAR-100, and ImageNet. Further to the aforementioned single modality-based deep neural networks; recently, multi-modal deep neural networks for multiple modalities based on signal processing tasks have been proposed from both Srivastava *et al.* [28] and Ngiam *et al.* [22]. As the aforementioned restriction, both these architectures are global image-based representations with some drawbacks. Moreover, these two architectures demand that the hidden states of the multiple modalities be the same. This is unacceptable for real applications where different modalities may, to some extent, be diverse.

2.2 Work Related to RGB-D Image Classification

In recent years, the growth of utilizing consumer RGB-D sensors has accelerated in computer vision research [7,13,27]. With the popularity of depth-sensing cameras, e.g. Microsoft Kinect, depth information can be readily accessed. These depth information facilitates characterize the 3D structure of an object and provide effective support for the inference of objects beyond the traditional RGB information. Significant effort has been made to effectively employ the depth information in the developed models. For example in scene understanding, Gupta *et al.* [9] use gPb like machinery to obtain long range grouping in non-overlapping superpixels to segmentation and recognition. Ren *et al.* [23] transform pixel-level similarity into descriptors based on kernel descriptors and then adopt context modeling to a hierarchical region based on a superpixel Markov Random Field (MRF). Silberman *et al.* [27] infer the overall 3D structure and estimate the supported relations based on jointly parsing images into separate objects. For the robotic vision community, Bo *et al.* [4] developed a hierarchical matching pursuit (HMP) based on sparse coding for new feature representations in an unsupervised manner. There are numerous papers on instance and image classification using RGB-D perception, combining color and depth channels from multiple scenes [3,4,15]. Motivated by the leading works, we develop a deep R^{2}ICA network by encoding the relationship between the gray-scale and depth images and utilize it for image representation.

3 Deep R^{2}ICA Framework

The basic building blocks of the proposed deep R^{2}ICA network consists of four modules: (i) data whitening, (ii) filter learning with R^{2}ICA and feature encoding,

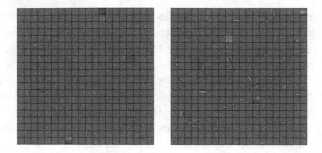

Fig. 2. Visualization of randomly sampled filters in layer 1 on RGB-D object benchmark [15]. Left: Filters learned with our proposed R^2ICA method. Right: Filters learned with RICA [17].

(iii) spatial pooling, and (iv) local contrast normalization (LCN) [14]. We propose stacking three such basic R^2ICA layers to construct the deep architecture. In the following subsections, we will explain each of these modules in detail.

Before exploiting the deep R^2ICA network-based image representation details, we need to mathematically define the variables that will be used in the following sections. We use $\{x_i^k\}_{i=1}^n \in \mathbb{R}^p$ to index the unlabeled gray-scale or depth image patches. The subscript i is used to index the number of patches and the superscript k is used to index whether the patch is a gray-scale or depth image patch. Specifically, x_i^1 corresponds to a gray-scale image patch; x_i^2 corresponds to a depth image patch. The size of each patch is $h \times h$. The gray-scale and depth patch with the same subscript, i.e., x_i^1 and x_i^2, correspond to the patches collected from the same regions of a gray-scale and depth image pair. In a deep R^2ICA network, we learn the features from the raw pixels, i.e., we stack all the pixels within each patch as the input to the network, the dimensionality of the input $p = h \times h$. We gather all the patches and organize them into a matrix form: $X = [x_1^1, \ldots, x_n^1, x_1^2, \ldots, x_n^2] \in R^{p \times 2n}$. Here n is the total number of gray-scale image patches or depth image patches. For the general gray-scale image, each x_i^1 is a feature corresponding to an image patch.

3.1 Data Preprocessing

Numerous studies in the machine learning community have shown that *whitening* is an important preprocess to de-correlate the data and is commonly used in building deep neural networks [6,19]. Therefore, we also whiten the input data before unsurprised learning the image representation. Specifically, each feature x_i^k is normalized by subtracting the mean of all its entries and then consequently dividing by their standard deviation. This whitening process is important for ensuring the effective performance of the proposed deep R^2ICA network. For example, we have found that whitening boosts the accuracy by 0.7 % on the 2D3D object recognition benchmark.

3.2   Filter Learning and Feature Encoding

We first simply introduce the basic auto-encoder (AE) [24], the encoder is to map each input[2] x to hidden representation with a mapping function

$$e = f_h(x) = \varphi_h(W^\top x + b_h), \tag{1}$$

where φ_h is a nonlinear activation function, i.e., a logistic sigmoid function, and the encoder is parametrized by a weight matrix W, and b_h is a bias function. Then, the decoder function f_r maps hidden representation back to a reconstruction r with the function $f_r(e) = \varphi_r(We) + b_r$, where φ_r is nonlinear activation function and a bias vector b_r. Following the single modality concept, given a set of input data X corresponding to the features of all the patches, Independent Components Analysis (ICA) [12] aims at learning filters in an unsupervised fashion. Its objective can be written as follows:

$$\min_W \sum_{i=1}^n \sum_{j=1}^m \sum_k \psi(W_j^\top x_i^k), \quad s.t \ \ W^\top W = \mathbf{I}, \tag{2}$$

where ψ is a nonlinear convex function such that L_1 penalty: $\phi(\cdot) = (\log \cosh(\cdot))$ in [17], m is the number of filters (components) and W is the weight matrix $W \in \mathbb{R}^{p \times m}$. However, the method has difficulty learning overcomplete filters because of the orthogonality constraint $W^\top W = \mathbf{I}$. The hard orthogonal constraint in ICA can be relaxed with a soft reconstruction cost. Then, we arrive at the objective function that can be written as follows:

$$\min_W \sum_k (\lambda \sum_{i=1}^n \sum_{j=1}^m \psi(W_j^\top x_i^k) + \frac{1}{n} \sum_{i=1}^n \|x_i^k - WW^\top x_i^k\|_2^2), \tag{3}$$

where W is the tied encoding and decoding weights. The smooth penalty in Eq. (3) is called *reconstruction cost* and the unconstraint problem can resolve the overcomplete problem in Eq. (2), meanwhile it can be optimized efficiently.

For improved image classification, recent advanced research in [3,4] utilizes the advantages of the RGB-D images to learn from the 3D features for object recognition. In this task, we propose a deep Regularized Reconstruction Independent Component Analysis network (R^{2}ICA) to discover the joint weights, i.e., *filters*, from both of the unlabeled gray-scale and depth images. To effectively construct the joint weights, we formulate the learning filter problem as the following objective function:

$$\min_W \sum_{i=1}^n \eta\|W^\top x_i^2 - W^\top x_i^1\|_2^2 + \lambda(\|W^\top x_i^1\|_2^2 + \|W^\top x_i^2\|_2^2)$$

$$\|x_i^1 - WW^\top x_i^1\|_2^2 + \|x_i^2 - WW^\top x_i^2\|_2^2, \tag{4}$$

where x_i^1 is a gray-scale image patch, x_i^2 is a depth image patch, λ and η are the parameters. For learning the joint weights W,[3] we adopt the L-BFGS algorithm

---

[2] Here, we only discuss one modality data and x is to represent an input.

[3] For simplification, we apply the same W to the gray-scale and depth patches. Experimental results show that the performance is promising.

with line search to resolve the unconstraint problem. It is important to note that the complexity of the proposed method is the same as [17, 18]. Therefore, the proposed R^{2}ICA formulation can be optimized efficiently. Figure 2 shows the visualization of 400 learned filters from the RGB-D object recognition dataset [15] from 20,000 randomly selected patches and compared with the Le *et al* method [17] based on whitening preprocessing. As can be seen, the proposed R^{2}ICA method yields additional sharp filters. This is because we impose the last term in Eq. (4). Many grayscale image patches (e.g., patches corresponding to object boundaries) are closely related to their corresponding depth patches. These boundaries represented by two maps should be similar for the same object and are important for object recognition. By forcing the outputs of the depth image and RGB image to be similar, the learned filters encode the edge correspondence and therefore the sharpness.

3.3   Spatial Pooling and Normalization

Once we have obtained the filters with the R^{2}ICA algorithm in one layer, we can simply map all the patches of an image to obtain a new image representation, $y_i^k = W^T x_i^k$. Then we subsequently use spatial maximum pooling [18] and local contrast normalization (LCN) [14] for the subsequent image processing. The spatial maximum pooling improves the robustness of the image representation to local translation. LCN is a practice inspired by the computational neuroscience models [21] and has demonstrated its effectiveness for DNN-based image representation. After filter learning and encoding, spatial pooling, and LCN, we can get a new sets of feature maps which corresponding to the gray-scale image and depth image, respectively. These new feature maps will serve as the input to the next layer or the image representation at the current layer.

3.4   Implementation Details

Because there are numerous training patches and these could cause memory issues, it is not feasible to use all the patches to learn W. For simplification, we randomly sample specific patches to learn the W in our deep neural networks. Once the W is learned, we apply it to both the gray-scale and depth image for image representation. We repeat the basic building block (R^{2}ICA, Pooling, and LCN) for three layers. Then a 1-vs.-all linear SVM is used to train the classifiers for label prediction.

4   Experiments

In this section, we evaluated the proposed method on two publicly available RGB-D object recognition datasets (RGB-D object dataset [15] (RGBDO) and 2D & 3D object dataset (2D3D) [7]) and one indoor scene dataset (NYU Depth V1 indoor scene segmentation dataset [13]). We also compared the proposed deep R^{2}ICA network with the following methods that are considered state-of-the-art for image classification. (1) Spatial Pyramid Matching (SPM) [16]. We adopted the spatial pyramid matching method with the standard experimental settings of [16] to represent the RGB and depth images. The dictionary size was set to 200. (2) RICA-based method [17]. We followed the standard experimental setting of [12] to combine the RGB images with the depth images as input for the unsupervised learning. (3) Hierarchical Matching Pursuit with sparse coding (HMP-S) [4]. This approach uses sparse coding to learn hierarchical feature representation from raw RGB-D images. (4) We also compared our work with *CKM Desc* [3], *NIPS11* [6], and *RICA* [17] because of the close relationship between the proposed method and these approaches. In the proposed deep R^2ICA network, we set the depth of our network at 3 layers on all datasets and report the performance based on using the combined image representation, i.e., each filter has been extracted from different layers for image representation. In all of the experiments, the images are resized to 200×200 pixels and each patch is extracted using an *overlapped patch size* equal to 1 pixel, where the overlapped patch size indicates the distance between two neighboring patches. We randomly sampled $500,000$ image patches for the unsupervised filter learning and set the numbers of filters in W to 200, 400, and 400 for layer1, layer2, and layer3, respectively. Furthermore, we preprocessed the input data before the unsupervised learning[4]. To determine the appropriate parameters, we varied the values of λ and η during the unsupervised learning and selected the optimal values based on five random training/testing splits. For evaluation, we employed linear SVM to train the classifiers for image classification. Moreover, we evaluated the performance of the proposed deep R^2sICA with different settings by varying the patch and pooling sizes in each task.

4.1   RGB-D Object Recognition Benchmark [15]

We first tested our proposed method on the RGB-D object recognition benchmark [15] that contains 300 physically distinct objects with different viewpoints. This dataset consists of 51 different object categories varying from fruits and coffee mugs to scissors and soda cans under large changes in lighting conditions, and the total number of RGB-D images is $41,877$. Since the proposed method can handle single and multiple layers feature representation, we also reported the performance of our method with different layers.

Based on the experiment settings in [15], we evaluated the performance of the different methods with two types of object recognition tasks, i.e., category recognition and instance recognition. For the category recognition, we randomly selected one object instance per category for testing and utilized the remaining objects for training. We average the classification accuracies over 5 random trials as the performance measure for the category classification. For the evaluation of the instance recognition (leave-sequence-out [15]), we tested the images of $45°$ angle using the training images captured from $30°$ and $60°$ elevation angles. In

---

[4] To de-correlate the input data, it was individually normalized by subtracting the mean and dividing by the standard deviation of the high dimensional data before our unsupervised filter learning.

Table 1. Performance comparisons (%) with the baseline methods on the RGB-D object recognition benchmark.

RGB-D		Compared Methods					Our Approach
		SPM [16]	RICA [17]	CKM Desc [3]	NIPS11 [6]	HMP-S [4]	Three Layers
Category	RGB	73.2 ± 2.6	84.1 ± 2.9	N/A	74.7 ± 2.5	82.4 ± 3.1	$\mathbf{85.65 \pm 2.7}$
	Depth	66.5 ± 3.6	79.7 ± 3.1	N/A	70.3 ± 2.2	81.2 ± 2.3	$\mathbf{83.94 \pm 2.8}$
	RGB-D	79.1 ± 4.1	86.7 ± 2.7	86.4 ± 2.3	82.1 ± 3.3	87.5 ± 2.9	$\mathbf{89.59 \pm 3.8}$
Instance	RGB	82.3	88.3	82.9	75.8	92.1	**92.43**
	Depth	47.9	49.6	N/A	39.8	51.7	**55.69**
	RGB-D	84.7	89.7	90.4	78.9	92.8	**93.23**

this task, the patch size and spatial pooling size were 8×8 and 5×5, respectively. The average classification accuracy over all 51 object categories in the test set was used as the evaluation metric.

Category classification. Table 1 summarizes the performance of the different methods for category classification. We also included the results from [3,4,6]. From Table 1, we can observe that:

- The combination of RGB with depth achieves higher accuracy than that based on the RGB image only for all methods, confirming the usefulness of depth image information.
- The proposed R^2ICA approach significantly outperforms the Hierarchical Matching Pursuit with sparse coding (HMP-S) [4] and RICA [17] methods, verifying that the effectiveness of enforcing gray-scale and depth images to have similar representation.
- R^2ICA with three layers outperforms R^2ICA with only one layer (see Fig. 5) demonstrating the effectiveness of the deep architecture for image represen tation.
- The proposed method with three layers outperforms the baseline methods, i.e., HMP-S, RICA, and NIPS11, by 2.09 %, 2.89 %, and 7.49 %, respectively. The improvement is significant confirming the effectiveness of the proposed deep R^2ICA network for RGB-D image representation.

Instance classification. In this test, we used the same evaluation settings as the category classification. It is also worth noting that the performance gap between the instance and category classification was not as significant as that in the work [15](3.64 % in our paper vs. 5.3 % in [15]). The rationale may be that color information, which is more important for identifying the same object in instance classification than the category classification, is not used in the proposed R^2ICA framework. Moreover, Fig. 5 also indicates that the performance improvement of 2-layer R^2ICA over 1-layer R^2ICA is marginal. This may be because the number of filters in the second layer is not sufficiently large, and as shown in [29], additional filters usually improve the performance. In real applications, we can determine the number of filters based on the characteristics of

Table 2. Performance comparisons (%) with the baseline methods on the 2D3D object recognition benchmark.

RGB-D	Compared Methods					Our Approach
		SPM [16]	RICA [17]	Ev2D3D [7]	HMP-S [4]	Three Layers
Category	RGB	60.7	85.1	66.6	83.7	**87.9**
	Depth	75.2	87.3	74.6	87.6	**89.2**
	RGB-D	78.3	91.5	82.8	91.0	**92.7**

the data we are processing. Furthermore, we also determined that vegetables and fruits were more frequently misclassified in our experiments because color information is more important in this environment, however, not used in our setting. By excluding the instances from these two categories, the performance of the proposed method can attain up to 97.2 % for instance classification.

4.2 2D3D Object Dataset

We evaluated our approach on the 2D3D object dataset [7]. This dataset contained 18 kinds of objects varying from bottles and coffee pots to cups, and all the objects were highly textured. For each object in the dataset, images corresponding to 36 views are recorded, with the angle between two different views was 10 10° along the vertical axis. The total number of objects was 154 with 154 × 36 views. Then all these images were categorized into 14 different categories. It is worth noting this 2D3D dataset was very challenging for object recognition due to the large variance of views. The image size in this dataset was smaller than that in the RGB-D Object dataset, therefore we resized the image size to 250 × 250 pixels. In the experiments, the patch size for extracting features and size of spatial pooling were fixed to be 8 × 8 and 5 × 5, respectively. In the experiment, 800, 000 patches were randomly sampled to learn the filters. Following the experimental setting in [7], we chose 18 views for training and use the remaining views for testing.

We reported the average classification accuracy over the 14 categories of different methods in Table 2. It can be seen that our proposed method R^2ICA yields 92.7 % accuracy for category classification, which outperforms the HMP-S [4] and Ev2D3D [7] by 1.7 % and 9.9 %, respectively.

We also evaluated the performance of the proposed deep R^2ICA network by varying the patch size and overlapped patch size as illustrated in Figs. 3 and 4. As can be seen in Fig. 3, the classification accuracy of all layers increased with the increase of patch size when the patch size was smaller than 8 × 8. When the patch size was equal to 16 × 16, the performance decreased. The reason may be that the limited number of filters was not sufficient to preserve the information in the larger patches resulting in information loss for the image representation and a decline in the performance. Figure 4 confirms that the performance decreases when we increase the size of the overlapped patch size. This observation agrees with CNN concept that by using all the local patches sampled at every pixel

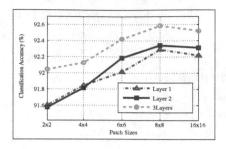
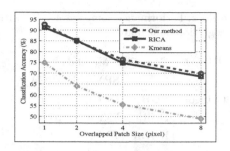

Fig. 3. The comparative effects of different patch sizes on the 2D3D object recognition dataset. This figure is best viewed in color (Color figure online).

Fig. 4. The comparative effects of various overlapped patch sizes on the 2D3D object recognition dataset. This figure is best viewed in color (Color figure online).

Table 3. Performance comparisons (%) with the baseline methods on the NYU Depth V1 indoor scene dataset.

RGB-D	Compared Methods			Our Approach
	SPM [16]	RICA [17]	ScSPM [31]	Three Layers
Category RGB	52.8 ± 3.2	74.5 ± 2.9	71.6 ± 3.2	**75.9 ± 2.9**
Depth	53.2 ± 2.7	64.7 ± 2.1	64.5 ± 2.7	**65.8 ± 2.7**
RGB-D	63.4 ± 2.9	74.5 ± 3.5	73.1 ± 3.6	**76.2 ± 3.2**

for an image representation, additional useful information can be discovered and preserved, thus boosting the classification accuracy. In addition, based on our observation, the number of filters should be determined based on the content complexity of the patches. This content complexity is also related to the patch size. A larger patch size increases the content complexity of the patch, and therefore, more filters are required to characterize these patches.

Figure 6 presents the classification performance under different values of λ and η for recognition, where we set the number of filters and patch size to 400, and 8×8 pixels, respectively. As can be seen, we obtained the highest accuracy when the λ and η were equal to 0.1. Furthermore, even though the λ parameter had a larger performance variation than η, the maximum difference was within 1.1 %. Therefore, in our case, the parameters may not have been an influencing factor.

4.3   NYU Depth V1 Indoor Scene Benchmark

We evaluated our method on indoor scene segmentation on NYU Depth V1 [26]. This dataset was composed of 108, 617 unlabeled frames, including 64 different indoor environment and 7 scene types such as living room, bedroom, and kitchen, etc. Each scene consisted of 41 to 781 images, and the image size was 640 by 480. Following the image classification protocol in [26], we removed the "Cafe"

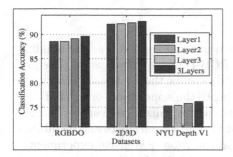
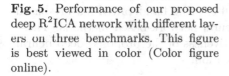
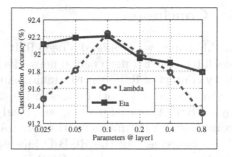

Fig. 5. Performance of our proposed deep R^2ICA network with different layers on three benchmarks. This figure is best viewed in color (Color figure online).

Fig. 6. RGB-D Performance comparison (%) with different values of λ and η on the 2D3D object recognition benchmark. This figure is best viewed in color (Color figure online).

scene images in our experiment. We randomly split each scene into disjoint training/testing sets of equal size. It is worth noting that the indoor segmentation scene dataset contains various objects in one scene, this makes the dataset very challenging to scene classification.

For the scene classification on this dataset, to reduce the computational cost, we resized the image to 150×150 and respectively set patch size, spatial pooling size by 8×8 and 3×3. The number of patches chosen for learning the filters was $500,000$. For the baseline methods, i.e., SPM method, we followed the setting in [16] for SIFT descriptor extraction in both RGB and depth images. The sizes of maximum pooling in a 3-level spatial pyramid were partitioned into 1×1, 2×2, 4×4 sub-regions and dictionary size was set to 200. The representation of the RGB-D image was concatenated RGB image and depth image to one feature vector. For sparse coding SPM (ScSPM), we utilized the experimental setting from Yang et al. [31] and set the vocabulary size of the codebook to 1024.

Table 3 indicates the performance of different methods on this dataset. As can be seen, the proposed method R^2ICA achieves 76.2 % classification accuracy, which outperformed the baseline methods, i.e., RICA [17], ScSPM [31] and HMP-S [4] by 1.7 %, 3.1 % and 3.4 %, respectively. To verify the contribution of local contrast normalization (LCN), we trained the network by removing the LCN process. The performance presented that the classification accuracy decreased to 75.1 %. We had the consistent observation with previous important studying of local contrast normalization [14]. Figure 5 showed the performance of each layer on the three datasets. As we can see, the combined 3 layers representation obtained better performance than using each individual layer. This makes sense intuitively due to the representation taking the advantage of layer1, layer2 and layer3, simultaneously. The experimental results in NYU Depth V1 have only around 76 % classification accuracy, since the dataset originally designed for indoor scene segmentation, which contained various objects in one category rather than a single object for each category.

5   Conclusion

In this paper, we proposed a deep R^2ICA network and applied it as the building block to construct deep neural networks for RGB-D image classification. The primary concept of R^2ICA is to simultaneously determine the relationships between the gray-scale and depth images corresponding to the same object or scene. Employing R^2ICA, spatial pooling, and local contrast normalization, features learned from these deep neural networks were robust to common variances and facilitated the enhancement of the RGB-D image representation. Extensive experimental results on publicly available RGB-D image classification benchmarks confirmed that the proposed method outperformed all existing handcrafted feature-based image representation and baseline deep neural network-based methods. These encouraging results demonstrated the effectiveness of the proposed deep neural network structure for RGB-D image classification.

Acknowledgements. This work was supported by grant MOST 103-2911-I-001-531.

References

1. Banerjee, J., Moelker, A., Niessen, W.J., van Walsum, T.: 3D LBP-based rotationally invariant region description. In: Park, J.-I., Kim, J. (eds.) ACCV Workshops 2012, Part I. LNCS, vol. 7728, pp. 26–37. Springer, Heidelberg (2013)
2. Bariya, P., Novatnack, J., Schwartz, G., Nishino, K.: 3D geometric scale variability in range images: features and descriptors. IJCV **99**, 232–255 (2012)
3. Blum, M., Springenberg, J., Wlfing, J., Riedmiller, M.: A learned feature descriptor for object recognition in RGB-D Data. In: ICRA (2012)
4. Bo, L., Ren, X., Fox, D.: Unsupervised feature learning for RGB-D based object recognition. In: Desai, J.P., Dudek, G., Khatib, O., Kumar, V. (eds.) ISER 2012. STAR, vol. 88, pp. 387–402. Springer, Heidelberg (2012)
5. Bo, L., Lai, K., Ren, X., Fox, D.: Object recognition with hierarchical kernel descriptors. In: CVPR (2012)
6. Bo, L., Ren, X., Fox, D.: Hierarchical matching pursuit for image classification: architecture and fast algorithms. In: NIPS (2011)
7. Browatzki, B., Fischer, J., Graf, B., Blthoff, H.H., Wallraven, C.: Going into depth: evaluating. 2D and 3D cues for object classification on a new, large-scale object dataset. In: ICCV Workshop (2011)
8. Frome, A., Huber, D., Kolluri, R., Bülow, T., Malik, J.: Recognizing objects in range data using regional point descriptors. In: Pajdla, T., Matas, J.G. (eds.) ECCV 2004. LNCS, vol. 3023, pp. 224–237. Springer, Heidelberg (2004)
9. Gupta, S., Arbelaez, P., Malik, J.: Perceptual organization and recognition of indoor scenes from RGBD images. In: CVPR (2013)
10. Hinton, G.E., Osindero, S., Teh, Y.-W.: A fast learning algorithm for deep belief nets. Neural Comput. **18**(7), 1527–1554 (2006)
11. Krizhevsky, A., Sutskever, I., Hinton, G.E.: ImageNet classification with deep convolutional neural networks. In: NIPS (2012)
12. Hyvarinen, A., Karhunen, J., Oja, E.: Independent Component Analysis. Wiley Interscience, New York (2001)

13. Janoch, A., Karayev, S., Jia, Y., Barron, J.T., Fritz, M., Saenko, K., Darrell, T.: A category-level 3-D object dataset: putting the kinect to work. In: ICCV Workshop (2011)
14. Jarrett, K., Kavukcuoglu, K., Ranzato, M.A., LeCun. Y.: What is the best multi-stage architecture for object recognition? In: ICCV (2009)
15. Lai, K., Bo, L., Ren, X., Fox, D.: A large-scale hierarchical multi-view RGB-D object dataset. In: ICRA (2011)
16. Lazebnik, S., Schmid, C., Ponce, J.: Beyond bags of features: spatial pyramid matching for recognizing natural scene categories. In: CVPR (2006)
17. Le, Q.V., Karpenko, A., Ngiam, J., Ng, A.Y.: ICA with reconstruction cost for efficient overcomplete feature learning. In: NIPS (2011)
18. Le, Q.V., Ranzato, M.A., Monga, R., Devin, M., Chen, K., Corrado, G.S., Dean, J., Ng, A.Y.: Building high-level features using large scale unsupervised learning. In: ICML (2012)
19. Le, Q.V., Ngiam, J., Chen, Z., Chia, D., Koh, P., Ng, A.Y.: Tiled convolutional neural networks. In: NIPS (2010)
20. LeCun, Y., Boser, B., Denker, J.S., Henderson, D., Howard, R.E., Hubbard, W., Jackel, L.D.: Backpropagation applied to handwritten zip code rsecognition. Neural Comput. 1(4), 541–551 (1989)
21. Lyu, S., Simoncelli, E.: Nonlinear image representation using divisive normalization. In: ICCV (2009)
22. Ngiam, J., Khosla, A., Kim, M., Nam, J., Lee, H., Ng, A.Y.: Multimodal deep learning. In: ICML (2011)
23. Ren, X., Bo, L., Fox, D.: RGB-(D) scene labeling: features and algorithms. In: CVPR (2012)
24. Rifai, S., Vincent, P., Muller, X., Glorot, X., Bengio, Y.: Contractive auto-encoders: explicit invariance during feature extraction. In: ICML (2011)
25. Socher, R., Huval, B., Bhat, B., Manning, C.D., Ng, A.Y.: Convolutional-recursive deep learning for 3D object classification. In: NIPS (2012)
26. Silberman, N., Fergus R.: Indoor scene segmentation using a structured light sensor. In: ICCV Workshop (2011)
27. Silberman, N., Hoiem, D., Kohli, P., Fergus, R.: Indoor segmentation and support inference from RGBD images. In: Fitzgibbon, A., Lazebnik, S., Perona, P., Sato, Y., Schmid, C. (eds.) ECCV 2012, Part V. LNCS, vol. 7576, pp. 746–760. Springer, Heidelberg (2012)
28. Srivastava, N., Salakhutdinov, R.: Multimodal learning with deep boltzmann machines. In: NIPS (2012)
29. Vincent, P., Larochelle, H., Lajoie, I., Bengio, Y., Manzagol, P.-A.: Stacked denoising autoencoders: learning useful representations in a deep network with a local denoising criterion. JMLR 11(5), 3371–3408 (2010)
30. Wang, N., Yeung, D.-Y.: Learning a deep compact image representation for visual tracking. In: NIPS (2013)
31. Yang, J., Yu, K., Gong, Y., Huang, T.: Linear spatial pyramid matching using sparse coding for image classification. In: CVPR (2009)
32. Zeiler, M., Krishnan, D., Taylor, G., Fergus, R.: Deconvolutional networks. In: CVPR (2010)

Non-maximum Suppression for Object Detection by Passing Messages Between Windows

Rasmus Rothe[1]([✉]), Matthieu Guillaumin[1], and Luc Van Gool[1,2]

[1] Computer Vision Laboratory, ETH Zurich, Zurich, Switzerland
{rrothe,guillaumin}@vision.ee.ethz.ch
[2] ESAT - PSI/IBBT, K.U. Leuven, Leuven, Belgium
luc.vangool@esat.kuleuven.be

Abstract. Non-maximum suppression (NMS) is a key post-processing step in many computer vision applications. In the context of object detection, it is used to transform a smooth response map that triggers many imprecise object window hypotheses in, ideally, a single bounding-box for each detected object. The most common approach for NMS for object detection is a greedy, locally optimal strategy with several hand-designed components (*e.g.*, thresholds). Such a strategy inherently suffers from several shortcomings, such as the inability to detect nearby objects. In this paper, we try to alleviate these problems and explore a novel formulation of NMS as a well-defined clustering problem. Our method builds on the recent Affinity Propagation Clustering algorithm, which passes messages between data points to identify cluster exemplars. Contrary to the greedy approach, our method is solved globally and its parameters can be automatically learned from training data. In experiments, we show in two contexts – object class and generic object detection – that it provides a promising solution to the shortcomings of the greedy NMS.

1 Introduction

Non-maximum suppression (NMS) has been widely used in several key aspects of computer vision and is an integral part of many proposed approaches in detection, might it be edge, corner or object detection [1–6]. Its necessity stems from the imperfect ability of detection algorithms to localize the concept of interest, resulting in groups of several detections near the real location.

In the context of object detection, approaches based on sliding windows [2–4] typically produce multiple windows with high scores close to the correct location of objects. This is a consequence of the generalization ability of object detectors, the smoothness of the response function and visual correlation of close-by windows. This relatively dense output is generally not satisfying for understanding the content of an image. As a matter of fact, the number of window hypotheses at this step is simply uncorrelated with the real number of objects in the image. The goal of NMS is therefore to retain only one window per group, corresponding

Electronic supplementary material The online version of this chapter (doi:10. 1007/978-3-319-16865-4_19) contains supplementary material, which is available to authorized users.

© Springer International Publishing Switzerland 2015
D. Cremers et al. (Eds.): ACCV 2014, Part I, LNCS 9003, pp. 290–306, 2015.
DOI: 10.1007/978-3-319-16865-4_19

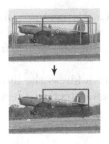 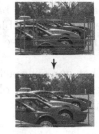 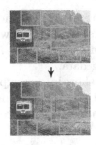

(a) The top-scoring box may not be the best fit. (b) It may suppress nearby objects. (c) It does not suppress false positives.

Fig. 1. Examples of possible failures when using a greedy procedure for NMS. [NB: All our figures are best viewed in color.] (Color figure online)

to the precise local maximum of the response function, ideally obtaining only one detection per object. Consequently, NMS also has a large positive impact on performance measures that penalize double detections [7,8].

The most common approach for NMS consists of a greedy iterative procedure [2,3], which we refer to as *Greedy NMS*. The procedure starts by selecting the best scoring window and assuming that it indeed covers an object. Then, the windows that are too close to the selected window are suppressed. Out of the remaining windows, the next top-scoring one is selected, and the procedure is repeated until no more windows remain. This procedure involves defining a measure of similarity between windows and setting a threshold for suppression. These definitions vary substantially from one work to another, but typically they are manually designed. Greedy NMS, although relatively fast, has a number of downsides, as illustrated in Fig. 1. First, by suppressing everything within the neighborhood with a lower confidence, if two or more objects are close to each other, all but one of them will be suppressed. Second, Greedy NMS always keeps the detection with the highest confidence even though in some cases another detection in the surrounding might provide a better fit for the true object. Third, it returns all the bounding-boxes which are not suppressed, even though many could be ignored due to a relatively low confidence or the fact that they are sparse in a subregion within the image.

As these problems are due to greediness and hard-thresholding, in this paper we propose to consider NMS as a clustering problem that is solved globally, where the hard decisions taken by Greedy NMS are replaced with soft penalties in the objective function. The intuition behind our model is that the multiple proposals for the same object should be grouped together and be represented by just one window, the so-called *cluster exemplar*. We therefore adopt the framework of Affinity Propagation Clustering (APC) [9], an exemplar-based clustering algorithm, which is inferred globally by passing messages between data points.

However, APC is not directly usable for NMS. We need to adapt it to include two constraints that are specific to detection. First, since there are false positives, not every window has to be assigned to a cluster. Second, in certain scenarios it is beneficial to encourage a diverse set of proposals and penalize selecting exemplars that are very close to each other. Hence, our contributions are the following: (i) we extend APC to add repellence between cluster centers; (ii) to model false positives, we relax the clustering problem; (iii) we introduce weights between the terms in APC, and show how these weights can be learned from training data.

We show in our experiments that our approach helps to address the limitations of Greedy NMS in two different contexts: object class detection (Sect. 4) and generic object detection (Sect. 5).

2   Related Work

NMS is a widely used post-processing technique in several computer vision applications. For edge, corner and interest point detection, its role is to find the local maxima of a function defined over a pixel scale-space pyramid, and it is common to simply suppress any pixel which is not the maximum response in its neighborhood [1,10].

Similarly, for object detection, many approaches have been proposed to prune the set of responses that score above the detection threshold. The Viola-Jones detector [4] partitions those responses in disjoint sets, grouping together responses as soon as they overlap, and propose, for each group with enough windows, a window whose coordinates are the group average. Recently, a more common approach has been to adopt a greedy procedure [2,3,11] where the top-scoring window is declared an object, then neighboring windows are removed based on a hand-tuned threshold of a manually-designed similarity (distance between centers when the size ratio is within $0.5 - 2$ in [2,11]; relative size of the intersection of the windows with respect to the selected object window in [3]). Most current object category detection pipelines [12–14], but also generic object detection ones [7], use such a greedy procedure. As explained in the introduction, a greedy approach with manually-set parameters is not fully satisfactory.

Several alternatives have been considered. A first line of work considers the detector response as a distribution, and formulates the goal of NMS as that of finding the modes of this distribution. For instance, mean-shift for a kernel density estimation [15] and mixtures of scale-sensitive Gaussians [16] have been proposed. Although principled, these approaches still select only local maxima and fail to suppress false positive detections.

A second line of approaches includes iterative procedures to progressively remove extraneous windows. In [17], a re-ranking cascade model is proposed where a standard greedy NMS is used at every step to favor sparse responses. In [18], the authors also adopt an iterative procedure. From a base detector model, a more powerful detector is built using local binary patterns that encode the neighborhood of window scores in the target image. The procedure is iterated several times until saturation of the detector. This is very similar to the idea of contextual boosting [19]. These iterative procedures are rather time-consuming, as they involve re-training object detectors at each iteration.

For the special case of object detection performed through voting, NMS can be done implicitly by preventing a vote to be taken multiple times into account. For instance, with Hough Forests [20–22], patches vote for the location of the object center. The location with maximum response is selected as the object, and the votes within a given radius that contribute to the selected center are removed from the Hough space hence preventing double detections.

The same idea applies to part-based voting for detection [23]. However, these approaches are not generic and do not apply to every object detection framework. In [24,25], the authors propose to include repulsive pairwise terms into the search for high-scoring windows, so as to avoid performing NMS as a post-processing step. The search is performed using branch-and-bound techniques.

As mentioned earlier, Greedy NMS has the potential shortcoming of suppressing occluding or nearby instances. Several works aim at solving this problem in particular. For the problem of pedestrian detection, [26] proposed to learn detection models for couples of person. Unfortunately, this idea scales very unfavorably with the number of elements in a group, and creates new problems for NMS: what should be done when a double-detection and two single detections are found nearby?

A related field of research generalizes the idea of NMS to the problem of detecting multiple object classes at the same time. This is often referred to as *context rescoring* [3,27]. Those approaches explicitly model co-occurrence and mutual exclusion of certain object classes, and can incorporate NMS and counts for a given object class [27]. Several works go even further and also model scene type and pixel-level segmentation jointly [28,29].

To the best of our knowledge, our work is the first to view NMS as a message passing clustering problem. Clustering algorithms like k-means [30], k-medoids [31] and spectral clustering [32] are not well suited because they return a fixed number of clusters. However, the number of objects and therefore ideal number of clusters is an unknown prior and thus should not have to be fixed in advance. This inflexibility results in poor performance as shown in the experiments. We overcome these limitations by building our approach upon Affinity Propagation Clustering (APC), an exemplar-based clustering approach by Frey [9]. APC has been applied to a variety of problems [33–36] and extended in multiple ways. Reference [37] uses hard cannot-link constraints between two data points which should not be in the same cluster. Our repellence is much weaker and hence more flexible: it penalizes only when two data points are simultaneously cluster centers, resulting in an significantly different formulation than [37].

3 A Message-Passing Approach for NMS

We start in Sect. 3.1 by presenting Affinity Propagation Clustering (APC) [9] using its binary formulation [38], which is the most convenient for our extensions. In Sect. 3.2, we discuss how we have adapted APC for NMS with a novel inter-cluster repellence term and a relaxation of clustering to remove false positives. We show how the messages must be updated to account for these extensions. Finally, in Sect. 3.3, we propose to use a Latent Structured SVM (LSSVM) [39] to learn the weights of APC.

3.1 Affinity Propagation: Binary Formulation and Inference

Let N be the number of data points and $s(i, j)$ the similarity between data points i and $j \in \{1, \ldots, N\}$. APC is a clustering method that relies on data similarities to identify exemplars such that the sum of similarities between exemplars and cluster members is maximized. That is, $s(i, j)$ indicates how well j would serve as an exemplar for i, usually with $s(i, j) \leq 0$ [9]. Following [38], we use a set of N^2 binary variables c_{ij} to encode the exemplar assignment, with $c_{ij} = 1$ if i is represented by j and 0 otherwise. To obtain a valid clustering, the following constraints must hold: (i) each point belongs to exactly one cluster, or equivalently is represented by a single point: $\forall i : \sum_j c_{ij} = 1$; (ii) when j represents any other point i, then j has to represent itself: $\exists i \neq j : c_{ij} = 1 \Rightarrow c_{jj} = 1$. These constraints can be included directly in the objective function of APC:

$$E_{APC}(\{c_{ij}\}) = \sum_{i,j} S_{ij}(c_{ij}) + \sum_i I_i(c_{i1}, \ldots, c_{iN}) + \sum_j E_j(c_{1j}, \ldots, c_{Nj}), \quad (1)$$

where S_{ij}, I_i and E_j have the following definitions:

$$S_{ij}(c_{ij}) = \begin{cases} s(i, j) & \text{if } c_{ij} = 1 \\ 0 & \text{otherwise,} \end{cases} \quad (2)$$

$$I_i(c_{i1}, \ldots, c_{iN}) = \begin{cases} -\infty & \text{if } \sum_j c_{ij} \neq 1 \\ 0 & \text{otherwise,} \end{cases} \quad (3)$$

$$E_j(c_{1j}, \ldots, c_{Nj}) = \begin{cases} -\infty & \text{if } c_{jj} = 0 \text{ and } \exists i \neq j \text{ s.t. } c_{ij} = 1 \\ 0 & \text{otherwise.} \end{cases} \quad (4)$$

Here I_i enforces (i) while E_j enforces (ii). The *self-similarity* $s(i, i)$ favors certain points to be chosen as an exemplar: the stronger $s(i, i)$, the more contribution it makes to Eq. (1).

The inference of Eq. (1) is performed by the max-sum message-passing algorithm [9,38], using two messages: the *availability* α_{ij} (sent from j to i) reflects the accumulated evidence for point i to choose point j as its exemplar, and the *responsibility* ρ_{ij} (sent from i to j) describes how suited j would be as an exemplar for i:

$$\alpha_{ij} = \begin{cases} \sum_{k \neq j} \max(\rho_{kj}, 0) & \text{for } i = j \\ \min(0, \rho_{jj} + \sum_{k \notin \{i,j\}} \max(\rho_{kj}, 0)) & \text{for } i \neq j \end{cases} \quad (5)$$

$$\rho_{ij} = s(i, j) - \max_{q \neq j}(s(i, q) + \alpha_{iq}). \quad (6)$$

3.2 Adapting Affinity Propagation for NMS

We use the windows proposed by the object detector as data points for APC. The self-similarity, or preference to be selected as an exemplar, is naturally chosen as a function of the score of the object detector: the stronger the output, the more likely a data point should be selected. The similarity between two

1. Detector Output   2. Similarity Space   3. Clustering   4. Final Proposals

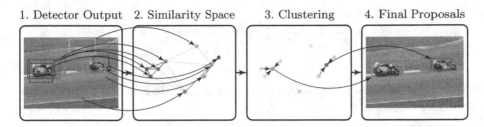

Fig. 2. Illustration of our NMS pipeline. *1. Detector Output:* the detector returns a set of object window hypotheses with scores. *2. Similarity Space:* the windows are mapped into a similarity space expressing how much they overlap. The intensity of the node color denotes how likely a given box is chosen as an exemplar, the edge strength denotes the similarity. *3. Clustering:* APC now selects exemplars to represent window groups, leaving some windows unassigned. *4. Final Proposals:* the algorithm then returns the exemplars as proposals and removes all other hypotheses.

windows is based on their *intersection over union (IoU)*, as $s(i,j) = \frac{|i \cap j|}{|i \cup j|} - 1$. Here the indices refer to the area of the windows. This expresses the degree of common area they cover in the image compared to the total area covered which is a good indicator of how likely they describe the same object. To perform competitively, in the following subsections we will extend APC to better suit our needs and present the contributions of this paper. The resulting processing pipeline is depicted in Fig. 2.

Identifying False Positives. False positives are object hypotheses that belong in fact to the background. Therefore, they should not be assigned to any cluster or chosen as an exemplar. This forces to relax constraint (i). To avoid obtaining only empty clusters, this relaxation must be compensated by a penalty for not assigning a data point to any cluster. We do this by modifying Eq. (3):

$$\tilde{I}_i(c_{i1}, \ldots, c_{iN}) = \begin{cases} -\infty & \text{if } \sum_j c_{ij} > 1 \\ \lambda & \text{if } \sum_j c_{ij} = 0 \\ 0 & \text{otherwise.} \end{cases} \tag{7}$$

Note how this updated term in Eq. (1) is equivalent to adding an extra *background* data point that has similarity λ to all the other data points and 0 self-similarity. In the following, the term $\tilde{I}_i$ will be weighted, hence we can set $\lambda = -1$ without loss of generality.

Inter-Cluster Repellence. In generic object detection the detector precision is much lower compared to detectors trained for a specific object class. To still achieve a high recall it is beneficial to propose a diverse set of windows that covers a larger fraction of the image. However by default, APC does not explicitly penalize choosing exemplars that are very close to each other, as long as they represent their respective clusters well. To encourage diversity among the windows, we therefore propose to include such a penalty by adding an extra term to Eq. (1).

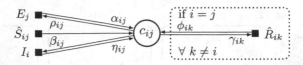

Fig. 3. The 6 messages passed between variables in our extension of Affinity Propagation are α, β, ρ, η, γ and ϕ.

While this term will favor not selecting windows in the same neighborhood, it will not preclude it strictly either. This will still allow APC to select multiple objects in close vicinity. We denote by $R = \sum_{i \neq j} R_{ij}(c_{ii}, c_{jj})$ the new set of *repelling* local functions, where, for $i \neq j$:

$$R_{ij}(c_{ii}, c_{jj}) = \begin{cases} r(i,j) & \text{if } c_{ii} = c_{jj} = 1 \\ 0 & \text{otherwise.} \end{cases} \tag{8}$$

In other words, we have added a new term for every pair of data points which is active only if both points are exemplars. We penalize this pair by the amount of $r(i,j)$, a *repellence cost*. Again, we base the *repellence cost* between two windows on their *intersection over union*, as $r(i,j) = -\frac{|i \cap j|}{|i \cup j|}$. Note that R_{ij} and R_{ji} refer to the same local function. However we keep both notations for simplicity.

Weights and Message Passing. Linearly combining all the above local functions gives us the following new objective function for APC:

$$\widetilde{E}_{APC} = w_a \sum_i S_{ii} + w_b \sum_{i \neq j} S_{ij} + w_c \sum_i \widetilde{I}_i + w_d \sum_{i<j} R_{ij} + \sum_j E_j. \tag{9}$$

We have omitted the c_{ij} variables for the sake of clarity, and we have further separated data similarities and self-similarities. Note that the local functions are defined so that all weights are expected to be positive.

Weights are only added to the 4 finite terms and only their relative weight matters for inference. Similar to the original APC, we perform inference, *i.e.*, find the values of $\{c_{ij}\}$ that maximize Eq. (9) using message-passing. In short, the new terms in Eq. (9), especially the repellence ones, lead to new messages to be passed between windows. For the sake of space, we show the factor graph corresponding to Eq. (9) and the full derivation of the 6 corresponding messages in the supplementary material. We illustrate them in Fig. 3.

The 6 messages (α, β, ρ, η, γ and ϕ) are reduced to 4 (α, ρ, γ and ϕ) by using substitution and integrating the weights back into the local functions. We view the *background* data point as the N+1-th entry in the similarity matrix and can thereby further simplify the derivation for the message passing. Then we have 2 messages for all variables c_{ij}:

$$\rho_{ij} = \begin{cases} \hat{s}(i,i) - \max\limits_{q \neq i}(\hat{s}(i,q) + \alpha_{iq}) + \sum_{l \neq i} \phi_{il} & \text{for } i = j \\ \hat{s}(i,j) - \max(\max\limits_{q \notin \{i,j\}}(\hat{s}(i,q) + \alpha_{iq}), \hat{s}(i,i) + \alpha_{ii} + \sum_{l \neq i} \phi_{il}) & \text{for } i \neq j, \end{cases} \tag{10}$$

$$\alpha_{ij} = \begin{cases} \sum_{k \neq j} \max(\rho_{kj}, 0) & \text{for } i = j \\ \min(0, \rho_{jj} + \sum_{k \notin \{i,j\}} \max(\rho_{kj}, 0)) & \text{for } i \neq j. \end{cases} \tag{11}$$

Additionally, we have 2 messages essentially resulting from the new R_{ij} term which only exist between the subset $\{c_{ii}\}$ of variables:

$$\gamma_{ik} = \hat{s}(i,i) + \alpha_{ii} - \max_{q \neq i}(\hat{s}(i,q) + \alpha_{iq}) + \sum_{l \notin \{i,k\}} \phi_{il} \qquad (12)$$

$$\phi_{ik} = \max(0, \gamma_{ki} + \hat{r}(i,k)) - \max(0, \gamma_{ki}). \qquad (13)$$

Following the original message-passing algorithm for APC [9,38], we initialize all messages with 0. We then iteratively update the messages until convergence.

3.3   Structured Learning for Affinity Propagation

We address now the problem of learning the weights w_a, w_b, w_c and w_d of Eq. (9) from training data so as to maximize the performance of the NMS procedure. The training data consists of images with N object window hypotheses and K ground-truth bounding-box annotations for the corresponding object category. The best possible output $\{c_{ij}^*\}$ of APC for those ground-truth bounding-boxes is to keep the proposal with the highest overlap for each ground-truth bounding-box as long as its IoU is at least 0.5. All other proposal should be discarded. This directly determines the target values c_{ii}^* of all c_{ii}. However, correctly setting target values for the remaining c_{ij} $(i \neq j)$ is not straightforward, as we cannot automatically decide which object was detected by this imprecise localization, or whether this window is better modeled as a false positive. Hence, we treat c_{ij} for $i \neq j$ as latent variables. This splits the set of variables in two subsets for each image n: $y_n = \{c_{11}^n, c_{22}^n, ..., c_{NN}^n\}$ are the observed variables, with their target y_n^*, and $z_n = \{c_{12}^n, ..., c_{1N}^n, c_{21}^n, c_{23}^n, ..., c_{N-1,N}^n\}$ the latent ones.

We can now rewrite our objective function for image n as: $\widetilde{E}_{APC}^n(y_n, z_n; \boldsymbol{w}) = \boldsymbol{w}^\top \boldsymbol{\Psi}_n(y_n, z_n)$, where $\boldsymbol{\Psi}_n$ is the concatenation of the terms in Eq. (9) in a vector, and $\boldsymbol{w} = [w_a, w_b, w_c, w_d, 1]^\top$. To learn $\boldsymbol{w}$, we resort to Structured-output SVM with latent variables (LSSVM) [39]. This consists of the following optimization problem:

$$\operatorname{argmin}_{\boldsymbol{w} \in \mathbb{R}^D, \xi \in \mathbb{R}_+^n} \frac{\lambda}{2} \|\boldsymbol{w}\|^2 + \sum_n \xi^n$$
$$\text{s.t. } \forall n, \max_{\hat{z}_n} \widetilde{E}_{APC}^n(y_n^*, \hat{z}_n; \boldsymbol{w}) \geq \max_{y_n, z_n} \left(\widetilde{E}_{APC}^n(y_n, z_n; \boldsymbol{w}) + \Delta(y_n, y_n^*) \right) - \xi^n, \qquad (14)$$

where ξ^n are slack variables, and Δ is a loss measuring how y_n differs from y_n^*. This is equivalent to finding a $\boldsymbol{w}$ which maximizes the energy of APC for the target variables y_n^*, by a margin Δ, independent of the assignment of z_n. Following [39], we solve Eq. (14) using the concave-convex procedure (CCCP) [40] and the Structured-output SVM implementation by [41]. We define Δ:

$$\Delta(y, y^*) = \sum_i \nu[c_{ii} - c_{ii}^* < 0] + \pi \left(1 - \max_{\text{obj}} \frac{|i \cap obj|}{|i \cup obj|} \right) [c_{ii} - c_{ii}^* > 0]. \qquad (15)$$

where $\nu \geq 0$ is the cost for not choosing a window as an exemplar although it is the best candidate for one of the objects. When a box is chosen as an exemplar even though it is not the best candidate it is considered as a false positive. This is smoothly penalized by $\pi \geq 0$ by considering the overlap with the ground-truth object it most overlaps with. The values for π and ν are chosen depending on the application, usually $\nu/\pi > 1$. Using CCCP additionally implies that we are able to perform loss-augmented inference (*i.e.*, find (y_n, z_n) that maximizes the right-hand side of the constraints in Eq. (14)), and partial inference of z_n (*i.e.*, the left-hand side of the constraint). For the left-hand side, $\mathrm{argmax}_{\hat{z}} \widetilde{E}_{APC}(y^*, \hat{z}; w)$ can be computed directly. Given the cluster centers y_n^* we just assign all other boxes which are not cluster centers to the most similar clusters. For false positives, this could also be the *background* data point depending on the current value for w_c. This results in a valid clustering which maximizes the total similarity for the given exemplars.

Concerning the right-hand side, we can easily incorporate Δ as an extra term in Eq. (9), and use message passing to obtain the corresponding (y_n, z_n). When incorporating the loss term into the message passing, only the similarity $\hat{s}$ needs to be modified, leading to $\hat{s}_\Delta$:

$$
\hat{s}_\Delta(i,j) = \begin{cases} \hat{s}(i,j) - \nu & \text{for } i=j \text{ and } c_{ii}^n = 1 \\ \hat{s}(i,j) + \pi \left(1 - \max_{obj} \frac{|i \cap obj|}{|i \cup obj|}\right) & \text{for } i=j \text{ and } c_{ii}^n = 0 \\ \hat{s}(i,j) & \text{otherwise.} \end{cases} \tag{16}
$$

4   Experiments on Object Class Detection

To compare the proposed exemplar based clustering framework to Greedy NMS, we measured their respective performance for object class detection. We are especially interested in the cases we presented in Fig. 1 where Greedy NMS fails, and we will present insights why our proposed method handles these better. A detailed analysis will address localization errors (Fig. 1a), close-by labeled objects (Fig. 1b), precision as well as detections on background (Fig. 1c). This is in line with Hoiem's [42] in-depth analysis of the performance of a detector, not only giving a better understanding of its weaknesses and strengths but also showing that specific improvements are necessary to advance in object detection.

4.1   Implementation Details

In this section the clustering is applied to Felzenszwalb's [3] (release 5) object class detector based on a deformable parts model (DPM). Performance is measured on the widely used Pascal VOC 2007 [8] dataset composed of 9,963 images containing objects of 20 different classes. We keep the split between training and testing data as described in [3]. The DPM training parameters are set to their default values. We keep all windows with a score above a threshold which is determined for each class during training but at most 250 per image. The similarity between two windows is based on their *intersection over union*, as described in Sect. 3. As the score of the Felzenszwalb boxes p is not fixed to a range, it is scaled to $[-1, 0]$ by a sigmoidal function $s(i, i) = \frac{1}{1+e^{-p}} - 1$. The presented results for APC are trained following Sect. 3.3 on the validation set. For a fair comparison, the ratio ν/π was set to yield a total number of windows similar to Greedy NMS.

4.2 Results

The results are presented in separate subsections that compare the performance of APC and Greedy NMS with emphasis on the specific issues presented in Fig. 1.

Can APC Provide Better Fitting Boxes Than Greedy NMS (Fig. 1a)?
Here we show that solving NMS globally through clustering can help to select better fitting bounding-boxes compared to Greedy NMS. We look at the detection rate for different IoU thresholds with the object for detection. The upper bound is determined by the detection rate of the detector when returning all windows, *i.e.* without any NMS.

The quantitative results in Fig. 4 confirm that APC recovers more objects with the same number of boxes compared to Greedy NMS, especially performing well when a more precise location of the object is required ($IoU \geq 0.7$). We then evaluated the area under the curve in Fig. 4 for each class separately (normalized to 1), whose values are shown in Table 1. Here we perform better across all classes with an increase between 0.17 for the *diningtable* class and 0.03 for the *tvmonitor* class. On average the AUC can be increased from 0.34 to 0.44. Even though selecting the right boxes from the output of the detector could have led up to an AUC of 0.65, APC was still able to narrow the gap by almost a third.

This is also confirmed by the qualitative results in Fig. 5: whereas NMS proposes several boxes for the same bike (e.g. (b), (c)) and even sometimes proposes

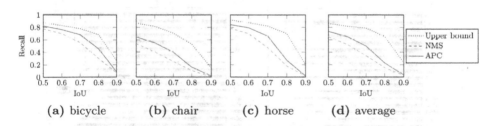

(a) bicycle   (b) chair   (c) horse   (d) average

Fig. 4. Object class detection: IoU vs. recall for a selection of classes (a-c) as well as the average across all (d). Our method consistently outperforms Greedy NMS for different IoU thresholds.

Table 1. Object class detection: area under curve (AUC) for IoU vs. recall.

	aeroplane	bicycle	bird	boat	bottle	bus	car	cat	chair	cow	diningtable
Upper bound	0.592	0.716	0.495	0.476	0.482	0.744	0.663	0.718	0.641	0.600	0.788
NMS	0.303	0.494	0.170	0.187	0.288	0.450	0.432	0.335	0.259	0.312	0.391
APC	0.426	0.589	0.297	0.260	0.333	0.552	0.498	0.432	0.361	0.426	0.556

	dog	horse	motorbike	person	pottedplant	sheep	sofa	train	tvmonitor		average
Upper bound	0.685	0.740	0.727	0.620	0.508	0.497	0.855	0.707	0.702		0.648
NMS	0.265	0.439	0.422	0.320	0.170	0.200	0.470	0.394	0.482		0.339
APC	0.336	0.540	0.522	0.418	0.303	0.322	0.584	0.533	0.510		0.440

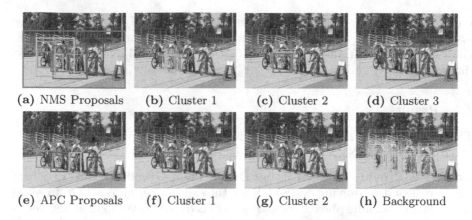

(a) NMS Proposals   **(b)** Cluster 1   **(c)** Cluster 2   **(d)** Cluster 3

(e) APC Proposals   **(f)** Cluster 1   **(g)** Cluster 2   **(h)** Background

Fig. 5. Object class detection: qualitative results. These figures show an example of the proposed windows. The colored box are the exemplars for the gray boxes. Upper row: Greedy NMS. Lower row: APC.

one box covering two objects (d), our method returns one box per bike ((f), (g)). These boxes are the exemplars of clusters only containing boxes which tightly fit the bikes – the others are collected in the background cluster (h).

Does APC Avoid to Suppress Objects in Groups (Fig. 1b)? Two (or more) objects form a group if they at least touch each other ($IoU > 0$). Thus we remove from the ground-truth the objects that do not overlap with any other object of the same class, and compute the recall (with $IoU = 0.5$) on the remaining objects for the same number of proposed windows as shown in Fig. 6a. On average APC recovers 62.9 % objects vs. 50.2 % for Greedy NMS, with an

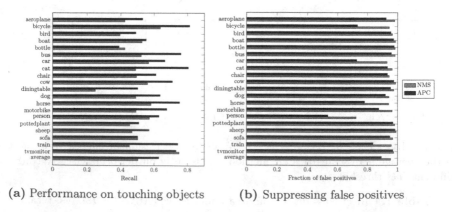

(a) Performance on touching objects   **(b)** Suppressing false positives

Fig. 6. Object class detection: in-depth analysis. (a) compares the recall of Greedy NMS and APC on pairs of objects ($IoU > 0$ between objects) – APC recovers significantly more of these rather difficult objects. (b) shows the fraction of false positives – windows that do not touch any object: APC on average reduces the fraction of false positives, with a significant reduction for some classes, *i.e. bicycle, car, person.*

increase of up to 31.7 % for individual classes. Noting that these objects are especially difficult to detect, APC is more robust at handling nearby detector responses. This is a clear advantage of the proposed clustering based approach.

Can APC Suppress More False-Positives (Fig. 1c)? Already the qualitative results in Fig. 5h suggest that the clustering relaxation proposed in Sect. 3.2 helps to remove extraneous boxes with low scores which do not describe any object. For a quantitative analysis, we look again at the results of APC and Greedy NMS when both return the same number of windows. Noting that both post-processing algorithms are provided with exactly the same windows by the detector as input, we now evaluate which method is better at suppressing false positives. In this context we define false positives as all boxes which do not touch any object ($IoU = 0$). These boxes are nowhere near detecting an object as usually at least $IoU \geq 0.5$ is required for detection. As shown in Fig. 6b APC is able to reduce the fraction of false positives proposed from 95.5 % for NMS to 89.4 % with consistent improvement across all classes. For some classes like *bicycle, car* and *person* whose objects often occur next to each other, APC shows significant false positive reduction of up to 21.6 %, proposing more relevant windows which also reflects in the recall in Fig. 4.

What is the Precision of APC Compared to NMS and k-medoids? We now vary the ratio of the training parameters ν/π. APC returns a fixed set of boxes, ranging from less than a box up to several hundreds per image depending on the clustering parameters which are obtained through training by setting this ratio for the specific application. These boxes, although they

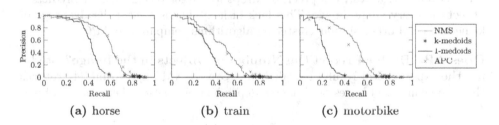

| | (a) horse | (b) train | (c) motorbike |

Fig. 7. Object class detection: precision vs. recall. The precision-recall curves reveal that APC performs competitively compared to Greedy NMS at a similar precision but higher recall while significantly outperforming k-medoids.

Table 2. Object class detection: average precision NMS vs. APC

		aeroplane	bicycle	bird	boat	bottle	bus	car	cat	chair	cow	diningtable
IoU 0.5	NMS	0.332	0.593	0.103	0.157	0.266	0.520	0.537	0.225	0.202	0.243	0.269
	APC	0.298	0.511	0.108	0.107	0.130	0.369	0.428	0.197	0.149	0.168	0.235
IoU 0.8	NMS	0.101	0.198	0.091	0.023	0.096	0.135	0.123	0.021	0.057	0.048	0.036
	APC	0.090	0.222	0.091	0.091	0.092	0.114	0.112	0.093	0.093	0.092	0.100

		dog	horse	motorbike	person	pottedplant	sheep	sofa	train	tvmonitor	mAP	"mAP"
IoU 0.5	NMS	0.126	0.565	0.485	0.433	0.135	0.209	0.359	0.452	0.421	0.332	
	APC	0.129	0.579	0.432	0.363	0.116	0.143	0.259	0.449	0.175		0.267
IoU 0.8	NMS	0.004	0.061	0.126	0.106	0.006	0.030	0.105	0.044	0.144	0.078	
	APC	0.091	0.122	0.128	0.111	0.091	0.091	0.115	0.104	0.107		0.108

cover the objects well, do not follow any kind of ranking as they altogether form the result of a globally solved problem. Since AP is designed to measure the performance of a ranking system, it is simply not appropriate for APC, as that would require that one can select the best possible subset of the proposed boxes. Still, we computed a proxy to AP by linearly interpolating the precision for points of consecutive recall (which need not be consecutive values of the varied parameter). This results in a "mAP" for APC of 0.27 compared to a real mAP of 0.33 for greedy NMS as shown in Table 2. AP is mostly influenced by the highest scored detections, so greedy NMS at an IoU of 0.5 is hard to beat with the same underlying detector. However, as such, AP does not reward methods with more precise object localizations than 0.5 and overall better recall. These are precisely areas where greedy NMS can be improved, and therefore we resorted to a deeper analysis. As a matter of fact, if we set a more difficult detection criterion of, e.g., 0.8 IoU, then APC outperforms greedy NMS with a "mAP" of 0.11 compared to 0.08. This is another aspect where APC shows superior performance compared to greedy NMS. As each clustering has a well-defined precision and recall, we can have a scatter plot to compare it to Greedy NMS. Figure 7 shows that APC achieves a similar precision at low recall but better recall at low precision.

We also compared APC to a k-medoids clustering baseline using the same similarity as for APC. To account for the score of the proposals, the self-similarity of the k selected cluster centers (varied from 1 to 10) was added to the overall cost function to favor boxes with better scores. k-medoids leads to similar precision-recall scatter plots as shown in Fig. 7. Additionally, we plot the precision-recall curve for $k = 1$ (*1-medoids*) by ranking the cluster centers with their original scores. As shown in Fig. 7 already in the case of *1-medoids* many objects are recovered. However, the precision drops for larger recalls since it predicts k objects in every single image. This lack of flexibility is a clear disadvantage of k-medoids and other similar clustering algorithms compared to APC.

Does APC Better Predict the Number of Objects in the Image? Studying the experimental results revealed that Greedy NMS approximately returns the same number of boxes per image independent of whether there was an object

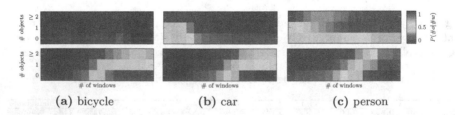

(a) bicycle   (b) car   (c) person

Fig. 8. Object class detection: predicting the number of objects. Greedy NMS approximately returns the same number of boxes independent of the number of objects in the image. Therefore the posterior $P(\#\ \text{objects} \mid \#\ \text{windows})$ remains uninformative about the object count. In contrast, APC is very flexible and adjust the number of windows being returned depending on how many objects there are in the image.

in the image. In contrast, for APC it greatly varied between images. Therefore, we simply measured the posterior probability $P(\#$ objects $\mid \#$ windows).
Figure 8 depicts this probability for both Greedy NMS and APC for a selection of
classes. For Greedy NMS (upper row in Fig. 8) the number of proposed windows
is mostly uninformative regarding how many objects there are in the image. In
comparison for APC (lower row in Fig. 8), there is a strong correlation between
the number of windows proposed and the likelihood that there are 1 or more
objects: given the number of windows APC proposes we can estimate how many
objects there are in the image.

5 Experiments on Generic Object Detection

We apply APC to generic object detection which gained popularity in recent
years as a preprocessing step for many state-of-the-art object detectors [13,14].
We use the objectness measure introduced by [43] which is the only one to
provide a probability p with the window it proposes, unlike [14,44,45].

5.1 Implementation Details

Performance is again evaluated on Pascal VOC 2007 where we split the dataset
in the same way as in [7] and used the classes *bird, car, cat, cow, dog, sheep*
for training the objectness algorithm as well as the clustering and the remaining 14 classes for testing. Images which had occurrences of both training and
testing classes were dropped and in contrast to [7] we also kept objects marked
as difficult and truncated. The self-similarity is based on the probability of containing an object $s(i,i) = p(i) - 1$ and the similarity between boxes is defined
by the overlap. We sampled 250 windows with multinomial sampling which still
allows to recover a large fraction of the objects. As presented in [7], Greedy
NMS significantly improved the detection rate for objectness. This motivates
our experiments where we compare Greedy NMS against APC.

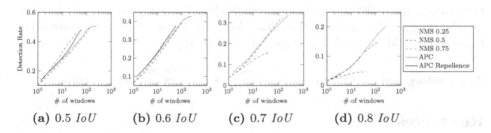

(a) 0.5 *IoU*   (b) 0.6 *IoU*   (c) 0.7 *IoU*   (d) 0.8 *IoU*

Fig. 9. Generic object detection: Greedy NMS requires to adopt the parameter for
suppression for different *IoU* thresholds to always perform competitively. In contrast,
APC performs consistently well, beating Greedy NMS especially for precise object
detection (*IoU* $\geq$ 0.7). Introducing a repellence helps to boost performance for less
precise object detection by enforcing diversity among the proposed windows.

5.2   Results

After training APC, we compare its detection rate with Greedy NMS for different IoU thresholds with the object. For APC we show the performance both without and with repellence; for NMS we varied the threshold for suppression. Looking at Fig. 9, we make 3 observations: (i) when proposing very few windows per image (< 10) APC typically performs better than Greedy NMS. (ii) for an $IoU \geq 0.7$ the standard NMS threshold of 0.5 performs significantly worse than APC. This requires that Greedy NMS re-runs with a higher threshold for suppression. In comparison our method is much more consistent across varying IoU. (iii) for APC diversity can be enforced by activating the inter-cluster repellence which avoids having cluster centers close-by each other. This boosts our performance for $IoU \leq 0.6$ by close to up to 5 % from 42.9 % to 47.5 % for $IoU = 0.5$.

6   Discussion

We presented a novel clustering-based NMS algorithm based on Affinity Propagation. We showed that it successfully tackles shortcomings of Greedy NMS for object class and generic object detection.

Specifically we show that our method – whose parameters can be learned automatically depending on the application – yields better fitting bounding-boxes, reduces false positives, handles close-by objects better and is better able to predict the number of objects in an image, all at a competitive precision compared to Greedy NMS. Given that APC tries to find a global solution to the NMS problem it is however computationally more complex and still relatively slow taking approximately 1 s to cluster 250 bounding-boxes. In the future, we therefore plan to explore approximative solutions.

APC could also be expanded to multi-class object detection integrating context and holistic knowledge. The newly introduced repellence could be based not only on the overlap between the boxes but rather the similarity in appearance expressing how likely the two windows cover the same object. In future work, we want to learn the window similarity potentially including visual features that may help to distinguish between multiple detections of the same object or nearby objects. We are convinced that APC can be of interest for many other areas where NMS is used, *e.g.* edge detection [1, 46].

Acknowledgement. The authors gratefully acknowledge support by Toyota.

References

1. Canny, J.: A computational approach to edge detection. TPAMI **8**(6), 679–698 (1986)
2. Dalal, N., Triggs, B.: Histograms of oriented gradients for human detection. In: CVPR (2005)

3. Felzenszwalb, P., Girshick, R., McAllester, D., Ramanan, D.: Object detection with discriminatively trained part based models. TPAMI **32**(9), 1627–1645 (2010)
4. Viola, P., Jones, M.: Robust real-time object detection. IJCV **57**(2), 137–154 (2004)
5. Girshick, R., Donahue, J., Darrell, T., Malik, J.: Rich feature hierarchies for accurate object detection and semantic segmentation. In: CVPR (2014)
6. Cheng, M.M., Zhang, Z., Lin, W.Y., Torr, P.H.S.: BING: binarized normed gradients for objectness estimation at 300fps. In: CVPR (2014)
7. Alexe, B., Deselaers, T., Ferrari, V.: Measuring the objectness of image windows. TPAMI **34**(11), 2189–2202 (2012)
8. Everingham, M., Van Gool, L., Williams, C.K.I., Winn, J., Zisserman, A.: The pascal visual object classes (VOC) challenge. IJCV **88**(2), 303–338 (2010)
9. Frey, B.J., Dueck, D.: Clustering by passing messages between data points. Science **315**(5814), 972–976 (2007)
10. Mikolajczyk, K., Schmid, C.: Scale & Affine invariant interest point detectors. IJCV **1**(60), 63–86 (2004)
11. Schneiderman, H., Kanade, T.: Object detection using the statistics of parts. IJCV **56**(3), 151–177 (2004)
12. Cinbis, R.G., Verbeek, J., Schmid, C.: Segmentation driven object detection with fisher vectors. In: ICCV (2013)
13. Szegedy, C., Toshev, A., Erhan, D.: Deep neural networks for object detection. In: NIPS (2013)
14. Uijlings, J.R.R., van de Sande, K.E.A., Gevers, T., Smeulders, A.W.M.: Selective search for object recognition. IJCV **104**(2), 154–171 (2013)
15. Dalal, N.: Finding people in images and videos. Ph.D. thesis, Institut National Polytechnique de Grenoble (2006)
16. Wojcikiewicz, W.: Probabilistic modelling of multiple observations in face detection. Technical report, Humboldt Universität zu Berlin (2008)
17. Blaschko, M.B., Kannala, J., Rahtu, E.: Non maximal suppression in cascaded ranking models. In: Kämäräinen, J.-K., Koskela, M. (eds.) SCIA 2013. LNCS, vol. 7944, pp. 408–419. Springer, Heidelberg (2013)
18. Chen, G., Ding, Y., Xiao, J., Han, T.X.: Detection evolution with multi-order contextual co-occurrence. In: CVPR (2013)
19. Ding, Y., Xiao, J.: Contextual boost for pedestrian detection. In: CVPR (2012)
20. Razavi, N., Gall, J., Van Gool, L.: Backprojection revisited: scalable multi-view object detection and similarity metrics for detections. In: Daniilidis, K., Maragos, P., Paragios, N. (eds.) ECCV 2010, Part I. LNCS, vol. 6311, pp. 620–633. Springer, Heidelberg (2010)
21. Barinova, O., Lempitsky, V., Kholi, P.: On detection of multiple object instances using hough transforms. TPAMI **34**(9), 1773–1784 (2012)
22. Wohlhart, P., Donoser, M., Roth, P.M., Bischof, H.: Detecting partially occluded objects with an implicit shape model random field. In: Lee, K.M., Matsushita, Y., Rehg, J.M., Hu, Z. (eds.) ACCV 2012, Part I. LNCS, vol. 7724, pp. 302–315. Springer, Heidelberg (2013)
23. Wu, B., Nevatia, R.: Detection and segmentation of multiple, partially occluded objects by grouping, merging, assigning part detection responses. IJCV **82**(2), 185–204 (2009)
24. Blaschko, M.B., Lampert, C.H.: Learning to localize objects with structured output regression. In: Forsyth, D., Torr, P., Zisserman, A. (eds.) ECCV 2008, Part I. LNCS, vol. 5302, pp. 2–15. Springer, Heidelberg (2008)

25. Blaschko, M.B.: Branch and bound strategies for non-maximal suppression in object detection. In: Boykov, Y., Kahl, F., Lempitsky, V., Schmidt, F.R. (eds.) EMMCVPR 2011. LNCS, vol. 6819, pp. 385–398. Springer, Heidelberg (2011)

26. Tang, S., Andriluka, M., Schiele, B.: Detection and tracking of occluded people. In: BMVC (2012)

27. Desai, C., Ramanan, D., Fowlkes, C.C.: Discriminative models for multi-class object layout. IJCV **95**(1), 1–12 (2011)

28. Ladický, L., Sturgess, P., Alahari, K., Russell, C., Torr, P.H.S.: What, where and how many? combining object detectors and CRFs. In: Daniilidis, K., Maragos, P., Paragios, N. (eds.) ECCV 2010, Part IV. LNCS, vol. 6314, pp. 424–437. Springer, Heidelberg (2010)

29. Yao, J., Fidler, S., Urtasun, R.: Describing the scene as a whole: joint object detection, scene classification and semantic segmentation. In: CVPR (2012)

30. MacQueen, J., et al.: Some methods for classification and analysis of multivariate observations. In: Proceedings of the Fifth Berkeley Symposium on Mathematical Statistics and Probability, vol. 1(14), pp. 281–297 (1967)

31. Kaufman, L., Rousseeuw, P.: Clustering by means of medoids. In: Dodge, Y. (ed.) Statistical Data Analysis Based on the L1-Norm and Related Methods. North-Holland, Amsterdam (1987)

32. Von Luxburg, U.: A tutorial on spectral clustering. Stat. Comput. **17**(4), 395–416 (2007)

33. Dueck, D., Frey, B.J.: Non-metric affinity propagation for unsupervised image categorization. In: ICCV (2007)

34. Dueck, D., Frey, B.J., Jojic, N., Jojic, V., Giaever, G., Emili, A., Musso, G., Hegele, R.: Using affinity propagation. In: RECOMB (2008)

35. Lazic, N., Frey, B.J., Aarabi, P.: Solving the uncapacitated facility location problem using message passing algorithms. In: AISTATS (2010)

36. Givoni, I.E., Chung, C., Frey, B.J.: Hierarchical affinity propagation. In: The 27th Conference on Uncertainty in Artificial Intelligence (UAI) (2011)

37. Givoni, I.E., Frey, B.J.: Semi-supervised affinity propagation with instance-level constraints. In: AISTATS (2009)

38. Givoni, I.E., Frey, B.J.: A binary variable model for affinity propagation. Neural Comput. **21**(6), 1589–1600 (2009)

39. Yu, C.N.J., Joachims, T.: Learning structural svms with latent variables. In: ICML (2009)

40. Yuille, A.L., Rangarajan, A.: The concave-convex procedure. Neural Comput. **15**(4), 915–936 (2003)

41. Vedaldi, A.: A MATLAB wrapper of SVMstruct (2011)

42. Hoiem, D., Chodpathumwan, Y., Dai, Q.: Diagnosing error in object detectors. In: Fitzgibbon, A., Lazebnik, S., Perona, P., Sato, Y., Schmid, C. (eds.) ECCV 2012, Part III. LNCS, vol. 7574, pp. 340–353. Springer, Heidelberg (2012)

43. Alexe, B., Deselaers, T., Ferrari, V.: What is an object? In: CVPR (2010)

44. Manén, S., Guillaumin, M., Van Gool, L.: Prime object proposals with randomized Prim's algorithm. In: ICCV (2013)

45. Ristin, M., Gall, J., Van Gool, L.: Local context priors for object proposal generation. In: Lee, K.M., Matsushita, Y., Rehg, J.M., Hu, Z. (eds.) ACCV 2012, Part I. LNCS, vol. 7724, pp. 57–70. Springer, Heidelberg (2013)

46. Dollar, P., Zitnick, C.L.: Structured forests for fast edge detection. In: ICCV (2013)

Stable Radial Distortion Calibration by Polynomial Matrix Inequalities Programming

Jan Heller[1]([⊠]), Didier Henrion[1,2,3], and Tomáš Pajdla[1]

[1] Faculty of Electrical Engineering, Czech Technical University in Prague,
166 27 Praha 6, Technická 2, Czech Republic
hellej1@cmp.felk.cvut.cz
[2] CNRS-LAAS, 7 Avenue du Colonel Roche, 31077 Toulouse, France
[3] Université de Toulouse, 31077 Toulouse, France

Abstract. Polynomial and rational functions are the number one choice when it comes to modeling of radial distortion of lenses. However, several extrapolation and numerical issues may arise while using these functions that have not been covered by the literature much so far. In this paper, we identify these problems and show how to deal with them by enforcing nonnegativity of certain polynomials. Further, we show how to model these nonnegativities using polynomial matrix inequalities (PMI) and how to estimate the radial distortion parameters subject to PMI constraints using semidefinite programming (SDP). Finally, we suggest several approaches on how to incorporate the proposed method into the overall camera calibration procedure.

1 Introduction

Radial distortion modeling is the most important non-linear part of the camera calibration process [9]. The first works on the topic came from the photogrammetric community [4,5,14]. Since then, a plethora of models has been suggested in the literature [16]. Among the proposed models, the ones based on polynomial and rational functions are the most popular. This popularity undoubtedly stems from the fact that these function are easily manipulated and yet provide sufficient fitting power for wide range or distortions. Unfortunately, the extrapolation qualities of polynomials can be quite unpredictable in situations where little or no data is available. However, even if data points are missing, the overall shape of the distortion is known *a priori* in many calibration scenarios, *e.g.*, the lens introduces barrel or pincushion distortions. Based on such *a priori* information, the shape of the polynomial and rational distortion functions can be controlled by enforcing nonnegativity of certain polynomials. For example, in the case of pincushion distortion we can accomplish the desired shape by enforcing nonnegativity of the first and the second derivatives of the distortion function on the whole field of view of the camera.

In this paper, we propose a radial distortion calibration procedure where a polynomial cost function, *e.g.*, reprojection error, is minimized subject to such shape constraints. This shape optimization procedure is designed to stabilize the

© Springer International Publishing Switzerland 2015
D. Cremers et al. (Eds.): ACCV 2014, Part I, LNCS 9003, pp. 307–321, 2015.
DOI: 10.1007/978-3-319-16865-4_20

shape of the distortion function. It is based on polynomial matrix inequalities (PMI) programming and can be easily incorporated into an existing camera calibration procedure.

In Sect. 2, we formally introduce the radial distortion function and present several extrapolation issues arising while using polynomial and rational distortion models. Next, in Sect. 3 we provide a minimal theoretical background needed for our shape stabilization approach. In Sect. 4, we demonstrate the proposed method on three types of radial distortion shapes and models and show how to incorporate the method into an overall camera calibration procedure. Finally, in Sect. 5 we experimentally validate our approach and show that the method guarantees the correct shape of a distortion function without compromising the quality of the overall camera calibration as measured by the reprojection error.

2   Camera Radial Distortion

Let us suppose that a set of scene points $\mathbf{X}_i \in \mathbb{R}^3$, $i = 1, \ldots, n$ is observed by a camera. If $\mathtt{R} \in SO(3)$, $\mathbf{t} \in \mathbb{R}^3$ are the camera extrinsic parameters, a scene point $\mathbf{X}_i$ gets projected into an image point $(x_i, y_i, 1)^\top$:

$$\lambda_i (x_i, y_i, 1)^\top = \mathtt{R}\mathbf{X}_i + \mathbf{t}, \ \lambda_i \in \mathbb{R}.$$

In reality, some amount of radial distortion is always present and the camera observes a point $(\hat{x}_i, \hat{y}_i, 1)^\top$ which does not coincide with the ideal (and unobservable) point $(x_i, y_i, 1)^\top$. In pixel coordinates, the camera observes a point $\mathtt{K}(\hat{x}_i, \hat{y}_i, 1)^\top$, where $\mathtt{K} \in \mathbb{R}^{3 \times 3}$ is the matrix of intrinsic camera parameters, the so-called calibration matrix. *Radial distortion function* $L \colon \mathbb{R} \to \mathbb{R}$ is a function of radius $r = \sqrt{x_i^2 + y_i^2}$ that models the radial displacement of the ideal image point position from the center of the radial distortion as

$$\begin{pmatrix} \hat{x}_i \\ \hat{y}_i \end{pmatrix} = L(r) \begin{pmatrix} x_i \\ y_i \end{pmatrix}. \tag{1}$$

The function $L(r)$ is only defined for $r > 0$ and $L(0) = 1$, $L(r) > 0$. For the purposes of demonstration of the proposed shape optimization procedure, we will use $L(r)$ defined as follows

$$L(r) = \frac{f(r)}{g(r)} = \frac{1 + k_1 r + k_2 r^2 + k_3 r^3}{1 + k_4 r + k_5 k^2 + k_6 r^3}, \tag{2}$$

where $\mathbf{k} = (k_1, k_2, \ldots, k_6)$ is the vector of model parameters. This definition accommodates several models already proposed in the literature [12]. However, we will see that the shape optimization procedure holds for any rational function.

2.1   Extrapolation Issues of Radial Distortion Calibration

Let us motivate the need for the radial distortion shape optimization by demonstrating two examples of extrapolation issues arising while using polynomial and rational distortion models.

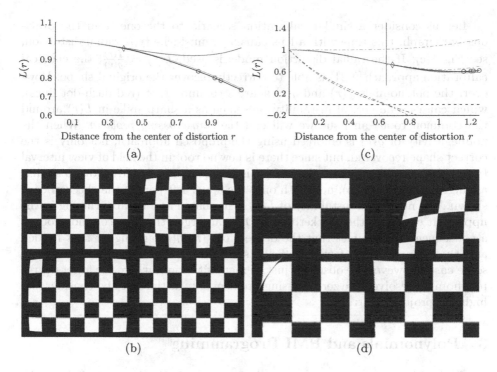

Fig. 1. *Calibration issues.* Examples of issues arising while using polynomial and rational function for radial distortion calibration. See text for details (Color figure online).

First, let's suppose a calibration scenario where images of a calibration target were taken, but the image projections of the known 3D points lie close to the center of the images with no points covering the corners of the images. Figure 1(a) shows in black the graph of the amount of barrel distortion introduced by the camera lens as a function of the distance from the center of the radial distortion. When a polynomial distortion model $L(r) = f(r)$ is used, see Eq. 2, in combination with an unconstrained calibration method [2, 21] (in red), the real distortion is fitted successfully near the center of the image on intervals where the data points are available (left of the diamond symbol). However, the recovered polynomial quickly drifts away elsewhere (red circles depict the distances of the projections of the image corners). In green, a polynomial recovered by the method proposed in this paper is shown. Here, the negativity of the first and the second derivatives of the polynomial on the whole field of view was enforced. This caused the model to fit the original distortion much closer on the whole field of view. Figure 1(b) shows a synthetic checkerboard image (the upper left corner) and the same image distorted by the original barrel distortion (the upper right corner). In the lower left corner, the image is undistorted back using the polynomial recovered by [2, 21]. In the lower right corner, the image successfully undistorted by the polynomial recovered using the proposed shape optimization method is shown.

Let us consider a similar calibration scenario to the one from the previous paragraph, this time with a lens causing a mustache type radial distortion, see Fig. 1(c). If the radial distortion model is used, $L(r) = \frac{f(r)}{g(r)}$, the classical calibration approach [2, 21] is able to correctly recover the original shape. However, the polynomials $f(r)$ and $g(r)$ share a common root (red dash-dot lines), which causes a numerical instability presented as a sharp spike in $L(r)$ around the common root—an issue we will call the *zero-crossing problem*. When the nonnegativity of $g(r)$ is enforced using the proposed approach, not only is the correct shape recovered, but since there is now no root in the field of view interval (green dash-dot lines), the spike in $L(r)$ is also gone. Figure 1(d) shows a similar arrangement as Fig. 1(b), now with only the upper left part of the checkerboard shown. The numerical instability of $L(r)$ is presented as a notable ringing in the upper left corner of the checkerboard. One can argue that the common root is a consequence of the fact that the degrees of $f(r), g(r)$ are higher that needed and that a model with fewer coefficients should be used. This may be true in some cases, however, we observed just as many situations where the lower degree polynomials resolved the zero-crossing problem only at the cost of a considerably higher reprojection error.

3   Polynomials and PMI Programming

In this section, we present a minimal theoretical background needed for the proposed shape optimization procedure.

3.1   Polynomials and Polynomial Matrices

An univariate polynomial $p(x) \in \mathbb{R}_n[x]$ of degree $n \in \mathbb{N}$ is a real function defined as

$$p(x) = p_n x^n + p_{n-1} x^{n-1} + \cdots + p_1 x + p_0 = \mathbf{p}^\top \boldsymbol{\psi}_n(x),$$

where $\mathbf{p} = (p_0, p_1, \ldots, p_n)^\top \in \mathbb{R}^{n+1}$ is the vector of coefficients with a nonvanishing coefficient p_n and $\boldsymbol{\psi}_n(x) = (1, x, x^2, \ldots, x^n)^\top$ is the canonical basis. Let $q(x) \in \mathbb{R}_{2n}[x]$. A symmetric matrix $\mathbf{Q} \in \mathbb{R}^{n' \times n'}$, $\mathbf{Q} = (q_{i,j})$, where $n' = n + 1$, is called *Gram matrix* associated with $q(x)$ and the basis $\boldsymbol{\psi}_n(x)$ [6] if

$$q(x) = \boldsymbol{\psi}_n^\top(x) \, \mathbf{Q} \, \boldsymbol{\psi}_n(x). \tag{3}$$

Generally, there is more than one Gram matrix associated with a polynomial $q(x)$ and we will denote the set of such matrices as $\mathcal{G}(q(x))$. The polynomial $q(x)$ can be expressed in the elements of $\mathbf{Q}$ by simply expanding the right hand side of Eq. 3 and by comparing the coefficients.

Let $\mathbf{x} = (x_1, x_2, \ldots, x_d) \in \mathbb{R}^d$ be a real vector and $\boldsymbol{\alpha} = (\alpha_1, \alpha_1, \ldots, \alpha_d) \in \mathbb{N}^d$ an integer vector. A *monomial* of degree $n = \sum \alpha_i$ is defined as $\mathbf{x}^{\boldsymbol{\alpha}} = \prod_{i=1}^n x_i^{\alpha_i}$.

A multivariate polynomial $p(\mathbf{x}) \in \mathbb{R}_n[\mathbf{x}]$ of degree $n \in \mathbb{N}$ is a mapping from $\mathbb{R}^d$ to $\mathbb{R}$ defined as a linear combination of monomials up to degree n,

$$p(\mathbf{x}) = \sum_{|\alpha| \leq n} p_\alpha \mathbf{x}^\alpha = \sum_{|\alpha| \leq n} p_\alpha x_1^{\alpha_1} x_2^{\alpha_2} \cdots x_d^{\alpha_d} = (p_\alpha)_{|\alpha| \leq n}^\top (\mathbf{x}_\alpha)_{|\alpha| \leq d} = \mathbf{p}^\top \boldsymbol{\psi}_n(\mathbf{x}),$$

where $\mathbf{p} \in \mathbb{R}^m$ is the vector of coefficients and $\boldsymbol{\psi}_n(\mathbf{x})$ is the canonical basis of $m = \binom{d+n}{d}$ monomials up to degree n. By a polynomial matrix we will understand a symmetric matrix whose elements are polynomials. In the next, $\mathbb{S}^n(\mathbb{R}[\mathbf{x}])$ will denote the set of $n \times n$ symmetric polynomial matrices. The degree of $\mathsf{P} = (p_{i,j}(\mathbf{x})) \in \mathbb{S}^n(\mathbb{R}[\mathbf{x}])$ is the largest degree of all the polynomial elements of P, $\deg \mathsf{P} = \max_{i,j} \deg p_{i,j}(\mathbf{x})$.

Besides parameterizing polynomials by the associated Gram matrices, we will also need to "linearize" them, i.e., to substitute every monomial $\mathbf{x}^\alpha$ by a new variable $y_\alpha \in \mathbb{R}$. To do this, we define the *Riesz functional* $\ell_\mathbf{y} : \mathbb{R}_n[\mathbf{x}] \to \mathbb{R}[\mathbf{y}]$, a linear functional that for a d-variate polynomial of degree n, $p(\mathbf{x}) = \sum_\alpha p_\alpha \mathbf{x}^\alpha$, returns an m-variate polynomial of degree one, $\ell_\mathbf{y}(p(\mathbf{x})) = \sum_\alpha p_\alpha y_\alpha$, $m = \binom{d+n}{d}$. With a slight abuse of notation, we will also use $\ell_\mathbf{y}$ as a matrix operator acting on $\mathbb{S}^n(\mathbb{R}[\mathbf{x}])$: if $\mathsf{P} \in \mathbb{S}^n(\mathbb{R}[\mathbf{x}])$, then $\mathsf{P}' = \ell_\mathbf{y}(\mathsf{P})$ if and only if $p'_{i,j}(\mathbf{y}) = \ell_\mathbf{y}(p_{i,j}(\mathbf{x}))$.

3.2   Polynomials Positive on Finite Intervals

The shape optimization procedure presented in this paper is based on enforcing nonnegativity of certain polynomials. Since most of the real cameras have limited fields of view, we only need to control the behavior of $L(r)$ for values $r \in [0, \bar{r}]$, where $\bar{r}$ is the maximal distance between the center of the radial distortion and an (undistorted) image point. For this, we need to characterize the set of univariate polynomials nonnegative on finite intervals. In [13], based on Markov-Lukacs theorem, Nesterov showed how to characterize such a set using positive semidefinite Gram matrices:

Theorem 1. *Let* $\alpha < \beta$, $p(x) \in \mathbb{R}[x]$ *and* $\deg p(x) = 2n$. *Then* $p(x) \geq 0$ *for all* $x \in [\alpha, \beta]$ *if and only if*

$$p(x) = s(x) + (x - \alpha)(\beta - x)t(x),$$

where $s(x) = \boldsymbol{\psi}_n^\top(x)\,\mathsf{S}\,\boldsymbol{\psi}_n(x)$, $t(x) = \boldsymbol{\psi}_{n-1}^\top(x)\,\mathsf{T}\,\boldsymbol{\psi}_{n-1}(x)$, *such that* $\mathsf{S}, \mathsf{T} \succeq 0$ *(i.e.,* $\mathsf{S} \in \mathcal{G}(s(x))$, $\mathsf{T} \in \mathcal{G}(t(x))$ *are positive semidefinite Gram matrices of polynomials* $s(x)$ *and* $t(x)$, *respectively).*

If $\deg p(x) = 2n + 1$, *then* $p(x) \geq 0$ *for all* $x \in [\alpha, \beta]$ *if and only if*

$$p(x) = (x - \alpha)s(x) + (\beta - x)t(x),$$

where $s(x) = \boldsymbol{\psi}_n^\top(x)\,\mathsf{S}\,\boldsymbol{\psi}_n(x)$, $t(x) = \boldsymbol{\psi}_n^\top(x)\,\mathsf{T}\,\boldsymbol{\psi}_n(x)$, *such that* $\mathsf{S}, \mathsf{T} \succeq 0$.

Even though Theorem 1 is an equivalence, we will only use it as an implication: as long as we will have matrices S, T that are positive semidefinitive, Theorem 1 guarantees that a polynomial $p(x)$ constructed using these matrices will be nonnegative on a given interval.

3.3 Polynomial Matrix Inequalities

According to Theorem 1, a polynomial is nonnegative on an interval as long the matrices S, T are positive semidefinite. By combining these constraints with a polynomial cost function, we get a problem of polynomial matrix inequalities (PMI) programming. A PMI program can be formally defined as follows:

Problem 1. (Polynomial matrix inequalities program)

$$minimize \ p(\mathbf{x})$$
$$subject \ to \ G_i(\mathbf{x}) \succeq 0, \ i = 1, \ldots, m,$$
$$where \ p(\mathbf{x}) \in \mathbb{R}[\mathbf{x}], G_i \in \mathbb{S}^{n_i}(\mathbb{R}[\mathbf{x}]).$$

In general, Problem 1 is a hard non-convex problem. Note however, that if the cost function $p(\mathbf{x})$ and the matrices $G_i(\mathbf{x})$, $i = 1, \ldots, m$ have degree one, then Problem 1 reduces to a linear matrix inequality (LMI) program and as such is a semidefinite program (SDP) solvable by any available SDP solver. In fact, most of the time the shape optimization problems in this paper lead to such a program.

Sometimes still, $G_i(\mathbf{x})$ will not be linear. In such cases, we will use the relaxation approach suggested by Henrion and Lasserre [10]. In [10], the authors proposed a hierarchy of LMI programs $\mathcal{P}_1, \mathcal{P}_2, \ldots$ that produces a monotonically non-decreasing sequence of lower bounds $p(\mathbf{x}_1^*) \leq p(\mathbf{x}_2^*) \leq \ldots$ on Problem 1 that converges to the global minimum $p(\mathbf{x}^*)$. Practically, the series converges to $p(\mathbf{x}^*)$ in finitely many steps, i.e., there exists $j \in \mathbb{N}$, such that $p(\mathbf{x}_j^*) = p(\mathbf{x}^*)$. The authors also showed how this situation can be detected and how the value of $\mathbf{x}^*$ can be extracted from the solution of the relaxation by the tools of linear algebra.

Let us show here how to construct $\mathcal{P}_\delta$, i.e., the LMI relaxation of Problem 1 of order δ; see [10] for the technical justification of this procedure. Let $G \in \mathbb{S}^n(\mathbb{R}[\mathbf{x}])$, $n = \sum_{i=1}^m n_i$ denote a block diagonal matrix with matrices G_i on it's diagonal. Since $(\forall i: G_i(\mathbf{x}) \succeq 0) \Leftrightarrow G(\mathbf{x}) \succeq 0$, we can replace the PMI constraints $G_i(\mathbf{x}) \succeq 0$ with one PMI constraint $G(\mathbf{x}) \succeq 0$. Next, we construct the so-called *moment matrix* $M_\delta(\mathbf{y})$ and *localizing matrix* $M_\delta(G, \mathbf{y})$ *of* G, defined as

$$M_\delta(\mathbf{y}) = \ell_{\mathbf{y}}(\psi_\delta(\mathbf{x})\psi_\delta^\top(\mathbf{x})),$$
$$M_\delta(G, \mathbf{y}) = \ell_{\mathbf{y}}((\psi_\delta(\mathbf{x})\psi_\delta^\top(\mathbf{x})) \otimes G),$$

where $\otimes$ denotes the Kronecker product [10]. Let $\gamma = 1$ if $\deg G \leq 2$, $\gamma = \frac{\lceil \deg G \rceil}{2}$ otherwise. Now, we can formally write the relaxation $\mathcal{P}_\delta$ as

Problem 2. (LMI relaxation $\mathcal{P}_\delta$ of order δ)

$$minimize \ \ell_{\mathbf{y}}(p(\mathbf{x}))$$
$$subject \ to \ M_{\delta-\gamma}(G, \mathbf{y}) \succeq 0,$$
$$M_\delta(\mathbf{y}) \succeq 0.$$

As the Riesz functional $\ell_{\mathbf{y}}$ was used to "linearize" both the cost function and the constraints, we can easily see that Problem 2 is an LMI program.

4   Shape Optimization for Radial Distortion Calibration

In this section, we show how to combine the results presented in Sect. 3 into the radial distortion shape optimization procedure. Technically, the procedure consists of minimization of a polynomial cost function in the vector of radial distortion parameters $\mathbf{k}$ subject to PMI constraints enforcing nonnegativity of certain polynomials in the radius r. Such a minimization problem is a PMI program that can be dealt with using the approach from Sect. 3.3.

As mentioned in Sect. 3.2, we only need to control the shape of $L(r)$ on the interval $[0, \bar{r}]$. Note, that $\bar{r}$ is the maximal distance between the center of the radial distortion and *undistorted* image points, *i.e.*, the value of $\bar{r}$ is not known prior to the actual calibration. The value of $\bar{r}$ is therefore a user supplied parameter. Fortunately, the proposed method is not very sensitive to the value of this parameter and even a gross overestimate yields minima identical to the ground truth value.

4.1   Unconstrained Radial Distortion Calibration

There are several ways how to determine the vector of parameters $\mathbf{k}$ of the distortion function $L(r)$ [9, 17]. All we need for our shape optimization approach is a polynomial cost function. Here, we will define and use one of such possible cost functions. Let us rewrite Eq. 1 using $L(r)$ from Eq. 2 as

$$ g(r) \begin{pmatrix} \hat{x}_i \\ \hat{y}_i \end{pmatrix} - f(r) \begin{pmatrix} x_i \\ y_i \end{pmatrix} = \begin{pmatrix} g(r)\,\hat{x}_i & f(r)\,x_i \\ g(r)\,\hat{y}_i & f(r)\,y_i \end{pmatrix} = \mathbf{0}. $$

By factoring out the vector of parameters $\mathbf{k}$ and by denoting

$$ \mathsf{A}_i = \begin{pmatrix} -r\,x_i & -r^2\,x_i & -r^3\,x_i & \hat{x}_i\,r & \hat{x}_i\,r^2 & \hat{x}_i\,r^3 \\ -r\,y_i & -r^2\,y_i & -r^3\,y_i & \hat{y}_i\,r & \hat{y}_i\,r^2 & \hat{y}_i\,r^3 \end{pmatrix}, \quad \mathbf{b}_i = \begin{pmatrix} x_i - \hat{x}_i \\ y_i - \hat{y}_i \end{pmatrix}, $$

we get a linear system $\mathsf{A}_i \mathbf{k} = \mathbf{b}_i$. Now, we can stack $\mathsf{A} = (\mathsf{A}_1^\mathsf{T}, \mathsf{A}_2^\mathsf{T}, \ldots, \mathsf{A}_n^\mathsf{T})^\mathsf{T}$, $\mathbf{b} = (\mathbf{b}_1^\mathsf{T}, \mathbf{b}_2^\mathsf{T}, \ldots \mathbf{b}_n^\mathsf{T})^\mathsf{T}$ and estimate the radial distortion parameters $\mathbf{k} = (k_1, k_2, \ldots, k_6)$ as a solution to an overdetermined system $\mathsf{A}\mathbf{k} = \mathbf{b}$ in the least square sense, *i.e.*, by minimizing $\|\mathsf{A}\mathbf{k} - \mathbf{b}\|^2$. Note that for polynomial model, *i.e.*, $g(x) = 1$, this corresponds to the minimization of the reprojection error.

Let us now express the minimization of $\|\mathsf{A}\mathbf{k} - \mathbf{b}\|^2$ as an LMI program. By expanding

$$ \|\mathsf{A}_i\mathbf{k} - \mathbf{b}_i\|^2 = (\mathsf{A}_i\mathbf{k} - \mathbf{b}_i)^\mathsf{T}(\mathsf{A}_i\mathbf{k} - \mathbf{b}_i) = \mathbf{k}^\mathsf{T}\mathsf{A}_i^\mathsf{T}\mathsf{A}_i\mathbf{k} - 2\mathbf{b}_i^\mathsf{T}\mathsf{A}_i\mathbf{k} + \mathbf{b}_i^\mathsf{T}\mathbf{b}_i $$

and by denoting $\mathsf{M} = \sum_{i=1}^n \mathsf{A}_i^\mathsf{T}\mathsf{A}_i$, $\mathbf{m} = -2\sum_{i=1}^n \mathsf{A}_i^\mathsf{T}\mathbf{b}_i$, $c = \sum_{i=1}^n \mathbf{b}_i^\mathsf{T}\mathbf{b}_i$, we can write the polynomial form of the cost function as

$$ \|\mathsf{A}\mathbf{k} - \mathbf{b}\|^2 = \mathbf{k}^\mathsf{T}\mathsf{M}\mathbf{k} + \mathbf{m}^\mathsf{T}\mathbf{k} + c. \tag{4} $$

As expected, Eq. 4 is a quadratic polynomial in $\mathbf{k}$ and by construction $M \succeq 0$, *i.e.*, M is a positive semidefinite matrix. Even though the cost function is quadratic, it can be converted into a linear function using the Schur complement trick [3]:

$$F = \begin{pmatrix} I & Lk \\ k^\top L^\top & -m^\top k - c + \gamma \end{pmatrix} \succeq 0 \Leftrightarrow k^\top L^\top Lk + m^\top k + c - \gamma \leq 0.$$

By decomposing M as $M = L^\top L$, *e.g.*, using the Cholesky or the spectral decomposition [7] (recall that $M \succeq 0$), we can rewrite the minimization of Eq. 4 as the following LMI program:

Problem 3. (Unconstrained radial distortion calibration)

$$minimize \ \gamma$$
$$subject \ to \ F = \begin{pmatrix} I & Lk \\ k^\top L^\top & -m^\top k - c + \gamma \end{pmatrix} \succeq 0.$$

4.2   Barrel Distortion and the Polynomial Model

As we can see from the example of barrel radial distortion in Fig. 1(a), this type of distortion can be characterized by the negativity of the first and the second derivatives:

$$\forall r \in [0, \bar{r}]: L'(r) \leq 0 \ \& \ L''(r) \leq 0, \tag{5}$$

where $[0, \bar{r}]$ spans the field of view of the camera. If we consider the polynomial model $L(r) = f(r)$, the constraints above mean that we need to enforce nonnegativity of polynomials

$$-f'(r) = -k_1 - 2k_2 r - 3k_3 r^2, -f''(r) = -2k_2 - 6k_3 r$$

on the interval $[0, \bar{r}]$. According to Theorem 1, $-f'(r) \geq 0$ for $\forall r \in [0, \bar{r}]$ iff

$$-f'(r) = -k_1 - 2k_2 r - 3k_3 r^2 = \psi_1(r)^\top S_1 \psi_1(r) + r(\bar{r} - r) T_1, \tag{6}$$

where

$$S_1 = \begin{pmatrix} s_{11} & s_{12} \\ s_{12} & s_{13} \end{pmatrix} \succeq 0, T_1 = (t_{11}) \succeq 0.$$

By expanding the right hand side of Eq. 6 and by comparing the polynomial coefficients, we get a parameterization of $\mathbf{k}$ in the elements of S_1 and T_1:

$$\left.\begin{array}{l} -k_1 = s_{11} \\ -2k_2 = 2s_{12} + \bar{r} t_{11} \\ -3k_3 = s_{13} - t_{11} \end{array}\right\} \Rightarrow k = (-s_{11}, -s_{12} - \tfrac{1}{2}\bar{r}t_{11}, \tfrac{1}{3}(t_{11} - s_{13}), 0, 0, 0). \tag{7}$$

Let's apply Theorem 1 to $-f''(r)$ to get the following constraint:

$$-f''(r) = -2k_2 - 6k_3 r = r \, S_2 + (\bar{r} - r)T_2, S_2 = (s_{21}) \succeq 0, T_2 = (t_{21}) \succeq 0. \tag{8}$$

By combining Eqs. 7 and 8, we can express the entries of S_2 and T_2 in the entries of S_1, T_1:

$$\left.\begin{array}{c} -2k_2 = \bar{r}\, t_{21} \\ -6k_3 = s_{21} - t_{21} \end{array}\right\} \Rightarrow \left\{\begin{array}{l} s_{21} = \frac{1}{\bar{r}}\left(2s_{12} + 2\bar{r}\, s_{13} - \bar{r}t_{11}\right) \\ t_{21} = \frac{2}{\bar{r}}\left(s_{12} + \frac{1}{2}\bar{r}t_{11}\right) \end{array}\right. \tag{9}$$

Now, we have four PMI constraints on the shape of $L(r)$. If we combine these constraints along with the parameterization of $\mathbf{k}$ from Eq. 7 with Problem 3, we get a radial distortion calibration problem that enforces a barrel type distortion shape of the resulting distortion model:

Problem 4. (Barrel distortion calibration)

$$minimize\ \gamma$$
$$subject\ to\ \mathbf{F} \succeq 0,\ \mathbf{S}_1 \succeq 0,\ \mathbf{T}_1 = (t_{11}) \succeq 0,$$
$$\mathbf{S}_2 = \left(\tfrac{1}{\bar{r}}\left(2s_{12} + 2\bar{r}\, s_{13} - \bar{r}t_{11}\right)\right) \succeq 0,$$
$$\mathbf{T}_2 = \left(\tfrac{2}{\bar{r}}\left(s_{12} + \tfrac{1}{2}\bar{r}t_{11}\right)\right) \succeq 0.$$

Problem 4 is a PMI program in 5 variables $\gamma, s_{11}, s_{12}, s_{13}, t_{11}$. Since both the cost function and the PMI constraints have degree one, Problem 4 is in fact an SDP problem. Once it is solved, the unknown distortion parameters $\mathbf{k}$ can be easily recovered using Eq. 7.

4.3 Pincushion Distortion and the Division Model

Let us make an analogous analysis for the pincushion distortion shape and the division model $L(r) = \frac{1}{g(r)}$. This type of distortion is characterized by the non-negativity of the first and the second derivatives of $L(r)$ on the field of view of the camera $[0, \bar{r}]$. From the first derivative we get the following constraint on the polynomial denominator $g(r)$:

$$L'(r) = \frac{-g'(r)}{g^2(r)} \quad \Rightarrow \quad L'(r) \geq 0 \Leftrightarrow -g'(r) \geq 0.$$

The second derivative yields a bit more complicated constraint:

$$L''(r) = \frac{g(r)h(r)}{g^4(r)} = \frac{h(r)}{g^3(r)} \Rightarrow L''(r) \geq 0 \Leftrightarrow \left\{\begin{array}{c} (g(r) \geq 0\,\&\,h(r) \geq 0)\ \vee \\ (g(r) \leq 0\,\&\,h(r) \leq 0), \end{array}\right.$$

where $h(r) = 2(g'(r))^2 - g(r)g''(r)$. However, since we know that $L(r) > 0$ by definition, we only need to consider the constraints $g(r) \geq 0, h(r) \geq 0$. Let us start with the constraint $g(r) \geq 0$. According to Theorem 1, $g(r) \geq 0$ for $\forall r \in [0, \bar{r}]$ iff

$$g(r) = 1 + k_4 r + k_5 r^2 + k_6 r^3 = \boldsymbol{\psi}_1(r)^\top \mathbf{S}_1 \boldsymbol{\psi}_1(r) + (\bar{r} - r)\,\boldsymbol{\psi}_1(r)^\top \mathbf{T}_1 \boldsymbol{\psi}_1(r), \tag{10}$$

where

$$S_1 = \begin{pmatrix} s_{11} & s_{12} \\ s_{12} & s_{13} \end{pmatrix} \succeq 0, \, T_1 = \begin{pmatrix} t_{11} & t_{12} \\ t_{12} & t_{13} \end{pmatrix} \succeq 0.$$

This leads to the following parameterization of $\mathbf{k}$ as well as to a constraint on the variable t_{11}:

$$\left.\begin{array}{l} 1 = \bar{r} t_{11} \\ k_4 = s_{11} - t_{11} + 2\bar{r} t_{12} \\ k_5 = 2s_{12} - 2t_{12} + \bar{r} t_{13} \\ k_6 = s_{13} - t_{13} \end{array}\right\} \Rightarrow \left\{\begin{array}{l} \mathbf{k} = (0, 0, 0, s_{11} - t_{11} + 2\bar{r} t_{12}, \\ \qquad 2s_{12} - 2t_{12} + \bar{r} t_{13}, s_{13} - t_{13}) \\ t_{11} = \frac{1}{\bar{r}} \end{array}\right. \qquad (11)$$

By applying Theorem 1 to the constraint $-g'(r) \geq 0$, we get

$$-g'(r) = -k_4 - 2k_5 r - 3k_6 r^2 = \psi_1(r)^\top S_2 \psi_1(r) + r (\bar{r} - r) T_2, \qquad (12)$$

where

$$S_2 = \begin{pmatrix} s_{21} & s_{22} \\ s_{22} & s_{23} \end{pmatrix} \succeq 0, \, T_2 = (t_{21}) \succeq 0.$$

As in the case of the barrel distortion optimization, we can express the entries of S_2 and T_2 in the entries of S_1, T_1. This time, however, we have more variables than equations and we have to set one of the entries free—we chose s_{22}:

$$\left.\begin{array}{l} -3k_4 = s_{21} \\ -2k_5 = 2s_{22} + \bar{r} t_{21} \\ -3k_6 = s_{23} - t_{21} \end{array}\right\} \Rightarrow \left\{\begin{array}{l} s_{21} = t_{11} - s_{11} - 2\bar{r} t_{12} \\ s_{23} = -\frac{1}{\bar{r}}(s_{12} + 2s_{22} - 4t_{12} + \bar{r}(3s_{13} - t_{13})) \\ t_{21} = -\frac{1}{\bar{r}}(2s_{12} + s_{22} - 2t_{12} + \bar{r} t_{13}) \end{array}\right. \qquad (13)$$

The final constraint is the most complicated because of the quadratic monomials in $\mathbf{k}$: $h(r) > 0$ for $\forall r \in [0, \bar{r}]$ iff

$$\begin{aligned} h(r) &= (6k_6 r^2 + 4k_5 r + 2k_4)(3k_6 r^2 + 2k_5 + k_4) - \\ &\quad - (2k_5 + 6k_6 r)(k_6 r^3 - k_5 r^2 + k_4 r + 1) \\ &= \psi_2(r)^\top S_3 \psi_2(r) + (\bar{r} - r) \, \psi_1(r)^\top T_3 \psi_1(r), \end{aligned} \qquad (14)$$

where

$$S_3 = \begin{pmatrix} s_{31} & s_{32} & s_{33} \\ s_{32} & s_{34} & s_{35} \\ s_{33} & s_{35} & s_{36} \end{pmatrix} \succeq 0, \, T_3 = \begin{pmatrix} t_{31} & t_{32} \\ t_{32} & t_{33} \end{pmatrix} \succeq 0.$$

Equation 14 gives us 5 constraints on 9 entries of S_3 and T_3. We chose to set free variables $s_{32}, s_{34}, s_{36}, t_{32}$; System 15 shows the form of the remaining 5 variables. Finally, we can combine these 6 PMI constraints, Problem 3 and the parameterization of $\mathbf{k}$ from Eq. 11 into a radial distortion calibration problem that enforces a pincushion type distortion shape:

Problem 5. (Pincushion distorion calibration)

$$minimize \, \gamma$$
$$subject \, to \, F \succeq 0, S_1 \succeq 0, T_1 \succeq 0, S_2 \succeq 0, T_2 \succeq 0, S_3 \succeq 0, T_3 \succeq 0.$$

$$\left.\begin{array}{rcl}
12k_6^2 &=& s_{36}-t_{33} \\
16k_5k_6 &=& 2s_{35}-2t_{32}+\bar{r}t_{33} \\
6k_5^2+6k_4k_6 &=& 2s_{33}+s_{34}-t_{31}+2\bar{r}t_{32} \\
6k_4k_5-6k_6 &=& 2s_{32}+\bar{r}t_{31} \\
2k_4^2-2k_5 &=& s_{31}
\end{array}\right\} \Rightarrow \left\{\begin{array}{rcl}
s_{31} &=& 4t_{12}-s_{12}-2\bar{r}t_{31}+2(s_{11}-t_{11}+2\bar{r}t_{12})^2 \\
s_{33} &=& -\frac{1}{2\bar{r}}(6s_{13}+2s_{32}-6t_{13}+\bar{r}s_{34} \\
&& -6\bar{r}(2s_{12}-2t_{12}+\bar{r}t_{13})^2+2\bar{r}^2t_{32}- \\
&& -6(s_{11}-t_{11}+2\bar{r}t_{12}) \\
&& (2s_{12}-2t_{12}+\bar{r}t_{13}+\bar{r}s_{13}-\bar{r}t_{13})) \\
s_{35} &=& t_{32}-\frac{2}{\bar{r}}s_{36}+6\bar{r}(s_{13}-t_{13})^2+ \\
&& +8(s_{13}-t_{13})(2s_{12}-2t_{12}+\bar{r}t_{13}) \\
t_{31} &=& -\frac{2}{\bar{r}}(3s_{13}+s_{32}-3t_{13}- \\
&& 3(2s_{12}-2t_{12}+\bar{r}t_{13})(s_{11}-t_{11}+2\bar{r}t_{12})) \\
t_{33} &=& s_{36}-12(s_{13}-t_{13})^2
\end{array}\right. \tag{15}$$

Problem 5 is a PMI program in 11 variables γ, s_{11}, s_{12}, s_{13}, t_{12}, t_{13}, s_{22}, s_{32}, s_{34}, s_{36}, and t_{32}. Since S_3 and T_3 are polynomial matrices of degree 2, Problem 5 has to be dealt with using the relaxation scheme from Sect. 3.3.

4.4 Zero-Crossing Problem of the Rational Model

Also the zero-crossing problem of the rational model $L(r) = \frac{f(r)}{g(r)}$ can be dealt with using the proposed shape optimization technique. A sufficient condition for avoiding a common root of the polynomials $f(r)$ and $g(r)$ on the interval $[0, \bar{r}]$ is to force at least one on them to have no root. Here, we decided on enforcing the constraint

$$\forall r \in \langle 0, \bar{r}\rangle : g(r) - p \geq 0, \text{ where } p > 0. \tag{16}$$

Since Theorem 1 guarantees only nonnegativity of a polynomial, we need a strictly positive parameter p to enforce strict positivity of $g(r)$. Even though parameter p must be user supplied, the method is not overly sensitive to its value; in our experiments, we set $p = 0.1$. By applying Theorem 1 to the above constraint and the interval $[0, \bar{r}]$, we get

$$g(r) - p = 1 - p + k_4r + k_5r^2 + k_6r^3 = \psi_1(r)^\top S_1\psi_1(r) + (\bar{r}-r)\,\psi_1(r)^\top T_1\psi_1(r),$$

where

$$S_1 = \begin{pmatrix} s_{11} & s_{12} \\ s_{12} & s_{13} \end{pmatrix} \succeq 0, \; T_1 = \begin{pmatrix} t_{11} & t_{12} \\ t_{12} & t_{13} \end{pmatrix} \succeq 0.$$

This yields a parameterization of $\mathbf{k}$ as well as a constraint on t_{11}:

$$\left.\begin{array}{l}
1-p=\bar{r}\,t_{11} \\
k_4=s_{11}-t_{11}+2\bar{r}t_{12} \\
k_5=2s_{12}-2t_{12}+\bar{r}t_{13} \\
k_6=s_{13}-t_{13}
\end{array}\right\} \Rightarrow \left\{\begin{array}{l}
\mathbf{k}=(k_1,k_2,k_3,s_{11}-t_{11}+2\bar{r}t_{12}, \\
\qquad 2s_{12}-2t_{12}+\bar{r}t_{13},s_{13}-t_{13}) \\
t_{11}=\frac{1-p}{\bar{r}}
\end{array}\right. \tag{17}$$

Again, by combining the two PMI constraints with Problem 3 and the parameterization of $\mathbf{k}$ from Eq. 17, we get a radial distortion calibration problem that eliminates the zero-crossing problem:

Problem 6. (Zero-crossing distortion calibration)

$$minimize\ \gamma$$
$$subject\ to\ \mathsf{F} \succeq 0,\ \mathsf{S}_1 \succeq 0,\ \mathsf{T}_1 \succeq 0.$$

Problem 6 is an LMI program in 9 variables $\gamma, s_{11}, s_{12}, s_{13}, t_{12}, t_{13}, k_1, k_2, k_3$.

4.5 Shape Optimization in Camera Calibration Procedure

All of the calibration problems presented in this paper expect the projection coordinates x_i, y_i, $\hat{x}_i$, and $\hat{y}_i$ to be known, see Eq. 1. This assumes a known calibration target $\mathbf{X}_i \in \mathbb{R}^3$ as well as known camera parameters $\mathsf{R} \in SO(3)$, $\mathbf{t} \in \mathbb{R}^3$, and the calibration matrix $\mathsf{K} \in \mathbb{R}^{3 \times 3}$. A straightforward idea how to fold the shape optimized radial distortion calibration into the camera calibration procedure is to first perform "classical" camera calibration [8,18,20,21], including radial distortion estimation. Once the projection coordinates are known, the shape optimized radial distortion calibration can be performed to replace the radial distortion parameters estimated by a classical method. One might argue that the quality of such a solution could be compromised, since different error functions may be considered by the camera and the shape optimization calibration methods. To mitigate this problem, we suggest an alternating approach to "shape-optimize" the results of the classical camera calibration: first, the shape optimization procedure is performed, followed by a bundle adjustment [19] step where the radial distortion parameters are fixed. This can be repeated in a loop for a fixed number of times, or until desired convergence is reached.

5 Experiments

To validate the proposed approach, this section presents several experimental results on synthetic as well as real world datasets. We implemented Problems 4, 5, and 6 in MATLAB using Yalmip toolbox [11] with SeDuMi [15] as the underlying SDP solver. Yalmip toolbox is a modeling language that can be used to solve LMI as well as PMI programs, which it automatically translates into LMI relaxations using the scheme presented in Sect. 3.3. All of the resulting SDP programs were solved under a second on an Intel i7 3.50 GHz based desktop computer running Linux and 64 bit MATLAB.

Synthetic Experiment. In the synthetic experiment, we studied the performance of the proposed method with respect to the image noise. We generated a synthetic 16×16 planar calibration target. A scene consisted of 9 random 640×480 pixel cameras randomly positioned on a hemisphere around the target and rotated to face its center. The focal length was set to approx. 540 px and the distances of the camera centers from the target were set up so that the target (calibration data point set) covered only the middle part of the field of view, approx 50 %. For each of the three model-shape problem combinations, we

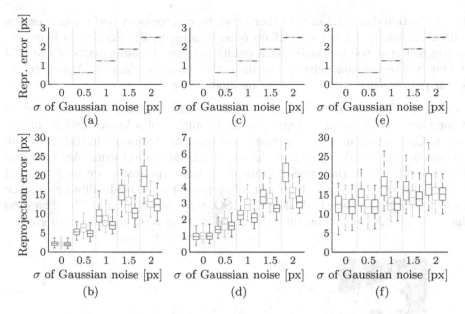

Fig. 2. *Image noise experiment.* Methods BA, SO, and ASO in red, green, and blue, respectively, on calibration and validation data point sets. (a–b) barrel distortion, (c–d) pincushion distortion (e–f) zero-crossing problem (Color figure online).

generated 100 scenes and corrupted the projections of the calibration target by an increasing amount of Gaussian image noise in 5 levels, standard deviation $\sigma \subset [0,2]$ px in $1/2$ px steps. We calibrated all scenes with OpenCV [2] made to disregard the radial distortion component. We compare three methods: the first method (BA) is the bundle adjustment method that included the respective radial distortion model performed together with the OpenCV calibration results, the second method (SO) is the respective shape-optimization method performed after the BA step, and the last method (ASO) is the alternating approach from Sect. 4.5, fixed to 10 iterations.

Barrel Distortion. First, we experimented with the barrel distortion and the polynomial model $L(r) = f(r)$. Figure 2(a) shows the mean of the reprojection errors on the calibration data point set for methods BA, SO, and ASO using MATLAB function boxplot. The methods show identical performance, however when a validation data set of points covering the whole field of view is used, see Fig. 2(a), we see both SO and ASO outperforming the classical BA approach.

Pincushion Distortion. Next, Figs. 2(c–d) show the analogous measure for the pincushion distortion and the division model $L(r) = \frac{1}{g(x)}$. Here, both BA and shape-optimization methods perform significantly better on the validation data point set. Still, we can see superior performance of SO and ASO as the noise increases.

Zero-Crossing. Finally, we experimented with the rational model $L(r) = \frac{f(r)}{g(r)}$ and the mustache type distortion. Figure 2(d) shows identical performance on the calibration dataset. On the other hand, we can see poor performance on the validation data point set even if no noise is present, Fig. 2(e). This is caused by the fact that too few calibration points were on the outer parts of the field of view where the convexity of the distortion function changes. Again, we see better performance of SO and ASO methods.

Real Experiment. In the real experiment, we calibrated a 2 MPix camera from Point Grey's Ladybug 3 system [1] using 12 images of a known 28×20 planar target. Calibration using BA method and the rational model introduced quite noticeable zero-crossing problem. As expected, calibration using ASO method does not suffer from this type of problem. In this experiment, we set $\bar{r} = 4$ and $p = 0.1$. Figure 3(a) shows the upper left corner of a rectified calibration image using **k** provided by methods BA and ASO, respectively. Figure 3(b) shows the shape of the BA calibration function in red and the ASO calibration in green.

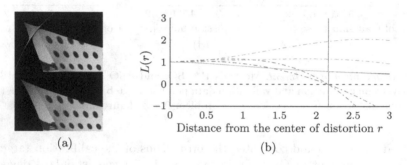

(a)   (b)

Fig. 3. *Real Experiment.* Correction of the zero-crossing problem of the rational model.

6   Conclusion

The aim of this work was not to argue for a specific radial distortion model, but to point out extrapolation problems inherent to all polynomial and rational models. We solved these problems by enforcing a predetermined shape of the distortion function. For most shapes and models, the proposed approach leads to small semidefinite programming problems that can be solved fast and globally optimally. We also showed how to deal with shapes and models that lead to PMI problems using a LMI relaxation scheme. We showed experimentally that in terms of the reprojection error on the known data points the proposed approach provides radial distortion models that are equivalent to those provided by the classical bundle adjustment approach, yet with the added value of having the correct shape that mollifies or completely removes all extrapolation issues.

Acknowledgments. The authors were supported by the EC under project FP7-SPACE-2012-312377 PRoViDE.

References

1. Ladybug 3 camera. http://www.ptgrey.com/products/ladybug3
2. Open source computer vision library. www.opencv.org
3. Boyd, S., Vandenberghe, L.: Convex Optimization. Cambridge University Press, Cambridge, March 2004
4. Brown, D.C.: Decentering distortion of lenses. Photometric Eng. **3**, 444–462 (1966)
5. Brown, D.C.: Close-range camera calibration. Photogrammetric Eng. **37**, 855–866 (1971)
6. Choi, M.-D., Lam, T.Y., Reznick. B.: Sums of squares of real polynomials. In: Proceedings of Symposia in Pure mathematics, vol. 58, pp. 103–126. American Mathematical Society (1995)
7. Golub, G.H., Van Loan, C.F.: Matrix computations (2012)
8. Hartley, R., Kang, S.B.: Parameter-free radial distortion correction with center of distortion estimation. IEEE Trans. Pattern Anal. Mach. Intell. **29**(8), 1309–1321 (2007)
9. Hartley, R., Zisserman, A.: Multiple view geometry in computer vision, 2nd edn. Cambridge University, Cambridge (2003)
10. Henrion, D., Lasserre, J.-B.: Convergent relaxations of polynomial matrix inequalities and static output feedback. IEEE Trans. Autom. Control **51**(02), 192–202 (2006)
11. Löfberg, J.: YALMIP: A toolbox for modeling and optimization in MATLAB. In: Proceedings of the CACSD Conference, Taipei, Taiwan (2004)
12. Ma, L., Chen, Y., Moore, K.: Rational radial distortion models of camera lenses with analytical solution for distortion correction. Int. J. Inf. Acquis. **1**(02), 135–147 (2004)
13. Nesterov, Y.: Squared functional systems and optimization problems. In: Frenk, H., Roos, K., Terlaky, T., Zhang, S. (eds.) High Performance Optimization, vol. 33, pp. 405–440. Springer, Heidelberg (2000)
14. Slama, C.C., Theurer, C., Henriksen, S.W., et al.: Manual of Photogrammetry, 4th edn. American Society of photogrammetry, New York (1980)
15. Sturm, J.F.: Using SeDuMi 1.02, a MATLAB toolbox for optimization over symmetric cones. Optim. Methods Softw. **11–12**, 625–653 (1999)
16. Sturm, P., Ramalingam, S., Tardif, J.-P., Gasparini, S., Barreto, J.: Camera models and fundamental concepts used in geometric computer vision. Found. Trends Comput. Graph. Vis. **6**(1–2), 1–183 (2011)
17. Szeliski, R.: Computer vision: algorithms and applications. Texts in Computer Science, vol. XX, p. 812. Springer, Heidelberg (2011)
18. Tardif, J.-P., Sturm, P., Trudeau, M., Roy, S.: Calibration of cameras with radially symmetric distortion. IEEE Trans. Pattern Anal. Mach. Intell. **31**(9), 1552–1566 (2009)
19. Triggs, B., McLauchlan, P.F., Hartley, R.I., Fitzgibbon, A.W.: Bundle adjustment - a modern synthesis. In: ICCV '99: Proceedings of the International Workshop on Vision Algorithms, pp. 298–372 (2000)
20. Tsai, R.Y.: An efficient and accurate camera calibration technique for 3D machine vision. In: Conference on Computer Vision and Pattern Recognition (1986)
21. Zhang, Z.: A Flexible new technique for camera calibration. IEEE Trans. Pattern Anal. Mach. Intell. **22**(11), 1330–1334 (2000)

Pedestrian Verification for Multi-Camera Detection

Scott Spurlock$^{(\boxtimes)}$ and Richard Souvenir

University of North Carolina at Charlotte, Charlotte, NC 28223, USA
{sspurloc,souvenir}@uncc.edu

Abstract. In this paper, we introduce an approach to multi-camera, multi-object detection that builds on low-level object localization with the targeted use of high-level pedestrian detectors. Low-level detectors often identify a small number of candidate locations, but suffer from false positives. We introduce a method of *pedestrian verification*, which takes advantage of geometric and scene information to (1) drastically reduce the search space in both the spatial and scale domains, and (2) select the camera(s) with the highest likelihood of providing accurate high-level detection. The proposed framework is modular and can incorporate a variety of existing detection methods. Compared to recent methods on a benchmark dataset, our method improves detection performance by 2.4 %, while processing more than twice as fast.

1 Introduction

Detection and tracking of multiple people from video has many important applications, including automated surveillance, crowd modeling, and sports analysis. As the number of people in the scene increases, occlusions become a major challenge. Compared with single-camera approaches (e.g., [1,2]), by making use of multiple, overlapping cameras, several recent methods [3–6] have shown robustness to occlusion in these types of crowded scenes with low-level detectors that measure 3D occupancy. Typically these approaches require a trade-off between speed and accuracy. Of recently developed approaches to multi-camera, multi-object (MCMO) detection, the most accurate involve expensive computation not suited to real-time application. The fastest methods tend to be less accurate, providing only probability maps and delaying final localization to a subsequent tracking phase.

In parallel, recent methods for pedestrian detection have shown promising results for identifying individual people in images. At low resolutions and in the presence of occlusion, however, even the best detectors perform poorly. Further, while detector speed has improved significantly in recent years, these methods are not designed to be used for multi-camera person detection in real-time at typical resolutions using the common approach of sliding windows at multiple scales and locations.

In this paper, we propose a hybrid approach that uses fast low-level detection and targeted high-level verification, achieving high accuracy at real-time speed.

© Springer International Publishing Switzerland 2015
D. Cremers et al. (Eds.): ACCV 2014, Part I, LNCS 9003, pp. 322–334, 2015.
DOI: 10.1007/978-3-319-16865-4_21

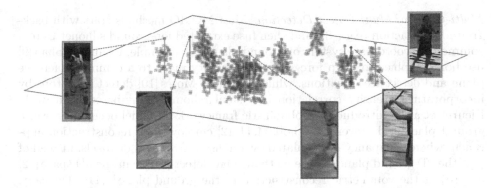

Fig. 1. MCMO detectors based on low-level features are prone to "ghosts" (red lines), or false positives, caused by shadows, occlusions, and projective effects among the true positive detections (green lines). Our method incorporates high-level image-based features from the camera(s) with the best view to verify actual people (Color figure online).

Our framework is modular, consisting of low, medium, and high-level detection steps. The modularity of the design allows our framework to incorporate new or pre-existing detector implementations as needed. With each successive step more computationally expensive than the previous, the goal is to discard as many hypotheses as possible using computationally inexpensive methods, and only use high-level detectors to *verify* uncertain earlier hypotheses. Figure 1 illustrates the idea. A low-level occupancy detector identifies 3D foreground voxels, shown as gray cuboids. A mid level aggregation step localizes objects, finding both true detections (green lines) as well as false positives (red lines), known as ghosts. For high-level pedestrian verification, image patches are extracted corresponding to locations to be verified. The goal is for a pedestrian detector to accurately evaluate the presence of a person in the image patch. However, in a multi-camera environment, certain viewpoints may be preferable to others, in terms of the expected accuracy of the detector.

Our main contribution is a multi-stage, coarse-to-fine framework for MCMO detection, which includes a probabilistic model for selecting the optimal camera(s) with respect to expected detection accuracy. The targeted use of high-level verification keeps computational cost low while keeping accuracy high. We evaluate our method on a challenging benchmark dataset for MCMO detection and tracking. Our results show the efficacy of our real-time approach, outperforming recent methods in both detection accuracy and computational efficiency. Note that while our focus in this paper is on MCMO detection, the method can easily be incorporated into any end-to-end tracking system, directly benefiting tracking performance.

2   Related Work

Detecting people from images and video has been well-covered over many years [7]. Our focus is on multi-camera methods that incorporate low-level features for occupancy estimation.

Multi-Camera, Multi-Object Detection. Most MCMO methods start with background subtraction (e.g., [8]) and then fuse extracted foreground silhouettes to a common 3D coordinate system or ground plane. For example, Khan and Shah [9] use homographies to warp foreground probability maps to a common reference plane and detect feet locations, while Eshel and Moses [10] detect head tops by incorporating intensity correlation in a similar homography-based framework. Fleuret et al. [5] introduce a probabilistic framework to model occupancy over a ground plane grid. Several methods [4,11,12] employ a 3D reconstruction approach, where occupancy is calculated over a discrete 3D grid of voxels, instead of just the 2D ground plane. These methods may detect people in the 3D space [12] or project the volumetric reconstruction to the ground plane [4,11]. Typically, exact localization is delayed to a later tracking phase based on, e.g., graph cuts [9] or dynamic programming [5] over temporal windows.

Reducing False Positive Detections. Some recent MCMO detection methods have explicitly incorporated schemes to address ghosts. Alahi et al. [3] model ground plane occupancy estimation as a sparse optimization problem. A sparsity constraint is intended to rule out false positives during the detection phase. While this method achieves high detection accuracy, the authors' implementation takes 10 s per frame, making it unsuitable for real-time applications. Peng et al. [6] incorporate a graphical model that explicitly encodes occlusion relationships among discretized ground-plane locations. An iterative algorithm finds the occupancy configuration that best explains the camera foreground images. The method reduces the occurrence of ghost detections due to the occlusion reasoning, but takes 3 s per frame in the authors' implementation. Other methods incorporate simple rules to reduce ghosts, such as fixing a priori the number of objects to be detected [13].

Our framework, which includes concepts common to MCMO methods, incorporates pedestrian verification directly into the detection stage rather than a subsequent tracking step or with ad hoc rules. The verification step relies on selecting the best viewpoints for image-based pedestrian detection. However, compared to the sliding window approach commonly employed for single image pedestrian detectors, our method drastically reduces the search space by only evaluating selected image patches. Viewed in this light, the low-level detection step provides geometric context similar to approaches (e.g., [14]) that use scene context to reduce false positives. By combining efficient low-level detection, mid-level aggregation, and targeted use of high-level verification, our framework is capable of real-time multi-person detection in multi-camera networks.

3   Base Detector

Our pedestrian verification approach could be used with any low- or mid-level MCMO detector. In this section, we describe our base detector implementation.

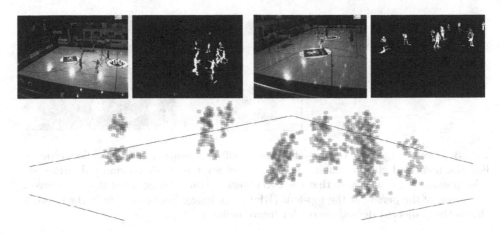

Fig. 2. Example input frames and extracted foreground silhouettes used to perform a coarse 3D reconstruction for our low-level detector.

3.1 Low-Level Detection

As shown in Fig. 2, our low-level detector performs change detection on C cameras viewing the scene in order to create a coarse 3D reconstruction of the visual hulls of moving objects. The scene volume is discretized into a voxel grid, $V = \{v_1, v_2, \ldots, v_n\}$, where each voxel is identified as either background or foreground by a straightforward voting scheme:

$$v_i = \begin{cases} 1 & \text{if } \sum_k \pi(v_i, k) \geq \gamma \\ 0 & \text{otherwise} \end{cases} \tag{1}$$

where $\pi(v_i, k)$ indicates whether voxel v_i projects to foreground in camera k, and γ is the threshold for the number of cameras in the network that must agree for a positive voxel detection. To implement the voxel-image occupancy function, π, other MCMO detectors (e.g., [4]) employ *point sampling*, where the voxel center is projected to a single pixel in an image. For greater robustness to noisy foreground extraction, we employ *area sampling*, where the 3D extent of the voxel is projected to a bounding box in an image. Then, we define the voxel-image occupancy function as:

$$\pi(v_i, k) = \begin{cases} 1 & \text{if } \rho(v_i, k) \geq \beta \\ 0 & \text{otherwise} \end{cases} \tag{2}$$

where ρ represents the proportion of pixels in the associated bounding box in image k corresponding to foreground and β is a system-specific threshold that can be tuned based on the noise level of the foreground segmentation process. The voxel-image occupancy function with area sampling can be implemented efficiently using the integral image technique [15] with the foreground mask image.

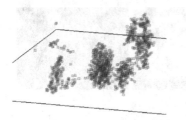 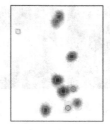 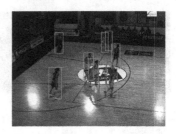

Fig. 3. Given foreground voxels (left), mean shift clustering (middle) localizes objects. For the identified cluster centers, green squares are true positives and red circles are false positives (ghosts). Note that the two ghosts are more pronounced than the correct detection of the person at the top-left. (Right) An image from a camera in the network shows the projected detections (Color figure online).

3.2   Mid-Level Aggregation

The next stage is aggregation of voxel detections to objects, illustrated in Fig. 3. Our approach relies on mean shift clustering (MSC) [16] for this step. MSC is a non-parametric clustering approach that can find non-uniform or narrow modes in a distribution, which, in our case, correspond to potential object locations in the scene. MSC is well-suited to the problem because no prior knowledge about the number or location of objects is needed.

Let $\{\mathbf{x}_i\}$ be the set of points in $\mathbb{R}^3$ corresponding to the centers of the identified foreground voxels. We define the kernel density estimator [16] for occupancy at a point $\mathbf{x}$ as

$$\hat{f}(\mathbf{x}) \propto \sum_i K_{\mathbf{H}}\left(\mathbf{x} - \mathbf{x}_i\right) \tag{3}$$

where $K_{\mathbf{H}}(\mathbf{x}) = |\mathbf{H}|^{-1/2} K\left(\mathbf{H}^{-1/2}\mathbf{x}\right)$. Here $\mathbf{H}$ is a d × d bandwidth matrix and K is the unit flat kernel [17]

$$K(x) = \begin{cases} 1 & \text{if } \|x\|_\infty \leq 1 \\ 0 & \text{otherwise} \end{cases} \tag{4}$$

where $\|\cdot\|_\infty$ is the infinity norm, which implies an axis-aligned, box-shaped kernel with dimensions controlled by bandwidth matrix, $\mathbf{H}$, a diagonal matrix, where each element along the diagonal is the squared bandwidth for a dimension of the box. For person detection, we choose $\mathbf{H}$ to approximate the dimension of an upright person, i.e., $h_1 = h_2 = h_3/4$. While MSC implementations typically incorporate the smoothly differentiable Epanchnikov or Gaussian kernels, our choice of an axis-aligned box kernel allows for faster computation and works well in practice.

Each cluster is scored based on the proportion of foreground voxels within the bandwidth to total bandwidth volume

$$s_d(\delta_m) = \frac{\hat{f}(\delta_m)}{\prod_{j=1}^d h_j} \tag{5}$$

where δ_m is the d-dimensional cluster mean (for our application, $d = 3$). The cluster score can be thresholded to discard low-scoring detections, which often correspond to ghosts. However, care must be taken to avoid rejecting valid detections. Figure 3 shows an example where a valid detection scores lower than two ghost detections. In the next section, we describe how pedestrian detection can help distinguish between correct and incorrect detections.

4 Pedestrian Verification

In some systems [3,5,6], the output from low- and/or mid-level stages are directly used as output detections. However, some of these may actually be "ghosts," or false positive detections due to shadows, reflections, or occlusions. These errors become increasingly common as crowd density increases, and, in complex scenes, significantly degrade overall system accuracy. Figure 3 shows two examples of ghost detections in red. Our high-level detection stage, pedestrian verification, is aimed at identifying and eliminating these false detections without filtering out correct detections.

4.1 Predicting Verification Accuracy

For a given cluster, represented by center location, δ_m, the 3D bounded region corresponds to an image patch in each camera. For each candidate patch, we compute the *Expected Detection Accuracy (EDA)*, $E[Q|\Theta]$, where Q is a continuous random variable representing accuracy of a pedestrian detector under the conditions encoded by the vector, Θ. Ideally, the model attributes would be features that are efficient to compute following the low-level detection phase. A recent survey [18] provides an evaluation of the performance of numerous detectors as a function of occlusion and scale. The best performing detectors work well for near-scale (at least 80 pixels high) examples, with rapid performance decrease as pedestrian size decreases. Additionally, all of the detectors were sensitive to occlusion; even partial occlusion (<35 %) led to a log-average miss rate of 73 % for the best detector. To estimate the predictive power of a pedestrian detector from a given viewpoint, our model incorporates occlusion, scale, and also verticality, a measure of how upright a person appears from a particular viewpoint. For a candidate location and corresponding image patches, these three features can be computed using the projection of the 3D bounding boxes.

4.2 Model Attributes

We define the bounding box for detection m projected into camera k as the (rectangular) area of pixels, r_m^k. For the candidate detection, the up vector, U_m^k, is the projection of a 3D vector pointing up along the positive Z-axis from the candidate ground location, m, to the target's estimated height, as viewed in camera k.

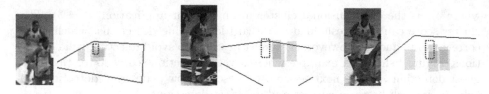

Fig. 4. The occlusion value is estimated by calculating the overlap of the candidate bounding box (dashed blue rectangle) with other, closer detections (gray boxes). For the views shown, occlusion is 0.82, 0.00, and 0.56, respectively (Lower is better.) (Color figure online).

Occlusion. In order to estimate an occlusion ratio for each detection based on the other (potential) detections in the scene, we adapt the painter's algorithm [19] from computer graphics. The idea is to order the detections by proximity to the camera center, and project a synthetic bounding box, r_j^k, into a 2D accumulator for each detection that is closer to the camera than r_m^k. The occlusion ratio measures the overlap of other (potential) detections with the candidate location:

$$s_o(m, k) = \frac{\left|\left(\bigcup_j r_j^k\right) \cap r_m^k\right|}{|r_m^k|} \tag{6}$$

where $|\cdot|$ is the number of pixels in the box. Figure 4 shows an example of how occlusion is calculated for three different views of one example detection from the scene depicted in Fig. 3.

Verticality. Typically, pedestrian detectors are trained on examples containing mostly upright (vertical) people. So, rather than incur the cost of training many detectors or applying a warp to each image patch, we estimate how upright a person at a given 3D location will appear from a particular view. Verticality is computed as:

$$s_u(m, k) = \left\langle \frac{U_m^k}{\|U_m^k\|}, \frac{I_m^k}{\|I_m^k\|} \right\rangle \tag{7}$$

where I_m^k is a vector pointing in the up direction (along the positive Y axis) in the image and $\langle \cdot, \cdot \rangle$ indicates the inner product.

Height. One of the features most correlated with pedestrian detection accuracy is the pixel height of the pedestrian [18]. The height, in pixels, of a projected object is simply the magnitude of the projected up vector, $s_h(m, k) = \|U_m^k\|$.

4.3 Model

Given a set of training examples, we compute, for each attribute, the expected accuracy (true positive, true negative) using a binary logistic regression model. That is, we compute $E[Q \mid s_x]$ for each attribute. To model the joint expectation

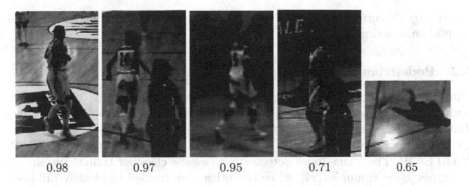

0.98   0.97   0.95   0.71   0.65

Fig. 5. The estimated detection accuracy (Eq. 8) for selected image patches. The first patch depicts an ideal case (unoccluded, upright, and near-field). The remaining patches show examples of slight occlusion, smaller height, moderate occlusion, and non-verticality, respectively.

for a given image patch, we make the Naive Bayes assumption of conditional independence between the features. This gives:

$$E[Q \mid \Theta] \propto E[Q \mid s_o] \cdot E[Q \mid s_u] \cdot E[Q \mid s_h] \tag{8}$$

Figure 5 shows some examples of the expected detection accuracy evaluated for selected patches. In the next section, we show how this value can be used to compare multiple image patches of the same object detection to select the best view(s) for pedestrian verification in a real-time MCMO detection framework.

5   Results

We evaluated our method on the APIDIS dataset[1], which contains footage from a basketball game captured by 7 calibrated, pseudo-synchronized cameras. The dataset contains people of similar appearance and heavy occlusions, as well as shadows and reflections on the court. In order to compare results with other recent work [3–6], we followed the most common protocol of measuring performance within the bounds of the left side of the basketball court, which is covered by the most cameras. For quantitative evaluation, we used precision and recall, where a true positive is a detection whose estimated location projects onto the ground plane is within a person-width of the ground truth, a false positive is a detection unmatched to an actual person, and a false negative is a missed detection.

5.1   Implementation Details

We set the minimum number of cameras for voxel occupancy voting, γ, to 3, and the foreground ratio threshold, β, to 0.25. For mean shift clustering, the bandwidth was $45 \times 45 \times 180$ cm. In the 3D occupancy grid, each voxel covered 10 cm^3.

---

[1] http://www.apidis.org/.

For change detection, our method uses a GPU implementation of adaptive background subtraction [20].

5.2 Pedestrian Detector Evaluation

Our method supports most image-based pedestrian detectors. We evaluated four commonly-used, pre-trained detectors: HOG [21], VJ, based on the Viola-Jones cascade classifier [15], and the Dollár et al. [22] detector, trained with the INRIA dataset [21] (DOLLAR-INRIA) and the CalTech dataset [23] (DOLLAR-CALTECH). The Viola-Jones detector is a cascade classifier trained specifically on upper body examples [24], while the others are trained to identify full-body pedestrians. Each of these pedestrian detectors provides a detection score, and a threshold is commonly applied to obtain the final result. For a set of image patches containing both positive (people) and negative (background) examples, we computed the ROC curve across a range of thresholds for each detector and used the Area Under the Curve (AUC) measure as a basis for comparison. HOG, VJ, DOLLAR-INRIA, and DOLLAR-CALTECH achieved 0.65, 0.56, 0.60, and 0.67, respectively. Overall, DOLLAR-CALTECH performed the best, and, unless otherwise specified, is the implementation we employed for subsequent experiments. These values are much higher than would be expected from the typical approach of pedestrian detection of sliding windows across multiple image scales and locations. Beyond the efficiency concerns, this approach leads to many false positives and false negatives. However, with a fixed location and scale (i.e., an image patch corresponding to a particular 3D location), such detectors can be quite accurate. This phenomenon was noted in a recent survey [18], which found that classifier performance on image patches is only weakly correlated with detection performance on full images.

5.3 Pedestrian Verification

To evaluate the effect of pedestrian verification on MCMO detection, we implemented the base detector, and performed experiments applying pedestrian verification from multiple cameras. We tested two schemes: (1) using the top-k cameras, and (2) selecting a variable number of cameras based on predicted accuracy. To combine the results from multiple cameras, the k detector scores are averaged, weighted by the expectation (Eq. 8), prior to thresholding. In the variable-camera scheme, all cameras with an EDA above .9 are included in the ensemble.

Figure 6 shows precision-recall curves for various verification schemes on the APIDIS dataset for two pedestrian detectors (HOG and DOLLAR-CALTECH). While increasing from $k = 0$ to $k = 2$ cameras improves the overall performance, adding a third or fourth camera does not. This result suggests that, for this particular dataset, there are many instances where two of the available cameras provide complementary suitable views of a particular location, but additional viewpoints are neither helpful and perhaps contradictory. Overall, using a variable number of cameras for each location performed best, although the effect is

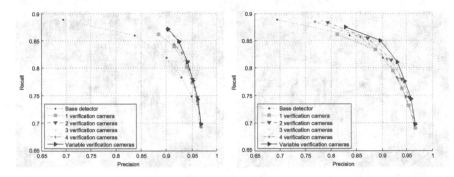

Fig. 6. Precision-recall curves for base detection with pedestrian verification with DOLLAR-CALTECH (left) and HOG (right) using both fixed and variable number of camera schemes.

more pronounced with the HOG detector than with DOLLAR-CALTECH. On average, the variable scheme resulted in 2.56 image patches evaluated for each candidate location.

5.4 Comparison with Other MCMO Methods

Table 1 compares the results of our method with several recently published approaches on the APIDIS dataset. For each method, the precision, recall, F-score, and frames-per-second (FPS) are shown. Excluding our method, the speed-accuracy trade-off is evident across the related approaches. To the best of our knowledge, our method using $k = 2$ verification cameras (base detector + verification) outperforms all other reported detection results on the APIDIS dataset, while performing at real-time speeds. Note that our detection method outperfroms approaches that also incorporate tracking. Figure 7 shows some examples from this experiment.

Table 1. Comparison of our method and several recent approaches using precision and recall rate on the APIDIS dataset. POM+KSP results are taken from [4] and POM results are from [3].

Method	Precision	Recall	F-Score	FPS
Base detector	0.84	**0.86**	0.85	13.13
Base detector + verification	**0.93**	0.85	**0.89**	10.40
Alahi [3]	0.92	0.82	0.87	0.1
Peng [6]	0.90	0.84	0.87	0.33
Posseger [4] (with tracking)	0.88	0.79	0.83	4.42
POM+KSP [5, 25] (with tracking)	0.80	0.73	0.76	0.03
POM [5]	0.51	0.63	0.56	**80.70**

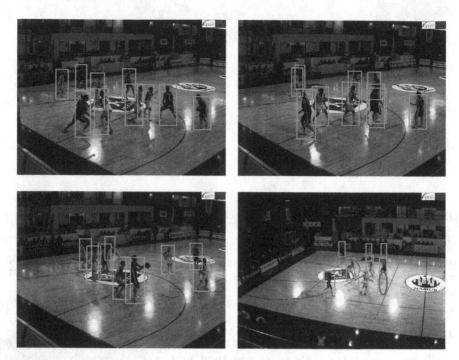

Fig. 7. The top two frames show examples of our correctly identifying the presence of multiple people (green rectangles). The bottom two frames show challenging cases where the selected pedestrian detector failed for a given patch (red oval) (Color figure online).

Precision, recall, and framerate (FPS) numbers for the other methods are taken from results reported in the respective papers. Timing numbers, in particular, may not be directly comparable due to differences in hardware and other implementation details. Our method was implemented in C++ with OpenCV and deployed on a 2.5 GHz PC with 8 GB RAM and a Tesla C2075 GPU. For the base detector with verification, processing time is roughly 73 %, 6 %, and 21 % for low-, medium-, and high-level detection, respectively.

6   Conclusions

We presented a framework for multi-camera, multi-object detection. Our multi-stage approach incorporates fast low-level detection and more accurate high-level pedestrian detection to verify uncertain hypotheses. The method is agnostic to any specific implementation of the base detector or verification method. This hybrid approach was shown to be effective in experiments on a challenging dataset, achieving state-of-the-art performance at real-time speeds. For the future, we plan to investigate a cost-sensitive scheme to choose which techniques to deploy in which situations to allow the speed-accuracy tradeoff to be explicitly controlled, depending on the requirements of the system.

References

1. Nakajima, C., Pontil, M., Heisele, B., Poggio, T.: Full-body person recognition system. Pattern Recognit. **36**, 1997–2006 (2003)
2. Zhao, T., Nevatia, R., Wu, B.: Segmentation and tracking of multiple humans in crowded environments. IEEE Trans. Pattern Anal. Mach. Intell. **30**, 1198–1211 (2008)
3. Alahi, A., Jacques, L., Boursier, Y., Vandergheynst, P.: Sparsity driven people localization with a heterogeneous network of cameras. J. Math. Imaging and Vis. **41**, 39–58 (2011)
4. Possegger, H., Sternig, S., Mauthner, T., Roth, P.M., Bischof, H.: Robust real-time tracking of multiple objects by volumetric mass densities. In: 2013 IEEE Conference on Computer Vision and Pattern Recognition (CVPR), pp. 2395–2402. IEEE (2013)
5. Fleuret, F., Berclaz, J., Lengagne, R., Fua, P.: Multicamera people tracking with a probabilistic occupancy map. IEEE Trans. Pattern Anal. Mach. Intell. **30**, 267–282 (2008)
6. Peng, P., Tian, Y., Wang, Y., Huang, T.: Multi-camera pedestrian detection with multi-view Bayesian network model. In: BMVC, pp. 69.1–69.12 (2012)
7. Yilmaz, A., Javed, O., Shah, M.: Object tracking: a survey. ACM Comput. Surv. **38**(4) (2006). Article No. 13
8. Stauffer, C., Grimson, W.: Adaptive background mixture models for real-time tracking. In: IEEE Conference on Computer Vision and Pattern Recognition, vol. 2 (1999)
9. Khan, S., Shah, M.: Tracking multiple occluding people by localizing on multiple scene planes. IEEE Trans. Pattern Anal. Mach. Intell. **31**(3), 505–519 (2008)
10. Eshel, R., Moses, Y.: Homography based multiple camera detection and tracking of people in a dense crowd. In: IEEE Computer Society Conference on Computer Vision and Pattern Recognition, pp. 1–8 (2008)
11. Liem, M., Gavrila, D.M.: Multi-person tracking with overlapping cameras in complex, dynamic environments. In: British Machine Vision Conference (BMVC), pp. 199–218. British Machine Vision Association (2009)
12. Canton-Ferrer, C., Casas, J.R., Pardàs, M., Monte, E.: Multi-camera multi-object voxel-based Monte Carlo 3D tracking strategies. EURASIP J. Adv. Sig. Process. **2011**, 1–15 (2011)
13. Delannay, D., Danhier, N., De Vleeschouwer, C.: Detection and recognition of sports(wo)men from multiple views. In: International Conference on Distributed Smart Cameras. pp. 1–7 (2009)
14. Hoiem, D., Efros, A., Hebert, M.: Putting objects in perspective. Int. J. Comput. Vis. **80**, 3–15 (2008)
15. Viola, P., Jones, M.: Rapid object detection using a boosted cascade of simple features. In: Proceedings of the 2001 IEEE Computer Society Conference on Computer Vision and Pattern Recognition, CVPR 2001, vol. 1, pp. 511–518. IEEE (2001)
16. Comaniciu, D., Meer, P.: Mean shift: a robust approach toward feature space analysis. IEEE Trans. Pattern Anal. Mach. Intell. **24**, 603–619 (2002)
17. Cheng, Y.: Mean shift, mode seeking, and clustering. IEEE Trans. Pattern Anal. Mach. Intell. **17**, 790–799 (1995)
18. Dollar, P., Wojek, C., Schiele, B., Perona, P.: Pedestrian detection: an evaluation of the state of the art. IEEE Trans. Pattern Anal. Mach. Intell. **34**, 743–761 (2012)

19. Hearn, D., Baker, P., Carithers, W.: Computer Graphics With OpenGL. Prentice Hall (2011)
20. Zivkovic, Z., van der Heijden, F.: Efficient adaptive density estimation per image pixel for the task of background subtraction. Pattern Recogn. Lett. **27**, 773–780 (2006)
21. Dalal, N., Triggs, B.: Histograms of oriented gradients for human detection. In: IEEE Computer Society Conference on Computer Vision and Pattern Recognition, CVPR 2005, vol. 1, pp. 886–893. IEEE (2005)
22. Dollár, P., Appel, R., Kienzle, W.: Crosstalk cascades for frame-rate pedestrian detection. In: Fitzgibbon, A., Lazebnik, S., Perona, P., Sato, Y., Schmid, C. (eds.) ECCV 2012, Part II. LNCS, vol. 7573, pp. 645–659. Springer, Heidelberg (2012)
23. Dollár, P., Wojek, C., Schiele, B., Perona, P.: Pedestrian detection: a benchmark. In: IEEE Conference on Computer Vision and Pattern Recognition, CVPR 2009, pp. 304–311. IEEE (2009)
24. Kruppa, H., Castrillon-Santana, M., Schiele, B.: Fast and robust face finding via local context. In: Joint IEEE Internacional Workshop on Visual Surveillance and Performance Evaluation of Tracking and Surveillance (VS-PETS), pp. 157–164 (2003)
25. Berclaz, J., Fleuret, F., Turetken, E., Fua, P.: Multiple object tracking using K-shortest paths optimization. IEEE Trans. Pattern Anal. Mach. Intell. **33**, 1806–1819 (2011)

Color Photometric Stereo Using a Rainbow Light for Non-Lambertian Multicolored Surfaces

Sejuti Rahman[1]([⊠]), Antony Lam[2], Imari Sato[3], and Antonio Robles-Kelly[4]

[1] Carnegie Mellon University, Pittsburgh, USA
sejutir@andrew.cmu.edu
[2] Saitama University, Saitama, Japan
antonylam@cv.ics.saitama-u.ac.jp
[3] National Institute of Informatics, Tokyo, Japan
imarik@nii.ac.jp
[4] National ICT Australia (NICTA), Canberra, Australia
antonio.robles-kelly@nicta.com.au

Abstract. This paper presents a novel approach for recovering the shape of non-Lambertian, multicolored objects using two input images. We show that a ring light source with complementary colored lights has the potential to be effectively utilized for this purpose. Under this lighting, the brightness of an object surface varies with respect to different reflections. Therefore, analyzing how brightness is modulated by illumination color gives us distinct cues to recover shape. Moreover, the use of complementary colored illumination enables the color photometric stereo to be applicable to multicolored surfaces. Here, we propose a color correction method based on the addition principle of complementary colors to remove the effect of illumination from the observed color. This allows the inclusion of surfaces with any number of chromaticities. Therefore, our method offers significant advantages over previous methods, which often assume constant object albedo and Lambertian reflectance. To the best of our knowledge, this is the first attempt to employ complementary colors on a ring light source to compute shape while considering both non-Lambertian reflection and spatially varying albedo. To show the efficacy of our method, we present results on synthetic and real world images and compare against photometric stereo methods elsewhere in the literature.

1 Introduction

Reconstructing 3D shape from multiple images has attracted ample attention from the computer vision community. Along these lines, one of the most popular approaches is photometric stereo (PS) [1], which reconstructs the object shape by varying the light direction across multiple images that share the same viewpoint. By assuming Lambertian reflectance and using calibrated lights, PS can recover the object shape and spatially varying albedo making use of three images.

On the other hand, color PS [2–4] augments conventional PS with the idea of multiplexing in the spectral domain. Rather than using three grayscale images, the method uses a single color image of a Lambertian surface being illuminated

© Springer International Publishing Switzerland 2015
D. Cremers et al. (Eds.): ACCV 2014, Part I, LNCS 9003, pp. 335–350, 2015.
DOI: 10.1007/978-3-319-16865-4_22

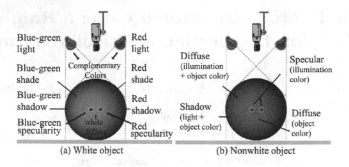

Fig. 1. Observed brightness under two complementary colored lights, (a) White colored object; (b) Non-white colored object (Color figure online).

by three different colored lights. This allows for its application to the reconstruction of deformable surfaces [5,6]. However, in general, color PS approaches [2–5,7] often assume constant object albedo and Lambertian reflectance. These assumptions can be overly restrictive in practice.

The aim of this paper is to extend color PS for non-Lambertian, multicolored surfaces. Here, we show that a ring light source with complementary colored lights has the potential to be effectively utilized for this purpose. The key observation is that, under a complementary colored light source, the observed color of an object surface varies with respect to different reflections (shown in Fig. 1). Therefore, analyzing how object color is modulated by illumination color gives us clues to estimate surface orientations. On top of that, the complementary colored illumination also allows the inclusion of multicolored surfaces in shape estimation. To deal with such surfaces, we propose a color correction method that exploits the addition principle of complementary colors to remove the effect of illumination from the observed color. This eases the estimation of object color and makes the method applicable to any number of chromaticities.

There have been a few approaches that consider scenes with varying chromaticity by either employing time multiplexing [8,9], applying regularization to the normal field [10], using extra information provided by a depth camera [11], or a two camera stereo system [6]. However, our approach has significant advantages over the previous approaches as we can deal with shadows and specular highlights which are almost unavoidable phenomena in the real world.

It is worth noting in passing that our work has been partially motivated by the work in [12], where the same light configuration is utilized for depth edge extraction based on shadow cue. However, our approach differs from this work in that, we employ a colored ring light for 3D shape reconstruction, not for depth edge, and we utilize shading, shadow, and specularity cues altogether. Our method is effective and requires only two input images taken under complementary colored lights. To the best of our knowledge, this is the first attempt that utilizes a complementary colored ring light for 3D reconstruction. The contributions of our paper are:

- We propose a new approach of color PS for non-Lambertian surfaces that utilizes the variation in observed surface color according to different reflections under complementary colored illumination.
- We present a color correction method based on the addition principle of complementary colors to render color PS applicable to multicolored surfaces.
- We show that the color difference between images under complementary illumination is useful for detecting diffuse, specular, and attached shadow reflections.

The rest of the paper is organized as follows. In Sect. 2, we summarize earlier research in PS for non-Lambertian, multicolored surfaces. In Sect. 3, we explain brightness variation under complementary illumination in different reflections, that we employ in Sect. 4 to develop theories to estimate shape. Experimental results and comparisons are presented in Sect. 5. Finally, in Sect. 6, we conclude on the developments presented here.

2 Related Work

Most of the surfaces around us are non-Lambertian. Conventional PS can not reliably reconstruct those, especially when deviation from the Lambertian assumption is large. Therefore, since the seminal work of Woodham [1], PS has received significant efforts to incorporate non-Lambertian phenomena. The existing approaches in this direction can be categorized into three broad classes.

The first approach is to model non-Lambertian surfaces using parametric models that are more complex than the Lambertian, e.g. Georghiades [13] uses a simplified Torrance-Sparrow (TS) model [14] to account for specular highlights but discards shadows as outliers; Goldman et al. [15] employ the Ward model [16] to include both shadow and highlights, but require more user inputs.

The second group [17, 18] assumes that the non-Lambertian phenomena, such as shadows and highlights, are restricted to small regions of an image. As a result, these can be treated as outliers and hence, removed from further consideration.

The third and more recent approach is to exploit general properties rather than assuming any specific reflectance model, e.g., radiance similarity [19], attached shadow codes [20], monotonicity and isotropy in diffuse reflectance [21], isotropy and reciprocity [22–24], reflectance monotonicity [25], and so on. However, approaches in the latter two categories use a large number of observations. Our method belongs to the first category as we utilize the TS model to include non-Lambertian surfaces. However, our method is a color PS approach and our novelty is that we exploit the potential of complementary colored illumination to extend the applicability of PS to non-Lambertian cases.

Apart from the non-Lambertian cases, we also develop a theory to incorporate multicolored surfaces, which is often ignored in color PS. It is known that given an image of a surface of uniform chromaticity, illuminated by three spectrally and spatially separated light sources, it is possible to estimate a surface normal at each pixel [2]. However, this is no longer possible for surfaces with multiple chromaticities as a change in pixel color could be caused by either a change in surface orientation or a change in chromaticity. Therefore, most of the color PS algorithms [2–5,7,26] are applicable to uniform colored surfaces. However, there are also a few works that consider scenes with varying chromaticity.

In [6,11], Anderson et al. assume a scene to be comprised of multiple piecewise constant chromaticity. To render the problem tractable, they segment the input image into regions of constant chromaticity before applying PS to estimate shape. To perform the segmentation, they require low resolution geometry of the scene provided by either a two-camera stereo system [6] or a depth camera [11].

In another approach, Janko et al. [10] apply color PS to estimate the shape of a dynamic and multicolored surface. To separate the contribution of surface orientation from that of albedo in observed color, the method exploits a constraint based on the temporal constancy in surface albedo. However, their method has two major drawbacks. Firstly, it enforces spatial smoothness on the surface normal over neighboring pixels, which, in turn, can cause over smoothing of fine shape details. Secondly, to estimate albedo, their method requires the surface to be dynamic enough and the input sequence to be long enough so that all normals turn towards each light source at least once.

Decker et al. [8] and Kim et al. [9] resort to time multiplexing to relax the assumption of constant chromaticity and apply color PS for dynamic scenes. The method in [9] accounts for time varying surface orientation and requires three images to recover shape at each frame. On the other hand, the method in [8] assumes surface normal to be constant across the frames and requires at least 2 input images to estimate shape. The method in [8], like ours, also utilizes complementary colored light to estimate object albedo.

However, all these color PS methods, including that in [8], assume Lambertian reflectance. In a related development, Hernández et al. [26] considers shadows by applying an integrability constraint, but limit their attention to monochromatic surfaces and disregards specular highlights.

Like ours, there have been several other PS approaches [22–24,27], that utilize the ring light setup. However, all these methods assume monochromatic lights and require a large number of input images. For example, the work in [22] requires 20–30 images to recover only partial reconstruction of isotropic surfaces and [23] requires much more (about 100). Zhou and Tan [27] recover Euclidean structure for multicolored, Lambertian surfaces using at least 5 images and 2 views. Based on a ring light setup and reflectance symmetry, Tan et al. [24] also recover Euclidean structure by extending the partial reconstruction developed in [22]. However, their method depends on the algorithm in [22] to compute the iso-depth contours and, therefore, requires a large number of images. This contrasts with our method, which only requires two images captured from a single view.

3   Brightness Under Complementary Colors

This section describes our observations on brightness under complementary illumination, that we will utilize later to develop our theory for recovering shape.

Under a ring of colored lights, the observed color of an object includes not only surface color but also illumination color. Analyzing how object color is modulated by illumination color gives us clues to estimate surface orientations. Let us first consider the simple case depicted in the left-hand panel of Fig. 1, where the target object has a neutral (white) color and is illuminated by two lights with complementary hues, red and blue-green.

This complementary light configuration provides significant information for each of the diffuse, specular, and attached shadow reflections:

- Diffuse: Depending on the surface orientation, brightness in diffuse pixels can be of two types, non-white shaded and white shaded. As shown in Fig. 1(a), when the surface normal is tilted towards one of the light sources, we see the shade of that particular light. On the other hand, when the surface normal is not biased towards any specific light source, both lights contribute the same. As the mixture of complementary colors in an additive color space results in white, these pixels appear white.
- Specular: It is well known that specularity is the mirror-like reflection of light observed when the direction of the incoming light and reflected light have equal angles with respect to the surface normal. In the case of a color ring light, the color of specular reflection depends on the surface orientation. For instance, in Fig. 1(a), we see red specularity at points where its mirror reflection is oriented towards the red light source.
- Shadow: Attached shadow appears in a pixel when the angle between the surface normal at that point and a light source is more than 90°. In this case, the surface does not receive any light from this light source and the pixel is colorized according to the contribution from the other light source with which the incident angle is less than 90°.

The discussion above can be extended to a continuous ring light that is formed as a maximally saturated complementary hue circle with same brightness. Under this light, we experience similar observations. As for diffuse reflection, the white shade appears when the surface normal is toward the camera and thus receives an equal amount of light from all lights on the ring. On the other hand, a nonwhite shade appears when the surface normal is tilted towards a specific light on the ring. In such cases, it is colored according to a weighted average of all light colors, where that particular light weights more than the rest.[1]

As for specular reflection, each specular pixel exhibits the color of a specific light on the ring when its mirror reflection is oriented towards that light. As already seen in the case of two lights, a shadow pixel is colorized according to the contributions from the visible light sources.

Note, however, that the scenario becomes more complex when the target object has a non-white surface color. As shown in the right-hand panel of Fig. 1, the shading and shadow are now a product of both, the illuminant and object color, whereas pure specular pixels show the illumination color. From the figure, we can understand that the separation of the illumination color from the object

---

[1] This follows Newton's geometrical weighting [28], which states that the additive mixture of any number of colors is determined as the weighted average of the positions of the original colors on the hue-saturation plane.

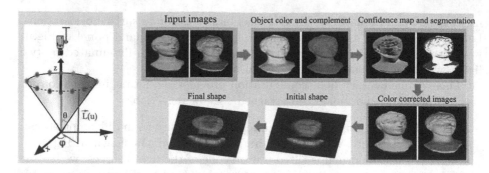

Fig. 2. Left-hand panel: illumination geometry for our colored ring light setup. Right-hand panel: a diagrammatic representation of our method (Color figure online).

color becomes a challenging task. Later, in Sect. 4.1, we show how complementary illumination can be used to perform color correction. This delivers an image where the object color has been effectively canceled out.

4   Shape from Complementary Colors

We start from the assumption of directional illumination and orthographic projection. We consider a ring light setup where the observer is fixed at direction v. The global coordinate system is selected such that the Z-axis is aligned with the viewer direction, i.e., $v = (0, 0, 1)^T$. We assume that the scene is being illuminated by a ring light source, where the lights are arranged in equidistance on a cone centered at the viewing direction (see left-hand panel of Fig. 2). We further assume that our coordinate system is aligned with the HSV space and select colors on the ring such that the colors form a complementary hue circle. Our assumptions on scene properties are: no cast shadows in the scene, uniform roughness over the surface, and brightness distribution is Gaussian.

The right-hand panel of Fig. 2 shows a diagrammatic representation of our method, where our algorithm uses two input images and computes their sum to obtain the object color. Once the surface color is in hand, a pair of color-corrected images is recovered for purposes of color PS.

Next we consider the cases where objects are composed of multicolored diffuse surfaces in Sect. 4.1, specular surfaces in Sect. 4.2, and surfaces with both colored diffuse and specular reflections in Sect. 4.3.

4.1   Multicolored Diffuse Reflection

Let us assume that the scene is being illuminated by a ring-light source made up of k lights, i.e., $L = \{L_1, ..., L_k\}$, each with a different hue from the set of hues, $H = \{H_1, ..., H_k\}$. Now, if we capture an input image M_1 under H, the color of each channel $c \in \{R, G, B\}$ for each diffuse pixel u, is in fact a linear combination of contribution from all the light sources, given as,

$$M_{1,c} = \sum_{i=1}^{k} (\boldsymbol{L}_i \cdot \boldsymbol{N}) \int \rho(\lambda) P_i(\lambda) Q_c(\lambda) d\lambda \tag{1}$$

where, the contribution of the i-th light source with power spectrum $P_i(\lambda)$ is integrated over the visible spectrum (380 nm–720 nm). $Q_c(\lambda) = \{\bar{r}(\lambda), \bar{g}(\lambda), \bar{b}(\lambda)\}$ is the camera spectral sensitivity function. $\boldsymbol{N}$ and $\rho(\lambda)$ denote surface normal and diffuse spectral reflectance at pixel u, respectively.

For the time being, let us assume that the surface is white and therefore has a constant spectral reflectance τ over all wavelengths. Following the scalar multiplication property and distributive law of dot products, we rewrite Eq. (1) as,

$$M_{1,c} = \tau \left(\sum_{i=1}^{k} (\boldsymbol{L}_i q_i(c)) \right) \cdot \boldsymbol{N} \tag{2}$$

where $q_i(c) = \int P_i(\lambda) Q_c(\lambda) d\lambda$. From Eq. (2), we can solve for surface normal as, $\boldsymbol{N} = A^{-1} b$, where $A = \sum_{i=1}^{k} \boldsymbol{L}_i q_i(c)$ and $b = [M_{1,c}]$. Thus our system of linear equations comprises of 3 equations to solve for 3 unknowns. Note that, we drop the term τ from our solution and assume that the surface normals are scaled by τ. This assumption is not exclusive to our method but rather common across other PS approaches [29].

To deal with nonwhite or multicolored surfaces, next we propose a color correction method that removes the contribution of object color to image brightness. For this, we need a second input image M_2, that we capture under the complementary set of H, denoted by $\bar{H} = \{\bar{H}_1, ..., \bar{H}_k\}$. The image brightness equation for M_2 is given by,

$$M_{2,c} = \sum_{i=1}^{k} (\boldsymbol{L}_i \cdot \boldsymbol{N}) \int \rho(\lambda) \bar{P}_i(\lambda) Q_c(\lambda) d\lambda \tag{3}$$

Note that, everything remains the same as in Eq. (1) except power spectrum of the i-th light $\bar{P}_i(\lambda)$ now corresponds to $\bar{H}_i$, i.e., the complementary hue of H_i.

Now if we add M_1 and M_2, this results in an image showing only object color devoid of illumination color, as $(P_i(\lambda) + \bar{P}_i(\lambda))$ is equivalent to unity,[2]

$$M_{1,c} + M_{2,c} = \sum_{i=1}^{k} (\boldsymbol{L}_i \cdot \boldsymbol{N}) \left(\int \rho(\lambda) P_i(\lambda) Q_c(\lambda) d\lambda + \int \rho(\lambda) \bar{P}_i(\lambda) Q_c(\lambda) d\lambda \right)$$

---

[2] We note that in practice, $(P_i(\lambda) + \bar{P}_i(\lambda))$ do not always perfectly sum to 1 at each wavelength. Despite this, since we ultimately examine RGB values in our method and not individual wavelengths, we found the amount of error introduced did not adversely affect our algorithm.

$$= \sum_{i=1}^{k} (\boldsymbol{L}_i \cdot \boldsymbol{N}) \left(\int \rho(\lambda) \left(P_i(\lambda) + \bar{P}_i(\lambda) \right) Q_c(\lambda) d\lambda \right)$$

$$= \sum_{i=1}^{k} (\boldsymbol{L}_i \cdot \boldsymbol{N}) \left(\int \rho(\lambda) Q_c(\lambda) d\lambda \right) \tag{4}$$

Now, if we assume that we have the complementary spectrum of $\rho(\lambda)$, we can generate a new image $\bar{M}_1$ whose equation in the RGB space is given by,

$$\bar{M}_{1,c} = \sum_{i=1}^{k} (\boldsymbol{L}_i \cdot \boldsymbol{N}) \int \bar{\rho}(\lambda) P_i(\lambda) Q_c(\lambda) d\lambda \tag{5}$$

where, in contrast to Eq. (1), ρ is now replaced by $\bar{\rho}$, which denotes the complementary spectrum of object color.

In practice, we use an RGB camera and do not have the complementary spectrum, so we utilize the HSV space to generate $\bar{M}_1$. As the hue of $M_1 + M_2$ corresponds only to the object hue in the HSV space, we use this to compute the complementary hue of the object as, $\bar{obj}_{hue} = mod(obj_{hue} + 0.5, 1)$ where the object hue is normalized to $[0, 1]$. Then we generate an image $(\bar{obj})_{HSV}$, that shows only complementary object color, by changing the hue value of $(M_1 + M_2)_{HSV}$ from obj_{hue} to $\bar{obj}_{hue}$, keeping saturation and brightness unchanged. Now, adding $(M_1)_{RGB}$ to $(\bar{obj})_{RGB}$ results in only illumination color. Let's denote it by $(light)_{RGB}$. As $\bar{M}_1$ is composed of complementary object and illumination color (Eq. (5)), therefore, we get $(\bar{M}_1)_{RGB} = (\bar{obj})_{RGB} + (light)_{RGB}$.

Now adding $\bar{M}_1$ to M_1, the term $(\rho(\lambda) + \bar{\rho}(\lambda))$ becomes unity, thus resulting in a brightness equation without the diffuse spectral reflectance term. This is given by,

$$M'_{1,c} = M_{1,c} + \bar{M}_{1,c} = \sum_{i=1}^{k} (\boldsymbol{L}_i \cdot \boldsymbol{N}) \left(\int \left(\rho(\lambda) + \bar{\rho}(\lambda) \right) P_i(\lambda) Q_c(\lambda) d\lambda \right)$$

$$= \sum_{i=1}^{k} (\boldsymbol{L}_i \cdot \boldsymbol{N}) \left(\int P_i(\lambda) Q_c(\lambda) d\lambda \right) \tag{6}$$

We name the image M'_1 as the color corrected image of M_1. Now with the color corrected image, we can use the solution presented earlier for white colored surfaces to multicolored surfaces without any loss of generality.

4.2   Specular Reflection

As described in Sect. 3, the observed color of a pure specular pixel corresponds to the illumination color. Therefore, we utilize the pixel's hue value to determine the illumination direction that causes the specular peak. As shown in the left-hand panel of Fig. 2, we define the illumination direction $\boldsymbol{L}$ at pixel u using two angles: slant θ and tilt ϕ, where θ is the opening angle of the cone of the ring light source. To compute tilt, we assume that our coordinate system is aligned with the HSV space, and use the hue value of u in HSV space to determine ϕ.

With the estimated illumination direction, we compute the surface normal using the half angle between the illumination and viewer direction. However, with the assumption of an idealized reflection direction, we miss off-specular reflections here. Therefore, we utilize the hue-based computations as initial shape estimates and update further using a coordinate descent [30] optimization scheme based on the simplified TS model [14]. According to this model, the image brightness equation for a specular pixel u can be expressed as,

$$M_{s,c} = \sum_{i=1}^{k} \left(\frac{1}{\cos \theta_s} \exp \left(-\frac{\theta_h^2}{2\sigma^2} \right) \right) \int P_i(\lambda) Q_c(\lambda) d\lambda \qquad (7)$$

where, θ_s, θ_h, and σ denote reflection angle, half-angle, and surface roughness.

It is worth noting in passing that, in this section, we assume M_1 to be the observed specular-only reflection. Our goal is to fit this observed data to Eq. (7) using the least square minimization. We formulate our cost function in terms of two variables, surface normal and roughness.

At the first step, our algorithm utilizes the initial hue-based estimation of shape to estimate the surface roughness. We assume uniform surface roughness and employ the following cost function,

$$\sigma = \arg\min_{\sigma} \sum_{u \in M_1} \left[M_{1,c} - M_{s,c}(\mathbf{N}, \sigma) \right]^2 \qquad (8)$$

We compute σ for each band separately and take the average if they are not the same. Once it estimates the optimal value for σ, the algorithm proceeds to the second step where the current estimate of σ is used to obtain surface normals. The cost function for $\mathbf{N}$ is given as,

$$\mathbf{N} = \arg\min_{\mathbf{N}} \sum_{c} \left[M_{1,c} - M_{s,c}(\mathbf{N}, \sigma) \right]^2 \qquad (9)$$

Thus the algorithm iterates between these two steps until none of the parameters change between two successive iterations or when a maximum number of iterations are completed.

4.3   A Unified Framework for Objects with both Diffuse and Specular Reflection

So far, we described our approach for diffuse-only and specular-only reflections. This section presents a unified approach that addresses surfaces with both diffuse and specular reflections.

We model the scene radiance as a linear combination of specular and diffuse reflectance based upon the TS reflectance model. Therefore, the image brightness at pixel u is given by,

$$M_{TS,c} = \sum_{i=1}^{k} \left[\max\left(0, (\boldsymbol{N} \cdot \boldsymbol{L_i})\right) \int \rho(\lambda) P_i(\lambda) Q_c(\lambda) d\lambda \right.$$
$$\left. + K_s \frac{1}{\cos\theta_s} \exp\left(-\frac{\theta_h^2}{2\sigma^2}\right) \int P_i(\lambda) Q_c(\lambda) d\lambda \right] \qquad (10)$$

Here, the first term on the right hand side denotes diffuse reflection where $\max(0, (\boldsymbol{N} \cdot \boldsymbol{L_i}))$ accounts for attached shadow, and the latter term denotes specular reflection with K_s as specular reflection coefficient at u.

From Eq. (10), we first show that our color correction process applies to surfaces with both diffuse and specular components. The image brightness equation for $M_1 + M_2$ is given as,

$$M_{1,c} + M_{2,c} = \sum_{i=1}^{k} \left[\max\left(0, (\boldsymbol{N} \cdot \boldsymbol{L_i})\right) \int \rho(\lambda) \left(P_i(\lambda) + \bar{P}_i(\lambda)\right) Q_c(\lambda) d\lambda \right.$$
$$\left. + K_s \frac{1}{\cos\theta_s} \exp\left(-\frac{\theta_h^2}{2\sigma^2}\right) \int \left(P_i(\lambda) + \bar{P}_i(\lambda)\right) Q_c(\lambda) d\lambda \right]$$
$$= \sum_{i=1}^{k} \left[\max\left(0, (\boldsymbol{N} \cdot \boldsymbol{L_i})\right) \int \rho(\lambda) Q_c(\lambda) d\lambda \right.$$
$$\left. + K_s \frac{1}{\cos\theta_s} \exp\left(-\frac{\theta_h^2}{2\sigma^2}\right) \int Q_c(\lambda) d\lambda \right] \qquad (11)$$

As shown in Eq. (11), illumination colors are canceled for both diffuse and specular reflection. Therefore, all pixels, except the pure specular ones, now show only object color.

It is worth noting that the specular-only pixels become white in $M_1 + M_2$, which is an important observation as this relates to the accuracy in estimating object color from $M_1 + M_2$. In this context, we would like to mention that this causes noticeable error in shape estimation at specular pixels in the color PS method in [8], that also utilizes complementary colored illumination to estimate object albedo. However, this does not affect our method as we deal with object color using our color correction method.

From the brightness equation of $M_1 + \bar{M}_1$, we see that our color correction process is applicable to surfaces with both reflection components,

$$M_{1,c}' = M_{1,c} + \bar{M}_{1,c} = \sum_{i=1}^{k} \left[\max\left(0, (\boldsymbol{N} \cdot \boldsymbol{L_i})\right) \int \left(\rho(\lambda) + \bar{\rho}(\lambda)\right) P_i(\lambda) Q_c(\lambda) d\lambda \right.$$
$$\left. + 2K_s \frac{1}{\cos\theta_s} \exp\left(-\frac{\theta_h^2}{2\sigma^2}\right) \int P_i(\lambda) Q_c(\lambda) d\lambda \right] \qquad (12)$$

As the albedo term is exclusive to the diffuse part, adding $\bar{M}_1$ to M_1, removes the object color from the diffuse part, while leaving the illumination color unchanged in the specular part.

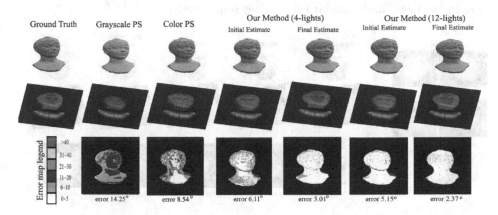

Fig. 3. Comparative results on 3D reconstruction for a synthetic shape. We present the RGB-encoded normal map and depth map for the ground truth data and that yielded by grayscale PS [1], color PS [8], our method with 4-lights and 12-lights, respectively. The bottom row shows error maps and average per-pixel angular error measures (in degrees) for the surface normals yielded by each of the methods under consideration as compared to the ground truth (Color figure online).

Next, we pose the shape estimation problem as an iterative minimization and fit the observed data to Eq. (10) to recover the parameters N, σ, and K_s.

Initialization. For initialization, we first segment image pixels into diffuse, specular, or shadows on the assumption that either they are purely diffuse, specular, or shadows based on the color difference between M_1 and M_2. Then we utilize the approaches in Sects. 4.1 and 4.2 to initialize surface normals in diffuse-only and specular-only pixels.

For shadow pixels, we employ a hue-based computation. The surface orientation at a shadow pixel u is defined using two angles: slant θ and tilt ϕ, where θ comes from the opening angle of the cone of the ring light source and ϕ is set according to the hue of u in the HSV space.

For segmentation, we compute the Euclidean distance between the images in the hue-saturation plane and name this the shadow-specularity confidence map. The distance has higher values in specular and shadow pixels and lower values in diffuse. This conforms to our observations in Sect. 3, where we see that the color difference between two input images are higher in these reflections than the diffuse. Moreover, the distribution of this distance is bimodal and, hence, we can apply Otsu's adaptive threshold method [31] to select D_{th}, a threshold on this distance, that can be employed to segment the specular and shadow pixels from diffuse pixels. Finally, we apply a threshold on brightness, V_{th} to separate shadows from specular highlights. Since we have considered the distribution of brightness to be Gaussian and specular pixels to occupy a minor portion of the scene, V_{th} should be on the right bottom rim of the bell curve for the distribution and can be computed as, $V_{th} = mean(V) + 1.5 * std(V)$, where $mean(\cdot)$ and $std(\cdot)$ denote the mean and standard deviation, respectively.

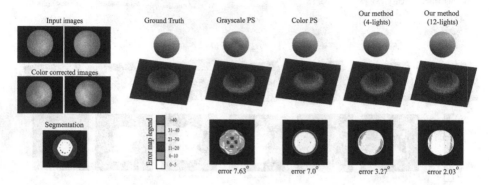

Fig. 4. The left-hand panel shows input images, color corrected images, and segmentation for a real-world sphere. The right-hand panel shows comparative results for 3D reconstruction. The top row presents the RGB-encoded normal maps and the middle row presents depth maps for the ground truth data (left) and that yielded, in turn, by grayscale PS [1], color PS [8], our method with 4 lights, and our method with 12 lights. The bottom row shows error maps and average per-pixel angular error (in degrees) for the surface normals yielded by each of the methods (compared to the ground truth) (Color figure online).

Iterative Updates. The coordinate descent approach comprises of three interleaved minimization steps. We write the cost functions using the TS model given in Eq. (10). Note that Eq. (10) shows the general form of the TS model, whereas the model we fit in assumes all $\rho(\lambda) = 1$, since our method allows for the ρ terms in Eq. (12) to sum to unity. Also, Eq. (12) shows $2K_s$ when Eq. (10) only shows K_s. In Eqs. (13–15), this scalar difference is accounted for during optimization.

At the first step, the algorithm solves for surface roughness over all pixels by using the initial estimates of shape as,

$$\sigma = \arg\min_{\sigma} \sum_{u \in M_1'} \left[M_{1,c}' - M_{TS,c}(K_s, \mathbf{N}, \sigma) \right]^2 \tag{13}$$

At the second step, with the current estimates of σ and $\mathbf{N}$, it minimizes the following cost function to obtain K_s at each pixel,

$$K_s = \arg\min_{K_s} \sum_c \left[M_{1,c}' - M_{TS,c}(K_s, \mathbf{N}, \sigma) \right]^2 \tag{14}$$

At the third step, it solves for $\mathbf{N}$ using the updated values of K_s and σ, by minimizing the following cost function,

$$\mathbf{N} = \arg\min_{\mathbf{N}} \sum_c \left[M_{1,c}' - M_{TS,c}(K_s, \mathbf{N}, \sigma) \right]^2 \tag{15}$$

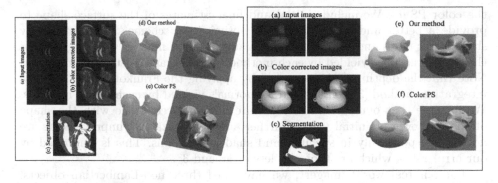

Fig. 5. The left-hand and right-hand panels show 3D reconstruction results for two real world objects, a squirrel and a duck, respectively. In each panel: (a) input images, (b) color corrected images, (c) segmentation, (d) and (e) present RGB-encoded normal maps and depth maps delivered by our method and color PS [8], respectively (Color figure online).

Thus once the former variables are at hand, we obtain optimal values for the latter ones. The algorithm iterates between these three steps, until convergence.

5   Experimental Results

We now illustrate the accuracy of our method for the purposes of 3D reconstruction using synthetic and real world data. To evaluate our method, we compare our results against ground truth data and two other PS approaches. As our method requires only two input images, we compare our results with those obtained by the methods that require a small number of images. The first of these is the PS method in [1], for which we use four images. To obtain these images, we turn on each of the 4 evenly distributed lights on the ring one by one.

The other of our alternatives is a closely related work, i.e., the color PS method in [8], that uses complementary illumination for estimating surface albedo to relax the assumption of constant object chromaticity. This method does not work for non-Lambertian surfaces and requires $(k+2)/3$ images over k lights. This contrasts with our method, which can be applied to non-Lambertian objects and to any number of light sources greater than or equal to two.

In fact, the accuracy of our estimated shape increases with the number of light sources on the ring. We illustrate this behavior in Fig. 3, where we show results for a synthetic shape for four and twelve lights. For both $k = 4$ and $k = 12$ cases, we evenly distribute the colored lights on the ring. The human face in Fig. 3 has been rendered (shown in Fig. 2) using the reflectance model in Eq. (10) and the albedo of a Aloe vera leaf obtained in house using a spectrometer. For the microfacet slope values, we have used a normal distribution with a mean of 2.0 and a standard deviation of 0.01.

In the figure, we also show the RGB encoded normal map and depth map delivered by our method and the two alternatives, i.e., the grayscale PS [1] and the color PS [8]. We include initial and final estimates of the surface shape to provide a better understanding of our optimization scheme. The bottom row shows error maps and average per-pixel angular error measures (in degrees) for the surface normals yielded by each method compared against the ground truth. Note that the depth map is recovered by applying the Frankott and Chellappa integration method [32] on the surface normals yielded by each of the methods. We can see that our surface normals are in good accordance with the shape of the face even at initial value. Further, after optimization, improvements are noticeable specifically in specular and shadowed regions. This is confirmed by our error rates, which are typically less or around 3°.

For our real world imagery, we have used three non-Lambertian objects. These are a glossy wooden sphere (Fig. 4), a squirrel figurine with a very specular surface (Fig. 5), and a plastic duck (Fig. 5). All the objects are multicoloured and include specular highlights and shadows.

For each object, we show input images, color corrected images, segmentation results, and reconstructed shape. In Fig. 4, we also show the ground truth data and provide error maps for surface normals estimated by our method and that by two other alternative methods. Our method outperforms the alternatives, which is evident in the qualitative results, i.e., normals maps and depth maps, and also in quantitative error measures.

Next we present shape reconstruction results for the squirrel and the duck in Fig. 5. As mentioned earlier, our method can take input images acquired using any number of illuminants. However, to make our method comparable to that in [8], in the following we only employ two input images with 4 light sources. For each object, we compare the RGB encoded normal map and depth map yielded by our method with that delivered by the color PS [8]. From the figures we can see that the color PS fails to estimate the correct shape in specular and shadowed pixels. This contrasts with our method, which delivers better surface detail, and, in turn, more accurate shapes.

6   Conclusion

In this paper, we have presented a novel method for recovering the 3D shape of a non-Lambertian, multicolored object by utilizing a ring light source. The underlying theory for our method is based on the properties of complementary colors and the brightness variations in diffuse, specular, and shadow reflections. This allows for the computation of a pair of color corrected images which can be used for purposes of color PS making use of an iterative optimization scheme. As far as we know, this is the first attempt to utilize colored illuminants on a ring to recover object shape. Moreover, our method can naturally process non-Lambertian, multicolored surfaces with unknown reflectance properties using only two input images. A future research direction would be to extend the theory for deformable surfaces and uncalibrated PS.

Acknowledgement. This research was supported in part by the Ministry of Education, Science, Sports and Culture Grant-in-Aid for Scientific Research on Innovative Areas.

References

1. Woodham, R.J.: Photometric method for determining surface orientation from multiple images. Opt. Eng. **19**, 139–144 (1980)
2. Drew, M., Kontsevich, L.: Closed-form attitude determination under spectrally varying illumination. In: IEEE Conference on Computer Vision and Pattern Recognition (1994)
3. Kontsevich, L., Petrov, A., Vergelskaya, I.: Reconstruction of shape from shading in color images. J. Opt. Soc. Am. A **11**, 1047–1052 (1994)
4. Woodham, R.J.: Gradient and curvature from photometric stereo including local confidence estimation. J. Opt. Soc. Am. A **11**, 3050–3068 (1994)
5. Brostow, G., Hernández, C., Vogiatzis, G., Stenger, B., Cipolla, R.: Video normals from colored lights. IEEE Trans. Pattern Anal. Mach. Intell. **33**, 2104–2114 (2011)
6. Anderson, R., Stenger, B., Cipolla, R.: Color photometric stereo for multicolored surfaces. In: IEEE International Conference on Computer Vision (2011)
7. Hernández, C., Vogiatzis, G., Brostow, G.J., Stenger, B., Cipolla, R.: Non-rigid photometric stereo with colored lights. In: IEEE International Conference on Computer Vision (2007)
8. Decker, B.D., Kautz, J., Mertens, T., Bekaert, P.: Capturing multiple illumination conditions using time and color multiplexing. In: IEEE Conference on Computer Vision and Pattern Recognition (2009)
9. Kim, H., Wilburn, B., Ben-Ezra, M.: Photometric stereo for dynamic surface orientations. In: European Conference on Computer Vision (2010)
10. Janko, Z., Delaunoy, A., Prados, E.: Colour dynamic photometric stereo for textured surfaces. In: Asian Conference on Computer Vision (2010)
11. Anderson, R., Stenger, B., Cipolla, R.: Augmenting depth camera output using photometric stereo. In: MVA (2011)
12. Taguchi, Y.: Rainbow flash camera: depth edge extraction using complementary colors. In: Fitzgibbon, A., Lazebnik, S., Perona, P., Sato, Y., Schmid, C. (eds.) ECCV 2012, Part VI. LNCS, vol. 7577, pp. 513–527. Springer, Heidelberg (2012)
13. Georghiades, A.: Incorporating the Torrance and Sparrow model of reflectance in uncalibrated photometric stereo. In: IEEE International Conference on Computer Vision (2003)
14. Torrance, K., Sparrow, E.: Theory for off-specular reflection from roughened surfaces. J. Opt. Soc. Am. A **57**, 1105–1114 (1967)
15. Goldman, D., Curless, B., Hertzmann, A., Seitz, S.: Shape and spatially-varying BRDFs from photometric stereo. IEEE Trans. Pattern Anal. Mach. Intell. **32**, 1060–1071 (2010)
16. Ward, G.: Measuring and modeling anisotropic reflection. Comput. Graph. **26**, 265–272 (1992)
17. Barsky, S., Petrou, M.: The 4-source photometric stereo technique for three dimensional surfaces in the presence of highlights and shadows. IEEE Trans. Pattern Anal. Mach. Intell. **25**, 1239–1252 (2003)

18. Wu, L., Ganesh, A., Shi, B., Matsushita, Y., Wang, Y., Ma, Y.: Robust photometric stereo via low-rank matrix completion and recovery. In: Kimmel, R., Klette, R., Sugimoto, A. (eds.) ACCV 2010, Part III. LNCS, vol. 6494, pp. 703–717. Springer, Heidelberg (2011)
19. Sato, I., Okabe, T., Yu, Q., Sato, Y.: Shape reconstruction based on similarity in radiance changes under varying illumination. In: IEEE International Conference on Computer Vision (2007)
20. Okabe, T., Sato, I., Sato, Y.: Attached shadow coding: estimating surface normals from shadows under unknown reflectance and lighting conditions. In: IEEE International Conference on Computer Vision (2009)
21. Higo, T., Matsushita, Y., Ikeuchi, K.: Consensus photometric stereo. In: IEEE Conference on Computer Vision and Pattern Recognition (2010)
22. Alldrin, N., Kriegman, D.: Toward reconstructing surfaces with arbitrary isotropic reflectance: a stratified photometric stereo approach. In: IEEE International Conference on Computer Vision (2007)
23. Alldrin, N., Zickler, T., Kriegman, D.: Photometric stereo with non-parametric and spatially-varying reflectance. In: IEEE Conference on Computer Vision and Pattern Recognition (2008)
24. Tan, P., Quan, L., Zickler, T.: The geometry of reflectance symmetries. IEEE Trans. Pattern Anal. Mach. Intell. **33**, 2506–2520 (2011)
25. Shi, B., Tan, P., Matsushita, Y., Ikeuchi, K.: Elevation angle from reflectance monotonicity: photometric stereo for general isotropic reflectances. In: Fitzgibbon, A., Lazebnik, S., Perona, P., Sato, Y., Schmid, C. (eds.) ECCV 2012, Part III. LNCS, vol. 7574, pp. 455–468. Springer, Heidelberg (2012)
26. Hernández, C., Vogiatzis, G., Cipolla, R.: Shadows in three-source photometric stereo. In: Forsyth, D., Torr, P., Zisserman, A. (eds.) ECCV 2008, Part I. LNCS, vol. 5302, pp. 290–303. Springer, Heidelberg (2008)
27. Zhou, Z., Tan, P.: Ring-light photometric stereo. In: Daniilidis, K., Maragos, P., Paragios, N. (eds.) ECCV 2010, Part II. LNCS, vol. 6312, pp. 265–279. Springer, Heidelberg (2010)
28. MacEvoy, B.: Color vision (2008). http://www.handprint.com/LS/CVS/color.html
29. Higo, T., Matsushita, Y., Joshi, N., Ikeuchi, K.: A hand-held photometric stereo camera for 3-d modeling. In: IEEE International Conference on Computer Vision (2009)
30. Friedman, J., Hastie, T., Hfling, H., Tibshirani, R.: Pathwise coordinate optimization. Ann. Appl. Stat. **1**, 302–332 (2007)
31. Otsu, N.: A threshold selection method from gray-level histogram. IEEE Trans. Syst. Man Cybern. **9**, 62–66 (1979)
32. Frankot, R., Chellappa, R.: A method for enforcing integrability in shape from shading algorithms. IEEE Trans. Pattern Anal. Mach. Intell. **10**, 439–451 (1988)

Predicting the Location of "interactees" in Novel Human-Object Interactions

Chao-Yeh Chen$^{(\boxtimes)}$ and Kristen Grauman

University of Texas at Austin, Austin, USA
chaoyeh@cs.utexas.edu

Abstract. Understanding images with people often entails understanding their *interactions* with other objects or people. As such, given a novel image, a vision system ought to infer which other objects/people play an important role in a given person's activity. However, while recent work learns about action-specific interactions (e.g., how the pose of a tennis player relates to the position of his racquet when serving the ball) for improved recognition, they are not equipped to reason about *novel* interactions that contain actions or objects not observed in the training data. We propose an approach to predict the localization parameters for "interactee" objects in novel images. Having learned the generic, action-independent connections between (1) a person's pose, gaze, and scene cues and (2) the interactee object's position and scale, our method estimates a probability distribution over likely places for an interactee in novel images. The result is a human interaction-informed saliency metric, which we show is valuable for both improved object detection and image retargeting applications.

1 Introduction

Understanding human activity is a central goal of computer vision with a long history of research. Whereas earlier work focused on precise body pose estimation and analyzed human gestures independent of their surroundings, recent research shows the value in modeling activity in the context of *interactions*. An interaction may involve the person and an object, the scene, or another person(s). For example, a person *reading* reads a book or paper; a person *discussing* chats with other people nearby; a person *eating* uses utensils to eat food from a plate. In any such case, the person and the **"interactee"** object (i.e., the book, other people, food and utensils, etc.) are closely intertwined; together they define the story portrayed in the image or video.

A surge of recent research in human action recognition aims to exploit this close connection [1–8]. Their goal is to improve recognition by leveraging human action (as described by body pose, appearance, etc.) in concert with the object being manipulated by the human. However, prior work is restricted to a closed-world set of objects and actions, and assumes that during training it is possible to learn patterns between a particular action and the particular object category it involves. For example, given training examples of *using a computer*, typical

© Springer International Publishing Switzerland 2015
D. Cremers et al. (Eds.): ACCV 2014, Part I, LNCS 9003, pp. 351–367, 2015.
DOI: 10.1007/978-3-319-16865-4_23

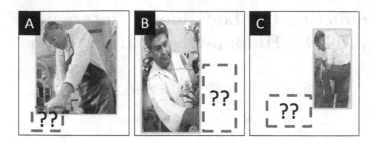

Fig. 1. Despite the fact we have hidden the remainder of the scene, can you infer where is the object with which each person is interacting? Our goal is to predict the position and size of such "interactee" objects in a *category-independent* manner, without assuming prior knowledge of the specification/object types.

poses for typing can help detect the nearby computer, and vice versa; however, in existing methods, this pattern would not generalize to help make predictions about, say, a person operating a cash register. Furthermore, existing work largely assumes that the interactions of interest involve a direct manipulation, meaning that physical contact occurs between the person and the interactee.

We seek to relax these assumptions in order to make predictions about novel, unseen human-object interactions. In particular, we consider the following question: *Given a person in a novel image, can we predict the location of that person's "interactee"—the object or person with which he interacts—even without knowing the particular action being performed or the category of the interactee itself?* Critically, by posing the question in this manner, our solution cannot simply exploit learned action-specific poses and objects. Instead, we aim to handle the open-world setting and learn generic patterns about human-object interactions. In addition, we widen the traditional definition of an interactee to include not only directly manipulated objects, but also untouched objects that are nonetheless central to the interaction (e.g., the poster on the wall the person is reading).

Why should our goal be possible? Are there properties of interactions that transcend the specific interactee's category? Figure 1 suggests that, at least for humans, it is plausible. In these examples, without observing the interactee object or knowing its type, one can still infer the interactee's approximate position and size. For example, in Fig. 1.A, we may guess the person is interacting with a small object in the bottom left.

We can do so because we have a model of certain pose, gaze, and scene layout patterns that exist when people interact with a person/object in a similar relative position and size. We stress that this is without knowing the category of the object, and even without (necessarily) being able to name the particular action being performed. The ability to predict *where* an interactee object is independent of *what* it is would be valuable to vision systems that must analyze novel interactions from arbitrary categories.

Based on this intuition, our idea is to learn from data how the properties of a person relate to the interactee localization parameters. Given instances labeled with both the person and interactee outlines—from a variety of activities and objects—we train a probabilistic model that can map observed features of the person to a distribution over the interactee's position and scale. Then, at test time, given a novel image and a detected person, we predict the most likely places the interactee will be found. Our method can be seen as an "interaction-informed" metric for object saliency: it highlights regions of the novel image most likely to contain objects that play an important role in summarizing the image's content.

The proposed approach addresses a number of challenges. They include designing a reliable data collection procedure to handle this somewhat unusual annotation task; developing a bank of descriptors to capture the "meta-cues" about human appearance that signal localized interactions; and presenting applications to exploit the interactee predictions. For the latter, we show that by focusing attention on regions in the image that are prominently involved in the human interaction, our method enables novel applications for priming object detectors and image retargeting. As we will see in Sect. 3.4, the ability to localize the object without categorizing it is precisely what enables these new tasks.

Our results on two challenging datasets, SUN and PASCAL Actions, demonstrate the practical impact. We show the advantages compared to an existing high-level "objectness" saliency method and a naive approach that simply looks for interactees nearby a person. Finally, we perform a human subject study to establish the limits of human perception for estimating unseen interactees.

2 Related Work

Human-object interactions for recognition. A great deal of recent work in human activity recognition aims to jointly model the human and the objects with which he or she interacts [1–8]. The idea is to use the person's appearance (body pose, hand shape, etc.) and the surrounding objects as mutual context—knowing the action helps predict the object, while knowing the object helps predict the action or pose. For example, the Bayesian model in [2] integrates object and action recognition to resolve cases where appearance alone is insufficient, e.g., to distinguish a spray bottle from a water bottle based on the way the human uses it. Similarly, structured models are developed to recognize manipulation actions [9] or sports activities [3,4] in the context of objects. Novel representations to capture subtle interactions, like playing vs. holding a musical instrument, have also been developed [5]. Object recognition itself can benefit from a rich model of how human activity [1] or pose [8] relates to the object categories. While most such methods require object outlines and/or pose annotations, some work lightens the labeling effort via weakly supervised learning [6,7].

While we are also interested in human-object interactions, our work differs from all the above in three significant ways. First, whereas they aim to improve object or action recognition, our goal is to predict the location and size of an interactee—which, as we will show, has applications beyond recognition. Second, we widen the definition of an "interactee" to include not just manipulated objects, but also those that are untouched yet central to the interaction. Third, and most importantly, the prior work learns the spatial relationships between the human and object in an *action-specific* way, and is therefore inapplicable to reasoning about interactions for any action/object unseen during training. In contrast, our approach is *action-* and *object-independent*; the cues it learns cross activity boundaries, such that we can predict where a likely interactee will appear even if we have not seen the particular activity (or object) before.

Carried object detection. Methods to detect carried objects (e.g., [10,11]) may be considered an interesting special case of our goal. Like us, the intent is to localize an interactee object that (in principle) could be from any category, though in reality the objects have limited scale and position variety since they must be physically carried by the person. However, unlike our problem setting, carried object detection typically assumes a static video camera, which permits good background subtraction and use of human silhouette shapes to find outliers. Furthermore, it is specialized for a single action (carrying), whereas we learn models that cross multiple action category boundaries.

Social interactions. Methods for analyzing social interactions estimate who is interacting with whom [12–14], or categorize the type of physical interaction [15]. The "interactee" in our setting may be another person, but it can also belong to another object category. Furthermore, whereas the social interaction work can leverage rules from sociology [12] or perform geometric intersection of mutual gaze lines [13,14], our task requires predicting a spatial relationship between a person and possibly inanimate object. Accordingly, beyond gaze, we exploit a broader set of cues in terms of body posture and scene layout, and we take a learning approach rather than rely only on spatial reasoning.

Object affordances. Methods to predict object affordances consider an object [16,17] or scene [18] as input, and predict which actions are possible as output. They are especially relevant for robot vision tasks, letting the system predict, for example, which surfaces are sittable or graspable. Our problem is nearly the inverse: given a human pose (and other descriptors) as input, our method predicts the localization parameters of the object defining the interaction as output. We focus on the implications for object detection and image retargeting tasks.

Saliency. Saliency detection, studied for many years, also aims to make class-independent predictions about what is important in an image. While many methods look at low-level image properties (e.g., [19]), a recent trend is to *learn* metrics for "object-like" regions based on cues like convexity, closed boundaries, and color/motion contrast [20–23]. Such metrics are category-independent by design: rather than detect a certain object category, the goal is to detect instances of *any* object category, even those not seen in training. In contrast, methods to predict the relative "importance" of objects in a scene [24–26] explicitly use knowledge about the object categories present. Different from any of the above, our method predicts *regions likely to contain an object involved in an interaction*. We compare it extensively to a state-of-the-art objectness metric [21] in our experiments, showing the advantages of exploiting human interaction cues when deciding which regions are likely of interest.

3   Approach

To implement our idea, we learn probabilistic models for interactee localization parameters. In the following, we first precisely define what qualifies as an interactee and interaction (Sect. 3.1) and describe our data collection effort to obtain annotations for training and evaluation (Sect. 3.2). Then, we explain the learning and prediction procedures (Sect. 3.3). Finally, we briefly overview two example applications that exploit our method's interactee predictions (Sect. 3.4).

3.1   Definition of Human-Interactee Interactions

First we must define precisely what a human-interactee[1] interaction is. This is important both to scope the problem and to ensure maximal consistency in the human-provided annotations we collect.

Our definition considers two main issues: (1) the interactions are not tied to any particular set of activity categories, and (2) an interaction may or may not involve physical contact. The former simply means that an image containing a human-object interaction of any sort qualifies as a true positive; it need not depict one of a predefined list of actions (in contrast to prior work [2–4,6,7,27,28]). By the latter, we intend to capture interactions that go beyond basic object manipulation activities, while also being precise about what kind of contact does qualify as an interaction. For example, if we were to define interactions strictly by cases where physical contact occurs between a person and object, then walking aimlessly in the street would be an interaction (interactee = road), while reading a whiteboard would not. Thus, for some object/person to be an interactee, the person ("interactor") must be paying attention to it/him and perform the interaction with a purpose.

Specifically, we say that an image displays a human-interactee interaction if either of the following holds:

1. The person is watching a specific object or person and paying specific attention to it. This includes cases where the gaze is purposeful and focused on some object/person within 5 m. It excludes cases where the person is aimlessly looking around.
2. The person is physically touching another object/person with a specific purpose. This includes contact for an intended activity (such as holding a camera to take a picture), but excludes incidental contact with the scene objects (such as standing on the floor, or carrying a camera bag on the shoulder).

An image can contain multiple human-interactee relationships. We assume each person in an image has up to one interactee. At test time, our method predicts the likely interactee location for each individual detected person in turn.

---

[1] An interactee refers to the thing a particular person in the image is interacting with; an interactee could be an object, a composition of objects, or another person.

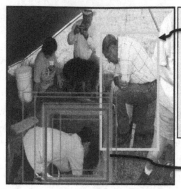

Q1: Is the person inside the yellow bounding box interacting with any object or other person in the image?

Q2: If an interaction is present, draw a bounding box on the object or person that the person in the given yellow bounding box is interacting with.

Multiple annotators' interactee estimates (orange) and the consensus ground truth (thick red).

Fig. 2. Example annotation task. Top right shows (abbreviated) annotator instructions to identify the interactee for the person in the yellow bounding box. Here we also display in orange the boxes provided by 7 MTurkers, from which we compute the ground truth interactee (thick red box) as described in the text (Color figure online).

3.2 Interactee Dataset Collection

Our method requires images of a variety of poses and interactee types for training. We found existing datasets that contain human-object interactions, like the Stanford-40 and PASCAL Actions [27,28], were somewhat limited to suit the category-independent goals of our approach. Namely, these datasets focus on a small number of specific action categories, and within each action class the human and interactee often have a regular spatial relationship. Some classes entail no interaction (e.g., *running, walking, jumping*) while others have a low variance in layout and pose (e.g., *riding horse* consists of people in fairly uniform poses with the horse always just below). While our approach would learn and benefit from such consistencies, doing so would essentially be overfitting, i.e., it would fall short of demonstrating action-independent interactee prediction.

Therefore, we curated our own dataset and gathered the necessary annotations. We use selected images from two existing datasets, SUN [29] and PASCAL 2012 [28]. SUN is a large-scale image dataset containing a wide variety of indoor and outdoor scenes. Using all available person annotations, we selected those images containing more than one person. The SUN images do not have action labels; we estimate these selected images contain 50–100 unique activities (e.g., *talking, holding, cutting, digging,* and *staring*). PASCAL is an action recognition image dataset. We took all images from those actions that exhibit the most variety in human pose and interactee localization—*using computer* and *reading*. We pool these images together; our method does not use any action labels. This yields a large number of unique activities.

We use Amazon Mechanical Turk (MTurk) to get bounding box annotations for the people and interactees in each image. The online interface instructs the annotators how to determine the interactee using the definition outlined above in Sect. 3.1. Figure 2 shows a condensed form; see Supp for more details. We get each image annotated by 7 unique workers, and keep only those images for which at least 4 workers said it contained an interaction. This left 355 and 754 images from SUN and PASCAL, respectively.

The precise location and scale of the various annotators' interactee bounding boxes will vary. Thus, we obtain a single ground truth interactee bounding box via an automatic consensus procedure. First, we apply mean shift to the coordinates of all annotators' bounding boxes. Then, we take the largest cluster, and select the box within it that has the largest mean overlap with the rest.

The interactee annotation task is not as routine as others, such as tagging images by the objects they contain. Here the annotators must give careful thought to which objects may qualify as an interactee, referring to the guidelines we provide them. In some cases, there is inherent ambiguity, which may lead to some degree of subjectivity in an individual annotator's labeling. Furthermore, there is some variability in the precision of the bounding boxes that MTurkers draw (their notion of "tight" can vary). This is why we enlist 7 unique workers on each training example, then apply the consensus algorithm to decide ground truth. Overall, we observe quite good consistency among annotators. The average standard deviation for the center position of bounding boxes in the consensus cluster is 8 pixels. See Fig. 5, columns 1 and 3, for examples.

3.3   Learning to Predict an Interactee's Localization Parameters

Training. For each training image, we are given the bounding boxes for each person and its interactee. From each person box, we extract a descriptor $f = [f_p, f_o, f_s]$, composed of the following three features:

Body pose, f_p: This feature captures the body pose of the person, which gives cues about how the person's posture and gesture relate to the interactee. For example, an extended arm may indicate that an interactee appears at the end of the reach; an extended leg may indicate an interactee is being kicked; a slouched torso may indicate holding a large object, while an upright torso may indicate holding a small light object, etc. We use a part-based pose representation called the *poselet activation vector* (PAV) [30]. A poselet is an SVM that fires on image patches with a given pose fragment (e.g., a bent leg, a tilted head). The PAV records how strongly each poselet is detected within the person bounding box. This yields a P-dim. vector for f_p, where P is the number of poselets.

Orientation of head and torso, f_o: These features capture the direction the person is looking or physically attending to. The head orientation is a proxy for eye gaze, and the torso orientation reveals how the person has situated his body with respect to an interactee. We predict both using the method of [30], which uses PAVs to train discriminative models for each of a set of discrete yaw intervals in $[-180°, 180°]$. This yields a 2-dimensional vector for $f_o = [\theta_{head}, \theta_{torso}]$ consisting of the two predicted angles.

Scene layout, f_s: This feature records the position of the person. It reflects the person in the context of the greater scene, which helps situate likely positions for the interactee. For example, assuming a photographer intentionally framed

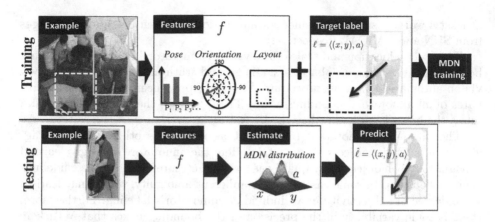

Fig. 3. Data flow in our approach. Top: training stage entails extracting features and target interactee positions/scales to learn a mixture density network (MDN). Bottom: testing stage entails estimating a mixture model from the learned MDN in order to predict the interactee's position/scale.

the photo to capture the interaction, then if the person is to the far right, the interactee may tend to be to the left. This yields a 2-dimensional vector for $f_s = [X, Y]$, where X, Y denotes the normalized image position of the person.

The target "label" for f consists of the localization parameters for its interactee box: $\ell = \langle (x, y), a \rangle$. The coordinates (x, y) specify the position, in terms of the vector from the person's center to the interactee's center. The area a specifies the size of the interactee. We normalize both components by the size of the person (height plus width).[2] See Fig. 3, top row. When there are multiple people in the training image, we record a set of features f for each one, separately, and pair it with that person's respective interactee label ℓ.

To build a predictive distribution for the interactee localization parameters, we want to represent a conditional probability density $P(\ell | f_k)$, for $k \in \{p, o, s\}$, where the subscript indexes the three features defined above. Since any given pose/gaze configuration may correspond to multiple feasible interactee localizations, we model this density as a mixture of Gaussians with m modes:

$$P(\ell | f_k) = \sum_{i=1}^{m} \alpha_i \mathcal{N}(f_k; \mu_i, \Sigma_i), \qquad (1)$$

where α_i denotes the prior mixing proportion for component i, μ is its mean, and Σ_i is its covariance matrix.

Offline, we use the N labeled training examples $\{(f^1, \ell^1), \ldots, (f^N, \ell^N)\}$ to train a Mixture Density Network (MDN) [31] for each feature k. An MDN is a neural network that takes as input the observed features (f_k), their associated parameters (ℓ), and the desired number of components m, and as output

---

[2] For this reason, it is not necessary to record scale in the scene layout feature above.

produces a network able to predict the appropriate Gaussian mixture model (GMM) parameters $(\boldsymbol{\alpha}, \boldsymbol{\mu}, \boldsymbol{\Sigma})$ for a novel set of observed features.[3]

We stress that our goal is to model interactions regardless of the type of the activity or the category of the interactee. Therefore, during training our method does not use any object or activity category labels.

Testing. Given a novel test image represented by $\boldsymbol{f}^t$, our goal is to estimate the interactee's bounding box. First, we extract the descriptors from the person bounding box in the novel image. Then, we use the learned MDN to generate the GMM $P(\boldsymbol{\ell}^t | \boldsymbol{f}_k^t)$ representing the most likely positions and scales for the target interactee. We get one GMM for each descriptor $\boldsymbol{f}_k$, where $k \in \{p, o, s\}$. Then, to fuse their predictions, we take the output of the model with the highest probability among all descriptors:

$$P(\boldsymbol{\ell}^t = \langle(\hat{x}, \hat{y}), \hat{a}\rangle \mid \boldsymbol{f}^t) = \max_{\boldsymbol{f}_k^t} P(\boldsymbol{\ell}^t \mid \boldsymbol{f}_k^t). \tag{2}$$

In this way, we can assign a probability to any candidate position and scale in the novel image.[4] To estimate the single most likely parameters $\boldsymbol{\ell}^*$ for $P(\boldsymbol{\ell}|\boldsymbol{f})$, we use the center of the mixture component with the highest prior (α_i), following [31]. The output interactee box is positioned by adding the predicted $(\hat{x}, \hat{y})$ vector to the person's center, and it has side lengths of $\sqrt{\hat{a}}$. See Fig. 3, bottom row.

While all training images consist of true human-interactee interactions, it is possible a test image would have a human performing no interaction. In that case, the probabilistic outputs above can be used to reject as non-interactions those images whose interactee estimates are too unlikely.

3.4   Applications of Interactee Prediction

Our method is essentially an object saliency metric that exploits cues from observed human-interactions. Therefore, it has fairly general applicability. To make its impact concrete, aside from analyzing how accurate its predictions are against human-provided ground truth, we also study two specific applications that can benefit from such a metric.

Interactee-Aware Contextual Priming for Object Detection. First, we consider how interactee localization can prime an object detector. The idea is to use our method to predict the most likely place(s) for an interactee, then focus an off-the-shelf object detector to prioritize its search around that area. This has potential to improve both object detection accuracy and speed, since one can

---

[3] We found it beneficial to model the two components of ℓ with separate MDNs, i.e., one for position and one for area. Thus, altogether we have six MDNs, and predict $(\hat{x}, \hat{y})$ and $\hat{a}$ using their respective distributions in the test image.

[4] We also attempted a logistic regression fusion scheme that learns weights to associate per feature, but found the max slightly superior, likely because the confidence of each cue varies depending on the image content.

avoid sliding windows and ignore places that are unlikely to have objects involved in the interaction. It is a twist on the well-known GIST contextual priming [32], where the scene appearance helps focus attention on likely object positions; here, instead, the cues we read from the person in the scene help focus attention. Importantly, in this task, our method will look at the person (to extract f^t), but will *not* be told which action is being performed; this distinguishes the task from the methods discussed in related work, which use mutual object-pose context to improve object detection for a particular action category.

To implement this idea, we run the Deformable Part Model (DPM) [33] object detector on the entire image, then we apply our method to discard the detections that are outside the 150 % enlarged predicted interactee box (i.e., scoring them as $-\infty$). (To alternatively save run-time, one could apply DPM to only those windows near the interactee.)

Interactee-Aware Image Retargeting. As a second application, we explore how interactee prediction may assist in image retargeting. The goal is to adjust the aspect ratio or size of an image without distorting its perceived content. This is a valuable application, for example, to allow dynamic resizing for web page images, or to translate a high-resolution image to a small form factor device like a cell phone. Typically retargeting methods try to avoid destroying key gradients in the image, or aim to preserve the people or other foreground objects. Our idea is to protect not only the people in the image from distortion, but also their predicted interactees. The rationale is that both the person and the focus of their interaction are important to preserve the story conveyed by the image.

To this end, we consider a simple adaption of the Seam Carving algorithm [34]. Using a dynamic programming approach, this method eliminates the optimal irregularly shaped "seams" from the image that have the least "energy". The energy is defined in terms of the strength of the gradient, with possible add-ons like the presence of people (see [34] for details). To also preserve interactees, we augment the objective to increase the energy of those pixels lying within our method's predicted interactee box. Specifically, we scale the gradient energy g within both person and interactee boxes by $(g + 5) * 5$.

4   Experimental Results

We evaluate four things: (1) how accurately do we predict interactees, compared to several baselines? (Sect. 4.1), (2) how well can humans perform this task? (Sect. 4.2), (3) does interactee localization boost object detection? (Sect. 4.3), and (4) does it help retargeting? (Sect. 4.4).

Baselines. No existing methods predict interactee locations in a category independent manner. Therefore, to gauge our results we compare to the following three methods: (1) OBJECTNESS (OBJ) [21], which is a state-of-the-art category-independent salient object detector. Like our method, it does not require information about the object category to detect; unlike our method, it does not

Table 1. Quantifying the accuracy of interactee localization with three metrics.

Metric	Dataset	OURS	NEAR PERSON	OBJ [21]	RANDOM
Position error	SUN	**0.2331**	0.2456	0.4072	0.6113
	PASCAL	**0.1926**	0.2034	0.2982	0.5038
Size error	SUN	**33.19**	39.51	257.25	126.64
	PASCAL	34.39	**31.97**	206.59	100.31
mAP accuracy	SUN	**0.1542**	0.1099	0.0975	0.0450
	PASCAL	**0.1640**	0.1157	0.1077	0.0532

exploit the interaction cues given by a person. We use the authors' code[5]. (2) NEAR PERSON, which assumes that the interactee is close to the person. Specifically, it returns a bounding box centered at the person's center, with the same aspect ratio, and a size 40 % of the person area (we optimized this parameter on training data). This is an important baseline to verify that interactee detection requires more sophistication than simply looking nearby the person. (3) RANDOM, which randomly generates an interactee location and size.

Implementation details. For each dataset, we use 75 % of the data for training and 25 % for testing, and resize images to 500 × 500 pixels. For both our method and NEAR PERSON, we use the true person bounding boxes for both training and testing, to avoid conflating errors in interactee prediction with errors in person detection. When evaluating mAP, all methods consider sliding window candidates with a 25-pixel step size and 20 scales, and declare a hit whenever normalized overlap exceeds 0.3. Our method sorts the windows by their overlap with l^*. For the MDNs, we use $m = 8$ and 10 mixture components on SUN and PASCAL, respectively, and use 10 hidden units. We use publicly available code[6] to compute the PAV vectors, which use $P = 1200$ poselets.

4.1   Accuracy of Interactee Localization

Table 1 compares the raw accuracy of interactee localization for all methods. We include three metrics to give a full picture of performance: position error, size error, and mean average precision (mAP). The errors are the absolute difference in position/area between the predicted and ground truth values, normalized by the person box size (height plus width) to prevent larger instances from dominating the result. The errors use only each method's most confident estimate (i.e., our l^*, and the highest scoring box according to OBJ and NEAR PERSON). The mAP quantifies accuracy when the methods generate a ranked list of window candidates.

Our method outperforms the baselines on both datasets and all metrics, in all but one case. We improve average precision by 40 % over the next competing

---

[5] http://groups.inf.ed.ac.uk/calvin/objectness/.
[6] http://ttic.uchicago.edu/~smaji/projects/action/.

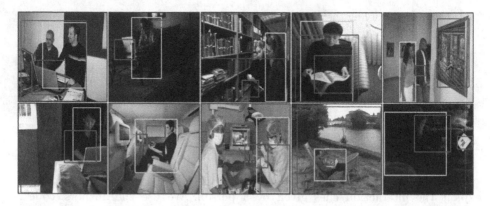

Fig. 4. Example interactee predictions for the given person (yellow), using our method (red) or OBJECTNESS [21] (green). NEAR PERSON predicts a box centered at the person with ~40% of its area (not shown for legibility). Note that there is no object detection involved in these predictions. Our method often accurately locates the interactee. OBJECTNESS can be distracted by the background or other objects (first four columns), while it works better than our method when the background is simple and the interactee is prominent (last column). NEAR PERSON does not handle complex interactions well, but succeeds when the interactee is handheld and small (e.g., reading, 4th column). Best viewed in color (Color figure online).

baseline. Our error reductions on size and position are also noticeable.[7] The NEAR PERSON baseline does reasonably well, but suffers compared to our method because it is unable to predict interactees that don't entail physical contact, or those that rely on gaze and other high-level patterns (see last two rows of Table 1). It does, however, beat our method in terms of size error on PASCAL. Upon inspection, we find this is due to its easy success on the *reading* instances in PASCAL; people usually hold the reading material in their hands, so the interactee is exactly in the center of the body. We find OBJECTNESS suffers on this data by often predicting too large of a window covering much of the image. Our advantage confirms the value in making interaction-informed estimates of object-like regions. Figure 4 shows example predictions.

4.2   Human Subject Experiment

Next we establish an "upper bound" on accuracy by asking human subjects on MTurk to solve the same task. Our method localizes an interactee without observing the background content (outside of the person box) and without knowing what category the interactee belongs to. Thus, we construct an interface forcing humans to predict an interactee's location with a similar lack of information. Figure 5, columns 2 and 4, illustrate what the human subjects see, as well as the responses we received from 10 people.

---

[7] To help interpret the normalized errors: an error in predicted position of 0.20 amounts to being about 100 pixels off, while an error in predicted size of 33 amounts to about 6% of the image area.

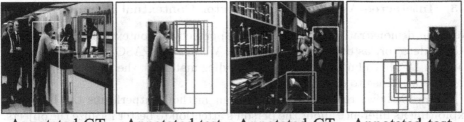

Annotated-GT   Annotated-test   Annotated-GT   Annotated-test

Fig. 5. We remove the background from the original image and ask human subjects to infer where the interactee might be. Red boxes denote their predictions, green box denotes consensus. Annotated-GT shows the full image (which is the format seen for ground truth collection, cf. Sect. 3.2). Annotated-test shows the human subject results. Naturally, annotators can more reliably localize the interactee when it is visible (Color figure online).

Table 2. Results of the human subject test

	Human subject			Ours		
	Position error	Size error	mAP	Position error	Size error	mAP
SUN w/o visible	0.1573	28.92	0.3523	0.2736	36.58	0.1086
PASCAL w/o visible	0.0952	40.84	0.5226	0.2961	43.27	0.1750

Table 2 shows the human subjects' results alongside ours, for the subset of images in either dataset where the interactee is not visible within the person bounding box (since those cases are trivial for the humans and require no inference).[8] The humans' guess is the consensus box found by aggregating all 10 responses with mean shift as before. The humans have a harder time on SUN than PASCAL, due to its higher diversity of interaction types. This study elucidates the difficulty of the task. It also establishes an (approximate) upper bound for what may be achievable for this new prediction problem.

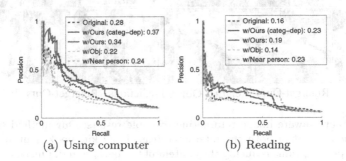

(a) Using computer   (b) Reading

Fig. 6. Interactee context helps focus the object detector. Numbers denote mAP.

---

[8] Since the test set here is a subset of the images, our numbers are not identical to our numbers in Table 1.

4.3 Interactee-Aware Object Detector Contextual Priming

Next we demonstrate the utility of our approach for contextual priming for an object detector, as discussed in Sect. 3.4. We use the PASCAL training images to train DPMs to find computers and reading materials, then apply our method and the baselines to do priming.

Figure 6 shows the results. We see our method outperforms the baselines, exploiting its inference about the person's attention to better localize the objects. While OURS uses action-independent training as usual, we also show a variant of our method where the MDN is trained only with images from the proper action class (see OURS (CATEG-DEP)). As expected, this further helps accuracy. Again, we see that NEAR PERSON fares well for the *reading* instances, since the book or paper is nearly always centered by the person's lap.

4.4 Interactee-Aware Image Retargeting

Finally, we inject our interactee predictions into the Seam Carving retargeting algorithm, as discussed in Sect. 3.4. Figure 7 shows example results. For reference, we also show results where we adapt the energy function using OBJECTNESS's top object region prediction. Both methods are instructed to preserve the provided person bounding box. We retarget the source 500×500 images to 300×300.

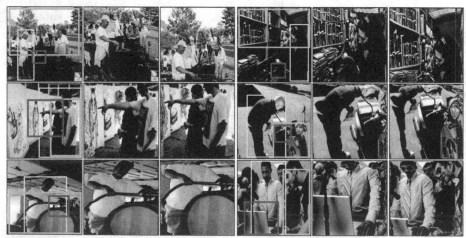

Predictions   Retarget-Ours   Retarget-Obj   Predictions   Retarget-Ours   Retarget-Obj

Fig. 7. Interactee-aware image retargeting example results. Our method successfully preserves the content of both the interactee (e.g., BBQ kit, book, painting of horse, laptop) and person, while reducing the content of the background. OBJECTNESS cannot distinguish salient objects that are and are not involved in the activity, and so may remove the informative interactees in favor of background objects. The bottom right example is a failure case for our method, where our emphasis on the interactee laptop looks less pleasing than the baseline's focus on the people. See Supp for more examples.

We see that our method preserves the content related to both the person and his interactee, while removing some unrelated background objects. In contrast, OBJECTNESS [21], unaware of which among the prominent-looking objects might qualify as an interactee, often discards the interactee and instead highlights content in the background less important to the image's main activity.

5 Conclusions

This work considers a new problem: how to predict where an interactee object will appear, given cues about a person's pose and gaze. While plenty of work studies action-specific object interactions, predicting interactees in an action-independent manner is both challenging and practical for various applications. The proposed method shows promising results to tackle this challenge. We demonstrate its advantages over multiple informative baselines, including a state-of-the-art object saliency metric, and illustrate the utility of knowing where interactees are for both contextual object detection and image retargeting. In future work, we are interested in exploring features based on more fine-grained pose and gaze estimates, and extending our ideas to video analysis.

Acknowledgements. This research is supported in part by DARPA CSSG and a PECASE award from ONR.

References

1. Peursum, P., West, G., Venkatesh, S.: Combining image regions and human activity for indirect object recognition in indoor wide-angle views. In: ICCV (2005)
2. Gupta, A., Kembhavi, A., Davis, L.: Observing human-object interactions: using spatial and functional compatibility for recognition. PAMI **31**, 1775–1789 (2009)
3. Desai, C., Ramanan, D., Fowlkes, C.: Discriminative models for static human-object interactions. In: Workshop on Structured Models in Computer Vision, Computer Vision and Pattern Recognition (SMiCV) (2010)
4. Yao, B., Fei-Fei, L.: Modeling mutual context of object and human pose in human-object interaction activities. In: CVPR (2010)
5. Yao, B., Fei-Fei, L.: Grouplet: A structured image representation for recognizing human and object interactions. In: CVPR (2010)
6. Ikizler-Cinbis, N., Sclaroff, S.: Object, scene and actions: combining multiple features for human action recognition. In: Daniilidis, K., Maragos, P., Paragios, N. (eds.) ECCV 2010, Part I. LNCS, vol. 6311, pp. 494–507. Springer, Heidelberg (2010)
7. Prest, A., Schmid, C., Ferrari, V.: Weakly supervised learning of interactions between humans and objects. PAMI **34**, 601–614 (2012)
8. Delaitre, V., Fouhey, D.F., Laptev, I., Sivic, J., Gupta, A., Efros, A.A.: Scene semantics from long-term observation of people. In: Fitzgibbon, A., Lazebnik, S., Perona, P., Sato, Y., Schmid, C. (eds.) ECCV 2012, Part VI. LNCS, vol. 7577, pp. 284–298. Springer, Heidelberg (2012)

9. Kjellström, H., Romero, J., Martínez, D., Kragić, D.: Simultaneous visual recognition of manipulation actions and manipulated objects. In: Forsyth, D., Torr, P., Zisserman, A. (eds.) ECCV 2008, Part II. LNCS, vol. 5303, pp. 336–349. Springer, Heidelberg (2008)

10. Haritaoglu, I., Harwood, D., Davis, L.: W4: real-time surveillance of people and their activities. PAMI **22**, 809–830 (2000)

11. Damen, D., Hogg, D.C.: Detecting carried objects in short video sequences. In: Forsyth, D., Torr, P., Zisserman, A. (eds.) ECCV 2008, Part III. LNCS, vol. 5304, pp. 154–167. Springer, Heidelberg (2008)

12. Bazzani, L., Cristani, M., Paggetti, G., Fossati, A., Bue, A.D., Menegaz, G., Murino, V.: Social interaction discovery by statistical analysis of f-formations. In: BMVC (2011)

13. Marin-Jimenez, M., Zisserman, A., Ferrari, V.: Here's looking at you kid. detection people looking at each other in videos. In: BMVC (2011)

14. Fathi, A., Hodgins, J., Rehg, J.: Social interactions: a first-person perspective. In: CVPR (2012)

15. Yang, Y., Baker, S., Kannan, A., Ramanan, D.: Recognizing proxemics in personal photos. In: CVPR (2012)

16. Koppula, H., Saxena, A.: Anticipating human activities using object affordances for reactive robotic response. In: RSS (2013)

17. Desai, C., Ramanan, D.: Predicting functional regions on objects. In: CVPR Workshop on Scene Analysis Beyond Semantics (2013)

18. Gupta, A., Satkin, S., Efros, A., Hebert, M.: From 3D scene geometry to human workspace. In: CVPR (2011)

19. Hou, X., Zhang, L.: Saliency detection: a spectral residual approach. In: CVPR (2007)

20. Liu, T., Sun, J., Zheng, N., Tang, X., Shum, H.: Learning to detect a salient object. In: CVPR (2007)

21. Alexe, B., Deselaers, T., Ferrari, V.: What is an object? In: CVPR (2010)

22. Endres, I., Hoiem, D.: Category independent object proposals. In: Daniilidis, K., Maragos, P., Paragios, N. (eds.) ECCV 2010, Part V. LNCS, vol. 6315, pp. 575–588. Springer, Heidelberg (2010)

23. Lee, Y.J., Kim, J., Grauman, K.: Key-segments for video object segmentation. In: ICCV (2011)

24. Spain, M., Perona, P.: Some objects are more equal than others: measuring and predicting importance. In: Forsyth, D., Torr, P., Zisserman, A. (eds.) ECCV 2008, Part I. LNCS, vol. 5302, pp. 523–536. Springer, Heidelberg (2008)

25. Hwang, S.J., Grauman, K.: Learning the relative importance of objects from tagged images for retrieval and cross-modal search. IJCV **100**, 134–153 (2012)

26. Berg, A., Berg, T., Daume, H., Dodge, J., Goyal, A., Han, X., Mensch, A., Mitchell, M., Sood, A., Stratos, K., Yamaguchi, K.: Understanding and predicting importance in images. In: CVPR (2012)

27. Yao, B., Jiang, X., Khosla, A., Lin, A.L., Guibas, L.J., Fei-Fei, L.: Action recognition by learning bases of action attributes and parts. In: ICCV (2011)

28. Everingham, M., Van Gool, L., Williams, C.K.I., Winn, J., Zisserman, A.: The pascal visual object classes (voc) challenge. IJCV **88**, 303–338 (2010)

29. Xiao, J., Hays, J., Ehinger, K.A., Oliva, A., Torralba, A.: SUN database: large-scale scene recognition from abbey to zoo. In: CVPR (2010)

30. Maji, S., Bourdev, L., Malik, J.: Action recognition from a distributed representation of pose and appearance. In: CVPR (2011)

31. Bishop, C.M.: Mixture density networks. Technical report (1994)
32. Torralba, A.: Contextual priming for object detection. IJCV **53**, 169–191 (2003)
33. Felzenszwalb, P.F., Girshick, R.B., McAllester, D., Ramanan, D.: Object detection with discriminatively trained part based models. PAMI **32**, 1627–1645 (2010)
34. Avidan, S., Shamir, A.: Seam carving for content-aware image resizing. ACM Trans. Graph. **26**, 10 (2007)

Robust Stereo Matching Using Probabilistic Laplacian Surface Propagation

Seungryong Kim[1], Bumsub Ham[2], Seungchul Ryu[1], Seon Joo Kim[1], and Kwanghoon Sohn[1]($\boxtimes$)

[1] Yonsei University, Seoul, Republic of Korea
{srkim89,ryus01,seonjookim,khsohn}@yonsei.ac.kr
[2] Inria, Paris, France
bumsub.ham@inria.fr

Abstract. This paper describes a probabilistic Laplacian surface propagation (PLSP) framework for a robust stereo matching under severe radiometric variations. We discover that a progressive scheme overcomes an inherent limitation for this task, while most conventional efforts have been focusing on designing a robust cost function. We propose the ground control surfaces (GCSs) designed as progressive unit, which alleviates the problems of conventional progressive methods and superpixel based methods, simultaneously. Moreover, we introduce a novel confidence measure for stereo pairs taken under radiometric variations based on the probability of correspondences. Specifically, the PLSP estimates the GCSs from initial sparse disparity maps using a weighted least-square. The GCSs are then propagated on a superpixel graph with a surface confidence weighting. Experimental results show that the PLSP outperforms state-of-the-art robust cost function based methods and other propagation methods for the stereo matching under radiometric variations.

1 Introduction

Stereo matching aims to extract 3D scene information by finding the correspondence between stereo pairs taken at different viewpoints of the same scene [1]. Nowadays, state-of-the-art methods provide satisfactory results under the color consistency condition, i.e., corresponding pixels have a similar color distribution. However, the color consistency assumption is often violated since the color of an image is the result of complex combinations of imaging pipelines. Specifically, various factors including illumination source variations, non-Lambertian surfaces, vignetting, device characteristics, and an image noise have an influence on the performance of the stereo matching [2]. Conventionally, to alleviate these problems, a number of methods have been proposed to develop a robust cost function that is insensitive to radiometric distortions [2–7]. However, for stereo images taken under challenging environments, e.g., severe radiometric variations, some pixels or regions cause erroneous local minima. In this case, a robust cost

---

Bumsub Ham—WILLOW project-team, Département d'Informatique de l'Ecole Normale Supérieure, ENS/Inria/CNRS UMR 8548.

© Springer International Publishing Switzerland 2015
D. Cremers et al. (Eds.): ACCV 2014, Part I, LNCS 9003, pp. 368–383, 2015.
DOI: 10.1007/978-3-319-16865-4_24

function approach cannot guarantee to estimate reliable correspondences. In addition, costly global optimizations on the Markov random field (MRF), including a graph-cut (GC) and a belief propagation (BP) [8], cannot also infer a fully reliable solution and even propagate errors under these circumstances.

We discover that a progressive framework can overcome such an inherent limitation for the stereo matching under severe radiometric variations. It is inspired by interactive image editing methods in computer graphics such as colorization [9] and segmentation [10], which propagate an initial seed to infer fully dense results. A number of methods employed the progressive scheme to formulate the stereo matching as a constrained optimization problem [11–13]. These methods find ground control points (GCPs) on reliable regions and propagate them to infer dense disparity maps, which shows satisfactory performance with low complexity. However, an inherent problem of progressive methods is the sensitivity to outliers in initial GCPs since they assume that the initial GCPs are fully reliable [11]. In addition, they induce an edge-blurring on discontinuity regions since a disparity itself is propagated into first-order neighboring pixels. Since the GCPs estimated from stereo images taken under severe radiometric variations cannot be liberated from a false correspondence, conventional progressive methods are not suitable for these tasks.

To alleviate these problems, this paper proposes a probabilistic Laplacian surface propagation (PLSP) framework, which infers an edge-preserved and accurate disparity map even for unreliable GCPs. The PLSP overcomes the limitations of conventional progressive methods by leveraging a superpixel scheme and a confidence weighting. In stereo matching, a superpixel scheme has been popularly incorporated based on the fact that the disparity map is often spatially smooth while its discontinuities are aligned with image edges [14–20]. It reduces an influence of outliers or disparity fluctuations within the superpixel and consolidates boundaries, which enables sharp and accurate disparity maps. However, since slanted-surfaces are defined as three continuous parameters, conventional superpixel based approaches require an inference in continuous MRFs or assign a predefined disparity plane only, which is not robust while demanding a high complexity. The PLSP, combining a progressive scheme and a superpixel scheme, can infer fully continuous slanted-surfaces efficiently. In other words, the PLSP overcomes the limitations of conventional progressive methods and conventional superpixel based methods, simultaneously. Moreover, a novel confidence measure is employed for stereo pairs under radiometric variations, based on the probability of correspondences from initial GCPs. Specifically, the PLSP estimates reliable slanted-surfaces, called the ground control surfaces (GCSs), on superpixels from initial GCPs using a weighted least-square, and propagates these surfaces on a superpixel graph. For the stereo matching under severely different radiometric distortions, the PLSP outperforms other state-of-the-art robust stereo matching methods and propagation methods.

The remainder of this paper is organized as follows. Section 2 introduces related works for the proposed method. Section 3 describes the PLSP framework for a robust stereo matching. Experimental results are given in Sect. 4. Finally, conclusion and suggestions for future works are given in Sect. 5.

2   Related Work

Our approach aims to estimate an accurate disparity map for stereo pairs taken under radiometric variations, and it incorporates a progressive scheme on a superpixel graph. This section describes related works for a robust stereo matching, a progressive stereo matching, and a superpixel based stereo matching.

Robust Stereo Matching. For a stereo matching under radiometric variations, a number of methods have been proposed to develop a robust cost function [2–7]. A Census transform [3] based on a local order of intensities is tolerant to local illumination variations. It, however, produces unsatisfactory performance on homogeneous or noisy regions where the local order of intensities is indistinct. Although normalized correlation based cost functions such as an adaptive normalized cross-correlation (ANCC) [4] and a Mahalanobis distance cross-correlation (MDCC) [5] show satisfactory results for linear variations, they provide limited performances under severe radiometric distortions. A mutual information (MI) based on the joint probability has been widely used due to its robustness [6,7]. Hirschmüller and Scharstein evaluated in detail the robustness of cost functions in a stereo matching with respect to various radiometric variations. [2]. Note that any cost function cannot estimate a fully reliable disparity map for stereo pairs taken under severe radiometric variations since there exist the pixels or regions that cause erroneous local minima.

Progressive Stereo Matching. To address the inherent ambiguities of the stereo matching in homogeneous and occluded areas, progressive approaches have been proposed [11–13]. These methods find reliable disparities on salient pixels, referred as GCPs, and propagate them to neighboring pixels. Sun *et al.* employed a scanline construction with local color and connectivity constraints to propagate reliable disparities [13]. Hawe *et al.* proposed the compressive sensing based propagation scheme [12]. A Laplacian propagation inspired by [9] has been a seminal work due to its robustness [11]. It tried to minimize the difference between a disparity of a center pixel and weighted average of disparities within neighboring pixels [11]. However, conventional progressive approaches have inherent limitations, e.g., they are sensitive to outliers in initial GCPs and induce an edge-blurring especially on discontinuity regions. It is worth noting that unlike these methods, our approach employs a superpixel scheme and a confidence weighting, which provides the edge-preserved disparity maps with the robustness to erroneous GCPs.

Superpixel Based Stereo Matching. In stereo matching, a superpixel has been popularly incorporated to provide explicit smoothness priors, enforcing all pixels within the superpixel to lie on the same 3D surface [14–20]. These methods first assign an unique slanted-surface for each superpixel by applying the surface fitting to an initial disparity map, such as RANSAC based methods [19], least-square based methods [17], and voting based methods [18,20]. Then, extracted surfaces are optimized using the BP [18] or the GC [17]. However, the surface

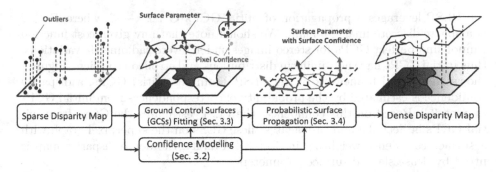

Fig. 1. Framework of the PLSP. The PLSP employs a confidence measure based on the probability of correspondences from initial sparse disparity map, and it is used to estimate a slanted-surface as GCSs and a confidence of GCSs itself. The PLSP estimates the GCSs on superpixels from sparse disparity map using a weighted least-square. These slanted-surface parameters are then propagated on a superpixel graph with a surface confidence weighting.

fitting is not an easy task when there exist errors on initial correspondences. In addition, since slanted-surfaces are defined as three continuous parameters, conventional superpixel based methods require an inference in continuous MRFs to estimate dense slanted-surface maps, which induces a dramatically high complexity [16]. Thus, most methods only assign the label from a predefined disparity plane set on each superpixel, which provides an inherent limitation. Compared to these methods, our approach estimates reliable slanted-surfaces and propagates them on a superpixel graph, which overcomes the limitations of conventional superpixel based methods.

Contributions of Our Approach. The contributions of this paper are summarized as follows. First, to the best of our knowledge, it is the first attempt to employ a progressive framework for the stereo matching under radiometric variations. Second, instead of propagating the GCPs itself on a pixel graph, our approach propagates the GCSs on a superpixel graph, which overcomes the limitations of conventional progressive methods and conventional superpixel based methods, simultaneously. Finally, a novel confidence measure is proposed for stereo pairs taken under different radiometric conditions based on the probability of correspondences from GCPs, weighted by SIFT features, and it is incorporated into a propagation framework.

3   Probabilistic Laplacian Surface Propagation

3.1   Problem Statement and Overview

Given stereo pairs $\mathbf{I}_L : \mathcal{I} \rightarrow \mathbb{R}^3$ and $\mathbf{I}_R : \mathcal{I} \rightarrow \mathbb{R}^3$ taken under different radiometric conditions, the PLSP aims to estimate a dense disparity map $\mathbf{D} : \mathcal{I} \rightarrow \mathcal{L}$ that assigns each pixel $\mathbf{m} = [x_{\mathbf{m}}, y_{\mathbf{m}}]^{\mathbf{T}} \in \mathcal{I}$ to a disparity $d_{\mathbf{m}} \in \mathcal{L}$, where $\mathcal{I} \subset \mathbb{N}^2$ is a dense discrete image domain and $\mathcal{L}$ is a discrete disparity candidate. To this end, the PLSP leverages a propagation of initial GCPs $\mathbf{G} : \mathcal{I}' \to \mathcal{L}$, where $\mathcal{I}' \subset \mathcal{I}$ is a sparse discrete image domain. We should note that any given cost function cannot find perfect GCPs for stereo images under severe radiometric variations, thus initial GCPs have non-uniform distributions and erroneous outliers. Figure 1 shows the overall framework of the PLSP. From the initial GCPs, a disparity confidence is estimated by the probability of correspondences from initial GCPs in Sect. 3.2. Based on this confidence, the PLSP estimates the GCSs from initial GCPs in Sect. 3.3 and propagates these GCSs on the superpixel graph with a surface confidence weighting in Sect. 3.4. Finally, the dense disparity map is fitted by dense slanted-surface parameters.

3.2   Confidence Modeling via Color Mapping Probability

In this section, a novel confidence measure is introduced for stereo pairs taken under different radiometric conditions. We argue that the confidence of a disparity at a pixel can be measured by the probability of correspondences between the pixel itself in the left image and the corresponding pixel in the right image. It assumes that there exists a one-to-one color mapping between stereo pairs, i.e., each color in the left image could be mapped into one color in the right image. This assumption explains many instances of color variation such as different camera and different camera setting. It can also explain illumination variations such as global lighting changes and even directional illumination changes [21].

To encode the confidence for a disparity, we leverage that initial GCPs, $\mathbf{G}$, provide the matching relationship between pixel $\mathbf{m} = [x_\mathbf{m}, y_\mathbf{m}]^\mathbf{T}$ in the left image and the corresponding pixel $\hat{\mathbf{m}} = [x_\mathbf{m} - d_\mathbf{m}, y_\mathbf{m}]^\mathbf{T}$ in the right image. For all disparities in initial GCPs, the probability of correspondences can be built by computing the joint probability density function (PDF). Since the space of possible color is much bigger than the color distribution of an image, $\mathbf{I}_L$ and $\mathbf{I}_R$ are quantized by $J_L \in \mathcal{J}$ and $J_R \in \mathcal{J}$, respectively, where $\mathcal{J}$ is a set of color indexes, in such a way that the color space is divided into fixed size bins. In addition, to encode a structural similarity between corresponding pixels, the joint PDF is weighted by the difference of SIFT features [22] similar to [7]. The SIFT-weighted joint PDF $p(j_L, j_R)$ is then defined by

$$p(j_L, j_R) = \frac{1}{|\mathcal{I}'|} \sum_{\mathbf{m} \in \mathcal{I}'} \psi(\mathbf{m}, \hat{\mathbf{m}}) T[(j_L, j_R) = (J_L(\mathbf{m}), J_R(\hat{\mathbf{m}}))], \qquad (1)$$

where $j_L \in J_L$ and $j_R \in J_R$. $T[\cdot]$ is a logistic operator providing 1 when the argument is true. $|\mathcal{I}'|$ is the total number of pixels in initial GCPs. $\psi(\cdot, \cdot)$ is a SIFT-weighting factor defined by

$$\psi(\mathbf{m}, \hat{\mathbf{m}}) = \exp(-\|\varepsilon_L(\mathbf{m}) - \varepsilon_R(\hat{\mathbf{m}})\|^2 / \lambda_\varepsilon), \qquad (2)$$

where λ_ε denotes a coefficient for the degree of structural similarity. $\varepsilon_L(\mathbf{m})$ and $\varepsilon_R(\hat{\mathbf{m}})$ are SIFT features for the pixel $\mathbf{m}$ in the left image and pixel $\hat{\mathbf{m}}$ in the right image, respectively.

Based on the SIFT-weighted joint PDF, a confidence $\mathcal{M}(\mathbf{m}, d_\mathbf{m})$ for a pixel $\mathbf{m}$ having a disparity $d_\mathbf{m}$ is defined by the bi-directional conditional probability of correspondences between $J_L(\mathbf{m})$ and $J_R(\hat{\mathbf{m}})$ as

$$\mathcal{M}(\mathbf{m}, d_\mathbf{m}) \triangleq p(J_L(\mathbf{m})|J_R(\hat{\mathbf{m}}))p(J_R(\hat{\mathbf{m}})|J_L(\mathbf{m})), \tag{3}$$

where $p(J_L(\mathbf{m})|J_R(\hat{\mathbf{m}}))$ and $p(J_R(\hat{\mathbf{m}})|J_L(\mathbf{m}))$ are computed using Baye's theorem and the marginalization as follows:

$$p(J_L(\mathbf{m})|J_R(\hat{\mathbf{m}})) = \frac{p(J_L(\mathbf{m}), J_R(\hat{\mathbf{m}}))}{p(J_R(\hat{\mathbf{m}}))}$$

$$= \frac{p(J_L(\mathbf{m}), J_R(\hat{\mathbf{m}}))}{\sum\limits_{\mathbf{k} \in \mathcal{J}} p(\mathbf{k}, J_R(\hat{\mathbf{m}}))}. \tag{4}$$

After estimating $p(J_R(\hat{\mathbf{m}})|J_L(\mathbf{m}))$ in a similar way, the confidence of disparity in Eq. 3 can be derived as follows:

$$\mathcal{M}(\mathbf{m}, d_\mathbf{m}) = \frac{p(J_L(\mathbf{m}), J_R(\hat{\mathbf{m}}))^2}{\sum\limits_{\mathbf{k} \in \mathcal{J}} p(\mathbf{k}, J_R(\hat{\mathbf{m}})) \sum\limits_{\mathbf{k} \in \mathcal{J}} p(J_L(\mathbf{m}), \mathbf{k})}. \tag{5}$$

This novel confidence measure estimates the reliability of disparity, and it is used to estimate a slanted-surface as GCSs and provides a confidence of GCSs itself for a propagation.

3.3 Ground Control Surfaces (GCSs)

In order to estimate a slanted-surface parameter of each superpixel from initial GCPs, a number of surface fitting methods can be used [17–20]. Among them, the least-square based approaches provides a slanted-surface fitting with a low computational load [17]. Since the cost function of this method is convex, a closed form solution can be easily found. However, this method is sensitive to outliers. The PLSP employs a weighted least-square for a slanted-surface fitting from initial GCPs on superpixels.

The PLSP uses a graph construction scheme such that every superpixel serves as a graph node and edge is placed between two superpixels if their boundaries have an overlap. Let us denote i-th superpixel as S_i and an index set of spatially adjacent superpixels for S_i as $\mathcal{N}_i$. Similar to other superpixel based methods, the PLSP leverages that a slanted-surface for a superpixel S_i represented as $\mathbf{f}_i = [f_i^\alpha, f_i^\beta, f_i^\gamma]^T \in \mathbb{R}^3$ enables an inference of a disparity value of pixel $\mathbf{m} \in S_i$ such that $d_\mathbf{m} = \mathbf{a}_\mathbf{m}^T \mathbf{f}_i$ where $\mathbf{a}_\mathbf{m} = [x_\mathbf{m}, y_\mathbf{m}, 1]^T$ [14]. The slanted-surface parameter $\mathbf{f}_i^*$ of GCSs is determined as minimizing errors between sparse disparities in initial GCPs and disparities estimated by a slanted-surface within superpixels. The PLSP employs the confidence weighting to reduce an influence of outliers in initial GCPs. In addition, to reduce outliers, a regularization term is employed. Thus, our energy function $\Phi_i(\mathbf{f})$ is defined as follows:

$$\Phi_i(\mathbf{f}) = \sum_{\mathbf{m} \in S_i \cap \mathcal{I}'} \mathcal{M}(\mathbf{m}, d_\mathbf{m})(d_\mathbf{m} - \mathbf{a}_\mathbf{m}^T \mathbf{f})^2 + \lambda_f \mathbf{f}^T \mathbf{f}, \tag{6}$$

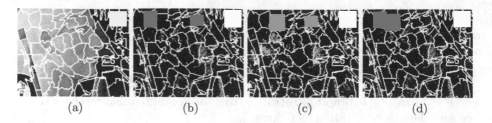

(a)　　　　　　　　(b)　　　　　　　　(c)　　　　　　　　(d)

Fig. 2. The GCSs fitting from initial GCPs for *Art* image pairs. (a) Superpixel decompositions for a reference image. (b) Initial GCPs **G** with the superpixel grid. (c) Confidence weights $\mathcal{M}(\mathbf{m}, d_{\mathbf{m}})$ for initial GCPs. The degree of the confidence is indicated as the brightness of green color. (d) The GCSs fitting as $\mathbf{f}_i^*$. The GCSs fitting on superpixels reduces the influence of erroneous GCPs. These GCSs can be a soft constraint for dense slanted-surface maps (Colour figure online).

where λ_f is a regularization parameter. It can be represented as the matrix-vector form as

$$\Phi_i(\mathbf{f}) = (\mathbf{D} - \mathbf{A}\mathbf{f})^{\mathbf{T}}\mathbf{M}(\mathbf{D} - \mathbf{A}\mathbf{f}) + \mathbf{f}^{\mathbf{T}}\Lambda\mathbf{f}, \tag{7}$$

where $\mathbf{M} = diag\{\mathcal{M}(\mathbf{m}, d_{\mathbf{m}})\}_{\mathbf{m} \in S_i \cap \mathcal{I}'}$, $\Lambda = diag\{\lambda_f\}$, $\mathbf{D} = \{d_{\mathbf{m}}\}_{\mathbf{m} \in S_i \cap \mathcal{I}'}$, and $A = \{\mathbf{a}_{\mathbf{m}}^{\mathbf{T}}\}_{\mathbf{m} \in S_i \cap \mathcal{I}'}$. The slanted-surface parameter, minimizing this energy function, can be estimated by $\nabla\Phi_i(\mathbf{f}) = 0$ as in Eq. 8.

$$\mathbf{f}_i^* = (\mathbf{A}^{\mathbf{T}}\mathbf{M}\mathbf{A} + \Lambda)^{-1}\mathbf{A}^{\mathbf{T}}\mathbf{M}\mathbf{D}. \tag{8}$$

In order to eliminate erroneous surface parameters, appearance neighbors are employed similar to [15]. Given a superpixel S_i, we search the neighboring superpixels having similar appearances by estimating a superpixel feature affinity, which will be described in the following section, within a predefined window. Let $\mathcal{N}_i^s$ is an index set of these superpixels. Our approach eliminates a non-reliable superpixel satisfying that

$$\left\| \mathbf{f}_i^* - \frac{1}{|\mathcal{N}_i^s|} \sum_{j \in \mathcal{N}_i^s} \mathbf{f}_j^* \right\| < \tau_s, \tag{9}$$

where $|\mathcal{N}_i^s|$ is the number of appearance neighbors, and τ_s is a threshold. Finally, the slanted-surface represented by a parameter $\mathbf{f}_i^*$ is defined as ground control surfaces (GCSs). We use these GCSs as initial sparse surfaces to provide the soft constraint for the propagation.

Figure 2 shows the GCSs fitting from initial GCPs for *Art* image pairs. As shown in GCPs, initial disparities are non-uniformly distributed with outliers. For the GCSs fitting, the reference image is decomposed as non-overlapping superpixels. Based on superpixels, the PLSP estimates a reliable slanted-surface on each superpixel with the confidence weighting, which consolidates disparity boundaries and reduces the influence of outliers in initial GCPs.

3.4 Optimization Framework

The PLSP formulates an inference of a set of piecewise continuous slanted-surfaces as a constrained optimization problem where the GCSs are interpreted as soft constraints. It formulates each energy function for slanted-surface parameters f_i^α, f_i^β, and f_i^γ and minimizes these functions, independently. Let $\mathbf{F} = \{f_i\}$ be the vector of all slanted-surface parameters for superpixels. The energy function of the PLSP is defined as follows:

$$\mathbf{E}(\mathbf{F}) = \mathbf{E}_{data}(\mathbf{F}) + \mathbf{E}_{smooth}(\mathbf{F}), \tag{10}$$

where a data term $\mathbf{E}_{data}(\mathbf{F})$ and a smoothness term $\mathbf{E}_{smooth}(\mathbf{F})$ are defined as

$$\mathbf{E}_{data}(\mathbf{F}) = \sum_i p_i(f_i - f_i^*)^2, \tag{11}$$

$$\mathbf{E}_{smooth}(\mathbf{F}) = \sum_i \sum_{j \in \mathcal{N}_i} \omega_{ij}(f_i - f_j)^2. \tag{12}$$

$\mathbf{E}_{data}(\mathbf{F})$ encodes the penalty for the dissimilarity of slanted-surface parameters f_i and corresponding parameters f_i^* for GCSs. In addition, it encodes a surface confidence weight p_i to reduce the influence of erroneous GCSs according to the reliability of surface. $\mathbf{E}_{smooth}(\mathbf{F})$ imposes the constraint that two adjacent superpixel i and j have similar slanted-surface parameters according to surperpixel feature affinity ω_{ij}, which will be detailed in the following section.

Confidence for Ground Control Surfaces. While conventional propagation methods impose an uniform confidence for initial seeds, the PLSP employs a confidence weighting for GCSs according to the reliability of GCSs. The GCSs represented as $\mathbf{f}_i^*$ enable an inference of the disparity value of pixels $\mathbf{m} \in S_i$ such that $\mathbf{a_m^T f}_i^*$. Thus, a confidence for pixels within a superpixel is computed as $\mathcal{M}(\mathbf{m}, \mathbf{a_m^T f}_i^*)$. In order to estimate a surface confidence weight p_i of GCSs, these confidence weights are aggregated within a superpixel S_i as

$$p_i = \frac{1}{|S_i|} \sum_{\mathbf{m} \in S_i} \mathcal{M}(\mathbf{m}, \mathbf{a_m^T f}_i^*), \tag{13}$$

where $|S_i|$ is the number of pixels within a superpixel S_i. This surface confidence weight enables the propagation of initial GCSs according to their reliability, thus reducing the influence of erroneous GCSs in a propagation procedure.

Superpixel Feature Affinity. A superpixel as a propagation unit can encode regional features, providing more robust affinity between adjacent superpixels compared to the intensity feature into first-order neighboring pixels in conventional methods [11]. The PLSP employs a superpixel feature composed of a color appearance, a SIFT feature, and a spatial feature. First, color appearance feature v_i^c describes statistical color information as the average and standard deviation for pixels within superpixels in RGB, Lab, and YCbCr color space [23]. Second,

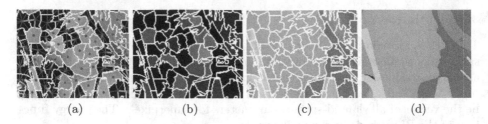

(a)   (b)   (c)   (d)

Fig. 3. Propagation of the GCSs in Fig. 2 on a superpixel graph. (a) The superpixel graph (blue dot: node, green line: edge with superpixel affinities ω_{ij}.) (b) Surface confidence weights p_i for GCSs. The degree of the confidence is indicated as the brightness of green color. (c) Results of the PLSP. (d) Ground truth. The PLSP propagates reliable GCSs on the superpixel graph with the surface confidence weighting, which provides an edge-preserved and accurate disparity map (Colour figure online).

in order to encode structural information, we adopt the SIFT feature v_i^s [22]. Specifically, dense SIFT features are extracted from pixels, and then, these features are aggregated within superpixels. Finally, spatial feature v_i^p is defined as a spatial centroid coordinate within superpixels.

Based on these superpixel features, a superpixel feature affinity ω_{ij} between adjacent superpixel i and j is computed as

$$\omega_{ij} \propto \exp(-\left\|v_i^c - v_j^c\right\|^2/\lambda_c - \left\|v_i^s - v_j^s\right\|^2/\lambda_s - \left\|v_i^p - v_j^p\right\|^2/\lambda_p), \qquad (14)$$

where λ_c, λ_s, and λ_p denote coefficients for the similarity degree measuring a coherence of neighboring superpixels. The larger ω_{ij} is, the more likely that two neighboring superpixels have same slanted-surfaces. The affinity ω_{ij} is normalized to have a unit sum such that

$$\sum_{j \in \mathcal{N}_i} \left\|\omega_{ij}\right\|^2 = 1. \qquad (15)$$

Solver. One strength of our approach is the low complexity since no costly global optimizations are required such as the GC and the BP [8]. The energy function $\mathbf{E(F)}$ in Eq. 10 can be expressed in matrix-vector form as

$$\mathbf{E(F)} = (\mathbf{F} - \mathbf{F}^*)^{\mathbf{T}}\mathbf{P}(\mathbf{F} - \mathbf{F}^*) + \mathbf{F^T}(\mathbf{L} - \mathbf{W})\mathbf{F}, \qquad (16)$$

where $\mathbf{F}^*$ is the vector of surface parameters of GCSs. The matrix $\mathbf{P}$ is a diagonal matrix whose diagonal elements with surface confidence weights such that $\mathbf{P}_{ii} = p_i$. The matrix $\mathbf{L}$ is an identity matrix. The matrix $\mathbf{W}$ is a weight matrix whose elements are pairwise affinities ω_{ij}.

The minimum of this discrete quadratic form can be obtained by setting $\nabla \mathbf{E(F)} = 0$, which amounts to solving the following linear system as

$$(\mathbf{P} + \mathbf{L} - \mathbf{W})\mathbf{F} = \mathbf{P}\mathbf{F}^*. \qquad (17)$$

This linear system with a laplacian matrix can be easily solved as conventional linear solvers [24]. Compared to propagation on a pixel graph [11], our approach can reduce the computational complexity of the linear solver with the proposition to the number of pixels within superpixels.

Figure 3(a) shows the superpixel graph constructed by superpixel feature affinities, and Fig. 3(b) shows the surface confidence weight. In the PLSP, the GCSs are propagated on the superpixel graph with the confidence weighting to infer dense disparity maps as in Fig. 3(c). The PLSP is summarized in Algorithm 1.

Algorithm 1. Probabilistic Laplacian Surface Propagation

    Input : stereo pairs $\mathbf{I}_L$, $\mathbf{I}_R$, and GCP $\mathbf{G}$.

    Output : dense disparity map $\mathbf{D}$.

1: Compute a confidence of disparity $\mathcal{M}(\mathbf{m}, d_\mathbf{m})$ as in Eq. (5) from GCPs $\mathbf{G}$.

2: Decompose the reference image $\mathbf{I}_L$ into superpixels S_i.

3: Estimate the parameter of GCSs $\mathbf{f}_i^* = [f_i^\alpha, f_i^\beta, f_i^\gamma]^\mathbf{T}$ as in Eq. (8).

4: Compute a Laplacian matrix $\mathbf{P} + \mathbf{L} - \mathbf{W}$ with surface confidence weights p_i in Eq. (13) and affinities ω_{ij} in Eq. (14).

5: Estimate the slanted-surface parameters by $\mathbf{F} = (\mathbf{P} + \mathbf{L} - \mathbf{W})^{-1} \mathbf{P} \mathbf{F}^*$ in Eq. (17) where $\mathbf{F}^* = [\mathbf{F}_\alpha^*, \mathbf{F}_\beta^*, \mathbf{F}_\gamma^*]$.

6: Estimate the dense disparity map $\mathbf{D}$ such that $d_\mathbf{m} = \mathbf{a}_\mathbf{m}^\mathbf{T} \mathbf{f}_i$ for all superpixels.

---

4 Experimental Results

In this section, the stereo matching performance is evaluated for the PLSP and other methods on the Middlebury datasets [2], where each dataset consists of stereo image pairs taken under varying illumination conditions indexed from 1 to 3 and exposure conditions indexed from 0 to 2. In order to evaluate the robustness to radiometric variations, stereo images were selected according to the index of illumination or exposure, e.g., "illumination combination 1/1" was defined as an index of illumination varying from 1 to 1 [2]. The PLSP was compared with the state-of-the-art robust stereo matching methods such as the MI [6], Census transform [3], the NCC [2], and the ANCC [4]. These methods were optimized with the graph-cut (GC) as in [4]. In addition, since the PLSP was designed to propagate initial GCPs to infer dense disparity map, it was also compared with other propagation methods for fixed GCPs, such as a weighted median filtering (WMF) with a hole filling [25], a Guided filtering (GF) based propagation [24,26], and a Laplacian propagation (LP) [11]. To evaluate the robustness of proposed confidence measure, the LP combined with a confidence weighting (PLP) was evaluated. To evaluate the robustness of the GCSs scheme, the Laplacian surface propagation (LSP)[1] was also evaluated. The parameters of each method were set to the same values from the original works. The evaluation criterion is the bad pixel error rate in the non-occluded areas of disparity maps since it has been popularly used in stereo literatures [4].

---

[1] In order to evaluate the robustness of only surface propagation, the LSP only expands the propagation unit as a superpixel without the confidence weighting for GCSs.

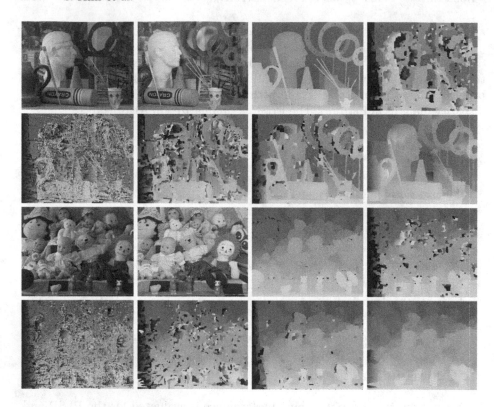

Fig. 4. Comparison of disparity estimation for *Art* and *Dolls* image pairs taken under illumination combination 1/3. (from left to right, from top to bottom) Left color image, right color image, and disparity maps for the ground truth, MI+GC [6], Census+GC [3], NCC+GC [2], ANCC+GC [4], and PLSP. Conventional robust cost functions cannot estimate a fully reliable correspondence even with a global optimization. In contrast, the PLSP estimates accurate disparity maps (Colour figure online).

In the experiments, similar to other methods detecting the GCPs [11–13], initial GCPs were estimated by a linear combination of cost functions, the NCC [2] and the Census [3], with a winner-takes-all (WTA) optimization and refined by left-right cross-check [13]. For the superpixel graph, the reference image was decomposed by a SLIC superpixel due to its compactness and regular shape [27], and the number of superpixels was set to from 1000 to 1500. The structural similarity coefficient was defined as $\lambda_\varepsilon = 1.3$. The color space was quantized as bin size $20 \times 20 \times 20$ in all experiments. For superpixel feature affinity, the parameters were empirically determined as $\{\lambda_c, \lambda_s, \lambda_p\} = \{0.036, 1.6, 12.8\}$.

4.1 Comparison with Robust Stereo Matching Methods

In order to evaluate the robustness for radiometric variations, disparity maps of the PLSP and other robust stereo matching methods were estimated for stereo pairs taken under radiometric variations. Figure 4 shows disparity maps for *Art*

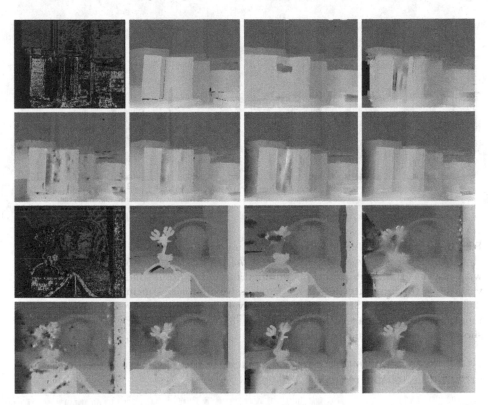

Fig. 5. Comparison of disparity propagation for GCPs from *Books* and *Reindeer* image pairs taken under illumination combination 1/3. (from left to right, from top to bottom) The initial GCPs and disparity maps for the ground truth, WMF with the hole filling [25], GF-based propagation [26], LP [11], PLP, LSP, and PLSP. Conventional methods show the limitation for unreliable GCPs. Disparity maps of PLP, LSP, and PLSP show that a superpixel scheme with the confidence weighting provides an edge-preserved and accurate disparity map.

and *Dolls* stereo images under the illumination combination 1/3, which is the most severe radiometric variation.

The performance of the MI-based method is degraded under local variations, since it is assumed that there are global variations. In addition, the Census transform provides poor results on homogeneous regions which have an indistinct order of intensities. The normalized correlation based methods such as the NCC and the ANCC show high performance compared to the Census transform. However, disparity maps of the NCC contain large errors in boundary regions since it does not encode the spatial structure. The ANCC improves the matching performance using weight distributions compared to the NCC. However, conventional approach for these tasks show the limitations. Pixels degraded by severe radiometric distortions are not estimated perfectly by robust cost functions even with a global optimization. In contrast, the PLSP outperforms conventional methods by addressing these problems. Since the PLSP propagates sparse and reliable

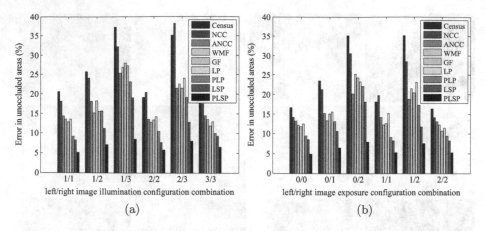

Fig. 6. Average bad pixel error rates in the un-occluded areas for disparity maps from *Art*, *Baby1*, *Books*, *Bowling2*, *Cloth3*, *Cloth4*, *Dolls*, *Moebius*, *Reindeer*, and *Wood1* with varying the combination of illumination and exposure index. (a) Illumination variations. (b) Exposure variations. Progressive approaches including WMF [25], GF [26], LP [11], PLP, LSP, and PLSP relatively outperform conventional robust cost function based approaches such as Census [3], NCC [2], and ANCC [4]. The PLSP shows the best performance with the lowest bad pixel error rates.

GCSs without estimating erroneous pixels, it fills these erroneous regions by propagating reliable regions.

4.2   Comparison with Robust Propagation Methods

In this section, the PLSP was compared with different robust propagation methods in terms of stereo matching under radiometric variations. For the fair comparison, the initial GCPs were fixed in all methods. Figure 5 shows disparity maps of different propagation methods for the GCPs estimated from *Books* and *Reindeer* image pairs under the illumination combination 1/3.

As shown in Fig. 5, initial GCPs have erroneous disparities and non-uniform distributions, which induces large hole regions on discontinuity regions. Although the WMF with the hole filling have shown the satisfactory performance in disparity refinements, it cannot estimate accurate dense disparity for erroneous GCPs, especially on large holes. The GF-based propagation provides more edge-preserved disparity maps compared to other methods. However, it is also sensitive to outliers of initial GCPs. In addition, since the GF uses a reference color image, the textures in the color image are also propagated in final disparity maps. As the most related method, the LP induces edge blurring and propagates erroneous initial GCPs, since it propagates disparity itself on a pixel graph without the consideration of the disparity confidence. In contrast, the LP with proposed confidence weighting, PLP, reduces an influence of the erroneous pixels. However, there still exists edge blurring problems. Compared to the pixel propagation, the Laplacian surface propagation, LSP, preserves disparity discontinuities. However, it cannot refine erroneous superpixels. The PLSP framework consisting of the surface propagation with the confidence weighting shows the best performance. It dramatically reduces an influence of errors in initial GCPs and provides edge-preserved disparity maps compared with other methods.

Figure 6 shows average bad pixel error rates of disparity maps from *Art*, *Baby1*, *Books*, *Bowling2*, *Cloth3*, *Cloth4*, *Dolls*, *Moebius*, *Reindeer*, and *Wood1* with varying the combination of illumination and exposure index. Most propagation methods relatively outperform robust cost function based methods since they propagate the GCPs without estimating erroneous pixels. However, since there still remain outliers on initial GCPs from stereo pairs under radiometric variations, conventional propagation methods provide the limited performance. In contrast, the PLSP shows the best performance with the lowest bad pixel error rates compared to other methods. In addition, the PLSP shows competitive performances for stereo pairs under normal conditions without radiometric variations. More experimental results are available in the supplementary materials.

5 Conclusion

The robust stereo matching framework called the PLSP has been proposed for the stereo matching under severe radiometric variations. We discover that a progressive framework overcomes the limitation of conventional approaches for these tasks. Instead of propagating the GCPs itself on the pixel graph, we introduced the GCSs as a propagation unit. To measure the confidence of a disparity for stereo pairs under radiometric variations, a novel confidence measure has been proposed based on the probability of correspondence from initial GCPs. The PLSP provides an edge-preserved disparity map while reducing the influence of outliers in initial GCPs. Experimental results have shown that the PSLP outperforms state-of-the-art robust stereo matching methods and propagation methods for stereo image pairs taken under severely different radiometric conditions.

For future work, the PLSP will be applied to address other correspondence problems under different radiometric conditions, such as optical flow or dense image alignment.

Acknowledgement. This research was supported by the MSIP(Ministry of Science, ICT and Future Planning), Korea, under the ITRC(Information Technology Research Center) support program (NIPA-2014-H0301-14-1012) supervised by the NIPA(National IT Industry Promotion Agency).

References

1. Scharstein, D., Szeliski, R.: A taxonomy and evaluation of dense two-frame stereo correspondence algorithms. IJCV **47**, 7–42 (2002)
2. Hirschmüller, H., Scharstein, D.: Evaluation of stereo matching costs on images with radiometric differences. TPAMI **31**, 1582–1599 (2009)

3. Zabih, R., Woodfill, J.: Non-parametric local transforms for computing visual correspondence. In: Eklundh, J.-O. (ed.) ECCV 1994. LNCS, pp. 151–158. Springer, Heidelberg (1994)

4. Heo, Y., Lee, K., Lee, S.: Robust stereo matching using adaptive normalized cross-correlation. TPAMI **33**, 807–822 (2011)

5. Kim, S., Ham, B., Kim, B., Sohn, K.: Mahalanobis distance cross-correlation for illumination invariant stereo matching. TCSVT **24**, 1844–1859 (2014)

6. Kim, J., Kolmogorov, V., Zabih, R.: Visual correspondence using energy minimization and mutual information. In: ICCV (2003)

7. Heo, Y., Lee, K., Lee, S.: Mutual information-based stereo matching combined with sift descriptor in log-chromaticity color space. In: CVPR (2009)

8. Szeliski, R., Zabih, R., Scharstein, D., Veksler, O., Kolmogorov, V., Agarwala, A., Tappen, M., Rother, C.: A comparative study of energy minimization methods for markov random fields. In: Leonardis, A., Bischof, H., Pinz, A. (eds.) ECCV 2006. LNCS, vol. 3952, pp. 16–29. Springer, Heidelberg (2006)

9. Levin, A., Lischinski, D., Weiss, Y.: Colorization using optimization. In: SIGGRAPH (2006)

10. Krishnan, D., Fattal, R., Szeliski, R.: Efficient preconditioning of laplacian matrices for computer graphics. In: SIGGRAPH (2013)

11. Wang, L., Yang, R.: Global stereo matching leveraged by sparse ground control points. In: CVPR (2011)

12. Hawe, S., Kleinsteuber, M., Diepold, K.: Dense disparity maps from sparse disparity measurements. In: ICCV (2011)

13. Sun, X., Mei, X., Zhou, M., Wang, H.: Stereo matching with reliable disparity propagation. In: 3DIMPVT (2011)

14. Yamaguchi, K., Hazan, T., McAllester, D., Urtasun, R.: Continuous Markov random fields for robust stereo estimation. In: Fitzgibbon, A., Lazebnik, S., Perona, P., Sato, Y., Schmid, C. (eds.) ECCV 2012, Part V. LNCS, vol. 7576, pp. 45–58. Springer, Heidelberg (2012)

15. Lu, J., Yang, H., Min, D., Do, M.: Patchmatch filter: Efficient edge-aware filtering meets randomized search for fast correspondence field estimation. In: CVPR (2013)

16. Bleyer, M., Rother, C., Kohli, P.: Surface stereo with soft segmentation. In: CVPR (2010)

17. Hong, L., Chen, G.: Segment-based stereo matching using graph cuts. In: CVPR (2004)

18. Klaus, A., Sormann, M., Karner, K.: Segment-based stereo matching using belief propagation and a self-adapting dissimilarity measure. In: ICPR (2006)

19. Sinha, S., Steedly, D., Szeliski, R.: Piecewise planar stereo for image-based rendering. In: ICCV (2009)

20. Wang, Z., Zheng, Z.: A region based stereo matching algorithm using cooperative optimization. In: CVPR (2008)

21. Hwang, Y., Lee, J., Kweon, I., Kim, S.: Color transfer using probabilistic moving least squares. In: CVPR (2014)

22. Lowe, D.: Distinctive image features from scale-invariant keypoints. IJCV **60**, 91–110 (2004)

23. Chia, A., Zhuo, S., Gupta, R., Tai, Y., Cho, S., Tan, P., Lin, S.: Semantic colorization with internet images. In: SIGGRAPH (2011)

24. Lang, M., Wang, O., Aydic, T., Smolic, A., Gross, M.: Practical temporal consistency for image-based graphics applications. In: SIGGRAPH (2012)

25. Ma, Z., He, K., Wei, Y., Sun, J., Wu, E.: Constant time weighted median filtering for stereo matching and beyond. In: ICCV (2013)

26. He, K., Sun, J., Tang, X.: Guided image filtering. In: Daniilidis, K., Maragos, P., Paragios, N. (eds.) ECCV 2010, Part I. LNCS, vol. 6311, pp. 1–14. Springer, Heidelberg (2010)
27. Achanta, R., Shaji, A., Smith, K., Lucchi, A., Fua, P., Susstrunk, S.: SLIC super-pixels compared to state-of-the-art superpixel methods. TPAMI **34**, 2274–2282 (2012)

Imposing Differential Constraints on Radial Distortion Correction

Xianghua Ying$^{(\boxtimes)}$, Xiang Mei, Sen Yang, Ganwen Wang, Jiangpeng Rong, and Hongbin Zha

Key Laboratory of Machine Perception (Ministry of Education),
School of Electronic Engineering and Computer Science, Peking University,
Beijing 100871, People's Republic of China
xhying@cis.pku.edu.cn

Abstract. Many radial distortion functions have been presented to describe the mappings caused by radial lens distortions in common commercially available cameras. For a given real camera, no matter what function is selected, its innate mapping of radial distortion is smooth, and the signs of its first and second order derivatives are fixed. However, such differential constraints have been never considered explicitly in existing methods of radial distortion correction for a very long time. The differential constraints we claimed in this paper are that for a given real camera, the signs of the first and second order derivatives of the radial distortion function should remain unchanged within the feasible domain of the independent variable, although over the whole domain, or outside of the feasible domain, the signs may change many times. Our method can be somewhat treated as a regularization of the distortion function within the viewing frustum. We relax the differential constraints by using a deliberate strategy, to yield the linear inequality constraints on the unknown coefficients of the radial distortion function. It seems that such additional linear inequalities are not difficult to deal with in recent existing methods of radial distortion correction. The main advantages of our method are not only to ensure the recovered radial distortion function satisfy differential constraints within the viewing frustum, but also to make the recovered radial distortion function working well in case of extrapolation, caused by the features used for distortion correction usually distributed only in the middle part, but rarely near the boundary of the distorted image. The experiments validate our approach.

1 Introduction

The ideal pinhole model is often employed in algorithms of 3D recovery from 2D images in the field of computer vision. Unfortunately, for common commercially available cameras, they usually do not strictly satisfy the ideal pinhole model, i.e., some deviations may exist. Such deviations can be more complex, and are called as lens distortions in literature [1]. There are many methods to model lens distortions. The most famous model was proposed by Brown [1] which described the radial, decentring and prism distortions. In fact, among these distortions,

© Springer International Publishing Switzerland 2015
D. Cremers et al. (Eds.): ACCV 2014, Part I, LNCS 9003, pp. 384–398, 2015.
DOI: 10.1007/978-3-319-16865-4_25

radial distortion is the most significant in recent cameras [2–12]. Other types of distortions are often little, and can be omitted in the calibration procedure of distortion correction.

Many kinds of radial distortion functions are presented to describe the radial distortion [2–12]. If we assume the center of radial distortion is known in advance, we can define the distance from the original distorted image point to the center of radial distortion as the distorted radius r_d, and the distance corresponding to the undistorted image point as the undistorted radius r_u. The radial distortion functions usually describe the relations between r_d and r_u, namely, $r_d = f(r_u)$ or $r_u = g(r_d)$ [1,2,13–17]. For some cases of metric calibration, the view angle θ corresponding to the undistorted image point is often chosen to replace of r_u. Now, radial distortion functions become $r_d = p(\theta)$ or $\theta = q(r_d)$ [5,12,18–20]. Basu and Licardie [14] proposed the logarithmic distortion model. Devernay and Faugeras [21] presented the field-of-view distortion model. Fitzgibbon [16] recommended the division model with a single parameter. Ying and Hu [3], Barreto and Daniilidis [4] extended the unified imaging model of central catadioptric cameras to describe the radial distortion. Claus and Fitzgibbon [17] constructed the rational function distortion model for a wide range of radial distortions. Hartley and Kang [6] utilized a nonparametric model for radial distortion.

For radial distortion functions of real lenses estimated using different methods [13,15,18–20,22–28], we can easily find a phenomenon that, the signs of their first and second order derivatives with respect to the radius (i.e., r_d or r_u) or the view angle (i.e., θ) should remain unchanged within the viewing frustum, namely, from zero to the maximum of the radius or the view angle within the feasible domain. However, such constraints are never considered explicitly in literature. One reason may be that someone may think such constraints can be satisfied automatically. Indeed, without the constraints, the signs may be changed within the feasible domain (Many examples often violated such constraints, such as, Figs. 3 and 7 in [26], and Fig. 8 in [22]). Another reason may be that to impose such constraints on existing methods of radial distortion correction may bring difficulties to optimizations. However, in fact, we demonstrate that if using a deliberate strategy, such constraints can often be relaxed to the linear inequality constraints on the unknown coefficients of the radial distortion functions. Here, we take the 3-order polynomial $r_u = g(r_d) = k_1 r_d + k_2 r_d^2 + k_3 r_d^3$ as a very easy instance (Other order polynomials can be dealt with in a very similar manner). If the original objective function in some recent existing method for radial distortion correction is $J = J(k_1, k_2, k_3)$, the solution is corresponding to the global minimum of the objective function:

$$\min_{k_1, k_2, k_3} J(k_1, k_2, k_3)$$

If we impose the differential constraints as claimed in this paper, the optimization problem becomes

$$\min_{k_1,k_2,k_3} J(k_1, k_2, k_3)$$

$$\text{subject to } k_1 + 2r_d k_2 + 3r_d^2 k_3 > 0 \text{ for all } 0 < r_d \le r_{dmax}$$

$$2k_2 + 6r_d k_3 > 0 \text{ for all } 0 < r_d \le r_{dmax}$$

where the first order derivative $g'(r_d) = k_1 + 2k_2 r_d + 3k_3 r_d^2 = k_1 + 2r_d k_2 + 3r_d^2 k_3$, the second derivative $g''(r_d) = 2k_2 + 6k_3 r_d = 2k_2 + 6r_d k_3$, and r_{dmax} is the maximum of r_d in a given distorted image taken by a real camera. The second derivative greater than zero means that the radial distortion is barrel (And the second derivative less than zero is corresponding to pincushion distortion). The above optimization problem seems more difficult to solve. We relax it as follows:

$$\min_{k_1,k_2,k_3} J(k_1, k_2, k_3)$$

$$\text{subject to } k_1 + 2r_{di} k_2 + 3r_{di}^2 k_3 > 0, i = 1, ..., n$$

$$2k_2 + 6r_{di} k_3 > 0, i = 1, ..., n$$

where r_{di} are some sample points lying in between 0 and r_{dmax}. The number of sample points n, can be selected easily as some reasonable number, e.g., 100. In this paper, we simply let $r_{di} = \frac{i}{n} r_{dmax}$, $i = 1, ..., n$. Obviously, now the constraints become the linear inequalities in the unknown coefficients. For pincushion distortion, it can be solved in a very similar manner.

Recently, the division model with one coefficient proposed in [16] and its extended versions with more coefficients are very popular and often employed for radial distortion correction [5, 7–11, 17, 29–32]. However, different from the polynomial models as discussed above, we cannot relax differential constraints in the division models in a direct way, since the constraints derived from differential constraints in the division models are no longer linear inequalities in the unknown coefficients. However, in this paper we use a deliberate strategy to show that such problems still can be relaxed to linear inequalities, which will be discussed in details in the main text.

Furthermore, we take the method proposed in [22] as an instance to show how to relax differential constraints in the extended division models, and what changes may be caused by imposing the additional linear inequalities on the process of optimization. In the original method proposed in [22], the unknown coefficients of radial distortion were solved by finding the Moore-Penrose pseudoinverse of a matrix, i.e., it is a linear method. After imposing the additional linear inequalities, the problem becomes a convex optimization. That means the novel method considering differential constraints can still be solved easily, since there are many software kits for convex optimization. It does not require initial values, and any local minimum must be a global minimum. Especially, by comparing the experimental results from the original method in [22] and our novel method with differential constraints, we can find out that our method is able not only to ensure the recovered radial distortion function satisfy differential constraints within the feasible domain, but also to make the recovered radial distortion function working well in case of extrapolation.

2 The Division Undistortion Model with Differential Constraints

The division undistortion model is firstly proposed by Fitzgibbon [16], which described the relations between r_d and r_u as follows:

$$r_u = g(r_d) = \frac{r_d}{1 + k_1 r_d^2} \tag{1}$$

There is only one coefficient k_1 in the radial distortion function. We can easily find out that, in general, $k_1 > 0$ is corresponding to pincushion distortion, and $k_1 < 0$ is corresponding to barrel distortion. However, from Fig. 1a, we can find that for some pincushion distortion, e.g., $k_1 = 1$, the first order derivative of $g(r_d)$ change the sign where $r_d = 1$. Note that for a real lens, it cannot have such curve.

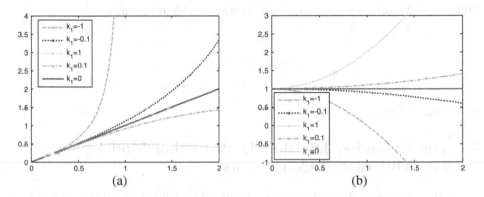

(a)   (b)

Fig. 1. (a) The curves of r_d vs. r_u under the division undistortion model, i.e., $r_u = \frac{r_d}{1+k_1 r_d^2}$, with different coefficient k_1 (Similar figure is shown as Fig. 2 in [31]). We can notice that for $k_1 = 1$, the sign of the first order differential of the curve changes where $r_d = 1$. Note that for a real lens, it cannot have such curve. (b) The curves for the denominator of the division undistortion model, i.e., $g_1(r_d) = 1 + k_1 r_d^2$ with different coefficient k_1.

The first order derivative of $g(r_d)$ is

$$g'(r_d) = \frac{1 - k_1 r_d^2}{(1 + k_1 r_d^2)^2} \tag{2}$$

and the second derivative of $g(r_d)$ is

$$g''(r_d) = \frac{-2k_1 r_d(3 - k_1 r_d^2)}{(1 + k_1 r_d^2)^3} \tag{3}$$

For barrel distortion, since $k_1 < 0$, $g'(r_d)$ and $g''(r_d)$ are automatically greater than zero in the feasible domain, i.e., $0 < r_d \le r_{dmax}$ (here we assume the denominator $1 + k_1 r_d^2$ not equal to zero, indeed such case means that the field of view of the real camera may be larger than 180 degrees, which will be discussed in the next section). Therefore, for barrel distortion with the division undistortion model, the optimization problem becomes

$$\min_{k_1} J(k_1)$$

$$\text{subject to } k_1 < 0$$

For pincushion distortion, $g'(r_d)$ should be greater than zero, and $g''(r_d)$ is less than zero. We cannot relax these differential constraints as the polynomial models described before, since the unknown coefficients of the radial distortion functions are no longer linear inequalities. We notice a fact that, $g'(r_d) > 0$ means that $1 - k_1 r_d^2 > 0$, since the denominator $(1 + k_1 r_d^2)^2$ is always greater than zero. Similarly, $g''(r_d) < 0$ means that $k_1 > 0$ and $3 - k_1 r_d^2 > 0$. Since $1 - k_1 r_d^2 > 0$ and $k_1 > 0$, must ensure that $3 - k_1 r_d^2 > 0$, for pincushion distortion with the division undistortion model, the optimization problem becomes

$$\min_{k_1} J(k_1)$$

$$\text{subject to } k_1 > 0$$

$$1 - r_{di}^2 k_1 > 0, i = 1, ..., n$$

where $r_{di} = \frac{i}{n} r_{dmax}$.

3 The Extended Division Undistortion Model with Differential Constraints

Since the division undistortion model proposed by Fitzgibbon [16] only has one coefficient, it is required to be extended with more coefficients to represent more complex radial distortion functions [5, 7–11, 29–32]:

$$r_u = g(r_d) = \frac{r_d}{1 + \sum_{i=1}^{m} k_i r_d^{2i}} \tag{4}$$

where $2m$ is the highest degree in the denominator. We indicate the denominator of $g(r_d)$ as

$$g_1(r_d) = 1 + k_1 r_d^2 + k_2 r_d^4 + k_3 r_d^6 \tag{5}$$

Obviously, it is an even-degree polynomial. Some curves of $g_1(r_d)$ corresponding to different m are shown in Fig. 2. Now, we take $m = 3$ as an instance (Other degrees can be dealt with in a very similar manner):

$$r_u = g(r_d) = \frac{r_d}{1 + k_1 r_d^2 + k_2 r_d^4 + k_3 r_d^6} \tag{6}$$

The first order derivative of $g(r_d)$ is

$$g'(r_d) = \frac{1 - k_1 r_d^2 - 3k_2 r_d^4 - 5k_3 r_d^6}{(1 + k_1 r_d^2 + k_2 r_d^4 + k_3 r_d^6)^2} \tag{7}$$

The second derivative of $g(r_d)$ is

$$g''(r_d) = \frac{-6k_1r_d + 2(k_1^2 - 10k_2)r_d^3 + (6k_1k_2 - 42k_3)r_d^5 + 12k_2^2r_d^7 + 34k_2k_3r_d^9 + 30k_3^2r_d^{11}}{(1 + k_1r_d^2 + k_2r_d^4 + k_3r_d^6)^3}$$

(8)

For barrel distortion, since $g'(r_d) > 0$ and $g''(r_d) > 0$ in the feasible domain (here we assume the denominator $1 + k_1r_d^2 + k_2r_d^4 + k_3r_d^6$ not equal to zero, indeed such case means that the field of view of the real camera may be larger than 180 degrees, which will be discussed later), we have

$$\min_{k_1,k_2,k_3} J(k_1, k_2, k_3)$$

$$\text{subject to } 1 - r_{di}^2 k_1 - 3r_{di}^4 k_2 - 5r_{di}^6 k_3 > 0, i = 1, ..., n$$

$$-6r_{di}k_1 + 2r_{di}^3(k_1^2 - 10k_2) + r_{di}^5(6k_1k_2 - 42k_3) + 12r_{di}^7 k_2^2 + 34r_{di}^9 k_2k_3 + 30r_{di}^{11} k_3^2 > 0$$

$$i = 1, ..., n$$

where $r_{di} = \frac{i}{n}r_{dmax}$. However, we notice that the constraints from $g'(r_d) > 0$ are linear inequalities in unknown coefficients, but the constraints from $g''(r_d) > 0$ are quadratic inequalities in unknown coefficients. As we know, in general, an optimization problem with quadratic inequalities is not easy to be solved. However, we find that the denominator of $g(r_d)$, i.e., $g_1(r_d)$, its first and second order derivatives, i.e., $g_1'(r_d) = 2k_1r_d + 4k_2r_d^3 + 6k_3r_d^5$ and $g_1''(r_d) = 2k_1 + 12k_2r_d^2 + 30k_3r_d^4$ may satisfy $g_1'(r_d) < 0$ and $g_1''(r_d) < 0$ for barrel distortion (see Fig. 3 in [26]). Therefore, for barrel distortion we have:

$$\min_{k_1,k_2,k_3} J(k_1, k_2, k_3)$$

$$\text{subject to } 1 - r_{di}^2 k_1 - 3r_{di}^4 k_2 - 5r_{di}^6 k_3 > 0, i = 1, ..., n$$

$$2r_{di}k_1 + 4r_{di}^3 k_2 + 6r_{di}^5 k_3 < 0, i = 1, ..., n$$

$$2k_1 + 12r_{di}^2 k_2 + 30r_{di}^4 k_3 < 0, i = 1, ..., n$$

(9)

where $r_{di} = \frac{i}{n}r_{dmax}$. If the field of view of a real camera is larger than 180 degrees, the denominator of $g(r_d)$, i.e., $g_1(r_d)$, can be equal to zero in some r_d corresponding to the view angle equal to 180 degrees, so $g'(r_d)$ and $g''(r_d)$ are undefined on this point. Therefore only $g_1'(r_d) < 0$ and $g_1''(r_d) < 0$ can be used here, i.e., for barrel distortion with the field of view larger than 180 degrees, we have

$$\min_{k_1,k_2,k_3} J(k_1, k_2, k_3)$$

$$\text{subject to } 2r_{di}k_1 + 4r_{di}^3 k_2 + 6r_{di}^5 k_3 < 0, i = 1, ..., n$$

$$2k_1 + 12r_{di}^2 k_2 + 30r_{di}^4 k_3 < 0, i = 1, ..., n$$

where $r_{di} = \frac{i}{n}r_{dmax}$. In Fig. 2b, we show some recovered curves estimated with differential constraints as claimed in this paper.

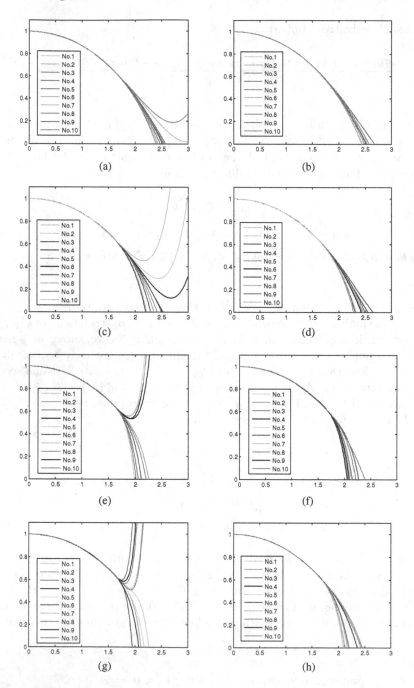

Fig. 2. (a)(c)(e)(g) Some recovered curves without differential constraints, for $g_1(r_d) = \sum_{i=1}^{m} k_i r_d^{2i}$ with different order m, where $m = 3, 4, 5, 6$, respectively (Similar figures are shown as Fig. 3 in [26]). (b)(d)(f)(h) Some recovered curves with differential constraints as claimed in this paper. Note that, the sample points are distributed within from 0 to 1.6. The portions of the curves with greater than 1.6 are the results of extrapolation.

4   Imposing Differential Constraints on Radial Distortion Correction Using the Constraints from the Images of Three Collinear Points

There are so many radial distortion correction methods in literature. Due to lack of space, we only show how to impose differential constraints on the method proposed in [22]. For a distorted image point $(u_d, v_d)^T$, if we establish the origin of the image coordinate system to the center of radial distortion, its corresponding undistorted image point $(u_u, v_u)^T$ under the extended division undistortion model with $m = 3$ may satisfies:

$$
\begin{bmatrix} u_u \\ v_u \\ 1 \end{bmatrix} \propto \begin{bmatrix} u_d \\ v_d \\ 1 + k_1 r_d^2 + k_2 r_d^4 + k_3 r_d^6 \end{bmatrix} \tag{10}
$$

where "$\propto$" denotes equality up to a scalar, and $r_d^2 = u_d^2 + v_d^2$. For three undistorted image points $(u_{ui}, v_{ui})^T$, $i = 1, 2, 3$, if they are collinear once rectified, we have

$$
\begin{vmatrix} u_{u1} & u_{u2} & u_{u3} \\ v_{u1} & v_{u2} & v_{u3} \\ 1 & 1 & 1 \end{vmatrix} = 0 \tag{11}
$$

From (9) and (10), we obtain [22],

$$
\begin{vmatrix} u_{d1} & u_{d2} & u_{d3} \\ v_{d1} & v_{d2} & v_{d3} \\ 1 + k_1 r_{d1}^2 + k_2 r_{d1}^4 + k_3 r_{d1}^6 & 1 + k_1 r_{d2}^2 + k_2 r_{d2}^4 + k_3 r_{d2}^6 & 1 + k_1 r_{d3}^2 + k_2 r_{d3}^4 + k_3 r_{d3}^6 \end{vmatrix} = 0 \tag{12}
$$

where $r_{di}^2 = u_{di}^2 + v_{di}^2$, $i = 1, 2, 3$. After some manipulations, and let

$$
a_1 = u_{d2}v_{d3}r_{d1}^2 - u_{d3}v_{d2}r_{d1}^2 + u_{d3}v_{d1}r_{d2}^2 - u_{d1}v_{d3}r_{d2}^2 + u_{d1}v_{d2}r_{d3}^2 - u_{d2}v_{d1}r_{d3}^2
$$
$$
a_2 = u_{d2}v_{d3}r_{d1}^4 - u_{d3}v_{d2}r_{d1}^4 + u_{d3}v_{d1}r_{d2}^4 - u_{d1}v_{d3}r_{d2}^4 + u_{d1}v_{d2}r_{d3}^4 - u_{d2}v_{d1}r_{d3}^4
$$
$$
a_3 = u_{d2}v_{d3}r_{d1}^6 - u_{d3}v_{d2}r_{d1}^6 + u_{d3}v_{d1}r_{d2}^6 - u_{d1}v_{d3}r_{d2}^6 + u_{d1}v_{d2}r_{d3}^6 - u_{d2}v_{d1}r_{d3}^6
$$
$$
b = u_{d2}v_{d3} - u_{d3}v_{d2} + u_{d3}v_{d1} - u_{d1}v_{d3} + u_{d1}v_{d2} - u_{d2}v_{d1}
$$

we have,

$$
a_1 k_1 + a_2 k_2 + a_3 k_3 = -b
$$

If there are s triplets of points, we may get s equations as follows:

$$
a_{1j} k_1 + a_{2j} k_2 + a_{3j} k_3 = -b_j
$$

where $j = 1, ..., s$. Then k_1, k_2, k_3 can be solved as follows:

$$
\mathbf{Ax} = \mathbf{b}
$$

where

$$\mathbf{A} = \begin{bmatrix} a_{11} \ a_{21} \ a_{31} \\ \vdots \\ a_{1s} \ a_{2s} \ a_{3s} \end{bmatrix}, \mathbf{x} = \begin{bmatrix} k_1 \\ k_2 \\ k_3 \end{bmatrix} \text{ and } \mathbf{b} = \begin{bmatrix} -b_1 \\ \vdots \\ -b_s \end{bmatrix}$$

Therefore, if $s > 3$, we can obtain an overdetermined least squares problem:

$$\min_{\mathbf{x}} \|\mathbf{Ax} - \mathbf{b}\|$$

The solution is:

$$\mathbf{x} = \mathbf{A}^+ \mathbf{b}$$

where $\mathbf{A}^+$ is the Moore-Penrose pseudoinverse of $\mathbf{A}$ [22]. If impose differential constraints on this optimization problem, we have

$$\min_{\mathbf{x}} \|\mathbf{Ax} - \mathbf{b}\|$$
$$\text{subject to } 2r_{di}k_1 + 4r_{di}^3 k_2 + 6r_{di}^5 k_3 < 0, i = 1, ..., n$$
$$2k_1 + 12r_{di}^2 k_2 + 30r_{di}^4 k_3 < 0, i = 1, ..., n$$

where $r_{di} = \frac{i}{n} r_{dmax}$. The above system represents a sparse convex quadratic program, and can be solved easily using a modern numerical package [33, 34].

5   Experiments

5.1   Simulation

We generate a mapping to simulate real radial distortion, and just select a part of the whole feasible domain of the independent variable to test the performances of methods with (i.e., our method) and without differential constraints (i.e., the method proposed in [22]). Gaussian noise with zero-mean and σ standard deviation is added to sample points of the mapping (Note that, the sample points are distributed within from 0 to 1.6. The portions of the curves with greater than 1.6 as shown in Fig. 2 are the results of extrapolation). We vary the noise level σ from 0 to 1 percent. The estimated results of the radial distortion functions with different degrees are shown in Fig. 2. It is not difficult to find out that our method with differential constraints is very suitable to make the recovered radial distortion function working well in case of extrapolation.

5.2   Real Data

A real image of a corridor was taken by a Basler PIA2400-17gc Color high resolution machine vision camera with Fujinon FE185C046HA-1 Fish-Eye Lens, as shown in Fig. 3a. The resolution of the image is 800×600. From this distorted

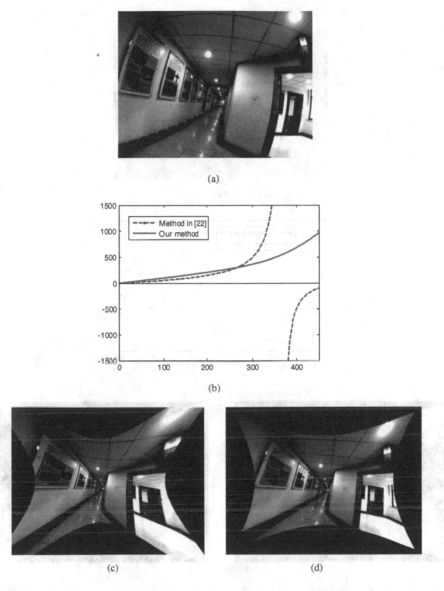

Fig. 3. (a) A real image of a corridor with radial distortion. (b) The recovered radial distortion functions with (i.e., our method) and without differential constraints (i.e., the method proposed in [22]). (c) The corrected image from the method without differential constraints [22]. (d) The corrected image from our proposed method with the differential constraints of (9). Note that [22] requires ten or more line images in a single image to obtain good results (see Fig. 10 in [22]). However, in this paper, with extremely less requirements, i.e., only some points lying on one line image, we can still obtain satisfactory results. From (b), we may find out that the recovered radial distortion function obtained from [22] maps some image points onto points at infinity, which obviously violated the differential constraints.

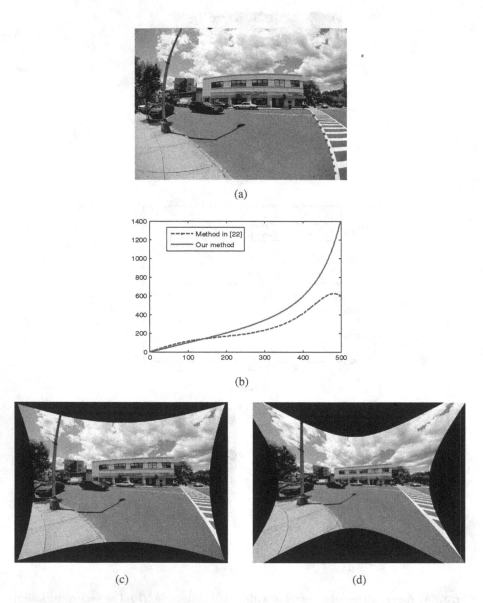

(a)

(b)

(c)   (d)

Fig. 4. (a) A real image of a street scene with radial distortion. (b) The recovered radial distortion functions with (i.e., our method) and without differential constraints (i.e., the method proposed in [22]). (c) The corrected image from the method without differential constraints [22]. (d) The corrected image from our proposed method with the differential constraints of (9). Note that [22] requires ten or more line images in a single image to obtain good results (see Fig. 10 in [22]). However, in this paper, with extremely less requirements, i.e., only some points lying on one line image, we can still obtain satisfactory results.

image, only about 10 sample points on an image curve of a space line are chosen. The corrected image is shown in Fig. 3cd. It is not difficult to find out that the correction results of all images of lines from our method look very reasonable. We also download some images with serious distortion from internet, and one of them is shown in Fig. 4a. We selected about 10 sample points on a single line image curve, and the corrected images are shown in Fig. 4cd. The corrected image from our method also looks very reasonable.

6   Discussions

Our approach seems able to be generalized to radial distortion models other than the polynomial and division models as discussed before. We take the distortion model used by Kanatani. Equation (5) in [12] as an example: $\theta = 2\tan^{-1}(c_0 r_d + c_1 r_d^3 + c_2 r_d^5 + \cdots)$. Our problem solving approach is based on a common-sense observation: Generally speaking, $c_0 r_d + c_1 r_d^3 + c_2 r_d^5 + \cdots$ should satisfy the differential constraints, otherwise, $2\tan^{-1}(c_0 r_d + c_1 r_d^3 + c_2 r_d^5 + \cdots)$ may "usually" violate the differential constraints. Note that, "$c_0 r_d + c_1 r_d^3 + c_2 r_d^5 + \cdots$ satisfies the differential constraints", is neither sufficient nor necessary condition for "$2\tan^{-1}(c_0 r_d + c_1 r_d^3 + c_2 r_d^5 + \cdots)$ satisfies the differential constraints". For a polynomial, which satisfies the differential constraints, we can easily convert it into linear inequalities as claimed in Sect. 1 of this paper. Even though such "simple" "relaxation" is not very "perfect" in mathematics, it seems to seek some better way to implement such differential constraints is very difficult. For other distortion functions, such as, log, sin, and etc., if they contain a polynomial(or even some function with a linear form with respect to distortion coefficients), we can also convert them into linear inequalities in the same manner. Especially, for the extended division model, the polynomial is in the denominator as discussed in Sect. 3.

7   Conclusions

Radial lens distortion is the most significant one among all kinds of lens distortions in recent cameras. Many models or called radial distortion functions with respect to the radius or the view angle are presented to describe radial lens distortion, and a lots of distortion correction methods are proposed by choosing the suitable one among these different radial distortion functions to accomplish their ideas. However, the differential constraints of these radial distortion functions were omitted in literature for a very long time. In this paper, we suggest the differential constraints should be imposed in the existing methods for radial distortion corrections. The constraints are that the signs of the first and second order derivatives of a radial distortion function with respect to the radius or the view angle should remain unchanged within the viewing frustum, or the feasible domain of the radius or the view angle, namely, from zero to the maximum of the radius or the view angle corresponding to the distorted image, although over the whole domain, the signs may be changed many times. Our method can be somewhat treated as a regularization of the distortion function within the viewing frustum.

To impose differential constraints on radial distortion correction, is very important and useful, since many examples often violated such constraints, such as, Figs. 3 and 7 in [26], and Fig. 8 in [22]. To impose differential constraints onto existing methods, is not trivial, but usually very, very difficult. We find some feasible approach to relax such differential constraints to linear inequality constraints on the unknown coefficients of the radial distortion functions. We imposed these constraints into the method proposed in [22] as an instance, which changes the original pseudo-inverse based linear method [22] into a novel convex optimization based method. It seems that to impose differential constraints on some existing methods of radial distortion correction may not bring too many difficulties into optimizations. Note that this paper just takes [22] as an example to show that we can implement differential constraints in some existing distortion correction methods. However, in fact, our basic idea is inspired from an observation: Some curves in Fig. 8 of [22], are very flat in some parts, look very strange, and do not satisfy the differential constraints. It is not difficult to incorporate the linear inequalities from differential constraints into the procedure of recovering the distortion center as proposed in [22]. Note that [22] requires ten or more line images in a single image to obtain good results (see Fig. 10 in [22]). However, in this paper, with extremely less requirements, i.e., only some points lying on a single line image, we can still obtain satisfactory results.

Acknowledgment. This work was supported in part by NKBPRC 973 Grant No. 2011CB302202, NNSFC Grant No. 61273283, NNSFC Grant No. 61322309, NNSFC Grant No. 91120004, and NHTRDP 863 Grant No. 2009AA01Z329.

References

1. Duane, C.B.: Close-range camera calibration. Photogram. Eng. **37**, 855–866 (1971)
2. Zhang, Z.: Flexible camera calibration by viewing a plane from unknown orientations. In: The Proceedings of the Seventh IEEE International Conference on Computer Vision, vol. 1, pp. 666–673. IEEE (1999)
3. Ying, X., Hu, Z.: Can we consider central catadioptric cameras and fisheye cameras within a unified imaging model? In: Pajdla, T., Matas, J. (eds.) ECCV 2004. LNCS, vol. 3021, pp. 442–455. Springer, Heidelberg (2004)
4. Barreto, J.P., Daniilidis, K.: Unifying image plane liftings for central catadioptric and dioptric cameras. Proc. OMNIVIS. **1**, 151–162 (2004)
5. Kannala, J., Brandt, S.S.: A generic camera model and calibration method for conventional, wide-angle, and fish-eye lenses. IEEE Trans. Pattern Anal. Mach. Intell. **28**, 1335–1340 (2006)
6. Hartley, R., Kang, S.B.: Parameter-free radial distortion correction with center of distortion estimation. IEEE Trans. Pattern Anal. Mach. Intell. **29**, 1309–1321 (2007)
7. Tardif, J.P., Sturm, P., Roy, S.: Plane-based self-calibration of radial distortion. In: IEEE 11th International Conference on Computer Vision, ICCV 2007, pp. 1–8. IEEE (2007)

8. Tardif, J.P., Sturm, P., Trudeau, M., Roy, S.: Calibration of cameras with radially symmetric distortion. IEEE Trans. Pattern Anal. Mach. Intell. **31**, 1552–1566 (2009)
9. Kukelova, Z., Pajdla, T.: A minimal solution to radial distortion autocalibration. IEEE Trans. Pattern Anal. Mach. Intell. **33**, 2410–2422 (2011)
10. Thirthala, S., Pollefeys, M.: Radial multi-focal tensors. Int. J. Comput. Vis. **96**, 195–211 (2012)
11. Kukelova, Z., Bujnak, M., Pajdla, T.: Real-time solution to the absolute pose problem with unknown radial distortion and focal length. In: Fifth IEEE International Conference on Computer Vision (2013)
12. Kanatani, K.: Calibration of ultrawide fisheye lens cameras by eigenvalue minimization. IEEE Trans. Pattern Anal. Mach. Intell. **35**, 813–822 (2013)
13. Stevenson, D., Fleck, M.M.: Nonparametric correction of distortion. In: TR 95–07, Computer Science, University of Iowa, Citeseer (1995)
14. Basu, A., Licardie, S.: Alternative models for fish-eye lenses. Pattern Recogn. Lett. **16**, 433–441 (1995)
15. Swaminathan, R., Nayar, S.K.: Nonmetric calibration of wide-angle lenses and polycameras. IEEE Trans. Pattern Anal. Mach. Intell. **22**, 1172–1178 (2000)
16. Fitzgibbon, A.W.: Simultaneous linear estimation of multiple view geometry and lens distortion. In: Proceedings of the 2001 IEEE Computer Society Conference on Computer Vision and Pattern Recognition, CVPR 2001, vol. 1, pp. I-125. IEEE (2001)
17. Claus, D., Fitzgibbon, A.W.: A rational function lens distortion model for general cameras. In: IEEE Computer Society Conference on Computer Vision and Pattern Recognition, CVPR 2005, vol. 1, pp. 213–219. IEEE (2005)
18. Shah, S., Aggarwal, J.: Intrinsic parameter calibration procedure for a (high-distortion) fish-eye lens camera with distortion model and accuracy estimation. Pattern Recogn. **29**, 1775–1788 (1996)
19. Xiong, Y., Turkowski, K.: Creating image-based vr using a self-calibrating fisheye lens. In: Proceedings of the 1997 IEEE Computer Society Conference on Computer Vision and Pattern Recognition, pp. 237–243. IEEE (1997)
20. Nave, T., Francos, J.M.: Global featureless estimation of radial distortions. In: 2nd International Conference on Signal Processing and Communication Systems, ICSPCS 2008, pp. 1–11. IEEE (2008)
21. Devernay, F., Faugeras, O.: Straight lines have to be straight. Mach. Vis. Appl. **13**, 14–24 (2001)
22. Tardif, J.-P., Sturm, P., Roy, S.: Self-calibration of a General Radially Symmetric Distortion Model. In: Leonardis, A., Bischof, H., Pinz, A. (eds.) ECCV 2006. LNCS, vol. 3954, pp. 186–199. Springer, Heidelberg (2006)
23. Barreto, J.P., Swaminathan, R., Roquette, J.: Non parametric distortion correction in endoscopic medical images. In: 3DTV Conference, 2007, pp. 1–4. IEEE (2007)
24. Hughes, C., Jones, E., Glavin, M., Denny, P.: Validation of polynomial-based equidistance fish-eye models. In: IET Irish Signals and Systems Conference (ISSC 2009), pp. 1–6. IET (2009)
25. Fujiki, J., Hino, H., Usami, Y., Akaho, S., Murata, N.: Self-calibration of radially symmetric distortion by model selection. In: 2010 20th International Conference on Pattern Recognition (ICPR), pp. 1812–1815. IEEE (2010)
26. Thirthala, S., Pollefeys, M.: The radial trifocal tensor: a tool for calibrating the radial distortion of wide-angle cameras. In: IEEE Computer Society Conference on Computer Vision and Pattern Recognition, CVPR 2005, vol. 1, pp. 321–328. IEEE (2005)

27. Cornelis, K., Pollefeys, M., Van Gool, K.: Lens distortion recovery for accurate sequential structure and motion recovery. In: Heyden, A., Sparr, G., Nielsen, M., Johansen, P. (eds.) ECCV 2002. LNCS, vol. 2351, pp. 186–200. Springer, Heidelberg (2002)

28. Gennery, D.B.: Generalized camera calibration including fish-eye lenses. Int. J. Comput. Vis. **68**, 239–266 (2006)

29. Byrod, M., Kukelova, Z., Josephson, K., Pajdla, T., Astrom, K.: Fast and robust numerical solutions to minimal problems for cameras with radial distortion. In: IEEE Conference on Computer Vision and Pattern Recognition, CVPR 2008, pp. 1–8. IEEE (2008)

30. Hughes, C., Denny, P., Glavin, M., Jones, E.: Equidistant fish-eye calibration and rectification by vanishing point extraction. IEEE Trans. Pattern Anal. Mach. Intell. **32**, 2289–2296 (2010)

31. Brito, J.H., Angst, R., Koser, K., Pollefeys, M.: Radial distortion self-calibration. In: 2013 IEEE Conference on Computer Vision and Pattern Recognition (CVPR), pp. 1368–1375. IEEE (2013)

32. Kukelova, Z., Bujnak, M., Pajdla, T.: Polynomial eigenvalue solutions to minimal problems in computer vision. IEEE Trans. Pattern Anal. Mach. Intell. **34**, 1381–1393 (2012)

33. Grant, M., Boyd, S., Ye, Y.: Disciplined Convex Programming. Springer, Heidelberg (2006)

34. Sturm, J.F.: Using sedumi 1.02, a matlab toolbox for optimization over symmetric cones. Optim. Methods Softw. **11**, 625–653 (1999)

Automatic Shoeprint Retrieval Algorithm for Real Crime Scenes

Xinnian Wang$^{(\boxtimes)}$, Huihui Sun, Qing Yu, and Chi Zhang

Dalian Maritime University, Dalian, China
wxn@dlmu.edu.cn

Abstract. This study is to propose a fully automatic crime scene shoeprint retrieval algorithm that can be used to link scenes of crime or determine the brand of a shoe. A shoeprint contour model is proposed to roughly correct the geometry distortions. To simulate the character of the forensic experts, a region priority match and similarity estimation strategy is also proposed. The shoeprint is divided into two semantic regions, and their confidence values are computed based on the priority in the forensic practice and the quantity of reliable information. Similarities of each region are computed respectively, and the matching score between the reference image and an image in the database is the weighted sum. For regions with higher confidence value, the similarities are computed based on the proposed coarse-to-fine global invariant descriptors, which are based on Wavelet-Fourier transform and are invariant under slight geometry distortions and interference such as breaks and small holes, etc. For regions with lower confidence value, similarities are estimated based on computed similarities of regions with higher confidence value. Parameters of the proposed algorithm have learned from huge quantity of crime scene shoeprints and standard shoeprints which can cover most practical cases, and the algorithm can have better performance with minimum user intervention. The proposed algorithm has been tested on the crime scene shoeprint database composed of 210,000 shoeprints provided by the third party, and the cumulative matching score of the top 2 percent is 90.87.

1 Introduction

It is generally understood that marks left by an offender's shoeprint at a crime scene may be helpful in the subsequent investigation of the crime [5]. According to statistics, 35 percent of crime scenes had footwear prints valuable in forensic science [11], and 30 percent of all burglaries provide valuable shoeprints [10]. Shoeprints are distinctive patterns that are often found at crime scenes and have been obtaining increasing importance in forensic investigations. The most challenging task for a forensic examiner is to work with highly degraded footwear marks and matching them to the most similar shoeprint available in the database.

Electronic supplementary material The online version of this chapter (doi:10. 1007/978-3-319-16865-4_26) contains supplementary material, which is available to authorized users.

© Springer International Publishing Switzerland 2015
D. Cremers et al. (Eds.): ACCV 2014, Part I, LNCS 9003, pp. 399–413, 2015.
DOI: 10.1007/978-3-319-16865-4_26

Some semiautomatic shoeprint retrieval methods based on various geometric patterns are reported in [3,10,20], and a series of patterns are chosen by human experts to classify the shoeprints. An automatic pattern classification method is proposed in [21], but it doesn't work well with debris and shadows.

Bouridane et al. [1,4] utilize fractals to represent the shoeprints and use a mean squared noise error as the similarity measure. Accuracy of the match is 88 % in classifying 145 images. This system does not attempt to answer the questions of partial, rotation or scale invariance.

Z. Geradts et al. [9] used the two-dimensional Fourier transform to classify those geometric shapes. Match was achieved with a neural network processing the Fourier transform coefficients and the positions of geometric shapes.

P. De Chazal et al. [8] use the power spectral density (PSD) to characterize the images for translational invariance, and the 2D correlation coefficient is used as the similarity measure. Results show that shoeprints are correctly matched in the top 5 % of the sorted DB patterns with an 85 % score. However, noisy images are not considered.

Fourier transforms modified phase only correlation (MPOC) is used in [12]. The reference DB consists of 100 different shoes available on the market and four sets of synthetic versions. The experimental result demonstrates a 100 % first rank recognition rate, but the system is not invariant under translation or rotation.

Hu's seven moments are employed in [2] in order to have translation, rotation and scale invariance. Hu's moments are used on a reference DB containing 500 shoeprints and their noisy rotated versions. Results show a sharp drop of accuracy to 5.4 % when the Gaussian noise variance is up to 0.2.

Gabor and Radon transform are used in [15] to extract multiresolution invariant features, and the first rank recognition rate can reach 91 %.

Maximally Stable Extremal Region (MSER) feature is used in [16] to identify the features of the shoeprint and the Scale Invariant Feature Transform (SIFT) descriptors are employed to describe them. The reference DB is made of 374 shoeprints. Each pattern class consists of two images, a reference set image containing a whole left and right print, while the test set is made of an image of either a complete left or right print. They reported a 94 % classification rate if viewing only 5 % of the database, but no tests are performed on noisy images.

An image retrieval algorithm combing the information of the phase and the power spectral density of the Fourier transform calculated on their Mahalanobis map is employed in [7] and [6]. The reference DB consists of 35 shoeprints and the system is tested on synthetic as well as on real shoeprints coming from crime scenes. They reported 91 % of the real case shoeprints found in the top 6.

Most of the above mentioned retrieval algorithms work well only with clear prints or synthetic shoeprints, but fail with crime scene shoeprints. The possible reasons are that they use features that are hard to be captured from the crime scene shoeprints, and the crime scene shoeprints are highly degraded and randomly partial. For example, (i) Real scene shoeprint images are always binarized to be separated from the backgrounds, but local invariant descriptors such as SIFT, MSER or SURF don't have good performance for binary images. (ii) There are many random extrusions, intrusions or breaks on the edges of patterns, and patterns are always randomly bridged. Fractal patterns and local invariant descriptors can be falsely extracted because of these interferences. (iii) Fourier based methods have better performance than fractal patterns and local invariant descriptors, but they are not well correlated with the human visual system.

2   Aim

In this paper, we propose a simple but efficient low quality shoeprint images retrieval algorithm, and the test images and shoeprint images in the database all come from real crime scenes without any synthetic shoeprints or generated partials. What the proposed algorithm differs from the other existing algorithms are on the capacity of the real crime scene database, Shoeprint Contour Model used for geometry correction, hybrid Wavelet-Fourier based global invariant feature descriptors and the robust matching strategy which has better correlation with the forensic experts.

3   Shoeprint Database

Two databases of shoeprint images are formed by more than 4,000 and 200,000 shoeprints provided by Dalian Everspry SCI &TECH CO., LTD, China. The first database consists of clear and full 4950 shoeprints created by taking impressions of footwear outsoles provided by footwear vendors, and in this paper, we refer this kind of shoeprints as standard shoeprints. The second databases is derived from the real crime scene and composed of variable quality left or right prints. Images from the second database possibly differ on position, orientation, scale, quantity of reliable information, quality and imaging conditions. Besides of some clear full prints, most images in the database are misaligned, incomplete and degraded prints interfered with debris, shadows or other artifacts. Some typical examples of both databases are shown in Fig. 1.

4   Methods

The proposed algorithm has two phases: on-line retrieval and off-line feature extraction. In the off-line feature extraction phase, every image in the constructed shoeprint database is firstly preprocessed to separate the shoeprint from backgrounds, and then Wavelet-Fourier based global invariant features of

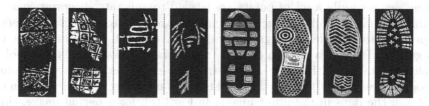

Fig. 1. Typical examples of shoeprints in the databases. The left four shoeprints are from real crime scenes, and the others are standard shoeprints.

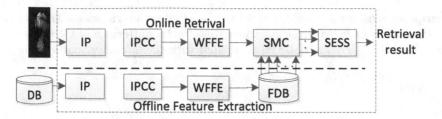

Fig. 2. The flow diagram of the proposed algorithm. IP, IPCC, WFFE, SMC, SESS, DB and FDB are abbreviations for Image Preprocessing, Image Partion and Confidence Computation, Wavelet-Fourier Based Feature Extraction, Similarity Measure Computation, Similarity Estimation and Score Sorting, Shoeprint Database and Feature Database, respectively.

each part are extracted, finally the features of each image are pooled into the shoeprint feature database prepared for print retrieval. In the on-line retrieval phase, confidence value and features of each part of every input image are computed, and then similarity measures of high confidence parts between the input image and an image in the database are computed, and similarity measures of low confidence parts are estimated based on computed similarity measures, and the similarity score between the input image and the image in the database is defined as the weighted sum of similarity measures of two parts, and finally outputs the ranked list of images based on the similarity score sorting. The flow diagram of the proposed algorithm is shown in Fig. 2.

4.1   Image Preprocessing

The goal of this stage is to separate the shoeprints from backgrounds and normalize the extracted shoeprints. Image preprocessing includes the following steps: (1) Shoeprint extraction: A local adaptive thresholding technique is used to extract the shoeprint images from backgrounds. We firstly split the image into a grid of cells and then apply a simple thresholding method (e.g. Otsu's method) on each cell to extract sub prints, and morphological operations are finally used to fill little holes and smooth edges. (2) Resolution normalization: The picture of the print is taken with a forensic scale near to the print and it is rescaled to a predefined dpi. (3) Orientation normalization: A Shoeprint Contour Model (SPCM) is proposed to normalize the shoeprint image.

The SPCM is to represent the shape of a shoeprint with a set of landmarks. Firstly enough shoeprint images with various shapes are collected to be as the training set. Secondly a set of points are labeled to annotate shoeprint contour, and finally dimensionality reduction technique are used to extract the average shoeprint contour model. In Fig. 3(a) and (b), given a full shoeprint image, the average SPCM model is used to estimate the initial positions, and a morphological close operation with larger size of structure element and an active contour method (e.g. Snake [22]) are used to find the best matching position between the model and the data in the input image. In Fig. 3(c), for a partial image, three points (front most point, rearmost point, and leftmost point) are marked interactively, and the shoeprint contour is estimated by the average SPCM model and the

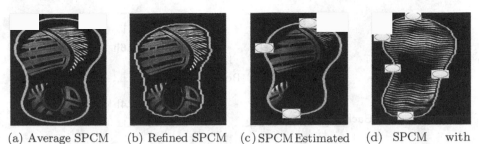

(a) Average SPCM   (b) Refined SPCM   (c) SPCM Estimated   (d) SPCM   with arch contour

Fig. 3. SPCM of the shoeprint images (White circles denote the landmarks)

landmarks. Once the contour of the input image is estimated, the shoeprint image can be aligned to the predefined orientation and position, and the scales can be refined. In practical applications, the region of foot arch usually can't be acquired from crime scenes, and the contour of foot arch just needs to be estimated coarsely. For accurate estimation of the foot arch, another two points besides of three points marked shown in Fig. 3(c) are needed to be labeled, and the two points are close to the maximum or minimum curvature points on the left or right boundary of the foot arch region respectively, which are shown in Fig. 3(d).

4.2   Image Partion and Confidence Computation

When an experienced forensic expert compares two shoeprints, he or she may divide a full shoeprint into toe section, sole section, instep (arch) section, heel section and back of heel section, and each section has a classification priority. The sole section has the highest priority, and the heel section has the second highest priority, and the arch section has the lowest priority. In the proposed algorithm, to simulate the character of the forensic experts, we define a confidence value which is biased toward those parts which: (i) have higher priority in the forensic practice and (ii) have much more reliable information.

Given a region $\mathbf{s}$, we define its confidence value $C(\mathbf{s})$ as the product of two terms:

$$C(\mathbf{s}) = P(\mathbf{s})H(\mathbf{s}) \tag{1}$$

We call $P(\mathbf{s})$ the priority term and $H(\mathbf{s})$ the information term. The confidence value of each region is used to be the weights of pooling region matching scores to be the total score. $C(\mathbf{s})$ is also used to judge whether the region can be used to retrieve shoeprints.

Based on thousands of crime scene shoeprints, we have found that patterns of the sole sections and the heel sections determine the retrieval results in most cases. Thus, the shoeprint is roughly divided into the top region and the bottom region. The top region mainly includes the toe section, sole section and parts of the arch section, and the bottom region mainly includes the other parts of the arch section, the heel section and the back of heel section. Each region is assigned a predefined priority value. The ratio of the top region height to the

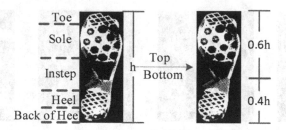

Fig. 4. Shoeprint partion

Table 1. Priority order of each section

Section number	Section of shoeprint	Rank order
1	Toe	3
2	Sole	1
3	Heel	2
4	Black of Heel	4
5	Instep	5

bottom region height is 3 to 2, which is learned from training samples. Details are shown in Fig. 4. The priority value is defined as:

$$P(\mathbf{s}) = 1 - \frac{\sum\limits_{j \in \mathbf{s}} R(j)}{\sum\limits_{i} R(i)} \tag{2}$$

where $\mathbf{s}$ represents the top region or the bottom region, $P(\mathbf{s})$ represents the priority value of region $\mathbf{s}$, $R(i)$ represents the priority order of each section. The priority orders of all sections are listed in Table 1.

Information value is used to measure the amount of reliable information of the two regions. For a region with all black pixels, the information value is set to 0. For a region with all white pixels, the information value is set to 1. The information value is defined as:

$$H(\mathbf{s}) = \frac{\sum\limits_{\mathbf{p} \in \mathbf{s}} \mathbf{I}(\mathbf{p})}{|\mathbf{s}|} \tag{3}$$

where $\mathbf{s}$ denotes the section, $|\mathbf{s}|$ is the area of $\mathbf{s}$, $\mathbf{p}$ is the pixel point, $\mathbf{I}$ represents the shoeprint image.

4.3 Wavelet-Fourier Feature Extraction

Three kinds of features which include fractal patterns, 2D Fourier Transforms or Fourier-Mellin Transform and local invariant descriptors have been commonly used to retrieve shoeprints in the literature. We have tested these features on more than 4 thousand kinds of standard shoeprints and 210 thousand real crime scene prints, and found that the three kinds of features work very well for standard shoeprints, synthetic prints or very clear and complete realcrime scene prints but failed for most of real crime scene prints.

Our perception of the universe uses different scales: Each category of observations is done in a proper scale. Using a larger scale, we can observe more details. Using a small scale, we can observe only macroscopic details of shoeprint patterns without seeing small holes, breaks, extrusions and intrusions. By changing the scale, we can observe or represent the object from coarse-to-fine. For these reasons, we use Wavelet transform [14] which represents both the spatial and frequency domain simultaneously to extract features of shoeprints across different scales. There is much redundant or irrelevant information contained in wavelet coefficients which are sensitive to translation, rotation and scaling, and Fourier-Mellin [13] transform is employed to extract discriminative invariant features in one or several special spatial-frequency subbands. We call this method Wavelet-Fourier transformation based global invariant descriptor. Since Fourier-Mellin transform can capture global invariant features, the proposed descriptor is not only global invariant under translation and rotation on each scale, but also has a multi-resolution matching ability.

The proposed feature extraction method has three steps. The first step is to transform a specified region of the input shoeprint $\mathbf{I(s)}$ to its wavelet domain, and $\mathbf{W}(l, h, v)$ is used to represent the wavelet coefficients where l denotes the level, h and v indicate the sub-bands of wavelet coefficients. The second step is to perform Fourier-Mellin transform on each band of wavelet coefficients and compute the power spectral density of the coefficients of Fourier-Mellin transform and filter out unnecessary coefficients. $\mathbf{M}(l, h, v)$ is used to represent the PSD of each band. The third step is to choose which bands of coefficients to be features. The flow diagram of the descriptor exaction is shown in Fig. 5.

The detailed steps of the feature extraction algorithm are as follows:

Step 1: Input the specified region $\mathbf{I(s)}$ with the confidence value greater than the predefined value. $\mathbf{I(s)}$ is decomposed using Haar Wavelet to a specified number of levels. At each level we will have one approximation subband and three details. The wavelet coefficients of $\mathbf{I(s)}$ can be described as:

$$\mathbf{W(s)} = \{\mathbf{W(l, h, v)}|0 \leq l \leq L, h, v = 0, 1\} \qquad (4)$$

where L is the maximum levels. To avoid merging the useful neighbor patterns, L should meet the critera: $2^{L-1} \leq D_{min}$, where D_{min} represents the minimum distance between two neighbor patterns which can be specified interactively.

Step 2: For each band of wavelet coefficients $\mathbf{W}(l, h, v)$, the Fourier-Mellin transform is applied, and the PSD of each band denoted as $\mathbf{M}(l, h, v)$ is computed. The processes are as follows:

Step 2.1: For a given band coefficients $\mathbf{W}(l, h, v)$, the PSD of its Fourier-Mellin transform is computed, and it is denoted as $\mathbf{P}(l, h, v)$ which is invariant under translation, rotation and scaling.

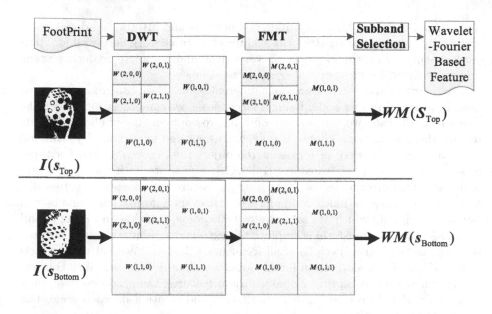

Fig. 5. Flow diagram of feature descriptor extraction

Step 2.2: In a shoeprint, large connected bridges between patterns appear in the PSD as very low-frequency components, and a high-pass filter $H(\xi, \eta)$ proposed in [18] is firstly used to weaken the effects of these components. Noises such as small holes, intrusions, extrusions and broken patterns appear in the PSD as very high-frequency components, and an ideal lowpass filter whose cut-off frequency is taken for 0.8 times of the highest frequency is then used to remove them. A band-pass filtered version of $\mathbf{M}(l, h, v)$ denoted as $\mathbf{P}(l, h, v)$ is finally obtained by previous two filters.

Step 3: This step is to determine which bands of coefficients to be the retrieval features. Each subband has different contribution to the retrieval results. For a highly degraded image, the approximation band is very important whereas details maybe interferences. For a shoeprint image with better quality, details can improve the accuracy. Subbands with rich information should be chosen intuitively. We use the standard deviation of $\mathbf{M}(l, h, v)$ to measure the information quantity, and choose the top k subbands to be the retrieval features:

$$\mathbf{WM(s)} = \{\hat{\mathbf{M}}^1(l, h, v) \cdots \hat{\mathbf{M}}^k(l, h, v)\} \tag{5}$$

where $\mathbf{WM(s)}$ represents the global invariance descriptor of region $\mathbf{s}$, $\hat{\mathbf{M}}^i(l, h, v)$ represents the ith subband ordered by the information quantity from the largest to the smallest value. For a highly degraded shoeprint, details are less important, and the approximation band of the highest level can directly be the features:

$$\mathbf{WM(s)} = \mathbf{M}(L, 0, 0) \tag{6}$$

The global invariance descriptors of the top region and the bottom region of the shoeprint with higher confidence can be computed, and they are denoted as

$\mathbf{WM}(\mathbf{s_T})$ and $\mathbf{WM}(\mathbf{s_B})$ respectively. These features are used to measure the similarities between two shoeprints. For shoeprints in the database, they are captured from different crime scenes with different quality, features of every suband are extracted for future use when constructing the feature database. For a shoeprint to be retrieved, the features are selected according to Eqs. (5) and (6).

4.4 Similarity Measure Computation

In order to compare a reference image with a database image, a measure of similarity between the images is required. The larger the measure of similarity between the reference image and the database image, the more similar the two images are. A reference image is compared to all images in the database and the similarity measure calculated for each comparison is used to rank the images in the database in a most similar to least similar order.

The similarity measure adapted in this paper is the 2D correlation coefficient [19]. For features $\mathbf{WM}_1$ and $\mathbf{WM}_2$, the correlation coefficient r is calculated using

$$
\begin{aligned}
\hat{\mathbf{W}}_1(\mathbf{s}) &= \mathbf{WM}_1'(\mathbf{s}) - \mathbf{W\bar{M}}_1'(\mathbf{s}) \\
\hat{\mathbf{W}}_2(\mathbf{s}) &= \mathbf{WM}_2'(\mathbf{s}) - \mathbf{W\bar{M}}_2'(\mathbf{s}) \\
r(\mathbf{s}) &= \frac{\hat{\mathbf{W}}_1(\mathbf{s})\hat{\mathbf{W}}_2(\mathbf{s})}{|\hat{\mathbf{W}}_1(\mathbf{s})||\hat{\mathbf{W}}_2(\mathbf{s})|}
\end{aligned}
\tag{7}
$$

where $\mathbf{WM}'(\mathbf{s})$ is the 1D vector representation of $\mathbf{WM}(\mathbf{s})$, $\mathbf{W\bar{M}}'(\mathbf{s})$ is the mean of $\mathbf{WM}(\mathbf{s})$, $\hat{\mathbf{W}}_1(\mathbf{s})$ and $\hat{\mathbf{W}}_2(\mathbf{s})$ represent features of region $\mathbf{s}$ from different shoeprints.

4.5 Similarity Estimation and Scores Computation

The shoeprint image is divided into the top and bottom regions. Similarities of each region are computed respectively, and the total similarity between the reference image and an image in the database is the weighted sum of the similarity measures of the two regions. For an input image, the similarity between its mirror version and an image in the database is also computed. The final score is the greater one, which is insensitive to the left print or the right print. The flow diagram of the matching score computation is shown in Fig. 6.

The matching score between the test shoeprint and the ith image in the database $g(i)$ is computed according to Eq. (8). For regions of higher confidence value, the similarity measure is computed directly according to Eq. (7). To weaken the effect of missing regions and regions of lower confidence value, the similarity measure of those regions can't be computed directly according to Eq. (7). If the confidence value of the specified region of the test shoeprint image is greater than the predefined threshold, and the confidence value of the image in the database is lower, the similarity measure is estimated from computed ones of images with higher confidence values, according to Eq. (17). If the confidence value of the specified region of the test image is also lower, the similarity measure is set to a predefined value. In order to let the full shoeprints of the same pattern in the

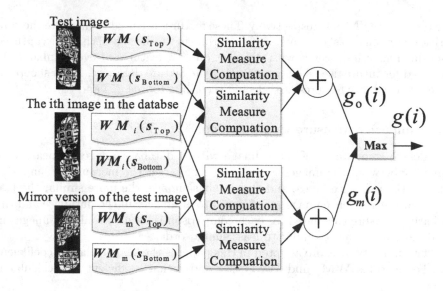

Fig. 6. Flow diagram of the matching score computation

database lie in front of the partial ones, the predefined value is not simply set
to 0, and it is obtained by means of trial and errors.

$$g(i) = \begin{cases} g_o(i) & g_o(i) > g_m(i) \\ g_m(i) & else \end{cases} \tag{8}$$

$$g_o(i) = T \bullet r_o(s_{Top}) + B \bullet r_o(s_{Bottom}) \tag{9}$$

$$g_m(i) = T \bullet r_m(s_{Top}) + B \bullet r_m(s_{Bottom}) \tag{10}$$

$$T = \frac{C(s_{Top})}{C(s_{Top}) + C(s_{Bottom})} \tag{11}$$

$$B = \frac{C(s_{Bottom})}{C(s_{Top}) + C(s_{Bottom})} \tag{12}$$

$$r_o(s_T) = \begin{cases} r(s_T) & C(s_T) > C_{th}(s_T), C_i(s_T) > C_{th}(s_T) \\ r_{oest}(s_T) & C(s_T) > C_{th}(s_T), C_i(s_T) < C_{th}(s_T) \\ r_{Top} & else \end{cases} \tag{13}$$

$$r_o(s_B) = \begin{cases} r(s_B) & C(s_B) > C_{th}(s_B), C_i(s_B) > C_{th}(s_B) \\ r_{oest}(s_B) & C(s_B) > C_{th}(s_B), C_i(s_B) < C_{th}(s_B) \\ r_{Bottom} & else \end{cases} \tag{14}$$

$$r_m(s_T) = \begin{cases} r(s_T) & C(s_T) > C_{th}(s_T), C_i(s_T) > C_{th}(s_T) \\ r_{oest}(s_T) & C(s_T) > C_{th}(s_T), C_i(s_T) < C_{th}(s_T) \\ r_{Top} & else \end{cases} \tag{15}$$

$$r_m(s_B) = \begin{cases} r(s_B) & C(s_B) > C_{th}(s_B), C_i(s_B) > C_{th}(s_B) \\ r_{oest}(s_B) & C(s_B) > C_{th}(s_B), C_i(s_B) < C_{th}(s_B) \\ r_{Bottom} & else \end{cases} \tag{16}$$

where $C_{th}(\mathbf{s}_T)$ and $C_{th}(\mathbf{s}_B)$ are the predefined thresholds, r_{Top} and r_{Bottom} are predefined default similarity values. After the similarities of regions with higher confidence values have been computed according to Eq. (7), $r_{oest}(\mathbf{s})$ is estimated from computed similarity measures:

$$r_{\text{oest}}(\mathbf{s}) = \frac{a(\mathbf{s}) + \varphi b(\mathbf{s})}{1 + \varphi} \tag{17}$$

$$a(\mathbf{s}) = \min_{i}(r_i(\mathbf{s})), s.t. C_i(\mathbf{s}) > C_{th}(\mathbf{s}) \tag{18}$$

$$b(\mathbf{s}) = \max_{i}(r_i(\mathbf{s})), s.t. C_i(\mathbf{s}) > C_{th}(\mathbf{s}) \tag{19}$$

where $r_i(\mathbf{s})$ represents the similarity measure, φ is the golden ratio which is 0.618.

5   Experiments and Results

5.1   Performance Evaluation Measure

The proposed algorithm is designed to sort shoeprint images of the database in response to a test image and present the ranked list to the user for final evaluation. An algorithm with higher performance will present fewer nonmatching images than an algorithm with lower performance. Cumulative Matching Characteristic Curve (CMC) is used to measure the accuracy performance of a retrieval algorithm operating in the closed-set identification task [17]. Images in the gallery set are compared and ranked based on their similarity with the test (probe) images. The CMC shows how often the probe image appears in the top n matches.

5.2   Test Images and Gallery Set

To evaluate the performance of the proposed algorithm, twelve groups of crime scene shoeprint images provided by the third party are used to be test images. Shoeprint images of each group have the same patterns, and have been acquired from different crime scenes with different image quality. The test images cover most patterns and possible cases that can be found in the real crime scenes. Each group has different number of images, and the total number of the test images is 72. Images from each group differ on position, orientation, scale, quantity of reliable information, quality and imaging conditions. In order to verify that the proposed algorithm is insensitive to geometry distortions, each test image is synthetically transformed into different translation, rotation and scaling versions, and another 432 images are inserted into the gallery sets.

Two gallery sets are constructed to test the performance. The first gallery set denoted as **GS$_1$** includes 72 test images, 432 generated geometry distortion versions of the test images and another 9592 crime scene shoeprints, and **GS$_1$** is often used by the third party to evaluate the performance of the retrieval algorithms. The second gallery set denoted as $\mathbf{GS_2}$ consists of about 210,000 real crime scene shoeprints of China. The proposed algorithm is used to retrieve the test images on these gallery sets and is evaluated by the CMC measure. It should be noted that many other shoeprints in the database have the same patterns with test images, but they aren't labeled, so the practical cumulative matching score of the proposed algorithm should be much higher than the experimental results.

5.3   Parameters Selection

The proposed algorithm has four main parameters, which are $C_{th}(\mathbf{s}_T)$, $C_{th}(\mathbf{s}_B)$, r_{Top} and r_{Bottom}. This experiment is to select the optimal value for every parameters, and the experiment is conducted on the gallery set $\mathbf{GS_1}$. The experimental result shows that the cumulative matching score can reach the highest one when the confidence value threshold is 0.03 and the estimated similarity is 0.3.

5.4   Performance of Anti-geometry Distortion

To verify the anti-geometry distortion ability of the proposed algorithm, 72 test images are respectively inputted into the retrieval algorithm, and statistically count the number of their synthetically generated geometry distortion versions lying in the top 7 in the ranked list of results. Since the gallery includes the test images, the first one in the sorted list is the test image itself. In theory, the transformed versions of the test image should be at the top of the sorted list, but in practice, the generated images may lose some information because of out of range, and some images of the same category may also lie in the top 7. Although the average percent is just more than 81 %, the left 19 % images are almost from the same classes. These results show the proposed algorithm is robust to geometry distortions.

5.5   Performance Comparisons with the State of Art Algorithms

Performance experiments are conducted on the two gallery sets $\mathbf{GS_1}$ and $\mathbf{GS_2}$ respectively, and the accuracies are shown in Table 2. The CMC curves are shown in Fig. 7. The experimental results show that the accuracy of top 2 % is more than 87.5 % on the gallery set $\mathbf{GS_1}$ and 90.87 % on the gallery set $\mathbf{GS_2}$. Furthermore,

Table 2. Retrieval performance of the proposed algorithm on $\mathbf{GS_1}$ and $\mathbf{GS_2}$

Datebase	Performance	Ranks of Retrieval Results						
		0.1 %	0.2 %	0.3 %	0.4 %	0.5 %	1 %	2 %
$\mathbf{GS_1}$	Accuracy (%)	45.2	64.1	69.4	73.8	75.8	81.8	87.5
	Cumulative Number	228	323	350	372	382	412	441
$\mathbf{GS_2}$	Accuracy (%)	68.7	75.2	77.6	80.0	80.8	84.7	90.9
	Cumulative Number	345	379	391	403	407	427	458

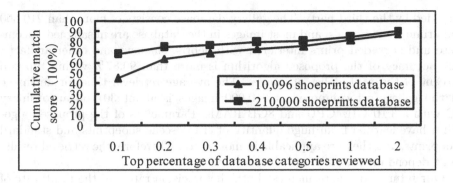

Fig. 7. CMC of the proposed algorithm on two gallery sets

Table 3. Comparison with other algorithms

Methods	Performance	Gallery set description
[4]	88 %	145 full-print images with no spatial or rotational variations
[8]	85 % (Top 5 %)	476 complete shoeprint images belonging to 140 pattern groups
[12]	100 % (the first rank)	100 shoeprint images and 6,400 generated images
[2]	99.4 % (Gaussian noise with variance 0.01)	500 clear and full shoeprints from shoe manufactures
[6,7]	91 % (Top 6)	35 shoeprints
Ours	45.2 % (Top 0.1 %)	10,096 crime scene shoeprints
	87.5 % (Top 2 %)	
	90.9 % (Top 2 %)	210,000 crime scene shoeprints
	94.1 % (Top 5 %)	

there are also a lot of unmarked same pattern images on the top 2 % of the ranked lists, and the accuracy of correct match would be much higher than the current accuracy.

As stated in introduction, most algorithms have better performance under their assumed conditions such as qualities of test images and capacity of the gallery set, etc. Due to lack of public evaluation databases and public available test softwares, comparisons just depend on what the literature reported, and the comparison results are listed in Table 3.

6   Conclusion

In this study, we proposed a simple but efficient low quality footprint images retrieval algorithm, and the proposed algorithm has been tested on the database provided by the third party. The gallery database consists of more than 210,000 real crime scene images, and most images in the database are misaligned, incomplete and degraded prints interfered with debris, shadows and other artifacts. The accuracy of the proposed algorithm is more than 90.87 % within top two percent of the ranked list of images. The average retrieval time for an image on the gallery set composed of 210,000 images is about 30 s on an ordinary PC with a 3.10 GHz CPU and 8GB RAMs. Parameters of the proposed algorithm have learned from huge quantity of crime scene shoeprints and standard shoeprints, and they are applicable in most cases. Therefore, the retrieval results don't depend on the skills of the operators.

Our future work is to increase both the precision rate and the recall rate of retrieving crime scene shoeprints with less reliable information.

Acknowledgement. This research has been supported by the Fundamental Research Funds for the Central Universities.

References

1. Alexander, A., Bouridane, A., Crookes, D.: Automatic classification and recognition of shoeprints. In: Proceedings of the International Conference on Image Processing and Its Applications vol. 2, pp. 638–641 (1999)
2. Algarni, G., Amiane, M.: A novel technique for automatic shoeprint image retrieval. Forensic Sci. Int. **181**, 10–14 (2008)
3. Ashley, W.: What shoe was that? The use of computerized image database to assist in identification. Forensic Sci. Int. **82**, 7–20 (1996)
4. Bouridane, A., Alexander, A., Nibouche, M., Crookes, D.: Application of fractals to the detection and classification of shoeprints. In: Proceedinds of the International Conference on Image Processing, vol. 1, pp. 474–477 (2000)
5. Bouridane, A.: Imaging for Forensics and Security: from Theory to Practice. Springer, New York (2009)
6. Cervelli, F., Dardi, F., Carrato, S.: An automatic footwear retrieval system for shoe marks from real crime scenes. In: Proceedings of the International Symposium on Image and Signal Processing and Analysis, pp. 668–672 (2009)
7. Dardi, F., Cervelli, F., Carrato, S.: A texture based shoe retrieval system for shoe marks of real crime scenes. In: Foggia, P., Sansone, C., Vento, M. (eds.) ICIAP 2009. LNCS, vol. 5716, pp. 384–393. Springer, Heidelberg (2009)
8. Chazal, P.D., Flynn, J., Reilly, R.B.: Automated processing of shoeprint images based on the Fourier transform for use in forensic science. IEEE Trans. Pattern Anal. Mach. Intell. **27**, 341–350 (2005)
9. Geradts, Z., Keijzer, J.: The image data rEBEZO for shoeprint with developments for automatic classification of shoe outsole designs. Forensic Sci. Int. **82**, 21–23 (1996)
10. Girod, A.: Computer classification of the shoeprint of burglar soles. Forensic Sci. Int. **82**, 59–65 (1996)
11. Girod, A.: Shoeprints - coherent exploitation and management. In: Proceedings of the European Meeting for Shoeprint Toolmark Examiners (1997)

12. Gueham, M., Bouridane, A., Crookes, D.: Automatic recognition of partial shoeprints based on phase-only correlation. In: Proceedings of the IEEE International Conference on Image Processing, vol. 4, pp. 441–444 (2007)
13. Gueham, M., Bouridane, A., Crookes, D., Nibouche, O.: Automatic recognition of shoeprints using Fourier-Mellin transform. In: Proceedings of the NASA/ESA Conference on Adaptive Hardware and Systems, pp. 487–491, 22–25 June (2008)
14. Neelamani, R.N., Hyeokho, C., Baraniuk, R.: Forward: Fourier-wavelet regularized deconvolution for ill-conditioned systems. IEEE Trans. Sig. Proc. **52**, 418–433 (2004)
15. Patil, P.M., Kulkarni, J.V.: Rotation and intensity invariant shoeprint matching using Gabor transform with application to forensic science. Pattern Recogn. **42**, 1308–1317 (2009)
16. Pavlou, M., Allinson, N.: Automated encoding of footwear patterns for fast indexing. Image Vis. Comput. **27**, 402–409 (2009)
17. Phillips, P.J., Moon, H., Rizvi, S.A., Rauss, P.J.: The FERET evaluation ethodology for face-recognition algorithms. IEEE Trans. Pattern Anal. Mach. Intell. **22**, 1090–1104 (2000)
18. Reddy, B.S., Chatterji, B.N.: An FFT-based technique for translation, rotation, and scale-invariant image registration. IEEE Trans. Image Process. **5**, 1266–1271 (1996)
19. Russ, J.C.: The Image Processing Handbook, 2nd edn. CRC Press, Boca Raton (1995)
20. Sawyer, N.: SHOE-FIT A computerized shoe print database. In: Proceedings of the European Convention on Security and Detection, pp. 86–89 (1995)
21. Tang, Y., Srihari, S.N., Kasiviswanathan, H., Corso, J.J.: Footwear print retrieval system for real crime scene marks. In: Sako, H., Franke, K.Y., Saitoh, S. (eds.) IWCF 2010. LNCS, vol. 6540, pp. 88–100. Springer, Heidelberg (2011)
22. Xu, C.Y., Prince, J.L.: Snakes, shapes, and gradient vector flow. IEEE Trans. Image Process. **7**, 359–369 (1998)

Lane Detection in Unstructured Environments for Autonomous Navigation Systems

Manh Cuong Le[✉], Son Lam Phung, and Abdesselam Bouzerdoum

School of Electrical, Computer and Telecommunications Engineering,
University of Wollongong, Wollongong, Australia
clm635@uowmail.edu.au

Abstract. Automatic lane detection is an essential component for autonomous navigation systems. It is a challenging task in unstructured environments where lanes vary significantly in appearance and are not indicated by painted markers. This paper proposes a new method to detect pedestrian lanes that have no painted markers in indoor and outdoor scenes, under different illumination conditions. Our method detects the walking lane using appearance and shape information. To cope with variations in lane surfaces, an appearance model of the lane region is learned on-the-fly. A sample region for learning the appearance model is automatically selected in the input image using the vanishing point. This paper also proposes an improved method for vanishing point estimation, which employs local dominant orientations of edge pixels. The proposed method is evaluated on a new data set of 1600 images collected from various indoor and outdoor scenes that contain unmarked pedestrian lanes with different types and surface patterns. Experimental results and comparisons with other existing methods on the new data set have demonstrated the efficiency and robustness of the proposed method.

1 Introduction

Lane detection plays a vital role in assistive navigation for blind people, autonomous vehicles and mobile robots. The aim of a lane detection system is to locate the lane region in each scene in front of the traveler. The system must cope with variations in the scene, the illumination condition, and the lane type. Automatically finding lanes using cameras is a popular approach for assistive navigation systems [1–3]. For autonomous cars, numerous vision-based algorithms of vehicle lane detection have been proposed [2,4–8]. However, there has been little work on pedestrian lane detection for assistive navigation of visually impaired people [1,9,10]. Furthermore, most existing pedestrian lane detection methods are designed to find pedestrian crossings, which are identified by painted markers [1,9–12]. To address this gap, this paper concentrates on vision-based detection of pedestrian lanes that have no painted markers for indoor and outdoor scenes, under varying illumination conditions and lane surfaces.

© Springer International Publishing Switzerland 2015
D. Cremers et al. (Eds.): ACCV 2014, Part I, LNCS 9003, pp. 414–429, 2015.
DOI: 10.1007/978-3-319-16865-4_27

Most existing methods for unstructured (i.e. unmarked) lane detection exploit the appearance properties (e.g. color and texture) of lane surfaces to classify the lane pixels from the background [6,13–15]. In these methods, the classifiers are trained off-line, and hence the detection performance is degraded when lane appearance differs from the training data (e.g. due to change in lane surface types or illumination conditions). In another approach, several algorithms detect the lane boundaries based on edge features (e.g. color and orientation) [2,16]. However, using only edges to identify the lane borders is sensitive to background clutter, and the detection performance is significantly affected by the robustness of edge detection.

This paper proposes a method for detecting unmarked pedestrian lanes, using appearance and shape information. In contrast to existing methods, the appearance model of the lane region is constructed on-the-fly employing the vanishing point, and therefore is invariant to varying illumination conditions and different lane surfaces. Furthermore, shape context [17] is used to model the shape of pedestrian lanes. The main contributions of the paper can be briefly described as follows:

- We propose an improved vanishing point estimation method, which is based on the votes of local orientations from color edge pixels. Using only edge pixels for voting the vanishing point is more efficient than using all pixels as in the existing methods [2,16]. Furthermore, to estimate robustly local orientations and edge pixels under severe illumination conditions, our method employs multiple color channels, instead of only the intensity channel.
- We propose using the vanishing point to identify a sample region on the input image for learning the appearance model of the pedestrian lane surface. The appearance model is thus adaptive to various types of lane surfaces. To make the appearance model invariant to different illumination conditions, a so-called illumination invariant space (IIS) is adopted.
- We propose a probabilistic model that combines both appearance and shape information for detecting unstructured pedestrian lanes. To evaluate pedestrian lane detection methods, we also create a new data set, collected from various indoor and outdoor environments with different types of unmarked lanes.

The remainder of the paper is organized as follows. Existing methods for lane detection in unstructured environments are reviewed in Sect. 2. The proposed method is described in Sect. 3. Experimental results are presented in Sect. 4. Finally, conclusions are given in Sect. 5.

2   Related Work

This section presents briefly vision-based approaches for unstructured lane detection. There are two major approaches: lane segmentation and lane border detection.

In the *lane segmentation* approach, off-line color models are used for classifying the lane pixels from the background [6,13,18,19]. The color models are first constructed from manually-selected sample regions, and then updated from the detected regions in the sequence frames. Different color spaces and color classifiers have been used. For example, Crisman and Thorpe use Gaussian models of red-green-blue (RGB) color components to represent the appearances of the road surface and background [6]. Tan *et al.* also use RGB components, but model the variability of the road surface by multiple histograms and the background by a single histogram [13]. Instead of using RGB components, Ramstrom and Christensen employ UV, normalized red and green components, and luminance to construct Gaussian mixture models for road surface and background classes. Sotelo *et al.* employ the hue-saturation-intensity (HSI) color space [18]. Because the color models are trained off-line, these methods do not cope well with the appearance variation of lane surfaces.

To address this problem, several algorithms construct the appearance model of the lane pixels directly from sample regions in the input image [7,20–22]. These algorithms determine the sample lane regions by different ways. For example, in [7,8], the sample lane regions are selected as small random areas at the bottom and middle parts of the input image. Miksik *et al.* initialize the sample lane region as a trapezoid area at the bottom and central part of the image, and then refine the sample region using the vanishing point [22]. He *et al.* determine the sample lane region from the potential lane boundaries, which are detected using the vanishing point and the width prior of lanes [20]. The performance of these algorithms depends on the quality of the sample regions, which in turns relies on the prior knowledge of the lanes.

In the *border detection* approach, the lane boundaries are determined using the vanishing point [2,16] or the predefined models of the lane boundaries [23]. In [16], the lane borders are detected simultaneously from edges directing to the vanishing point, employing the color difference between the lane region and non-lane regions. This method is effective only when the lane region is homogeneous and differs significantly in color from non-lane regions. Kong *et al.* also find the lane borders from edges directing to the vanishing point, except that their method uses the orientation and color cues of the edges [2]. Since this method is only based on edges for lane border detection, it is sensitive to background edges. In another method, the lane boundaries are located from the edges of homogeneous color regions, using the predefined models [23]. Recently, Chang *et al.* propose combining lane border detection and road segmentation for detecting the lane region [3]. Similarly to [2], their method detects lane borders using the vanishing point. The lane region is segmented using the color model learned from a homogeneous region at the bottom and middle part of the input image. Chang *et al.* 's method also relies on the prior knowledge of the lane location.

3   Proposed Method

The proposed method for detecting unstructured pedestrian lanes is based on the appearance and shape of the pedestrian lane. To make the detection method adaptive to different road surface structures, the appearance model of the lane region is learned automatically from a sample lane region, which is selected using the vanishing point. Shape context descriptor [17] is employed to model the shape of the lane region. The proposed method includes three main stages: vanishing point estimation, sample region selection, and lane detection. Each stage is described in the following subsections.

3.1 Vanishing Point Estimation

The vanishing point in an image is often found based on either line segments [4,24,25] or local orientations [2,26]. The algorithms using line segments are only suitable for structured environments where there exist straight edges. For unstructured environments, most existing vanishing point detection methods use local orientations [2,26,27]. These methods compute the local orientations of pixels using Gabor filters on the intensity channel, and therefore are not robust under challenging illumination conditions. Furthermore, the methods have high complexity and are sensitive to background clutter. To cope with the problems, we estimate the local orientations using the color tensors and detect the vanishing point employing the local orientations of edge pixels.

Given a color image $\mathbf{f}$, the tensor components are calculated on three color channels as in [28]:

$$
\begin{cases}
\mathbf{g}_{xx} = \sum_{k=1}^{3} \mathbf{g}_{xk}\mathbf{g}_{xk}, \\
\mathbf{g}_{yy} = \sum_{k=1}^{3} \mathbf{g}_{yk}\mathbf{g}_{yk}, \\
\mathbf{g}_{xy} = \sum_{k=1}^{3} \mathbf{g}_{xk}\mathbf{g}_{yk},
\end{cases}
\tag{1}
$$

where $\mathbf{g}_{xk} = \mathbf{w}*\mathbf{d}_x^k$ and $\mathbf{g}_{yk} = \mathbf{w}*\mathbf{d}_y^k$; $*$ denotes the convolution operator; $\mathbf{w}$ is the convolution kernel of a Gaussian filter; $\mathbf{d}_x^k$ and $\mathbf{d}_y^k$ denote the spatial derivatives of the color channel k. The local dominant orientation field is estimated as

$$
\theta = \frac{1}{2}\arctan\left(\frac{2\mathbf{g}_{xy}}{\mathbf{g}_{xx} - \mathbf{g}_{yy}}\right).
\tag{2}
$$

Figure 1(b) shows the local orientations of sampled pixels for the input image in Fig. 1(a).

To estimate the edge map of $\mathbf{f}$, we apply the color Canny edge detector, which is proposed in [28]. This edge detector computes the magnitude and orientation of pixels using the color tensor, and therefore is more robust than the conventional Canny edge detector using intensity gradients. Figure 1(c) shows the edge map detected from the input image in Fig. 1(a).

The vanishing point is determined by a voting scheme as follows. Each pixel location $v = (x_v, y_v)$ is considered as a vanishing point candidate, and voted by edge pixels $p = (x_p, y_p)$ that are below v. The voting score is computed as in [2]:

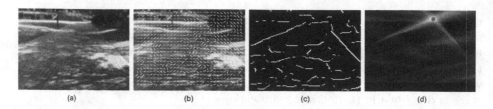

Fig. 1. Illustration of vanishing point estimation: (a) input image, (b) local orientations estimated by the color tensor for sampled pixels, (c) edge map, (d) voting map and the vanishing point (in red) (Colour figure online).

$$s(v,p) = \begin{cases} \frac{1}{1+(\delta\mu)^2} & \text{if } \delta \leq \frac{5}{1+2\mu}, \\ 0 & \text{otherwise.} \end{cases} \tag{3}$$

Here, δ is the difference between the local orientation $\theta(x_p, y_p)$ and the angle of the line L_{vp} connecting v and p; μ be the ratio between the length of L_{vp} and the diagonal length of the image. Equation (3) means that $s(v, p)$ is high when edge pixel p is close to v and is consistent in orientation with the line L_{vp}. The vanishing point is finally found as the point that has the highest sum of the voting scores. Figure 1(d) demonstrates the voting map and the vanishing point computed for the image in Fig. 1(a).

3.2   Sample Region Selection

Since the appearance (e.g. texture and color) of pedestrian lane regions is varied and strongly affected by illumination conditions, it is difficult to obtain an robust appearance model via off-line training. In our method, the appearance model is computed directly on the input image. Based on the vanishing point estimated in the previous step, a sample region of the pedestrian lane is automatically selected, and the appearance model is then constructed from the pixels in the sample region.

In existing methods (e.g. [8,21,22]), the sample region is chosen as a small region at the bottom and middle of the input image. However, the sample region selected in such a manner may include the background when the lane region is not located at the middle of the image. In our method, the sample region is automatically detected using the vanishing point and the geometric and appearance characteristics of the lane region.

Given the vanishing point estimated in the previous step, a set of N imaginary rays $\{r_1, r_2, ..., r_N\}$ is created as shown in Fig. 2(a). These rays are uniformly distributed in a fixed angle range $[\alpha_{\min}, \alpha_{\max}]$ relative to the horizontal direction. The training region is identified by finding a ray pair (r_i, r_j) that best represents the characteristics of the lane region. These characteristics include: (1) the lane direction φ estimated as the direction of the bisector between r_i and r_j; (2) the uniformity u of color pixels in the lane region R_{ij} formed by a ray pair (r_i, r_j) as shown in Fig. 2(b). The uniformity u is computed using the color histogram.

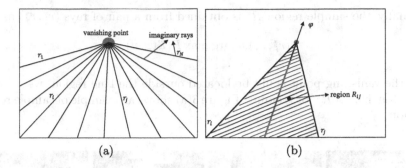

Fig. 2. Imaginary rays: (a) imaginary rays; (b) a pair of rays.

This is similar to [29], except that our method uses three color channels instead of intensity:

$$u = \sum_{m=1}^{M} \sum_{n=1}^{M} \sum_{k=1}^{M} h(m, n, k)^2. \tag{4}$$

Here, h is the normalized 3-D color histogram of R_{ij}, and M is the number of bins for each color channel.

Let $\mathcal{L}$ denote the lane class. The conditional probability of $\mathcal{L}$ for two features φ and u can be expressed as

$$P(\mathcal{L}|\varphi, u) \propto p(\varphi, u|\mathcal{L})P(\mathcal{L}) \propto p(\varphi|\mathcal{L})p(u|\mathcal{L}), \tag{5}$$

where $P(\mathcal{L})$ is prior probability, $p(\varphi|\mathcal{L})$ and $p(u|\mathcal{L})$ are the class-conditional probability density functions (*pdf*). Here, we assume that $p(\varphi, u)$ is uniform, $P(\mathcal{L})$ is constant, φ and u are statistically independent for a given $\mathcal{L}$.

We have found that the distribution of the lane directions φ in the training set is similar to a normal distribution. Therefore, $p(\varphi|\mathcal{L})$ is modeled as

$$p(\varphi_{ij}|\mathcal{L}) = \frac{1}{\sigma\sqrt{2\pi}} e^{-\frac{(\varphi-\overline{\varphi})^2}{2\sigma^2}}, \tag{6}$$

where $\overline{\varphi}$ and σ are the mean value and standard deviation of φ that are computed using the training data.

Our experiments have shown that lane regions have high uniformity and u varies in a range from 0 to 1. Based on these characteristics, we model $p(u|\mathcal{L})$ using the beta function as

$$p(u|\mathcal{L}) = \frac{1}{B(\alpha, \beta)} u^{\alpha-1}(1 - u)^{\beta-1}, \tag{7}$$

where $B(\alpha, \beta)$ is the beta function, α and β are positive parameters. These parameters are selected so that $p(u|\mathcal{L})$ is high when u is high, and vice versa.

Finally, the sample region R^* is obtained from a pair of rays (r_i^*, r_j^*) as

$$(r_i^*, r_j^*) = \arg\max_{r_i, r_j} P(\mathcal{L}|\varphi, u). \tag{8}$$

Since the vanishing point could be located outside the lane region, we use only the bottom half of R^* for training. Figure 3(a) shows an example of sample region selection.

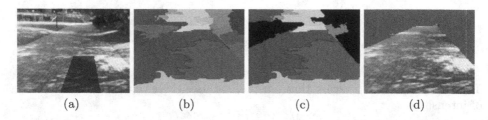

(a)   (b)   (c)   (d)

Fig. 3. Illustration of the proposed method for pedestrian lane detection: (a) training region (blue area) extracted from the vanishing point (red dot); (b) segmented regions using graph-based segmentation method [30]; (c) candidate regions considered in $\mathcal{R}'$ (background regions are marked in black); (d) detected walking lane (Colour figure online).

Given the sample region R^*, the appearance model of the lane region is represented as the class-conditional *pdf* $p(\mathbf{c}|\mathcal{L})$ of colors $\mathbf{c}$ for the lane class $\mathcal{L}$. The *pdf* $p(\mathbf{c}|\mathcal{L})$ is estimated using the color histogram of pixels in R^*. However, instead of using the RGB space which is sensitive to illumination conditions and shading, we convert colors from the RGB space to an illumination invariant space (IIS) [31] as

$$\begin{cases} C_1 &= \arctan\{R/\max(G, B)\}, \\ C_2 &= \arctan\{G/\max(R, B)\}, \\ C_3 &= \arctan\{B/\max(R, G)\}. \end{cases} \tag{9}$$

Figure 4 shows the color distribution of a lane region in the RBG and IIS space. The lane pixels have less variations in the IIS space than the RGB space.

3.3   Lane Detection

This subsection presents a method to detect the walking lane in the input image using both appearance and shape information. In our method, the input image is first segmented into homogeneous regions. The walking lane region is then determined by merging those image regions using appearance and shape criteria.

Let $\mathcal{R} = \{R_1, R_2, ...\}$ be the set of homogeneous regions obtained using the graph-based segmentation method in [30]. Figure 3(b) illustrates the homogeneous regions segmented from the input image in Fig. 3(a). The lane region is

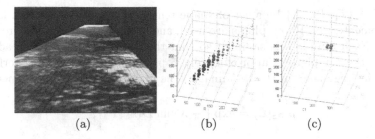

(a)   (b)   (c)

Fig. 4. Color distributions of lane pixels: (a) a sample lane region; (b) color distribution of lane pixels in the RGB space; (c) color distribution of lane pixels in the IIS space.

a combination of connected regions of $\mathcal{R}$. The two regions R_i and R_j are considered as connected if there exist two pixels $p_i \in R_i$ and $p_j \in R_j$ that are connected (e.g. 4-connected pixels). The lane region is the subset Z^* of $\mathcal{R}$ such that

$$
\begin{aligned}
Z^* &= \arg\max_{Z \subset \mathcal{R}} p(Z|\mathcal{L}) \\
&= \arg\max_{Z \subset \mathcal{R}} p(\bar{\mathbf{c}}_z, \mathbf{s}_z|\mathcal{L}) \\
&= \arg\max_{Z \subset \mathcal{R}} p(\bar{\mathbf{c}}_z|\mathcal{L}) p(\mathbf{s}_z|\mathcal{L}).
\end{aligned}
\tag{10}
$$

Here, $\bar{\mathbf{c}}_z$ is an appearance feature and $\mathbf{s}_z$ is a shape feature of region Z. It is also assumed that $\bar{\mathbf{c}}_z$ and $\mathbf{s}_z$ are statistically independent.

In (10), $\bar{\mathbf{c}}_z$ is defined as the mean color of all pixels in Z, and $p(\bar{\mathbf{c}}_z|\mathcal{L})$ is the *pdf* of the lane color and is learned from the sample region. For shape feature $\mathbf{s}_z$, we adopt the shape context descriptor proposed in [17]. Shape context descriptor is known for its robustness to local shape deformation and partial occlusion, and its invariance to scale and rotation. The shape context of a point p is the histogram of locations of points other than p in relative to p. The similarity between two shapes is computed as the matching cost between the corresponding sets of points on the two shapes.

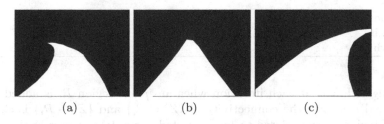

(a)   (b)   (c)

Fig. 5. Several shape templates of the lane region: (a) left-curved lane, (b) straight lane, (c) right-curved lane.

Let $\mathcal{T} = \{T_1, T_2, \ldots\}$ be a set of shape templates for the pedestrian lane. In our implementation, 10 templates are used, and some of the templates are shown in Fig. 5. Each template is sampled so that the distance between two adjacent points on the template is approximately 5 pixels. The sampling is performed similarly for regions Z in the test image. The likelihood $p(\mathbf{s}_z|\mathcal{L})$ is defined as

$$p(\mathbf{s}_z|\mathcal{L}) = \exp\left[-\lambda \min_{T \in \mathcal{T}} D(\mathbf{s}_z, T)\right], \tag{11}$$

where $D(\mathbf{s}_z, T)$ is the matching cost between the approximated outer contour $\mathbf{s}_z$ and a template T as in [17]. Note that the smaller is the matching cost $D(\mathbf{s}_z, T)$, the higher is the similarity between $\mathbf{s}_z$ and T, and therefore the likelihood $p(\mathbf{s}_z|\mathcal{L})$ is higher. In (11), λ is a positive scalar determined through training data.

Given the appearance likelihood $p(\bar{\mathbf{c}}_z|\mathcal{L})$ calculated from the sample region and shape likelihood $p(\mathbf{s}_z|\mathcal{L})$ defined in (11), the optimal set Z^* can be obtained with a computational complexity of $O(2^{|\mathcal{R}|})$ by exhaustively searching every possible sub-set of $\mathcal{R}$. To reduce the computational burden, we propose a greedy algorithm that generates Z^* by iteratively adding and removing regions. To further accelerate the algorithm, we only consider regions $R_i \in \mathcal{R}$ with $p(\bar{\mathbf{c}}_i|\mathcal{L})$ greater than or equal to τ_c, where $\bar{\mathbf{c}}_i$ is the mean color of all pixels in R_i and τ_c is a predefined threshold. The greedy algorithm is described in *Algorithm* 1.

Algorithm 1. Adding and moving regions for lane detection.

$\mathcal{R}' \leftarrow \{R_i \in \mathcal{R} \mid p(\bar{\mathbf{c}}_i|\mathcal{L}) \geq \tau_c\}$
$Z^* \leftarrow \arg\max_{R_i \in \mathcal{R}'} p(\bar{\mathbf{c}}_i|\mathcal{L})$
continue $\leftarrow$ TRUE
while (*continue*) **do**
    $\mathcal{R}_a \leftarrow \{R_i \in \{\mathcal{R}' - Z^*\}$ so that $Z^* \cup R_i$ is a connected set$\}$
    $R^+ = \arg\max_{R_i \in \mathcal{R}_a} p(\{Z^* \cup R_i\}|\mathcal{L})$
    $\mathcal{R}_r \leftarrow \{R_i \in Z^*$ so that $\{Z^* - R_i\}$ is a connected set$\}$
    $R^- = \arg\max_{R_i \in \mathcal{R}_r} p(\{Z^* - R_i\}|\mathcal{L})$
    if $p(\{Z^* \cup R^+\}|\mathcal{L}) \geq p(\{Z^* - R^-\}|\mathcal{L})$ **and** $p(\{Z^* \cup R^+\}|\mathcal{L}) > p(Z^*|\mathcal{L})$ **then**
        $Z^* \leftarrow Z^* \cup R^+$
    else if $p(\{Z^* - R^-\}|\mathcal{L}) > p(Z^*|\mathcal{L})$ **then**
        $Z^* \leftarrow \{Z^* - R^-\}$
    else
        continue $\leftarrow$ FALSE
    end if
end while

In Algorithm 1, at each iteration when an image region R_i is added to Z^* or removed from Z^*, the connectivity of $\{Z^* \cup R_i\}$ and $\{Z^* - R_i\}$ is checked. A set of regions is considered to be connected if any two regions in the set are connected. For example, supposed that set Z^* in Fig. 6 consists of regions 2, 6, 7, 8, and 10. Region 8 will not be removed from Z^* because doing so will break the connectivity of Z^*. Similarly, region 3 will not be added to Z^*.

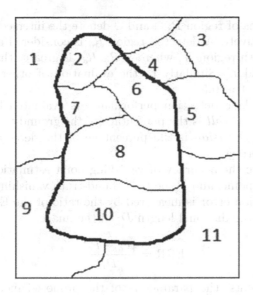

Fig. 6. Illustration of adding and removing regions.

Because the number of regions is finite and operators in Algorithm 1 are deterministic, the algorithm will converge. Figure 3(d) illustrates the result of lane detection using Algorithm 1 for the input image shown in Fig. 3(a).

4   Experimental Results

This section describes the image data, evaluation measures and parameters employed in the proposed method. It also presents experimental results for vanishing point estimation and pedestrian lane detection.

4.1   Experimental Methods

To evaluate the proposed method, we collected a data set of 1600 images in different indoor and outdoor scenes. The data set includes unmarked pedestrian lanes with various surface structures and shapes. In many cases, lane regions are affected by extreme illumination conditions (e.g. very low or high illumination). We manually annotated lane regions and determined the vanishing point in each image. In the experiments, we used 500 images for training, and 1100 images for testing. Note that the training set was employed only for estimating the orientation angles of lane regions and finding the parameters of the proposed method, it was not used for learning the appearance model.

To measure the detection performance, detected regions are compared with annotated regions. Let R_d denote a detected region and R_g denote a ground-truth region. The matching score between R_d and R_g is computed as

$$\chi(R_g, R_d) = \frac{|R_g \cap R_d|}{|R_g \cup R_d|}, \tag{12}$$

where $|R|$ is the area of region R, $\cap$ and $\cup$ denote the intersection and union of R_d and R_g, respectively. A detected region R_d is considered as *correct* if there exists a ground-truth region R_g where $\chi(R_g, R_d)$ is greater than or equal to an evaluation threshold τ_e. Similarly to the evaluation of other object detection systems [32], τ_e is set to 0.5.

The pedestrian lane detection performance is evaluated by two measures: recall and precision. *Recall* is the percentage of the ground-truth lanes that are detected correctly. *Precision* is the percentage of the detected lanes that are considered to be correct.

We also evaluate the accuracy of vanishing point estimation. Let P_d be the detected vanishing point, and P_g be the ground-truth vanishing point. Similarly to [27], the estimation error is measured by the ratio of the Euclidean distance from P_d to P_g and the diagonal length D_I of the image:

$$\text{ERR} = \frac{|P_d - P_g|}{D_I}. \tag{13}$$

In our experiments, the parameters of the proposed method were chosen based on analyzing the performance of the pedestrian lane detection on the training set. The window size $L \times L$ of $\mathbf{w}$ in Sect. 3.1 and the number of imaginary rays N in Sect. 3.2 are chosen as $N = 29$ and $L = 13$. Each color component in the IIS space is quantized into 180 bins. The parameters α and β in (7), λ in (11) and threshold τ_c in Sect. 3.3 are set as $\alpha = 2$, $\beta = 1$, $\lambda = 25$, and $\tau_c = 0.02$.

4.2   Experimental Results

The proposed vanishing point estimation (VPE) method was evaluated and compared with two existing algorithms: Hough-based method [4] and Gabor-based method [2]. The Hough-based method applies the Hough transform on the edge map to find line segments, and then computes the vanishing point by voting the intersections of line pairs in the Hough space [4]. The Gabor-based method employs Gabor filters for computing local orientations, and a local adaptive scheme for estimating the vanishing point [2].

Table 1 shows the performance of different VPE algorithms. The average error of the proposed method (0.057) was significantly lower than the Gabor-based method (0.086) and the Hough-based method (0.250). Furthermore, the average processing time per image (of size 100×140 pixels) of the proposed method (0.60 s) was significantly shorter than the Gabor-based method (3.00 s).

Table 1. Accuracy and speed of algorithms for vanishing point estimation.

Methods	Average error	Computational time (s)
Hough-based method [4]	0.250	0.06
Gabor-based method [2]	0.086	3.00
Proposed method	**0.057**	**0.60**

The Hough-based method had the shortest processing time, but it also had the lowest accuracy. Figure 7 shows several visual results of different VPE methods.

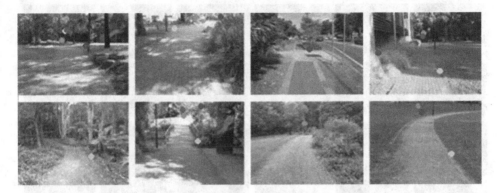

Fig. 7. Visual results of vanishing point (VP) detection: red dot is the ground-truth VP; green dot is the VP detected by the proposed method; yellow dot is the VP detected by Hough-based method [4]; blue dot is the VP detected by Gabor-based method in [2]. See electronic color image (Colour figure online).

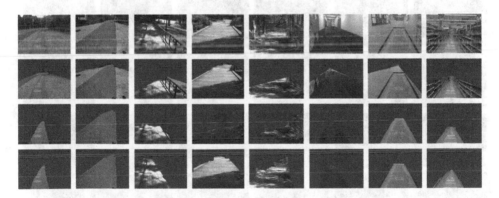

Fig. 8. Visual results of different methods for pedestrian lane detection. *Row 1*: input images. *Row 2*: pedestrian lanes detected by the method in [2]. *Row 3*: pedestrian lanes detected by the proposed method using the RGB color space. *Row 4*: pedestrian lanes detected by the proposed method using the IIS color space.

For pedestrian lane detection, we evaluated the proposed method using the IIS and RGB color space. In this comparison, the proposed VPE method was used for both color spaces. As shown in the last two rows of Table 2, using the IIS space, the proposed method achieved a recall rate of 94.8 % and a precision rate of 95.1 %. Using the RGB space, the recall and precision rate decreased to 91.2 % and 92.6 %, respectively.

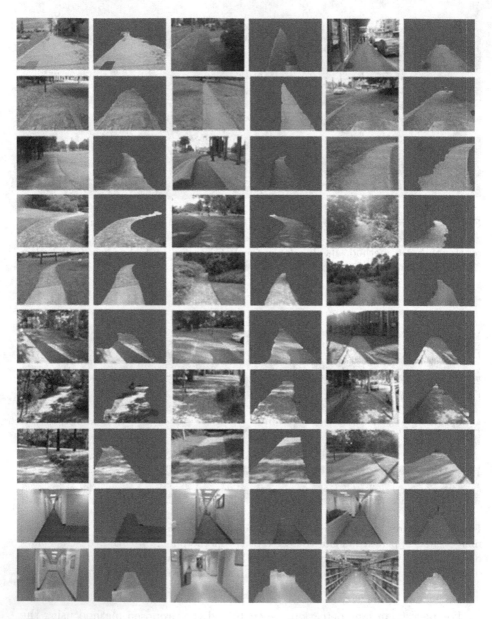

Fig. 9. Visual results of pedestrian lane detection. Column 1, 3 and 5:input images. Column 2, 4 and 6: detected lanes.

Table 2. Comparison of algorithms for pedestrian lane detection.

Methods	Recall (%)	Precision (%)	Processing time (s)
Lane border detection [2]	63.9	66.0	3.7
Proposed VPE + RGB	91.2	92.6	1.8
Proposed VPE + IIS	**94.8**	**95.1**	**1.8**

We also compared the proposed method with the lane border detection method of Kong *et al.* [2]. The method in [2] employs the vanishing point to determine the lane borders. As shown Table 2, the proposed method (recall rate of 94.8 % and precision rate of 95.1 %) outperformed significantly the method in [2] (recall rate of 63.9 % and precision rate of 66.0 %). Figure 8 shows several comparative results of different methods for pedestrian lane detection. These results demonstrate that the proposed method using the IIS color space is more robust than the proposed method using the RGB color space and the lane border detection method in [2].

Our MATLAB implementation took 1.8 s, on the average, to process an image of size 100 × 140 pixels. We consider speeding-up the method as future work. Several detection results of the proposed method are demonstrated in Fig. 9. The experimental results show that the proposed method detects robustly pedestrian lanes with various lane surface structures and shapes and under different illumination and weather conditions.

5   Conclusion

This paper presents a method for pedestrian lane detection in unstructured environments. The proposed method makes use the vanishing point to automatically determine a sample region from which an appearance model of the lane surface is constructed. Shape context descriptor is used to describe the shape of the lane region. The walking lane is then detected using both the appearance and shape features in a probabilistic approach. The proposed method is evaluated and compared with existing methods on a large data set collected from various environments. The experimental results have demonstrated that the proposed method is able to detect various types of unstructured pedestrian lanes under challenging environmental conditions. It also compares favorably with the existing methods.

References

1. Ivanchenko, V., Coughlan, J., Huiying, S.: Detecting and locating crosswalks using a camera phone. In: IEEE Conference on Computer Vision and Pattern Recognition, pp. 1–8 (2008)
2. Hui, K., Audibert, J.Y., Ponce, J.: General road detection from a single image. IEEE Trans. Image Process. **19**, 2211–2220 (2010)

3. Chang, C.K., Siagian, C., Itti, L.: Mobile robot monocular vision navigation based on road region and boundary estimation. In: IEEE/RSJ International Conference on Intelligent Robots and Systems, pp. 1043–1050 (2012)

4. Wang, Y., Teoh, E.K., Shen, D.: Lane detection and tracking using B-snake. Image Vis. Comput. **22**, 269–280 (2004)

5. Kim, Z.W.: Robust lane detection and tracking in challenging scenarios. IEEE Trans. Intell. Transp. Syst. **9**, 16–26 (2008)

6. Crisman, J.D., Thorpe, C.E.: Scarf: a color vision system that tracks roads and intersections. IEEE Trans. Robot. Autom. **9**, 49–58 (1993)

7. Alvarez, J.M., Lopez, A.M.: Road detection based on illuminant invariance. IEEE Trans. Intell. Transp. Syst. **12**, 184–193 (2011)

8. Alvarez, J.M., Gevers, T., LeCun, Y., Lopez, A.M.: Road scene segmentation from a single image. In: Fitzgibbon, A., Lazebnik, S., Perona, P., Sato, Y., Schmid, C. (eds.) ECCV 2012. LNCS, vol. 7578, pp. 376–389. Springer, Heidelberg (2012)

9. Uddin, M.S., Shioyama, T.: Bipolarity and projective invariant-based zebra-crossing detection for the visually impaired. In: IEEE Conference on Computer Vision and Pattern Recognition, pp. 22–30 (2005)

10. Le, M.C., Phung, S.L., Bouzerdoum, A.: Pedestrian lane detection for assistive navigation of blind people. In: International Conference on Pattern Recognition, pp. 2594–2597 (2012)

11. Le, M.C., Phung, S.L., Bouzerdoum, A.: Pedestrian lane detection for the visually impaired. In: International Conference on Digital Image Computing Techniques and Applications, pp.1–6 (2012)

12. Se, S.: Zebra-crossing detection for the partially sighted. In: IEEE Conference on Computer Vision and Pattern Recognition, pp. 211–217 (2000)

13. Tan, C., Tsai, H., Chang, T., Shneier, M.: Color model-based real-time learning for road following. In: IEEE Conference on Intelligent Transportation Systems, pp. 939–944 (2006)

14. Sha, Y., Zhang, G.y., Yang, Y.: A road detection algorithm by boosting using feature combination. In: IEEE Intelligent Vehicles Symposium, pp. 364–368 (2007)

15. Alvarez, J.M., Gevers, T., Lopez, A.M.: Vision-based road detection using road models. In: IEEE International Conference on Image Processing, pp. 2073–2076 (2009)

16. Rasmussen, C.: Texture-based vanishing point voting for road shape estimation. In: British Machine Vision Conference, pp. 470–477 (2004)

17. Belongie, S., Malik, J., Puzicha, J.: Shape matching and object recognition using shape contexts. IEEE Trans. Pattern Anal. Mach. Intell. **24**, 509–522 (2002)

18. Sotelo, M., Rodriguez, F., Magdalena, L., Bergasa, L., Boquete, L.: A color vision-based lane tracking system for autonomous driving on unmarked roads. Auton. Robot. **16**, 95–116 (2004)

19. Ramstrom, O., Christensen, H.: A method for following unmarked roads. In: IEEE Intelligent Vehicles Symposium, pp. 650–655 (2005)

20. He, Y., Wang, H., Zhang, B.: Color-based road detection in urban traffic scenes. IEEE Trans. Intell. Transp. Syst. **5**, 309–318 (2004)

21. Oh, C., Son, J., Sohn, K.: Illumination robust road detection using geometric information. In: International IEEE Conference on Intelligent Transportation Systems, pp. 1566–1571 (2012)

22. Miksik, O., Petyovsky, P., Zalud, L., Jura, P.: Robust detection of shady and highlighted roads for monocular camera based navigation of UGV. In: IEEE International Conference on Robotics and Automation, pp. 64–71 (2011)

23. Crisman, J., Thorpe, C.: Unscarf, a color vision system for the detection of unstructured roads. In: IEEE International Conference on Robotics and Automation, pp. 2496–2501 (1991)
24. Tardif, J.P.: Non-iterative approach for fast and accurate vanishing point detection. In: International Conference on Computer Vision, pp. 1250–1257 (2009)
25. Andaló, F.A., Taubin, G., Goldenstein, S.: Vanishing point detection by segment clustering on the projective space. In: Kutulakos, K.N. (ed.) Trends and Topics in Computer Vision. LNCS, vol. 6554, pp. 324–337. Springer, Heidelberg (2012)
26. Rasmussen, C.: Grouping dominant orientations for ill-structured road following. In: IEEE Conference on Computer Vision and Pattern Recognition, pp. 470–477 (2004)
27. Moghadam, P., Starzyk, J.A., Wijesoma, W.S.: Fast vanishing-point detection in unstructured environments. IEEE Trans. Image Process. 21, 425–430 (2012)
28. Weijer, J.V.D., Gevers, T., Smeulders, A.W.M.: Robust photometric invariant features from the color tensor. IEEE Trans. Image Process. 15, 118–127 (2006)
29. Gonzalez, R., Woods, R.: Digital Image Processing Using MATLAB. Prentice Hall, Englewood Cliffs (2004)
30. Felzenszwalb, P., Huttenlocher, D.: Efficient graph-based image segmentation. Int. J. Comput. Vis. 59, 167–181 (2004)
31. Gevers, T., A.W.M., S., Stokman, H.: Photometric invariant region detection. In: British Machine Vision Conference, pp. 659–669 (1998)
32. Everingham, M., Gool, L., Williams, C.K., Winn, J., Zisserman, A.: The pascal visual object classes (VOC) challenge. Int. J. Comput. Vis. 88, 303–338 (2010)

Multiple Stage Residual Model for Accurate Image Classification

Song Bai, Xinggang Wang, Cong Yao, and Xiang Bai[✉]

Department of Electronics and Information Engineering,
Huazhong University of Science and Technology,
Wuhan, People's Republic of China
{songbai,xgwang,xbai}@hust.edu.cn, yaocong2010@gmail.com

Abstract. Image classification is an important topic in computer vision. As a key procedure, encoding the local features to get a compact representation for image affects the final classification accuracy largely. There is no doubt that encoding procedure leads to information loss, due to the existence of quantization error. The residual vector, defined as the difference between the local image feature and its corresponding visual word, is the chief culprit that should be responsible for the quantization error. Many previous algorithms consider it as a coding issue, and focus on reducing the quantization error by reconstructing the feature with more than one visual words, or by the so-called soft-assignment strategy. In this paper, we consider the problem from a different view, and propose an effective and efficient model, which is called Multiple Stage Residual Model (MSRM), to make full use of the residual vector to generate a multiple stage code. Our proposed model is a generic framework, which can be built upon many coding algorithms and improves the image classification performance of the coding algorithms significantly. The experimental results on the image classification benchmarks, such as UIUC 8-Sport, Scene-15, Caltech-101 image dataset, confirm the validity of MSRM.

1 Introduction

Image classification is an important topic in computer vision with many applications, such as image retrieval [1,2], video retrieval and web content analysis [3]. Given an input image, the aim of image classification is to assign one or more class labels to it, or in other words, to determine its category. The Bag-of-Features (BoF) [4,5] model may be the most successful framework in image classification for its invariance to scale, translation and rotation.

The pipeline of a typical BoF image classification model is illustrated in Fig. 1. It consists of five basic steps: patch extraction, patch description, codebook learning, feature coding and feature pooling. With an input image in hand, the step of patch extraction is to generate lots of small patches via dense sampling, which are described by some local image descriptors in the patch description procedure. Various descriptors, such as SIFT [6] or HoG [7] can be used

© Springer International Publishing Switzerland 2015
D. Cremers et al. (Eds.): ACCV 2014, Part I, LNCS 9003, pp. 430–445, 2015.
DOI: 10.1007/978-3-319-16865-4_28

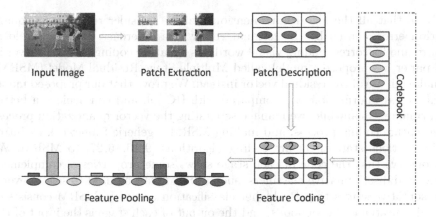

Fig. 1. The pipeline of general image classification framework

to describe these local patches. In the process of codebook learning, a subset of features randomly sampled in the training images are gathered to learn the codebook by some codebook learning algorithms (*e.g.* K-means [8]). Feature coding offers the way to generate the code for each local image descriptor, and in the feature pooling step, these codes are pooled together to get the final representation of an image.

Among the aforementioned five steps, feature coding plays an important role for its great impact on the accuracy and speed of image classification. Recently, many coding algorithms [9–23] have been proposed. The representative coding method is Hard-assignment Coding (HC) [9]. HC only accounts for the nearest visual word of a local feature for coding, which makes HC sensitive to the selection of the codebook. Localized Soft-assignment Coding (LSC) [11] adopts an "early cut-off" strategy, and assign the local feature to more than one visual words. The response coefficient for each visual word is determined by the distance between the local feature and the visual word. Different from voting-based algorithms like HC, Sparse Coding [18] shows its superiority gradually, but it is time-consuming. Locality-constrained Linear Coding (LLC) [10], as a typical sparse coding method, attaches more importance to locality than sparsity, and offers an efficient way to compute the approximate sparse code. Salient Coding (SC) [16] introduces the concept of "salience", and guarantees a salient representation without deviations.

After the codes of all local features are computed, the feature pooling step is adopted to integrate these codes together to generate an equal sized feature vector for each image in the database. The common used pooling methods are sum-pooling [9] and max-pooling [18]. A comprehensive analysis can be found in [24–26]. Meanwhile, in order to include the spatial information in the pooling step, Spatial Pyramid Matching (SPM) [9] is conducted via dividing the image into increasingly finer subregions. Each subregion is pooled individually, and all pooled features are concatenated to form the final feature vector of the whole image.

Note that all the algorithms mentioned above consider reducing the quantization error, caused by the residual vector (the difference between the local feature and its corresponding visual word), as a feature coding issue. However in this paper, we propose a model called Multiple Stage Residual Model (MSRM) to make full use of the residual vector instead. We prove that our proposed model leads to less information loss compared with HC [9], and can achieve a better performance. Meanwhile, we manage separating the vector quantization process from feature coding process, and making MSRM a generic framework by introducing various state-of-the-art coding algorithms [9,10,16,27] to MSRM. We also observe that the code of each stage shows some properties of complementarity, and discriminative classifiers, such as SVM, can be used to select several representative stages to get a higher classification accuracy. MSRM consists of several concatenated codebooks, and the output of each stage is the input of the next stage, which is simple and fast to compute.

The rest of this paper is organized as follows: In Sect. 2 we introduce some related work briefly. The introduction of MSRM is given in Sect. 3. In Sect. 4, we carry out several experiments on three benchmark datasets, and the experimental results prove the effectiveness of the proposed model. Conclusions are given in Sect. 5.

2   Related Work

Considering that MSRM is a generic model, in which many encoding methods can be embedded, we review some typical coding strategies recently proposed in the literature. These coding strategies act as a baseline, and a full comparison will be conducted in Sect. 4.

Based on the classification standard for coding methods in [28], these methods are grouped into five categories: voting-based methods, reconstruction-based methods, saliency-based methods, local tangent-based methods, and fisher coding-based methods.

Let $\mathcal{C} = \{c_1, c_2, \ldots, c_n\}$ $(1 \leq i \leq n, c_i \in \mathbf{R}^d)$ denote the codebook previously learned in the training set, and n represents the codebook size. In the case of extracting SIFT as the local image descriptor, the dimension d is usually 128. $x_i \in \mathbf{R}^d$ denotes the ith feature densely extracted in an image. Let w_i be the code of x_i, and w_{ij} be the response value of x_i with respect to c_j.

Hard-assignment coding (HC) [9] is a representative of voting-based methods. For each local descriptor x_i in an image, HC assigns it to the nearest visual word in the codebook under a certain metric. It means there is only one non-zero element in w_i. Locality-constrained Linear Coding (LLC) [10] is a typical example of reconstruction-based methods. Unlike traditional sparse coding methods, LLC emphasizes the importance of locality instead of sparsity, since locality must lead to sparsity but not necessary vice versa. A fast approximation of LLC is proposed in [10] to improve the computational efficiency. Salient Coding (SC) [16] is a representative method of saliency-based methods. SC deems that saliency is a fundamental property in coding, and define a "saliency" degree based on the nearest visual word c_j to x_i. Super Vector Coding (SVC) [15] is a representative of local tangent-based methods. Super Vector Coding considers feature coding as a manifold approximation using the visual words by assuming that all features constitute a smooth manifold. Improved Fisher Kernel(IFK) [14] is a representative of fisher coding-based methods. In IFK, the probability density distribution of the local features is described by the Gaussian mixture models. Vector of Local Aggregated Descriptors (VLAD) [27,29] aggregates the local features based on a locality criterion in feature space. It is known that VLAD is deemed as a simplified and non-probabilistic version of IFK, and becomes SVC if combined with BoF. Although VLAD is initially designed for large scale image retrieval, we prove it also effective in image classification as shown in Sect. 4. Considering the simpleness of VLAD, we adopts VLAD to get a compact representation for image throughout our experiments. The definitions of all the aforementioned coding algorithms are listed in Table 1.

Table 1. The coding algorithms used in our proposed model, and their corresponding definitions.

Algorithms	Definitions
HC [9]	$w_{ij} = \begin{cases} 1 & if \quad j = \underset{j=1,2,\ldots,n}{\arg\min} \|x_i - c_j\|_2^2 \\ 0 & otherwise \end{cases}$
LLC [10]	$w_i = \arg\min \|x_i - cw_i\| + \lambda \|d_i \odot w_i\|, \quad s.t. \ 1^T w_i = 1$
SC [16]	$w_{ij} = \begin{cases} 1 - \dfrac{\|x_i - c_j\|_2}{\frac{1}{K-1}\sum\limits_{k \neq j}^{K} \|x_i - c_k\|_2} & if \quad j = \underset{j=1,2,\ldots,n}{\arg\min} \|x_i - c_j\|_2^2 \\ 0 & otherwise \end{cases}$
VLAD [27,29]	$w_{ij} = \begin{cases} x_i - c_j & if \quad j = \underset{j=1,2,\ldots,n}{\arg\min} \|x_i - c_j\|_2^2 \\ 0 & otherwise \end{cases}$

Spatial Pyramid Matching (SPM) [9] has been proven to be effective in the pooling procedure with spatial information included. SPM starts with dividing an image into subregions, and obtains the histogram of each region via a pooling function $\mathcal{F}$. Usually, the pooling function $\mathcal{F}$ is max-pooling which selects the largest response value along each dimension of all the codes in a certain region, or sum-pooling that simply adds all the values. The "pyramid" means that the spatial division of image ranges from a global one, i.e., the entire image, to several local subregions. The final image representation is obtained by concatenating these histograms together. Other algorithms, such as Spatial Local Coding (SLC) [30], Feature Context [31], are also widely-used for modelling the spatial information.

Algorithm 1. Multiple Stage Codebook Learning with K-means

Input: The training features $\mathcal{X}$ for codebook learning; The codebook size n; The number of stage m.
Output: The learned codebook $\mathcal{C} = \{\mathcal{C}^1, \mathcal{C}^2, \ldots, \mathcal{C}^m\}$.
  1: **for** each $j \in [1, m]$ **do**
  2:     divide $\mathcal{X}$ into n clusters via K-means through Eq. 1 and Eq. 2;
  3:     and output the cluster centers $\mathcal{C}^j$;
  4:     **for** each $x \in \mathcal{X}$ **do**
  5:         compute the residual vector $r(x) = x - q(x)$;
  6:         $x = r(x)$;
  7:     **end for**
  8: **end for**

---

3   Multiple Stage Residual Model

Multiple Stage Residual Model has one codebook in each stage, and each stage will output a code with an encoder. The detail of MSRM is as follows.

3.1   Preliminary

Multiple Stage Vector Quantization (MSVQ) is a classic channel coding algorithm commonly used in Digital Voice Processing.

The theory of MSVQ is as follows: (1) Given an input signal represented by a vector x and the multiple stage codebook $\mathcal{C} = \{\mathcal{C}^1, \mathcal{C}^2, \ldots, \mathcal{C}^m\}$, where m is the number of stage. Each component $\mathcal{C}^j$ is the codebook in the jth stage of $\mathcal{C}$ with codebook size n (2) in the jth stage, the c_i^j with the minimum distortion is determined, and the subscript i, as well as the stage number j, is passed into channel (3) the input of the next stage, *i.e.* the $(j + 1)$th stage, is the residual vector $r(x) = x - c_i^j$. Following the same principle, c_i^{j+1} is determined again (4) the procedure of (2)(3) is iteratively conducted, until the final stage is reached (5) in the receiving terminal, the decoder reconstructs the signal by using the subscripts and the multiple stage codebook.

In this paper, we try to propose a specifically designed model similar to MSVQ for large scale image classification. One of our goals is the generality of the model, and we want to adapt as many as state-of-the-art feature coding methods to this model.

3.2   Codebook Learning in MSRM

Codebook learning is a necessary step before encoding the local features. There are various codebook learning algorithms in an unsupervised way [8], a weakly-supervised way [32], or a supervised way [33,34].

Among all the codebook learning algorithms, K-means may be the most widely used one for its simpleness and stableness. Given a randomly selected subset $\mathcal{X}$ of SIFT descriptors of the training set and the codebook size n, K-means seeks n vectors $C = \{c_1, c_2, \ldots, c_n\}$ iteratively, and minimizes the approximation error $\mathcal{E}$ defined as

$$\mathcal{E} = \sum_{x \in \mathcal{X}} \|x - q(x)\|^2 \tag{1}$$

$$x \to q(x) = arg\min_{c \in C} \|x - c\|^2 \tag{2}$$

Our proposed model also adopts K-means to learn the multiple stage codebook $\mathcal{C} = \{\mathcal{C}^j, 1 \le j \le m\}$. The pseudocode is presented in Algorithm 1.

3.3   Encoder in MSRM

As is presented in Sect. 2, many different coding strategies were proposed. In order to embed these coding strategies into our proposed model, we separate the vector quantization procedure from the feature coding procedure. Specifically, for a given local image descriptor x, on the one hand we only consider the nearest visual word to compute the residual vector $r(x) = x - q(x)$ according to Eq. 2 and pass the residual vector to the next stage, which is the new feature vector to be encoded in the future. On the other hand, we does not restrict the way and the number of the visual words used to generate the code for x, which is usually determined by the coding algorithm. For example, if LLC [10] is chosen as the encoder of MSRM, we use k (k is usually set to 5) visual words to encode x, and use only the nearest word to generate the residual vector. Our interpretation is that the nearest visual word to x captures its main pattern, and all the local image descriptors lying in the same cluster will eliminate the information redundancy if all of them are deprived with their common pattern. The operations of computing the residual vector and encoding the features are

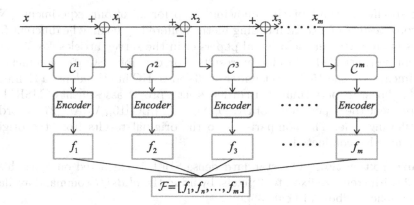

Fig. 2. The pipeline of Multiple Stage Residual Model. The input x is the local descriptor to be encoded. $\mathcal{C}^i$ ($1 \le i \le m$) is the ith stage codebook. The encoder can be various. f_j ($1 \le j \le m$) is the encoded feature via the encoder. The final representation for x is the concatenation of the output from all stages.

iteratively conducted until the final stage is reached. The pipeline of Multiple Stage Residual Model is illustrated in Fig. 2.

According to the taxonomy presented in [28], we introduce some typical algorithms as the encoder to our proposed model. Specifically, Hard-assignment Coding [9] is the representative of voting-based coding methods. Local-constrained Linear Coding [10] is the representative of reconstruction-based coding methods. Salient Coding [16] is the representative of saliency-based coding methods. Vector of Aggregated Local Descriptors [27] is used to replace the role of Super Vector-coding [15] (one of local tangent-based coding methods), and Improve Fisher Kernel [14] (one of fisher coding-based methods). When the stage number m is set to 1, our proposed model degenerates into the original encoding algorithms.

As shown in Sect. 4, the codes from different stages are greatly complementary to each other. If the classifier cannot give the image a right label prediction with the codes from a certain stage, the prediction can be revised with the usage of the codes from other stages in most cases.

4   Experiments

In this section, we first evaluate the effectiveness of MSRM on two benchmarks particularly collected for scene classification. We will give a comparison with the original algorithms to show the extent that MSRM can improve the baseline on Scene-15 dataset [9], UIUC 8-sport dataset [35]. An extra experiment is also conducted in Caltech-101 dataset [36] to evaluate the performance of MSRM in object recognition.

4.1   Implementation Details

If not specified, we adopt the following setup for all of our experiments. Note that some results of a certain coding method offered by us may be different from the results reported in the original papers or in the survey articles [28,37], since different settings lead to different results. For example, SC [16] conducts the experiment in Scene-15 dataset under 4096 codes, HC in [28] adopts a Hellingers kernel to boost its performance. In order to get a proper assessment of MSRM, we re-implement the experiments of HC [9], SC [16], LLC [10], VLAD [27] according the following rule. The comparisons to the original results from the original papers are also conducted.

Feature Extraction: The standard dense SIFT is extracted on a patch size 32×32, with step size fixed to 4 pixels, by using the vl_dsift command available in the public toolbox VLFeat [38].

Codebook Generation: Following the instruction described in Sect. 3.2, we learning a multiple stage codebook via k-means clustering. The codebook size depends on the coding algorithm that applied to MSRM. In particular, HC, LLC and SC adopt a relative larger codebook with a size of 1024, and 64 for VLAD respectively.

Coding and Pooling: As for the implementation of VQ, LLC and SC, we use the codes released by Huang in [28] to encode the local features. In order to include the spatial information, SPM [9] with 3 levels: 1×1, 2×2 and 4×4 is adopted with a same weight for each level. We use *vl_vlad* command in VLFeat for VLAD coding, and no spatial information is included. The max-pooling operation is performed with LLC and SC, and HC and VLAD use the sum-pooling operation.

Database Setup: Database images are resized to no more than 300×300 in all datasets except for UIUC 8-Sport, since images in this dataset have higher resolutions. We keep the maximum image size of UIUC 8-Sport dataset 400×400.

Classifier: Linear SVM, implemented by Liblinear toolbox [39], is used. We set the penalty parameter in SVM to 10.

4.2   Scene-15 Dataset

Scene-15 dataset [9] contains 15 categories and 4485 images, with 200–400 images per category. The categories vary from indoor scenes like bedrooms, to outdoor scenes like mountains. Based on the common experimental setting, 100 images per category are taken as training data, and the rest are used for testing.

Figure 3 presents the performance of MSRM with different encoders. As we can draw from Fig. 3, MSRM can significantly improve the performance compared with the original state-of-the-art coding algorithms. Generally, the classification accuracy improves as the stage number increases, and it gets saturated

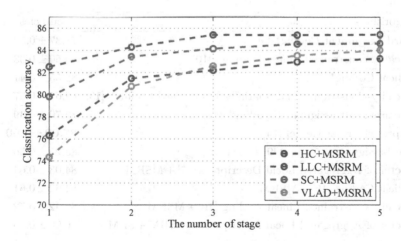

Fig. 3. The experimental results of MSRM with different encoders on Scene-15 dataset. The x-axis denotes the stage number m in MSRM, and the y-axis denotes the classification accuracy.

when the stage number comes to 5. The classification accuracy is increased by 6.94 % for HC [9], 2.90 % for LLC [10], 4.79 % for SC [16] and 9.67 % for VLAD [27] when MSRM sets the stage number to 5. As we can see, our proposed model is especially suitable for HC and VLAD. The reason might be that both HC and VLAD only consider the nearest visual word in the codebook to encode a local feature, and our proposed model can boost their performances largely by making use of the computed residual vector. In comparison, both LLC and SC take into account the contributions from more than one visual words, so the improvements of MSRM with LLC and SC are not as obvious as that with HC and VLAD, but are still convincing. The performance of MSRM is slightly lower than that of IFK [14] reported in [28]. However, the classification accuracy of MSRM with VLAD can be improved to 86.90 % if SPM [9] is used, which is comparable to IFK.

We also compare the performance of different coding methods in Table 2. As can be seen, the accuracy of our implementation for HC is much lower than that in [9], MSRM also enhances its discriminative ability, and even surpasses the original LLC and SC. As for SC, the original paper obtains a high performance since multi-scale dense sift and a larger codebook are used. VLAD is rarely used for scene classification, but usually applied to image retrieval. In this paper, we find VLAD also suitable to image classification. The results show that VLAD, integrated into MSRM, can achieve a superior performance to many state-of-the-art coding algorithms.

Table 2. The comparison of classification accuracies on Scene-15 dataset. (The tag "⋆" in the top right corner of a certain algorithm means that the classification accuracy of this algorithm is not implemented by us, but comes from the corresponding paper, or the survey articles.)

Algorithms	Accuracies (%)
Hard-assignment Coding⋆ [9]	78.87 ± 0.52
Locality-constrained Linear Coding⋆ [10]	80.50 ± 0.63
Salient Coding⋆ [16]	82.55 ± 0.41
Locality-Constrained and Spatially Regularized Coding⋆ [13]	82.67 ± 0.57
Localized soft-assignment Coding⋆ [11]	82.70 ± 0.39
Improved Fisher Kernel [14]	**87.00 ± 0.00**
Hard-assignment Coding [9] + MSRM	83.25 ± 0.50
Vector of Aggregated Local Descriptors [27] + MSRM	84.03 ± 0.64
Salient Coding [16] + MSRM	84.62 ± 0.61
Locality-constrained Linear Coding [10] + MSRM	85.42 ± 0.72
Vector of Aggregated Local Descriptors + MSRM + SPM	86.90 ± 0.45

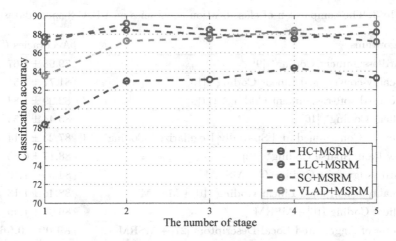

Fig. 4. The experimental results of MSRM with different encoders on UIUC 8-sport dataset. The x-axis denotes the stage number m in MSRM, and the y-axis denotes the classification accuracy.

4.3 UIUC 8-Sport Dataset

UIUC 8 Sport [35] is particularly collected for image-based event classification, and it consists of 1579 images grouped into 8 sport categories: badminton, bocce, croquet, polo, rock climbing, rowing, sailing and snow boarding. According to the standard setup for classification, we use 10 splits of the data, and random select 70 images from each category for training and 60 images for testing. The average accuracy, as well as the standard deviation, is reported.

The classification accuracies of MSRM with different encoders are illustrated in Fig. 4. We can also observe the positive effect on classification results brought by MSRM to various encoders. An exciting accuracy of **89.09 ± 0.96** is achieved by MSRM in conjunction with VLAD when the stage number is set to 5. The baseline of VLAD in UIUC 8-sport dataset is merely 83.56 ± 1.70, and is improved by nearly 6 % via MSRM.

We compare our proposed MSRM with some related algorithms in Table 3. The performance of MSRM is better than many coding methods [10,11,13,16], even outperforms Low Rank Sparse Coding [12], which achieves the state-of-the-art result recently.

4.4 Caltech-101 Dataset

We also evaluate our proposed model for object recognition in Caltech-101 dataset [36]. Caltech-101 dataset consists of 101 object categories including animals, faces, plants *etc.*, with 31–800 images per category. Following the standard experimental setting, we use 10 random splits of the data, while taking 30 random images per class for training and the rest for testing. Considering that Caltech-101 dataset is a relatively larger database, we extract dense sift at three

Table 3. The comparison of classification accuracies on UIUC 8-sport dataset.

Algorithms	Accuracies (%)
Hard-assignment Coding* [9]	79.98 ± 1.67
Locality-constrained Linear Coding* [10]	81.77 ± 1.51
Localized soft-assignment Coding* [11]	82.29 ± 1.84
Salient Coding* [16]	85.44 ± 1.54
Locality-Constrained and Spatially Regularized Coding* [13]	87.23 ± 1.14
Low Rank Sparse Coding* [12]	88.17 ± 0.85
Hard-assignment Coding [9] + MSRM	84.35 ± 1.16
Locality-constrained Linear Coding [10] + MSRM	88.46 ± 1.13
Salient Coding [16] + MSRM	89.07 ± 1.49
Vector of Aggregated Local Descriptors [27] + MSRM	**89.09 ± 0.96**

scales: 16×16, 24×24, 32×32. Since the spatial layout of object in the image is important in object recognition, we apply SLC [30] to VLAD coding.

In Fig. 5, we plot the performance of MSRM with different encoders under different stage number m. Similar to our experiments in the previous dataset, MSRM improves our selected encoders significantly, $i.e.$ HC [9] by 5.07 %, LLC [10] by 3.47 %, SC [16] by 5.33 %, VLAD [27] by 7.02 %. The performance of HC is much different from the results reported in [28], due to the usage of Hellinger kernel. We conduct the experiment of HC to make clear the effect of Hellinger kernel, and find that Hellinger kernel is extremely useful to HC in this dataset. A significant improvement of 13.25 % is observed.

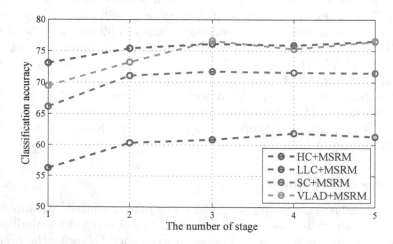

Fig. 5. The experimental results of MSRM with different encoders on Caltech-101 dataset. The x-axis denotes the stage number m in MSRM, and the y-axis denotes the classification accuracy.

Table 4. The comparison of classification accuracies on Caltech-101 dataset.

Algorithms	Accuracies (%)
Hard-assignment Coding* [9]	69.43 ± 0.52
Salient Coding* [16]	69.55 ± 0.83
Locality-constrained Linear Coding* [10]	71.67 ± 0.86
Localized soft-assignment Coding* [11]	72.58 ± 1.08
Locality-Constrained and Spatially Regularized Coding* [13]	73.23 ± 0.81
Low Rank Sparse Coding* [12]	75.02 ± 0.74
Hard-assignment Coding [9] + MSRM	61.88 ± 1.15
Salient Coding [16] + MSRM	71.73 ± 1.47
Locality-constrained Linear Coding [10] + MSRM	76.56 ± 0.90
Vector of Aggregated Local Descriptors [27] + MSRM	**76.59 ± 0.51**

We also list some excellent results reported by other algorithms in Table 4. Our proposed model also obtains competitive performance compared with many state-of-the-art algorithms.

4.5 Discussion

Information Loss: Average Quantization error is an important index in evaluating a feature coding algorithm, which is defined as

$$AQE = \frac{1}{N}\sum_{i=1}^{N} \|x_i - cw_i\|^2 \tag{3}$$

Large quantization error results in much information loss in the coding procedure, which impairs the classification accuracy heavily. The quantization error is brought in when we represent a local descriptor x by a visual word $q(x) \in \mathcal{C}$. Such a behaviour is simple, but also somehow harmful due to the existence of the residual vector $r(x) = x - q(x)$ between x and $q(x)$. Some previous methods [10,11,13] use more visual words to represent x to alleviate the problem.

In MSRM (we take Two Stage Residual Model with HC as example), the local descriptor x is represented by a tuple $(q_1(x), q_2(x - q_1(x)))$, where $q_i(x)$ is the nearest visual word of x in $\mathcal{C}^i$. The encoder applied to the tuple $(q_1(x), q_2(x - q_1(x)))$ generates the code for x.

We use Hard-assignment Coding (HC) [9] to show the way that MSRM reduces the quantization error. The AQE of HC is

$$AQE_{HC} = \frac{1}{N}\sum_{i=1}^{N} \|x_i - q_1(x_i)\|^2 \tag{4}$$

while the AQE of MSRM with HC is

$$AQE_{MSRM} = \frac{1}{N} \sum_{i=1}^{N} \|x_i - q_1(x_i) - q_2(x_i - q_1(x_i))\|^2 \tag{5}$$

It is straightforward that the energy of the residual vector $x - q(x)$ is relatively smaller than x itself. We compute the AQE of MSRM with HC in Scene-15 dataset, UIUC 8-sport dataset [35] and Caltech-101 dataset [36]. The result is presented in Table 5, and find that MSRM can significantly reduce the quantization error, which strongly explains why MSRM with HC as the encoder can improve the baseline.

Table 5. The Average Quantization Error in different datasets.

	Scene-15 dataset	UIUC 8-sport dataset	Caltech-101 dataset
HC [9]	2.16	3.02	3.02
HC + MSRM	1.01	1.43	1.73

Complementarity: We also observe that the output of each stage in MSRM is complementary to each other, and the powerful classifier SVM is able to select several distinctive stages to distinguish images from different categories.

In order to prove our conjecture, we conduct an interesting experiment shown in Fig. 6, that the features from each stage in MSRM with VLAD as the encoder form the input training set and testing set for SVM. We select one misclassified image per category, and find that although the classifier cannot give a correct judgement for the label of the image according to the features from $1st$ stage in MSRM, $i.e.$ the

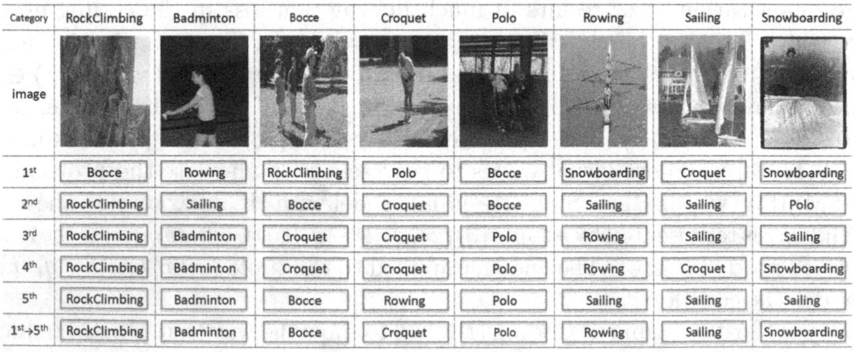

Fig. 6. Some misclassified images in UIUC 8-sport dataset. The "Category" in the first row indicates the ground truth of the image, and The third to the seventh row present the predicted label that SVM outputs based on the features of each stage in MSRM. The last row shows the result when we concatenate the features from all stages in MSRM. The red box means a false prediction, and the green box means a correct prediction.

original coding strategy, it can revise its prediction result with more complementary information from the latter stages in MSRM. For example, the image from Rowing category in the seventh column of Fig. 6, is misclassified as snowboarding in the first stage and sailing in the second stage, however, it obtains a correct labeling in the third stage and the fourth stage. When combining the features from all stages, the false prediction is corrected as shown in the last row. The last column presents an image from snowboarding is misclassified in the second, third and fifth stage, but is assigned a right label if the features from all the stages are combined together. This phenomena reveals the robustness of our proposed model.

To further confirm the complementarity between the features from each stage of MSRM, we compare our proposed MSRM with a single stage coding under the same feature dimension. Specifically, Scene-15 dataset is used, and VLAD is selected as the encoder. For MSRM, the codebook size in each layer of MSRM is 64, and the stage number m ranges from 1 to 5. Hence the feature dimension of MSRM for an image is $128 * 64 * m$. For the single stage coding, the codebook size is set to $64 * m$ ($1 \leq m \leq 5$). Hence the final feature dimension for an image is also $128 * 64 * m$. The results are presented in Table 6, which suggest that MSRM works significantly better than only single stage coding.

Table 6. The comparison of classification accuracy between MSRM and the single stage coding under the same feature dimension in Scene-15 dataset.

m	1	2	3	4	5
VLAD [27]	74.36 %	78.15 %	79.35 %	80.14 %	80.18 %
VLAD + MSRM	74.36 %	80.77 %	82.59 %	83.53 %	84.03 %

5   Conclusion

In this paper, we propose a generic model called Multiple Stage Residual Model (MSRM) to make full use of the residual vector, while many coding algorithms focus on reducing it. MSRM has been proved to be effective to improve the performance of many state-of-the-art coding algorithms further.

In the future, we will study how to introduce the spatial consistency to MSRM, and introduce more coding methods to MSRM in a proper way.

Acknowledgement. This work was primarily supported by National Natural Science Foundation of China (NSFC) (No. 61222308), and in part by NSFC (No. 61173120), Program for New Century Excellent Talents in University (No. NCET-12-0217), Fundamental Research Funds for the Central Universities (No. HUST 2013TS115). X.Wang was supported by Microsoft Research Asia Fellowship 2012.

References

1. Jégou, H., Zisserman, A., et al.: Triangulation embedding and democratic aggregation for image search. In: CVPR (2014)
2. Zheng, L., Wang, S., Liu, Z., Tian, Q.: Packing and padding: coupled multi-index for accurate image retrieval. In: CVPR (2014)
3. Kosala, R., Blockeel, H.: Web mining research: a survey. ACM Sigkdd Explor. Newslett. **2**, 1–15 (2000)
4. Csurka, G., Dance, C., Fan, L., Willamowski, J., Bray, C.: Visual categorization with bags of keypoints. In: ECCV (2004)
5. Fei-Fei, L., Perona, P.: A Bayesian hierarchical model for learning natural scene categories. In: CVPR (2005)
6. Lowe, D.G.: Distinctive image features from scale-invariant keypoints. IJCV **60**(2), 91–110 (2004)
7. Dalal, N., Triggs, B.: Histograms of oriented gradients for human detection. In: CVPR (2005)
8. Lloyd, S.: Least squares quantization in PCM. IEEE Trans. Inf. Theory **28**(2), 129–137 (1982)
9. Lazebnik, S., Schmid, C., Ponce, J.: Beyond bags of features: spatial pyramid matching for recognizing natural scene categories. In: CVPR (2006)
10. Wang, J., Yang, J., Yu, K., Lv, F., Huang, T., Gong, Y.: Locality-constrained linear coding for image classification. In: CVPR (2010)
11. Liu, L., Wang, L., Liu, X.: In defense of soft-assignment coding. In: ICCV (2011)
12. Zhang, T., Ghanem, B., Liu, S., Xu, C., Ahuja, N.: Low-rank sparse coding for image classification. In: ICCV (2013)
13. Shabou, A., Le Borgne, H.: Locality-constrained and spatially regularized coding for scene categorization. In: CVPR (2012)
14. Perronnin, F., Sánchez, J., Mensink, T.: Improving the Fisher kernel for large-scale image classification. In: Daniilidis, K., Maragos, P., Paragios, N. (eds.) ECCV 2010, Part IV. LNCS, vol. 6314, pp. 143–156. Springer, Heidelberg (2010)
15. Zhou, X., Yu, K., Zhang, T., Huang, T.S.: Image classification using super-vector coding of local image descriptors. In: Daniilidis, K., Maragos, P., Paragios, N. (eds.) ECCV 2010, Part V. LNCS, vol. 6315, pp. 141–154. Springer, Heidelberg (2010)
16. Huang, Y., Huang, K., Yu, Y., Tan, T.: Salient coding for image classification. In: CVPR (2011)
17. van Gemert, J.C., Geusebroek, J.-M., Veenman, C.J., Smeulders, A.W.M.: Kernel codebooks for scene categorization. In: Forsyth, D., Torr, P., Zisserman, A. (eds.) ECCV 2008, Part III. LNCS, vol. 5304, pp. 696–709. Springer, Heidelberg (2008)
18. Yang, J., Yu, K., Gong, Y., Huang, T.: Linear spatial pyramid matching using sparse coding for image classification. In: CVPR (2009)
19. Shaban, A., Rabiee, H.R., Farajtabar, M., Ghazvininejad, M.: From local similarity to global coding: an application to image classification. In: CVPR (2013)
20. Yu, K., Zhang, T., Gong, Y.: Nonlinear learning using local coordinate coding. Adv. Neural Inf. Process. Syst. **22**, 2223–2231 (2009)
21. Shen, W., Deng, K., Bai, X., Leyvand, T., Guo, B., Tu, Z.: Exemplar-based human action pose correction. IEEE Trans. Cybern. **44**, 1053–1066 (2014)
22. Zheng, L., Wang, S., Tian, Q.: Coupled binary embedding for large-scale image retrieval. IEEE Trans. Image Process. **23**, 3368–3380 (2014)
23. Shen, W., Deng, K., Bai, X., Leyvand, T., Guo, B., Tu, Z.: Exemplar-based human action pose correction and tagging. In: CVPR, pp. 1784–1791 (2012)

24. Boureau, Y.L., Ponce, J., LeCun, Y.: A theoretical analysis of feature pooling in visual recognition. In: ICML (2010)
25. Boureau, Y.L., Bach, F., LeCun, Y., Ponce, J.: Learning mid-level features for recognition. In: CVPR (2010)
26. Koniusz, P., Yan, F., Mikolajczyk, K.: Comparison of mid-level feature coding approaches and pooling strategies in visual concept detection. CVIU **117**(5), 479–492 (2013)
27. Jégou, H., Douze, M., Schmid, C., Pérez, P.: Aggregating local descriptors into a compact image representation. In: CVPR (2010)
28. Huang, Y., Wu, Z., Wang, L., Tan, T.: Feature coding in image classification: a comprehensive study. PAMI **35**(8), 1798–1828 (2013)
29. Arandjelovic, R., Zisserman, A.: All about VLAD. In: CVPR (2013)
30. McCann, S., Lowe, D.G.: Spatially local coding for object recognition. In: Lee, K.M., Matsushita, Y., Rehg, J.M., Hu, Z. (eds.) ACCV 2012, Part I. LNCS, vol. 7724, pp. 204–217. Springer, Heidelberg (2013)
31. Wang, X., Bai, X., Liu, W., Latecki, L.J.: Feature context for image classification and object detection. In: CVPR, IEEE, pp. 961–968 (2011)
32. Wang, X., Wang, B., Bai, X., Liu, W., Tu, Z.: Max-margin multiple-instance dictionary learning. In: ICML (2013)
33. Mairal, J., Bach, F., Ponce, J., Sapiro, G., Zisserman, A., et al.: Supervised dictionary learning. In: NIPS (2008)
34. Yang, J., Yu, K., Huang, T.: Supervised translation-invariant sparse coding. In: CVPR (2010)
35. Li, L.J., Fei-Fei, L.: What, where and who? classifying events by scene and object recognition. In: ICCV (2007)
36. Fei-Fei, L., Fergus, R., Perona, P.: Learning generative visual models from few training examples: an incremental Bayesian approach tested on 101 object categories. Comput. Vis. Image Underst. **106**(1), 59–70 (2007)
37. Chatfield, K., Lempitsky, V., Vedaldi, A., Zisserman, A.: The devil is in the details: an evaluation of recent feature encoding methods. In: BMVC (2011)
38. Vedaldi, A., Fulkerson, B.: VLFeat: an open and portable library of computer vision algorithms (2008). http://www.vlfeat.org/
39. Chang, C.C., Lin, C.J.: LIBSVM: a library for support vector machines. ACM Trans. Intell. Syst. Technol. (2011). Software available at http://www.csie.ntu.edu.tw/~cjlin/libsvm

Hybrid-Indexing Multi-type Features for Large-Scale Image Search

Qingjun Luo[1]([⊠]), Shiliang Zhang[2], Tiejun Huang[1], Wen Gao[1], and Qi Tian[2]

[1] School of Electronics Engineering and Computer Science, Peking University,
Beijing, People's Republic of China
qingjun.luo@pku.edu.cn
[2] Department of Computer Science, University of Texas at San Antonio,
San Antonio, USA

Abstract. Indexing local features with a vocabulary tree and indexing holistic features by compact hashing codes are two successful but separated lines of research. Both of the two indexing models are suited for specific features and are limited to certain scenarios like partial-duplicate search and similar image search, respectively. To conquer such limitations, we propose a novel hybrid-indexing strategy, which incorporates multiple similarity metrics into one inverted index file during off-line indexing. Hybrid-Indexing only requires the Bag-of-visual Words (BoWs) model as input for online query, but could obtain more satisfying retrieval results because the index file conveys hybrid similarities among images. Moreover, hybrid-indexing does not degrade the efficiency of classic BoWs based image search. Experiments on several public datasets manifest the effectiveness and efficiency of our proposed method.

1 Introduction

Though many successful image retrieval methods have been proposed in recent years, the existence of semantic gap still hinders the improvements of retrieval accuracy [1]. The major challenges come from two aspects, (1) it is not easy to capture the essential characteristic of an image by a single feature, if not impossible, and (2) it is hard to depict the actual search intention of the user.

Efforts to bridge the lack of coincidence between the extracted image information cues and the interpretation of human users are made in various ways. To obtain intrinsic descriptions of an image, different types of image features have been proposed. Local features and holistic features are two main categories. Not withdrawing their success, it has been more and more noticed that there is no a single type of feature which is optimal in all cases. For examples, local features with vocabulary trees are well suited to find partial duplicate objects, while global semantic attribute features aim to locate images that share similar semantic meanings. Different cues delineate distinct aspects of an image, and meet the users' various search intentions separately. Feature fusion is a reasonable option to leverage multiple cues [2,3]. Unfortunately, incompatibility issues arise accordingly because of the modality difference of the fused features. In the meanwhile,

© Springer International Publishing Switzerland 2015
D. Cremers et al. (Eds.): ACCV 2014, Part I, LNCS 9003, pp. 446–460, 2015.
DOI: 10.1007/978-3-319-16865-4_29

extracting various types of features during online retrieval stage would greatly increase the query time.

Another line of feasible methods to incorporate different cues is combining multiple retrieval results during online retrieval [4–7]. However, these methods suffer from either the difficulties of measuring and combining dramatically diverse features, or the computational expense which is introduced by online multiple feature extraction and fusion.

To the best of our knowledge, the effort on fusing different features or similarity metrics during the offline indexing is still limited. One of the original works is [8], which propose a semantic-aware co-indexing algorithm to jointly embed semantic attribute and local features in the inverted indices [9]. Packs semantic relevant images into an uniform unit, *i.e.*, superimage, and indexes these semantically compact units instead of single images, thus largely reduced the memory consumption while obtaining both semantically and visually relevant images at the same time.

As an important procedure in BoWs based image retrieval systems, off-line indexing organizes images sharing a common visual word together into one image list, *i.e.*, inverted list, which could be accessed by the ID of this visual word. The performance of BoWs based image retrieval may be affected by two factors, (1) feature detection failure, which fails to extract accurate local features, and (2) quantization error which assigns non-relevant local features into one visual word. This leads to two possible flaws of the reverted index, respectively, *i.e.*, the image list associating with a certain visual word misses entities that contains this visual word, and it also may contains images that are actually non-relevant.

In the meanwhile, images in the list are assumed to be visually relevant, but their overall distribution remains uninvestigated. Obviously, images that are not only visually similar but also share certain holistic consistencies should be reasonably organized together. That motivates us introduce holistic cues into the visually relevant image list.

In this paper, we introduce hybrid-indexing as a novel index fusion algorithm. Instead of extracting multiple image features during online retrieval or only consider two kinds of information cues such as co-indexing [8] or sharper image [9], our method incorporates multiple cues *simultaneously* into the inverted index. We investigate the consensus of images in various aspects and re-organize the index structure. The procedure only takes place off-line, and does not sacrifice online retrieval efficiency. Specifically, for each image lists that associating with a certain visual word, we build several directed graphs according to different holistic neighboring relationships. Then multiple graphs built by different cues are fused together by consolidating edges. A link analysis on the resulting graph is conducted to obtain the PageRank vector, which can be considered as a measurement of the image consistencies to each other. We remove the *isolated* images that are dissimilar to the others, and for the *significant* images with higher PageRank values, we replace them with their affiliating superimages [9]. The generated hybrid-indexing serves as the updated inverted index file, and can be accessed with the classic BoWs based retrieval model without any further modifications. The flowchart of the proposed method is illustrated in Fig. 1.

The main contribution of the proposed approach can be summarized as follows. (1) To our best knowledge, this is one of the few works on fusing different cues during off-line indexing period. (2) The proposed framework does not limit the quantity of fused cues and allow simultaneous consideration of local features and multiple holistic features, which may be infeasible in former works. (3) Our method does not need to extract multiple features during online retrieval, but manages to obtain consistent images not only are partially duplicated but also share a similar holistic characteristic.

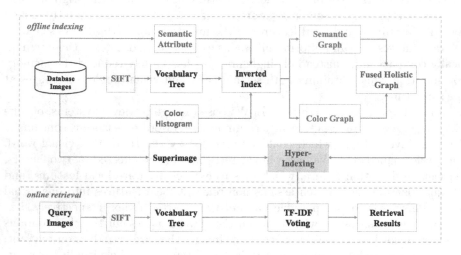

Fig. 1. Framework of the proposed method.

2   Related Work

There are two major categories of scalable image retrieval algorithms: searching for exact or near-duplicated images by indexing local features with vocabulary trees, and hashing holistic image features to binary codes to find similar images. We briefly review the two lines of retrieval strategies and the efforts have been made to combine them.

Local Features with Vocabulary Trees. Conventional BoWs model based image retrieval systems have been proven to be a great success in the past few years. By quantizing [10] local invariant image features [11–14] with vocabulary trees [15], an image is converted into a BoWs vector. The vocabulary tree is usually hierarchically trained on lots of local descriptors, and each of the leaf nodes is considered as a visual word. BoWs based retrieval systems commonly employ inverted index files to organize images [15], and in this file, each visual word is associated with a list of images containing this visual word. Retrieved candidates are further improved by spatial verification [16,17], query expansion [18], hamming embedded [19], high-order features [20]. Because the images are essentially described by local features, BoWs model is well suited for near-duplicate image search, while the results may show less global consensus due to lack of holistic depictions.

Holistic Features with Hashing Methods. Unlike local features, holistic features such as color histogram and GIST [21], aim to delineate overall distributions of an image, hence could capture certain aspects of the image global characteristics. Recent developments in large scale image recognition and classification also contribute to provide semantic-aware image features [22,23]. The outcomes of multi-class classifiers, often referred as semantic attributes [22–24], present a strong cue to find semantically relevant images. Holistic features are often indexed by locality sensitive hashing [25], and the resulting hash codes can be efficiently compared using Hamming distances. Since holistic features are not as invariant as local features, thus the retrieved candidates often miss near-duplicate objects.

Local Feature and Holistic Features Based Retrieval Fusion. Near-duplicate image retrieval using local features and similar image retrieval with holistic features are two lines of research. Although the limitation of individual retrieval schema is obvious, efforts made to fuse multiple features are rare. Combining local and holistic features can be conducted on the early feature fusion stage [2] or the later retrieved results fusion stage [4,6]. However, for image feature fusion, it is difficult to leverage various modalities of the fused feature. When it comes to ranking level fusion, multiple feature extraction and online re-ranking computation often introduce dramatic query time increasement. For example, [6] conducts query specific fusion during online retrieval and achieves a decent precision while consuming much memory overhead and query time. Works to fuse local features and holistic features in off-line indexing stage is either not optimal in identifying isolated images [8] or only could deal with one holistic feature at a time [9]. Our work shares some common properties with [8]. The differences are we involve more features and propose a more principled ranking strategy to spot and delete isolated images. Compared with [8], we achieve a more significant improvement over the baseline BoWs model.

3   Proposed Approach

We propose to fuse multiple image cues to build hybrid-indexing which embraces both local and multiple holistic features simultaneously. Various holistic features are extracted and superimages are constructed firstly, which is described in Sect. 3.1. In an inverted index file, images containing a common visual word form a short image list. We hence perform the following steps for each of the image lists throughout the whole index structure. For each of such lists, according to the kNN(k-Nearest Neighbor) relationships in every individual holistic feature space which is obtained in Sect. 3.1, multiple directed graph are built up, then these graphs are fused by consolidating edges to obtain a final graph (Sect. 3.2). PageRank values are computed on this graph to rank these images. For images with low rank values, we identified them as *isolated* images and remove them from the image list. For the *significant* images with high rank values, we replace them with their affiliating superimages [9]. This procedure is described in detail in Sects. 3.3 and 3.4.

3.1   Holistic Feature Extraction and Superimage Generation

The proposed method is not restricted to the usage of the type and quantity of holistic features. In our current implementation, we employ two commonly used holistic features, *i.e.*, semantic attributes and color histograms.

Semantic attributes are commonly computed as the classification scores of object classifiers. We follow the method of [8] to learn 1000 object SVM classifiers from the training images in LSVRC 10 [26], which is a subset of ImageNet dataset. Dense HOG and LBP features are extracted and further encoded by local coordinate coding. The margin scores of these SVMs are used as semantic attribute features. Our test sets are independent with ImageNet, hence we do not implicitly assume the query or the dataset are related to one object category in these semantic attributes. Distance of the 1000-dimensional features are measured by *cosine* distances, a common distance metric for floating-point features.

Colors are important visual cues to represent the image content. We employ distribution statistics from the HSV color space as image descriptors. Following the method of [3], we only focus on the saliency regions instead of extracting features from the whole image. Spectral Residual Model (SRM) is employed to automatically extract saliency regions, which are independent from any prior knowledge. The resulting color descriptor shows higher robustness than considering the whole image [3]. The dimension of the HSV color histogram is 48. We also use *cosine* distance to measure the distances between color features.

We follow exactly the same experimental and parameter settings of [9] to generate superimages. Specifically, mutual-kNN graph is built first based on semantic distances between images. We employ semantic attributes to build these sparse graphs and Euclidean distances to measure their distances. Maximal cliques searching algorithm is then employed to generate superimage candidates, followed by a greedy ranking algorithm to rank and select the final superimages. Each superimage contains a single or multiple images which are semantically relevant to each other, and thus can be considered as a representation of a particular semantic meaning. The superimage generation process can be completed off-line efficiently. For each image, we maintain an index structure to record its affiliating superimage, *i.e.*, the superimage that contain it. Note that, the superimage index structure will be used only in the procedure of hybrid-indexing construction (Sect. 3.4), and is no need for online retrieval stage.

3.2   Graph Generation and Fusion

The inverted index files organize the corresponding relationship between visual words and images. A set of images containing a certain visual word can be regarded as a set of locally visual relevant images. However, the discriminative capacity of a single local descriptor is limited, and the consistency of images within the set may not be reliable enough consequently. Therefore, we turn to further investigate their relationships in holistic feature spaces. Based on the obtained multiple holistic features, we build several relationship graphs over them respectively. We define the image set I_v associating with the visual word v as:

$$I_v = \{i|i \in D, v \in i\} \tag{1}$$

where D denotes the whole image dataset. For each image i in I_v, we link it with its kNN(k-Nearest Neighbor), then we use I_v as the vertex set and the directed connections as edge set, a graph

$$G -< I_v, E >$$

depicting their relationships is obtained, where

$$E = \{< i, j >)|i \in kNN(j), i, j \in I_v\} \tag{2}$$

in which i and j are two images in the list and $kNN(j)$ denotes kNN set of image j.

Based on different types of holistic features, a series of graphs $G^h =< I_v, E^h >$ can be generated. To utilize the advantage of multiple holistic cues simultaneously, we fuse them together into one graph $G =< I_v, E >$ with the same vertex set I_v and $E = \bigcup_h E^h$. That means if image i is kNN of j in any holistic feature space, there is a directed link pointing from i to j in the fused graph. Links that occur in more than one individual holistic graph imply much reliable relationship between images, and they will be favored in the following link analysis step. Note that, the procedure does not restrict the type of fused holistic feature, or the quantity of holistic cues. If there is only one holistic feature, the fused graph is identical to the one which is built on it.

An illustration of the process of graph fusion is shown in Fig. 2.

3.3 Significant and Isolated Image Detection

Given a graph G either generated by a single holistic feature or fused by multiple relationship graphs, the connectivity of a node reflects its global consensus to the others. This motivates us to conduct a link analysis [27] on graph G to rank according to their node connectivity. PageRank is a commonly used ranking algorithm to weight the importance of nodes in a graph. Because the graph G is built according to their neighboring relationships, a node is more important or relevant if it is more likely to be visited. A $|I_v| \times |I_v|$ connection matrix M is defined as $M_{ij} = 1/\deg(i)$, if $< i, j > \in E$, and $M_{ij} = 0$ otherwise, where $deg(i)$ denotes degree of node i. Normally, PageRank algorithm adopts a damping factor to guarantee its convergence. We empirically set it as 0.85 in all experiments.

After several iteration steps, a PageRank vector is computed and each image is assigned with a rank value, which depicts its importance in the graph G. To a certain extent, the obtained rank value can be deemed as the confidence of an

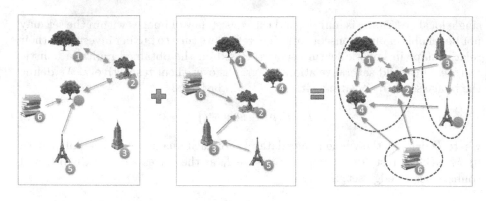

Fig. 2. An illustration of the process of multiple holistic graphs fusion. The toy example demonstrates two holistic graphs built over 6 images. A directed arrow represents that the end point is the kNN of the starting point ($k = 1$ in this example). The fused graph is constructed over the same vertex set and consolidated edges. It is can be observed that the fused graph captures more meaningful holistic distribution characteristic. PageRank algorithm is conducted on this fused graph to compute the rank value vector, and obtain the result: [0.2824, 0.3028, 0.0435, 0.3028, 0.0435, 0.0250]. Based the rank values, image 1, 2, and 4 are identified as *significant* images (red dotted circle), and image 6 is regarded as *isolated* image (black dotted circle) (Colour figure online).

image is relevant to this visual word. The images are ranked according to their PageRank values. Images with high values are considered as *significant* images, while the ones with low values are regarded as *isolated* images. Specifically, denote $PR(i)$ as the rank value of image i, α and β as the upper and lower threshold respectively, *significant* image set $\hat{I}_s$ is defined as

$$\hat{I}_s = \{i | i \in I_v, PR(i) > \alpha / |I_v|\} \tag{3}$$

and the *isolated* image set $\hat{I}_i$ is defined as

$$\hat{I}_i = \{j | j \in I_v, PR(j) < \beta / |I_v|\}. \tag{4}$$

In this way, images within the list I_v are divided into three categories, *i.e.*, *significant* images, *isolated* images, and the rest images. In the process of hybrid-indexing construction, images in different categories will be treated differently.

3.4   Hybrid-Indexing

Among all the images containing the visual word v, *significant* images are trusted to contain this visual word with certainty, and although v is also extracted on the *isolated* images, it is more likely that they may influenced by image noises or quantization errors. This motivates us to remove *isolated* images from the image set I_v and replace *significant* images with their affiliating superimages.

The concept of superimage is proposed in [9]. It consist of single or multiple compact semantic relevant images, and each image within is the mutual-kNN of each other. Once there is a *significant* image located, we replace it with its affiliating superimage. We maintain an index structure which is built in advance (Sect. 3.1) to record the superimage membership information. During the replacement process, the introduced superimages are unpacked into its affiliating images, thus for a *significant* i, the process is also equivalent to inserting images that share the same membership. The inserted images are assigned Term Frequency (TF) the same as image i. Note that, the size of superimages could be equal or greater than one. If the superimage size of i is one, in which case the superimage of i is identical to itself, image i in I_v remains unchanged. Apart from *significant* images and *isolated* images, the rest of the images also keep unchanged during the procedure. Specifically, a line of the constructed hybrid-indexing is obtained by

$$I_v{}^{new} = I_v - \hat{I}_i - \hat{I}_s + \{SI(i)|i \in \hat{I}_s\} \tag{5}$$

where $SI(i)$ is the affiliating superimage of i.

After the removal and replacement procedure, the image list I_v is updated by a new set $I_v{}^{new}$. Process all image lists in the inverted index file by order, hybrid-indexing with multi-type cues is generated. Image retrieval with the renewed hybrid-indexing does not need to alter the local feature extraction or the online retrieval stage, and it can be assembled with conventional BoWs model directly.

4   Experiments

4.1   Experimental Setup

Three different image retrieval tasks are conducted to evaluate the proposed method, *i.e.*, object search on UKbench [15], scene image search on INRIA Holidays [19], and large-scale image search on a dataset built by mixing MIRFLICKR-1M [28] collected from Flickr[1] with UKbench.

UKbench dataset contains 2,550 objects under 4 different viewpoints and illuminations. The retrieval performance is measured by the recall of top-4 retrieved images which is referred as N-S score. N-S score ranges from 0 to 4, indicting none or all of the relevant images are returned. INRIA holidays dataset includes 1,491 annotated personal holiday photos and 500 of them are served as queries. Performance on this dataset is measured by mAP (mean Average Precision). For large-scale image search, we use the public large dataset MIRFLICKR-1M [28] consisting 1 million real-world images as distractors, and mix it with UKbench dataset. Images from UKbench are employed as queries and N-S score is adopted as the performance metric.

4.2   Image Search

In this section, We test the proposed method with object search on UKbench and scene image search on INRIA Holidays. Different vocabulary trees are utilized to test if our method is sensitive to the vocabulary tree structures, which

---

[1] http://press.liacs.nl/mirflickr/.

usually result in different levels of quantization errors in classic BoWs based image search. We train a visual vocabulary tree with branch number $B = 10$ and layer number $L = 5$ (denoted as $T10^5$). It is trained against a separate data set consisting of 50,000 images randomly selected from ImageNet dataset. Besides of that, we also utilize the local features and the pre-computed visual words provided by the original authors of the two datasets for fair comparison. Despite of the authors of INRIA Holidays provide several varieties of vocabulary trees, for both of the two datasets, we employ vocabulary trees with $B = 10$ and $L = 6$ (denoted as $T10^6$) respectively. Retrieval performances of baseline approaches are summarized in Table 1.

Table 1. The retrieval performances of baseline methods

Dataset	UKBench(N-S Score)		Holidays(mAP)	
Performance	$T10^5$	$T10^6$	$T10^5$	$T10^6$
	2.8175	3.1664	58.3 %	66.5 %

Three parameters need to be decided during the process of constructing hybrid-indexing, *i.e.*, count of neighboring images k in Eq. 2, lower threshold α in Eq. 3, and upper threshold β in Eq. 4. We tune these three parameters on UKbench with $T10^6$, then apply them to the rest of our experiments.

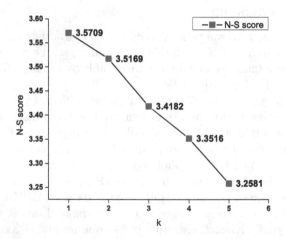

Fig. 3. The influence of the parameter k. Values larger than 1 yield less competitive results, thus we just search the nearest neighbor when constructing holistic feature graph.

We first fix α as 1 and β as 0, in which case no images will be identified as *significant* or *isolated* images, and investigate the influence of the count of neighboring images k in Eq. 2. Each image in Eq. 2 is linked to its k nearest neighbor, so the total count of edges in graph G is computed as $|E| = k * |I_v|$. That means larger k introduces more connections and makes the graph denser.

We demonstrate the influence of the parameter k on UKbench in Fig. 3. Interestingly, values larger than 1 yield less competitive precision than setting k as 1, i.e., only searching for the nearest neighborhood. The reason might be connecting excessive edges would introduce less stable relationships, thus is harmful to the performance. According to the tuning result, we set the count of neighboring images $k = 1$.

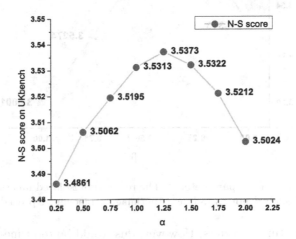

Fig. 4. The influence of the parameter α controlling the choice of *significant* images. It is clear that replacing *significant* images with their affiliating superimage improve the retrieval precision dramatically. With larger α, N-S score keeps increasing until a performance drop occurs.

Next, we keep setting β as 0, in which case the algorithm removes no *isolated* images and observe the impact of the choice of upper threshold α controlling the *significant* image selection. The experimental results are shown in Fig. 4. It can be seen that our algorithm shows significant improvement over the baseline (3.1664 of $T10^6$). The performance keeps increasing with reasonably lager α, indicating the benefit of embracing superimages is obvious. However, after a certain value, a performance drop occurs if we keep increasing α. The reason might be because larger α yield less *significant* images, thus not fully utilize the potential of the superimage replacement procedure. According to Fig. 4, in all of the following experiments, we set the upper threshold $\alpha = 1.25$.

After that, we fix the upper threshold and tune the lower threshold, i.e., β. The influence of the parameter β is demonstrated in Fig. 5. It proves the advantage of the procedure of isolated removal, although one can see that it does not help as much as superimage replacement. With increasing β, the algorithm removes more and more *isolated* images, and results in more compact index file and less memory consumption. The performance drops when excessive images are wrongly recognized as *isolated* images, and the precision is hindered consequently. Based on this observation, β is fixed as 0.25 in the following experiments.

Note that, in our current implementation, we adopt a simple parameter tuning strategy. Carefully evaluating the combinations of k, α and β would obtain

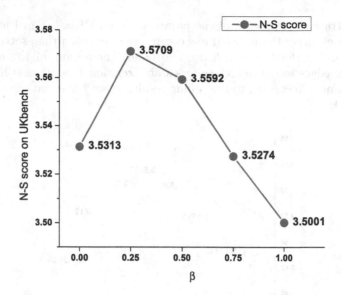

Fig. 5. The influence of the parameter β. The removal of isolated images does help the performance, although is not as well as superimage replacement procedure.

better parameter tuning results. However, this would be too time-consuming to conduct. Experimental results manifest that our current setting also yield decent performance.

As is described in Sect. 3.2, either single or multiple holistic features can be fused with local features to enhance the inverted index. We consider three cases on UKbench dataset, $i.e.$, employing semantic attribute only (SA), HSV color histogram only (HSV) and both of the two features (SA+HSV). Retrieval performances of the three different strategies are summarized in Fig. 6. It clearly proves that fusing multiple holistic features with our algorithm improves the retrieval precision dramatically. Quantitative study of the complementarity of holistic features and fuse them together guided by their complementarities is one of our future works.

We compare our method with recent retrieval approaches on UKbench and INRIA Holidays datasets, and summarize the results in Table 2. From the table, we can observe that the performance of our method is very competitive. The N-S score of UKbench increases 0.4 to 3.57 from 3.17, while on INRIA Holidays, mAP also has an improvement of 12.1 percent.

It is worthy to point out that we achieve the above performances in Table 2 without multiple feature extraction or re-ranking the results during online retrieval. Spatial verification or retrieval fusion, which introduce extra computations and memory costs, is adopted by some recent state-of-art retrieval systems, while our hybrid-indexing method deals with multi-type feature simultaneously totally during *off-line* stage. Our final performance is still decent considering we achieve them with a relatively low baseline. For example, [6] obtains a striking performance of N-S score on UKbench, but it is an increase of 0.23 based on a well implemented baseline which is 3.54.

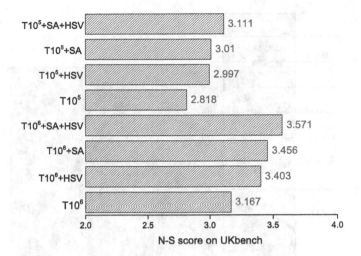

Fig. 6. Comparison of different fusion strategies. Complementarity of holistic features helps improvement of the retrieval precision on both baselines.

Another fact need to be stated is that compared with other indexing algorithms, memory consumption of hybrid-indexing is easily manageable. Indexed items of hybrid-indexing on UKbench counts to 7,869,590, while the conventional baseline indexes 5,712,698 items. That means an increase of 37.76 % memory overhead emerges with a series of the algorithm procedures. After the superimage replacement and isolated image removal, the inverted index file size of UKbench rise from 47.3M to 66.0M. As for INRIA Holidays, indexed items show an increase of 24.13 %, since less superimages are constructed on this dataset. Note that, some state-of-arts retrieval systems consume memory far more than ours, *e.g.*, Hamming Embedding [19] storage an 64 bits binary signature along with the image id for each indexed item. Even omit to store TF (normally 32 bits) in its implementation, it is still a 100 % memory consumption increase.

Some examples of retrieved images are presented in Fig. 7. It is obvious that our method is superior to retrieval algorithms that use single-type features.

Table 2. Comparison with the state-of-arts

Methods	Proposed	Baseline($T10^6$)	[8]	[29]	[30]	[16]	[19]	[6]
Ukbench, N-S	3.57	3.17		3.60	3.56	3.52	3.45	3.42	3.77
Holidays, mAP(%)	78.6	66.5		80.9	78.1	76.2	N/A	81.3	84.6

4.3   Large-Scale Image Search

To test the scalability of our approach, we also test our approach in the large-scale image search task. We employ a vocabulary tree with $B = 17$ and $T = 5$, which is trained on an independent large image dataset. We mix UKbench dataset with

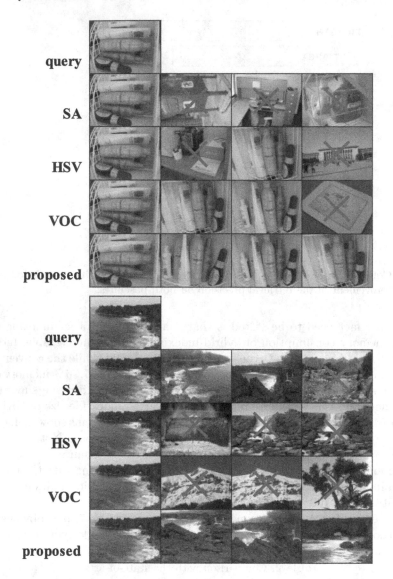

Fig. 7. Comparisons of retrieval results between our method and baseline methods, *i.e.*, image search with holistic feature semantic attribute (SA), color histogram (HSV) and BoWs retrieval baseline (VOC) on UKbench (*top*) and Holidays (*bottom*). The false results are marked by red crosses. The advantage of our method compared with any retrieval algorithms that use single-type features is evident (Colour figure online).

MIRFLICKR-1M [28] containing 1 million distraction images, and utilize images from UKbench as queries. Since our method is not restricted to the use of certain types of holistic features, we adopt Classemes [31] and HSV color histogram to fuse with local features to build hybrid-indexing. It is a more challenging task since superimages whose size larger than 1 on this dataset are rare due to its sparsity property. Despite of this, our method still improves the retrieval performance of baseline from 3.070 to 3.258 with a memory overhead of 19.7 %. Consequently, we could conclude that our approach is also scalable to retrieve images from million-scale datasets.

5   Conclusion

In this paper, we present a novel *off-line* indexing approach to fuse multi-type cues including local and various holistic features simultaneously. By introducing complementary holistic cues into the classic inverted index, the proposed hybrid-indexing algorithm effectively combines two separated image search schemas, thus the retrieved results not only contain locally similar objects but also images that share relevant holistic characteristics. Experimental results manifest the promising advantages of the proposed method and warrant further investigation in this direction.

Acknowledgement. This work was supported in part to Dr. Qi Tian by ARO grant W911NF-12-1-0057 and Faculty Research Awards by NEC Laboratories of America. This work was supported in part by National Science Foundation of China (NSFC) 61429201.

References

1. Smeulders, A.W., Worring, M., Santini, S., Gupta, A., Jain, R.: Content-based image retrieval at the end of the early years. TPAMI **22**, 1349–1380 (2000)
2. Gehler, P., Nowozin, S.: On feature combination for multiclass object classification. In: ICCV (2009)
3. Zhang, S., Huang, J., Huang, Y., Yu, Y., Li, H., Metaxas, D.N.: Automatic image annotation using group sparsity. In: CVPR, pp. 3312–3319. IEEE (2010)
4. Fagin, R., Kumar, R., Sivakumar, D.: Efficient similarity search and classification via rank aggregation. In: ACM SIGMOD (2003)
5. Jégou, H., Schmid, C., Harzallah, H., Verbeek, J.: Accurate image search using the contextual dissimilarity measure. TPAMI **32**, 2–11 (2010)
6. Zhang, S., Yang, M., Cour, T., Yu, K., Metaxas, D.N.: Query specific fusion for image retrieval. In: Fitzgibbon, A., Lazebnik, S., Perona, P., Sato, Y., Schmid, C. (eds.) ECCV 2012, Part II. LNCS, vol. 7573, pp. 660–673. Springer, Heidelberg (2012)
7. Ye, G., Liu, D., Jhuo, I.H., Chang, S.F.: Robust late fusion with rank minimization. In: CVPR (2012)
8. Zhang, S., Yang, M., Wang, X., Lin, Y., Tian, Q.: Semantic-aware co-indexing for image retrieval. In: ICCV (2013)
9. Luo, Q., Zhang, S., Huang, T., Gao, W., Tian, Q.: Superimage: packing semantic-relevant images for indexing and retrieval. In: ICMR (2014)
10. Zhou, W., Lu, Y., Li, H., Tian, Q.: Scalar quantization for large scale image search. In: Proceedings of the 20th ACM International Conference on Multimedia, pp. 169–178. ACM (2012)
11. Lowe, D.G.: Distinctive image features from scale invariant keypoints. IJCV **60**, 91–110 (2004)

12. Rublee, E., Rabaud, V., Konolige, K., Bradski, G.: ORB: an efficient alternative to sift or surf. In: ICCV (2011)
13. Zhang, S., Tian, Q., Huang, Q., Gao, W., Rui, Y.: USB: ultra short binary descriptor for fast visual matching and retrieval. IEEE Trans. Image Process. **23**(8), 3671–3683 (2014)
14. Tian, Q., Sebe, N., Loupias, E., Huang, T., Lew, M.: Image retrieval using wavelet-based salient points. J. Electron. Imaging **10**, 835–849 (2001)
15. Nistér, D., Stewénius, H.: Scalable recognition with a vocabulary tree. In: CVPR (2006)
16. Philbin, J., Chum, O., Isard, M., Sivic, J., Zisserman, A.: Object retrieval with large vocabularies and fast spatial matching. In: CVPR (2007)
17. Zhang, S., Tian, Q., Huang, Q., Rui, Y.: Embedding multi-order spatial clues for scalable visual matching and retrieval. IEEE J. Emerg. Sel. Top. Circuits Syst. **4**, 130–141 (2014)
18. Chum, O., Philbin, J., Sivic, J., Isard, M., Zisserman, A.: Total recall: automatic query expansion with a generative feature model for object retrieval. In: ICCV (2007)
19. Jegou, H., Douze, M., Schmid, C.: Hamming embedding and weak geometric consistency for large scale image search. In: Forsyth, D., Torr, P., Zisserman, A. (eds.) ECCV 2008, Part I. LNCS, vol. 5302, pp. 304–317. Springer, Heidelberg (2008)
20. Zhang, S., Tian, Q., Hua, G., Huang, Q., Gao, W.: Descriptive visual words and visual phrases for image applications. In: ACM Multimedia (2009)
21. Oliva, A., Torralba, A.: Modeling the shape of the scene: a holistic representation of the spatial envelope. IJCV **42**, 145–175 (2001)
22. Deng, J., Berg, A.C., Fei-Fei, L.: Hierarchical semantic indexing for large scale image retrieval. In: CVPR (2011)
23. Farhadi, A., Endres, I., Hoiem, D., Forsyth, D.: Describing objects by their attributes. In: CVPR (2009)
24. Douze, M., Ramisa, A., Schmid, C.: Combining attributes and fisher vectors for effcient image retrieval. In: CVPR (2011)
25. Andoni, A., Indyk, P.: Near-optimal hashing algorithms for approximate nearest neighbor in high dimensions. In: FOCS (2006)
26. Russakovsky, O., Deng, J., Su, H., Krause, J., Satheesh, S., Ma, S., Huang, Z., Karpathy, A., Khosla, A., Bernstein, M., Berg, A.C., Fei-Fei, L.: Imagenet large scale visual recognition challenge (2014)
27. Page, L., Brin, S., Motwani, R., Winograd, T.: The pagerank citation ranking: Bringing order to the web (1999)
28. Huiskes, M.J., Lew, M.S.: The mir flickr retrieval evaluation. In: MIR '08: Proceedings of the 2008 ACM ICMIR, ACM, New York (2008)
29. Wang, X., Yang, M., Cour, T., Zhu, S., Yu, K., Han, T.X.: Contextual weighting for vocabulary tree based image retrieval. In: ICCV (2011)
30. Shen, X., Lin, Z., Brandt, J., Avidan, S., Wu, Y.: Object retrieval and localization with spatially-constrained similarity measure and k-NN reranking. In: CVPR (2012)
31. Torresani, L., Szummer, M., Fitzgibbon, A.: Efficient object category recognition using classemes. In: Daniilidis, K., Maragos, P., Paragios, N. (eds.) ECCV 2010, Part I. LNCS, vol. 6311, pp. 776–789. Springer, Heidelberg (2010)

Look Closely: Learning Exemplar Patches for Recognizing Textiles from Product Images

Quoc Huy Phan[1]([✉]), Hongbo Fu[1], and Antoni B. Chan[2]

[1] School of Creative Media, City University of Hong Kong,
Kowloon, Hong Kong
quochuy.phan87@gmail.com
[2] Department of Computer Science, City University of Hong Kong,
Kowloon, Hong Kong

Abstract. The resolution of product images is becoming higher dues to the rapid development of digital cameras and the Internet. Higher resolution images expose novel feature relationships that did not exist before. For instance, from a large image of a garment, one can observe the overall shape, the wrinkles, and the micro-level details such as sewing lines and weaving patterns. The key idea of our work is to combine features obtained at such largely different scales to improve textile recognition performance. Specifically, we develop a robust semi-supervised model that exploits both *micro textures* and *macro deformable shapes* to select representative patches from product images. The selected patches are then used as inputs to conventional texture recognition methods to perform texture recognition. We show that, by learning from human-provided image regions, the method can suggest more discriminative regions that lead to higher categorization rates (+5-7%). We also show that our patch selection method significantly improves the performance of conventional texture recognition methods that usually rely on dense sampling. Our dataset of labeled textile images will be released for further investigation in this emerging field.

1 Introduction

Online shopping is changing the way people buy goods. It offers consumers the quickest way to check out a product's price and appearance without visiting an actual shop. In recent years, online fashion stores have provided high-resolution images to advertise their products, since users often pay attention to every detail, like materials, sewing lines, weaving quality, decorators, etc. Zoom-in functions may also be available to enable easy examination of the fine details of products. From a pattern recognition perspective, these high quality images are potentially useful for multiple tasks. For instance, one can use edge feature at macro scales to match products' global shape, while features at micro scales can be used for recognizing textures and details. More interestingly, one may combine features from different scales to reliably recognize objects.

One problem that might benefit from using a multi-scale approach is that of real-world textile recognition. Considering the case of leather, the best cue

© Springer International Publishing Switzerland 2015
D. Cremers et al. (Eds.): ACCV 2014, Part I, LNCS 9003, pp. 461–476, 2015.
DOI: 10.1007/978-3-319-16865-4_30

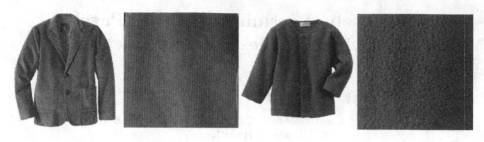

Fig. 1. Different scales reveal different characteristics of textiles. In this case, the micro scale exposes more discriminative features. Columns 1 and 2: Corduroy. Columns 3 and 4: Fleece.

to identify its instances is the macro shapes of the wrinkles, since leather has relatively smooth surface with few color patterns. Whereas, fur and fleece have rather rough micro structures with few or no wrinkles. To recognize these textiles, a better way should be to examine their texture features. See Fig. 1 for such an example, where macro shapes are largely similar while micro textures are very different. Motivated by this observation, we design a patch selection method that takes into account the evidences from two different scales (micro- and macro-scale) to identify discriminative patches in textile images. Having good patches identified, a number of related tasks such as retrieval and classification can be reliably carried out.

Despite the usefulness of higher resolution product images discussed above, existing works in the field of garment recognition (e.g., [1–4]) typically take small-sized images as input and thus ignore the information at micro scales. This limitation seriously restricts the understanding of garment textile, which is important to customers. On the other hand, texture recognition has been studied extensively in the field of computer vision. However, effective solutions (e.g., [5–7]) are typically demonstrated only on datasets of nicely cropped images. In contrast, real-world textures often appear at unknown positions and could be hidden in very large images. This makes it difficult to directly apply such solutions for recognizing textures in real-world contexts. One may expect that, applying these methods to a set of selective patches will improve the performance. However, as we will show in our experiments, existing patch selection methods (e.g., [8,9]) do not work well. In fact, the classification accuracies when using patches selected by these methods are even worse than those when using dense sampling on whole images. In contrast, our selection method provides patches that work well with traditional texture recognition methods, resulting in significantly higher accuracies.

In this paper, we introduce an efficient discriminative model to identify representative textured regions from product images. The key of our approach is an automatic patch selection process (Fig. 2 (A)), which is governed by both macro shape and micro texture. We assess the quality of the model by performing textile categorization on the patches selected by our method. Figure 2 (B) shows an overview of our categorization process. In experiments, categorization

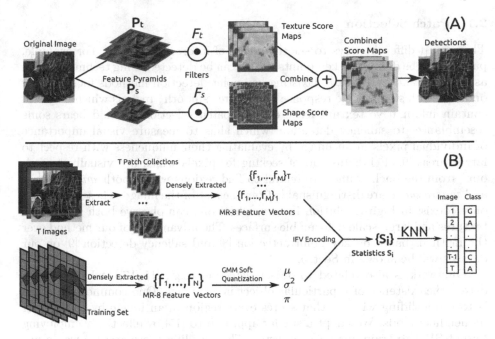

Fig. 2. (A) Patch selection process. First, two feature pyramids $\mathbf{P}_t$ and $\mathbf{P}_s$ are constructed. Next, they are convolved with two filters F_t and F_s to obtain two score maps. Finally, the score maps are combined and highly scored regions are selected. (B) texture categorization process. First, images in the training set are densely sampled and soft quantized to obtain (μ, σ^2 and π). Second, the patch selection algorithm chooses good patches for each image in the whole dataset. Third, feature vectors from those patches are densely extracted and encoded using IFV. Finally, the statistics $\{\mathbf{S}_i\}_{i=0}^T$ and the labels of the training data are used to classify novel images.

performance was significantly better when using our patch selection method, as compared to other methods like manual selection, SIFT detector selection [8], objectness measure [9], and dense sampling. We also introduce a simple texture feature that naturally fits into our framework, and has competitive performance when used with traditional classification models. To summarize, our findings are:

- An efficient discriminative model for texture-aware patch selection.
- A novel feature that is competitive with current state-of-the-art.
- A new textile dataset consisting of 480 samples (1000×1000 pixels), grouped into 8 classes and annotated with 9600 labels.

2   Related Work

This paper is connected to three different research fields: patch selection, texture recognition, and garment analysis.

2.1 Patch Selection

There exist different ways to select patches of interest in images. For example, patches can be defined at key points, which can be detected using techniques such as SIFT [8] and SURF [10]. Existing key point detection methods focus mainly on areas with strong edge response but ignore "smooth" regions which may still contain informative texture features. Our patch selection method bears some resemblances to saliency detection, which aims to measure visual importance of individual pixels in an image by evaluating their uniqueness with respect to larger areas [9, 11–14]. Instead of seeking for pixels which are visually "stand-out" from the background, we intend to find regions whose both *micro texture* and *macro shape* are distinguishable from the rest of the image. These properties only coexist in high resolution images, where one can observe both small-scale textures and large-scale deformable surfaces. The advantages of our method over the methods based on key point detection [8] and saliency detection [9] on our dataset will be shown in Sect. 5.

Our work is also related to object detection (e.g., [15–17]), which aims to detect the existence of a particular object in an image. One common approach is to use a sliding window that scores every region in an image by considering its neighborhoods. We adopt a similar approach to [15] by effectively employing Latent-SVM to train our patch selector. The key differences are: (a) we do not consider patch deformation with respect to a "root" filter, making our selector work on any type of object; (b) we simultaneously consider both texture and shape at different scales, which will be detailed in Sect. 4.1.

2.2 Texture Recognition

Texture recognition is already a mature field of computer vision. Dozens of techniques and datasets have been developed throughout the last decades. In terms of representation, one of the earliest works employs a bank of wavelets computed at various scales and rotations to capture the characteristics of textures [5, 18, 19]. Our work adopts the MR8 filter banks introduced by Varma and Zisserman [5] to represent textures. We choose this representation for its simplicity and compactness. Varma and Zisserman [20] challenged the role of filter banks by effectively replacing them with simple patches extracted densely on a grid. Approaches based on local binary patterns (LBP) [21, 22] also achieved great performance on standard datasets. Recently, Sifre and Mallat [6] used scattering convolutional network to extract very discriminative texture features and set the new state-of-the-art in texture classification (Rotation, Scaling and Deformation Invariant Scattering – RSDS). We will show the results of RSDS on our dataset in Sect. 5.

A common framework for texture recognition is the *texton* framework which has been first introduced by [18]. To describe texture, texton-based methods first build a dictionary of textons (visual words), which summarize basic components that make up texture appearance. Next, a histogram of visual words is constructed for every image by assigning a texton label to every pixel in that image. Recently Cimpoi et al. [7] presented a texture recognition method enabled by the Fisher Vector (FV). Instead of assigning hard labels to the pixels, the Fisher Vector uses soft labels and higher order statistics to describe texture. Their method achieves the state-of-the-art performance on very challenging datasets, such as FMD [23] and KTH-TIPS2 [24].

Researchers recently introduced the idea of texture *categorization* instead of *classification* [24,25]. While classification aims at recognizing instances of a texture, categorization generalizes them to a categorical level. Such generalizations enable the recognition of novel texture instances that do not appear in the training set. KTH-TIPS2 [24] is the first dataset to include different texture instances. We consider our work as texture categorization instead of classification.

Another trend is to recognize textures, since they appear in real-world contexts [25]. A prominent work of Liu et al. [26] is one of the first to address this problem. They introduced a very challenging dataset, namely the FMD dataset, which contains a wide range of texture images collected from Flickr. A significant contribution of their work is a psychological study on how humans recognize texture. They found that global shape is an equally important factor in texture recognition performance as local texture. Their finding forms a basis for our choice of using both shape and local texture for patch selection.

2.3 Garment Recognition

Garment understanding or recognition [27–29] has been an active research topic in recent years, and gives rise to many practical applications like product suggestions [4,30], genre classification [31], outfit recommendation [32], and clothing retrieval [1]. Our work is related to clothing attribute prediction [2,3]. Textile recognition is largely ignored in garment recognition, regardless of the fact that textile material plays a central role in customer decision making. For example Chen et al. [2] does not consider material at all. Liu et al. [1] uses material labels for performance measurement only. The work of [3] does include a limited number of materials as clothing attributes. However it does not show any textile prediction results and the reported classification rate is rather low (41 %).

3 Textile Dataset

We collected a large number of high-resolution images from online shopping and image sharing websites like Flickr, Polyvore and Amazon. The size of the images was at least 1000 pixels in both dimensions. While a large part of our dataset has relatively clean backgrounds, we chose to also include samples that contain objects as it appear in real-world contexts, e.g., with the human body and background. By doing so, we expect that our method should be able to distinguish between clothing and irrelevant regions such as skin, hair and other unaccounted materials. Although most of the objects are garments, we also included a number of non-garment objects like blankets and pillows. We then cropped and scaled all images to a regular size of 1000×1000 pixels (Fig. 3 (Left)). Images that contain different textile categories are removed to ensure fair testing and training. Unlike other real-world datasets like FMD [23], which provide masks to filter out unrelated regions, we assume there is a certain amount of noise in our samples. Finally, we had a collection of 480 high-resolution images which belong to

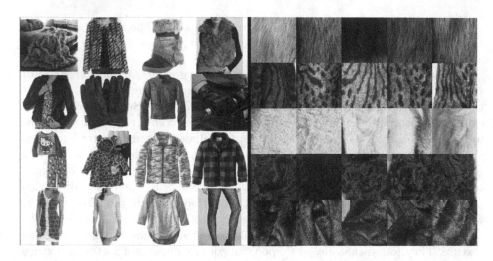

Fig. 3. (Left) Samples from Fur, Leather, Fleece and Lace (from top to bottom). (Right) Varieties of the Fur instances, with patches on the same row belonging to the same objects.

8 different textile categories: **Boucle, Fur, Leather, Lace, Knitted, Denim, Corduroy** and **Fleece** (60 samples per each).

Next, the images were contrast normalized and converted to grey-scale. All of our experiments are conducted on grey-scale images and do not consider color. Although color can be a good clue for texture recognition, it is also a source of confusion in the case of clothing since any color can be printed on any material with the current technologies. Figure 3 (Left) shows the diversity of our dataset. The Fleece category contains a wide range of printed patterns, while the Fur and Leather categories include samples from very different objects like gloves, blankets, shoes.

To supervise the recognition process, we manually labelled 20 patches of size 128×128 pixels in each image which contain representative textile instances. Figure 3 (Right) shows sample patches from the Fur category. It can be seen that different objects have very different appearance at both micro and macro levels even though they all belong to the same category. More challenging, object surfaces are not flat and vary largely with lighting conditions.

4   Model Learning and Patch Selection

We approach the problem of textile recognition[1] by treating each textile category as a mixture of textile instances. This idea came from the fact that a textile (with textured surface) has different appearances in the real world, depending on its functionality and context. Taking denim as an example, when denim is used to produce a jacket, it can be cut and sewed to make pockets, collars and

---

[1] We use the term "recognition" to refer to both patch selection and categorization.

sleeves which are apparently different from those elements on a pair of denim pants. By modelling each textile instance as a mixture component, we allow the components to compete with each other when fitting onto a novel image. If one of the components matches one part of the image with high confidence, we conclude that the whole item should belong to a specific textile category. This is intuitively natural to the way that human beings recognize textile: when we look at a piece of clothing and are not sure which material it is made of, we usually focus on the most distinctive part of it, e.g., regions without distracting decorations or details. In our recognition framework, both texture and shape are used for patch selection while only texture is used for categorization. Thus, the textile categorization step is simply *texture categorization* and we will use these two terms interchangeably.

Figure 2 (A) portrays the patch selection process. Starting from an image without annotations, we construct two feature pyramids $\mathbf{P}_t$ and $\mathbf{P}_s$, which represent texture and shape at multiple scales, respectively. The feature pyramids are then independently convolved with two filters F_t and F_s to obtain the score maps. The score maps are then combined into a final score map, which specifies good and bad regions to sample. Section 4.1 will discuss the score function in details.

Our textile recognition problem can be posed as a multi-instance learning problem, which can be addressed using different machine learning tools such as [33–35]. We employ the Latent-SVM [15] to train the filters F_t and F_s in a one-versus-all fashion.

Once we have selected the patches using the score map, it is straightforward to perform texture categorization. We use K-nearest neighbours in conjunction with bag-of-visual-words encoding to categorize textures. Sections 4.2 and 5 will explain the processes in details.

4.1   Learning Scheme

We use the Latent-SVM to learn the best filter parameters for each textile category. We next discuss the Latent-SVM, the associated score function, and our initialization procedure.

Multi-instance Learning with Latent-SVM. Since our patch selection problem is posed as a multiple-instance learning problem, we use Latent-SVM (L-SVM) [15] to learn the filter parameters F_t and F_s. Similar to a conventional SVM, L-SVM scores an example x with a function of the form

$$f_\beta(x) = \max_{z \in Z(x)} \langle \beta, \Phi(x, z) \rangle, \tag{1}$$

where β is a vector of model parameters (filters), z are latent values and Φ is a mapping from image space to feature space, i.e., the feature vector. In our model, β is a vectorized combination of F_t and F_s from all mixture components and will be discussed later. The inner product term in Eq. 1, $\langle \beta, \Phi(x, z) \rangle$, is called the score function. A binary label for x can be obtained by thresholding $f_\beta(x)$. The set $Z(x)$ defines the possible latent values for an example x. In our framework, z is the possible coordinates and scales of an image window in the feature pyramids. Unlike the model in [15], which contains one root and many parts, our method uses one window only. We also do not impose any spatial constraints on the windows and allow them to move freely to any place in the latent value space. Our patch selector thus works on any type of object.

The parameter vector β is learned from labelled examples $D = \{(x_i, y_i)\}_{i=1}^{n}$, $y_i \in \{-1, 1\}$, by minimizing the following objective function

$$L_D(\beta) = \frac{1}{2}\|\beta\|^2 + C \sum_{i=1}^{n} \max(0, 1 - y_i f_\beta(x_i)), \tag{2}$$

where $\max(0, 1 - y_i f_\beta(x_i))$ is the standard hinge loss and the parameter C controls the trade-off between penalizing the loss and maximizing the margins. Rather than optimizing $L_D(\beta)$ directly, L-SVM defines an auxiliary objective function $L_D(\beta, Z_p) = L_{D(Z_p)}(\beta)$, where $D(Z_p)$ is derived from D by restricting the latent values for positive examples which have latent values controlled by Z_p. Because $L_D(\beta) = \min_{Z_p} L_D(\beta, Z_p)$ the auxiliary objective function bounds the L-SVM objective. Please refer to [15] for more details. Subsequently, $L_D(\beta, Z_p)$ is minimized by using a 2-step iterative process:

– Relabel positive examples: Optimize $L_D(\beta, Z_p)$ over Z_p by selecting the highest scoring latent value for each positive example, $z_i = \text{argmax}_{z \in Z(x_i)} \beta \cdot \Phi(x_i, z)$.
– Optimize β: Optimize $L_D(\beta, Z_p)$ over β by solving the convex optimization problem defined by $L_{D(Z_p)}(\beta)$.

In our work, we use 1-vs-all training for each textile category, i.e., the samples from one category form the positive examples and the rest are negative examples.

Score Function. The score function is the inner product between the L-SVM parameter vector β and the feature vector Φ (see Eq. 1). The score function is used to score the latent values for positive examples (as in Step-1 of L-SVM optimization), to mine hard-negative examples and to perform patch selection. The patch selection process is discussed previously, and a hard-negative mining algorithm can be found in [15].

We compute the score by applying the filters to two feature pyramids $\mathbf{P}_s$ and $\mathbf{P}_t$, corresponding to the shape and texture of the textile. The texture feature pyramid is calculated at twice the resolution of the shape feature pyramid. The reason for computing texture features at higher resolution is to ensure that the local statistics are sufficient for discriminating different textiles. Whereas, shape feature at higher resolution will likely be less generic, i.e., it will not be sensitive to variations of a textile's macro deformable surfaces. Figure 4 shows the shape, texture and combined score maps from several images.

As mentioned earlier, we treat each textile category as a mixture model $M = (m_1, ..., m_N)$, where $\{m_i\}_{i=1}^{N}$ are the components of the mixture and N is the number of components. Each component represents an instance of the textile.

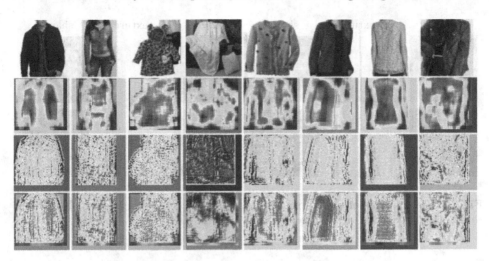

Fig. 4. Score maps from different categories. From top to bottom rows: original images, texture maps, shape maps, and combined score maps.

A textile instance hypothesis $\mathbf{h} = (i, z)$ for the mixture model specifies a component $i \in \{1, \cdots, N\}$ and a location $z = (u, v, l)$ for the filters of the component m_i, where l is the level in the feature pyramids and (u, v) is the spatial location. The score of hypothesis $\mathbf{h}$ is defined as:

$$Score(\mathbf{h}) = F_s^i \cdot \phi_s(\mathbf{P_s}, z) + F_t^i \cdot \phi_t(\mathbf{P_t}, z) + b_i, \qquad (3)$$

where F_s^i and F_t^i are the shape and the texture filters (as vectors) of the model i, respectively. $\phi_s(\mathbf{P_s}, z)$ and $\phi_t(\mathbf{P_t}, z)$ represent the respective shape and texture feature vectors, computed at level l of two feature pyramids $\mathbf{P_s}$, $\mathbf{P_t}$ and at location (u, v). The dot operator is the vector dot product, which is analogous to convolving the filter and feature vectors.

The score function in Eq. 3 can be written in inner product form, as in Eq. 1. β is formed by concatenating all filter parameters $\{F_s^i, F_t^i, b_i\}$ into a vector,

$$\beta = (F_s^1, F_t^1, b_1, ..., F_s^N, F_t^N, b_N). \qquad (4)$$

Similarly, a feature vector for each example (an image patch) is formed by concatenating shape and texture features extracted at location z in the feature pyramids,

$$\Phi_i(\mathbf{P_s}, \mathbf{P_t}, z) = (0, ..., 0, \phi_s(\mathbf{P_s}, z), \phi_t(\mathbf{P_t}, z), 1, ..., 0), \qquad (5)$$

where the zeros place the feature vectors in the position corresponding to the filters of the i-th mixture component, i.e., so that they are convolved with the correct filter entries in β.

After having β and Φ_i, we can measure the score of a hypothesis by simply taking a dot product $\langle \beta, \Phi_i(\mathbf{P_s}, \mathbf{P_t}, z) \rangle$.

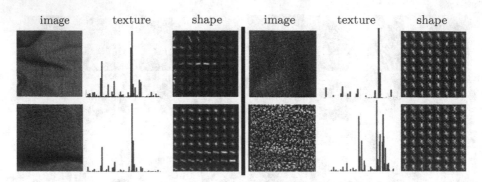

| image | texture | shape | image | texture | shape |

Fig. 5. Two scenarios of textile recognition. (Left) Texture filter fails but shape filter works. (Right) Shape filter fails and texture filter works.

Intuitively, the texture filter works as a texture detector that is sensitive to micro structures of a textile, whereas, the shape filter's role is to locate areas with similar macro shapes. Figure 5 shows two cases of textile recognition. In the first case (Left), the two texture histograms are very similar while the shapes (HOG) are obviously different. In contrast in the second case (Right), the two HOG maps are almost the same while the texture histograms are very discriminative.

Initialization Method. Initialization is a crucial part in training L-SVM. As noted by [15], β needs to be initialized carefully because the algorithm may select unreasonable latent values for the positive examples in the first iteration, causing bad models. In practice, we extract shape features from all the annotated regions in all training images. As introduced in Sect. 3, these annotations are patches identifying the interesting texture regions in each image. Recall that we want to build a mixture model $M = (m_1, ..., m_N)$ that represents N instances of the textile. We start with clustering all the image patches into N clusters by employing the K-means algorithm on the shape features. We do not consider texture as it did not show significant improvement in clustering quality. After the initialization, we have every region associated with a cluster label. The cluster label is used as the initial component assignment for each sample patch.

4.2   Categorization

Having the textile models in hand, we can either use the score assigned by L-SVM to directly classify the images, or use the highly-scored regions to extract the features and then learn another classifier. Experimental results show little difference between the two methods. We, however, choose the latter as this method often yields more stable results.

To proceed, we first perform a simple matching procedure. A mixture M_c is learned for each textile category, resulting in a set of mixtures $\{M_c\}_{c=1}^C$, where C is the number of categories. Given an image q we fit all mixtures $\{M_c\}_{c=1}^C$ on to the image by convolving the pair of filters from each component with it using Eq. 3. After this step, we obtain $\{\{p_{ic}\}_{i=1}^{N}\}_{c=1}^{C}$ candidate patches. We then calculate the score $\{s_c\}_{c=1}^{C}$ associated with each mixture,

$$s_c = \max_{i \in \{1,..,N\}} Score(p_{ic}),$$

where $Score(p_{ic})$ is computed using Eq. 3. In other words, the score for a given textile is the highest score among its mixture components. Feature vectors of the patches selected by the mixture with the largest s_c are then extracted and aggregated together to form a feature vector $\mathbf{f}$. Finally, textural statistics $\mathbf{S}$ is computed from $\mathbf{f}$ to form a descriptor for each query q:

$$\mathbf{d} = (\mathbf{S}_q, s_1, ..., s_C).$$

The concrete form of the textural statistics will be discussed in Sect. 5.

Next, a standard K-nearest neighbours classifier with Euclidean distance is used to assign labels to the testing samples. The number of neighbours is the same as the number of textile categories ($K = 8$). Figure 2(B) shows the whole categorization process.

5   Experiments

In this section we first give the implementation details and then discuss some experimental results.

5.1   Implementation Details and Experimental Set-Up

As mentioned earlier, our model consists of two parts: shape and texture. Our implementation uses histograms of oriented gradients (HOGs) [16] as the shape feature and improved Fisher vector (IFV) [36] with MR-8 Filter Banks [5] as the texture feature. The choice of using IFV fits well in our framework. First, it is shown theoretically in [37] that the distances between IFVs can be accurately measured by simply taking their dot products. Second, as a bag-of-words based method, IFV can effectively summarize textural statistics over multiple patches.

For the GMM soft quantization, we use $K = 200$ Gaussian modes. MR-8 descriptors are extracted densely for every pixel. Prior to extracting the MR-8, the images are normalized to have zero means and unit standard deviation. The parameter C of L-SVM is selected by cross-validation. Although it is possible to have higher accuracy by fine-tuning C for different mixtures, we choose to use the same C for all mixtures.

To train the model, we split the dataset into training and testing datasets with the ratios (35/25), (25/35), (15/45) and performed L-SVM training on each training set. We used $N = 20$ components for each mixture. We treated all images in the training set of a category as positive examples and all training images from other categories as negative examples. Additionally, we also used a set of 50 landscape images as negative examples; this is to make the model more robust against backgrounds. We conducted our experiments on all 8 categories: *Fleece, Fur, Corduroy, Denim, Knit, Leather, Boucle* and *Lace.*

To evaluate the effectiveness we compared our patch selection method with other selection schemes: manual selection, selection based on the SIFT detector [8], selection based on objectness measure (OM) [9] and dense sampling. All training and testing were performed individually on patches selected by each method. All patch selection and texture categorization tasks were repeated on 10 random splits. For SIFT, we computed MR-8 at the location (u, v) and scale l of 20 key-points. For OM, we used the software package provided by the authors with the default settings except for the color contrast cue, which was excluded for fair comparison with other methods. We trained OM on the same set of annotations from our dataset. Furthermore, we also include the results of the current state-of-the-art texture classification framework (RSDS) [6]. While all other methods were tested using the same framework as ours (IFV-MR8 and KNN), RSDS used the feature and the classifier provided by the authors [6].

5.2   Results

Sample Patch Selections. Figure 6 shows some sample images and the patches selected by both human and our method. The bottom-right example shows the difference between the human and machine patches. While the human annotator tends to choose the patches evenly over the object, our method selects patches around some certain areas. It is interesting to see that the pillow which was not noticed at all by the annotator is selected by our method. In contrast our method successfully avoids the rest of the image which contains the curtain and the wall. A similar conclusion is applicable to other examples. In the top-right example (i.e., red jacket), the hair is successfully avoided whereas there is only one misidentified patch in the top-left example.

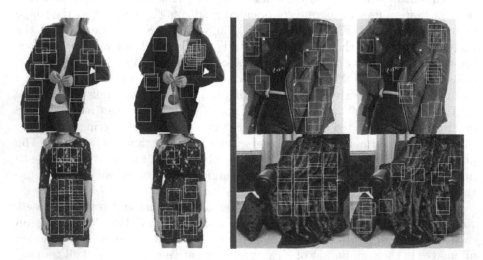

Fig. 6. Patch selection on novel images. In each example, the patches in the left image were human annotated and those in the right image were automatically selected by our method.

Categorization Results. Table 1 shows the categorization performance of the compared methods. Despite the diversity of the dataset and the simplicity of the feature our method achieved very promising results. The average accuracy when the model was trained with 35 samples was 64.6 %. In particular, the accuracies for the categories of Leather and Boucle were 77.8 % and 84.0 %, respectively. This is because Boucle and Leather often come with uniform patterns and decorations. The performance on the Fleece category was surprisingly good as we can see how diverse this category is in the dataset. It is worth noting that the differences between using 35, 25 and 15 training samples were not very large. This indicates that out method performs quite well even with a limited number of samples.

The categorization on human annotated patches was inferior to our method in almost all cases (Table 1), mainly because the L-SVM searches for the most discriminative patches. Since we treat the position of a patch as a latent value z, it is allowed to extensively search for better locations around the image. The search is constrained by two criterion: shape and texture. In cases like leather and chiffon that often exhibit little textural information at micro scales, the shape component computed at larger scales will play a major role. Whereas, textiles like fleece and fur have very vague macro shapes that do not contribute much to the discrimination. In these cases, the texture component will be "in charge". More importantly, by selecting patches with similar surfaces from different images, the texture comparison would be more accurate as the lighting condition and deformation are close.

The performance by SIFT and OM (Table 1) was consistently low for all the numbers of training samples. Since the SIFT-based detector and OM tend

Table 1. Categorization accuracies using patches selected by: Our method (Our), human (Man), SIFT detector, dense sampling (Dens), Objectness Measure (OM) and RSDS.

M	Fleece	Fur	Corduroy	Denim	Knit1	Leather	Boucle	Lace	Average
Number of training examples = 35									
Our	50.2 ± 6.8	59.6 ± 11.2	48.9 ± 7.5	**67.6** ± 5.5	63.6 ± 7.2	**77.8** ± 4.7	**84.0** ± 4.2	65.3 ± 8.2	**64.6** ± 2.3
Man	53.8 ± 5.7	57.3 ± 5.7	40.9 ± 8.2	52.0 ± 7.3	47.6 ± 14.2	74.2 ± 6.0	76.0 ± 8.6	48.0 ± 7.3	56.2 ± 3.5
SIFT	32.0 ± 6.0	46.7 ± 12.2	24.4 ± 12.0	41.3 ± 8.4	28.4 ± 6.9	64.0 ± 7.8	64.9 ± 8.0	55.1 ± 9.8	44.6 ± 3.3
Dens	36.0 ± 5.0	46.2 ± 11.2	28.4 ± 6.7	58.7 ± 8.4	46.7 ± 8.6	67.1 ± 3.7	77.3 ± 6.3	68.9 ± 10.3	53.7 ± 2.4
OM	44.9 ± 5.6	37.8 ± 7.1	26.7 ± 10.3	39.6 ± 8.3	36.0 ± 11.2	52.4 ± 7.4	58.2 ± 7.8	56.9 ± 9.2	44.1 ± 3.2
RSDS	**59.6** ± 9.3	**60.9** ± 10.9	**61.3** ± 10.4	53.8 ± 7.5	62.7 ± 7.2	45.3 ± 13.9	64.9 ± 7.4	**69.3** ± 9.4	59.7 ± 2.4
Number of training examples = 25									
Our	49.8 ± 9.3	53.3 ± 6.3	40.3 ± 5.5	**58.4** ± 7.5	56.2 ± 5.0	**81.9** ± 5.9	**86.0** ± 3.1	68.6 ± 4.5	**61.8** ± 2.4
Man	53.3 ± 6.6	**54.0** ± 9.4	37.5 ± 6.8	50.5 ± 8.7	47.0 ± 8.5	73.0 ± 4.5	75.6 ± 4.9	45.1 ± 8.6	54.5 ± 3.8
SIFT	23.5 ± 8.1	46.0 ± 8.6	28.9 ± 7.1	38.1 ± 6.0	28.3 ± 5.6	63.5 ± 5.7	64.4 ± 6.5	49.2 ± 10.4	42.7 ± 3.3
Dens	36.5 ± 4.4	44.1 ± 7.1	27.6 ± 8.6	58.7 ± 8.9	46.7 ± 7.9	64.8 ± 4.0	76.8 ± 6.7	62.5 ± 9.1	52.2 ± 2.8
OM	43.8 ± 6.2	38.1 ± 7.1	29.2 ± 8.2	35.9 ± 10.1	36.2 ± 8.4	45.7 ± 6.5	56.2 ± 5.0	55.9 ± 7.1	42.6 ± 1.7
RSDS	**55.6** ± 8.0	46.0 ± 10.7	**61.9** ± 13.2	42.5 ± 14.2	47.6 ± 10.6	49.2 ± 9.6	59.4 ± 6.5	67.6 ± 4.3	53.7 ± 2.8
Number of training examples = 15									
Our	32.6 ± 7.3	**52.8** ± 7.1	37.5 ± 6.9	55.6 ± 5.1	**56.5** ± 7.1	**73.1** ± 1.6	**76.8** ± 4.1	**64.4** ± 6.7	**56.2** ± 1.8
Man	41.7 ± 7.4	42.2 ± 7.9	38.3 ± 8.2	44.0 ± 3.4	50.1 ± 7.5	72.1 ± 6.2	72.1 ± 7.0	34.6 ± 7.8	49.4 ± 1.7
SIFT	24.0 ± 7.5	35.3 ± 8.3	27.4 ± 8.2	31.9 ± 7.6	28.9 ± 9.9	62.2 ± 8.2	60.5 ± 5.4	35.6 ± 9.2	38.2 ± 2.5
Dens	32.1 ± 6.5	38.5 ± 7.6	27.9 ± 7.8	**57.8** ± 12.7	46.7 ± 4.4	62.2 ± 6.2	75.6 ± 3.8	49.9 ± 8.6	48.8 ± 1.7
OM	39.0 ± 9.2	35.3 ± 7.1	26.7 ± 12.1	31.4 ± 9.0	34.1 ± 8.1	36.5 ± 5.7	53.8 ± 4.2	46.7 ± 8.2	37.9 ± 3.2
RSDS	**53.1** ± 14.5	41.7 ± 7.2	**50.9** ± 10.3	37.0 ± 11.2	51.1 ± 12.0	52.1 ± 10.4	42.7 ± 14.5	58.0 ± 12.5	48.3 ± 1.4

to select patches with strong edges, they mistakenly skip those "smooth" areas that may contain informative textural patterns. It is a surprise that both densely sampled IFV-MR8 and RSDS performed better than SIFT and OM, even though the features were computed over an entire image. Evidently, only our method selected patches better than dense sampling. When compared on the same feature, our method boosted the accuracy by 11 % (the case of 35 training examples, Table 1) and was 5–8 % better than the state-of-the-art method, RSDS.

Impact of Shape and Texture Components. To support our decision on choosing the components for patch detector, we show in Table 2 the categorization results when using shape-only and texture-only features for patch selection. Overall, the performance of the shape-only or texture-only method was clearly inferior to their combination. When using 35 training examples, patches selected with shape-texture features yielded 64.6 % accuracy, while the accuracies for shape-only and texture-only were only 41.1 % and 49.2 %, respectively. In addition, the performance of patches selected with texture features was generally lower than that of shape feature. However, texture feature is more robust in the cases of Fur, Lace and Boucle.

Table 2. Comparison of textile categorization using shape-only (Shape), texture-only (Tex) and shape-texture (Both) features for patch selection.

Method	Fleece	Fur	Corduroy	Denim	Knit1	Leather	Boucle	Lace	Average
Number of training examples = 35									
Both	50.2 ± 6.8	59.6 ± 11.2	48.9 ± 7.5	67.6 ± 5.5	63.6 ± 7.2	77.8 ± 4.7	84.0 ± 4.2	65.3 ± 8.2	64.6 ± 2.3
Tex	28.9 ± 7.5	50.7 ± 7.8	38.7 ± 4.2	48.4 ± 6.7	33.3 ± 7.8	59.6 ± 7.4	72.9 ± 5.9	61.3 ± 7.8	49.2 ± 2.2
Shape	33.3 ± 7.1	28.9 ± 7.5	24.9 ± 7.7	44.9 ± 9.9	41.3 ± 8.4	44.9 ± 7.7	66.7 ± 4.2	44.0 ± 8.0	41.1 ± 3.0
Number of training examples = 25									
Both	49.8 ± 9.3	53.3 ± 6.3	40.3 ± 5.5	58.4 ± 7.5	56.2 ± 5.0	81.9 ± 5.9	86.0 ± 3.1	68.6 ± 4.5	61.8 ± 2.4
Tex	33.7 ± 5.5	45.7 ± 9.3	34.6 ± 9.8	43.8 ± 5.4	31.7 ± 7.8	59.7 ± 10.6	68.6 ± 6.7	54.9 ± 8.3	46.6 ± 1.8
Shape	38.4 ± 4.3	47.0 ± 12.8	40.3 ± 6.4	45.1 ± 10.0	47.9 ± 9.0	58.4 ± 8.4	71.4 ± 3.3	59.7 ± 6.9	51.0 ± 2.0
Number of training examples = 15									
Both	32.6 ± 7.3	52.8 ± 7.1	37.5 ± 6.9	55.6 ± 5.1	56.5 ± 7.1	73.1 ± 1.6	76.8 ± 4.1	64.4 ± 6.7	56.2 ± 1.8
Tex	23.0 ± 5.5	38.5 ± 6.9	30.1 ± 6.4	35.6 ± 10.2	26.2 ± 6.7	54.1 ± 9.5	69.1 ± 6.9	53.3 ± 8.0	41.2 ± 2.4
Shape	26.9 ± 5.7	37.8 ± 6.5	29.4 ± 7.5	53.6 ± 6.3	49.9 ± 5.7	50.9 ± 10.9	61.7 ± 4.3	48.4 ± 7.3	44.8 ± 1.3

6   Conclusions

We have presented a novel model for textile recognition, consisting of patch selection and textile categorization. The patch selection process is carried out with Latent-SVM, an efficient learning method recently introduced into the world of object recognition, and uses both micro level texture and macro deformable shape to select representative patches. Our model is capable of detecting the most representative textural regions in an image, leading to significantly better textile categorization performance. An important property of our method is the ability of the machine to learn from human annotations patches and then refine them to produce more discriminative patches. We believe that by replacing the basic texture feature with more advanced ones our model could achieve even better performance.

References

1. Liu, S., Song, Z., Liu, G., Xu, C., Lu, H., Yan, S.: Street-to-shop: cross-scenario clothing retrieval via parts alignment and auxiliary set. In: IEEE Conference on Computer Vision and Pattern Recognition (CVPR), pp. 3330–3337 (2012)
2. Chen, H., Gallagher, A., Girod, B.: Describing clothing by semantic attributes. In: Fitzgibbon, A., Lazebnik, S., Perona, P., Sato, Y., Schmid, C. (eds.) ECCV 2012, Part III. LNCS, vol. 7574, pp. 609–623. Springer, Heidelberg (2012)
3. Bossard, L., Dantone, M., Leistner, C., Wengert, C., Quack, T., Van Gool, L.: Apparel classification with style. In: Lee, K.M., Matsushita, Y., Rehg, J.M., Hu, Z. (eds.) ACCV 2012, Part IV. LNCS, vol. 7727, pp. 321–335. Springer, Heidelberg (2013)
4. Wang, X., Zhang, T.: Clothes search in consumer photos via color matching and attribute learning. In: Proceedings of the 19th ACM International Conference on Multimedia, pp. 1353–1356 (2011)
5. Varma, M., Zisserman, A.: A statistical approach to texture classification from single images. Int. J. Comput. Vis. **62**, 61–81 (2005)
6. Sifre, L., Mallat, S.: Rotation, scaling and deformation invariant scattering for texture discrimination. In: IEEE Conference on Computer Vision and Pattern Recognition (CVPR), pp. 1233–1240 (2013)
7. Cimpoi, M., Maji, S., Kokkinos, I., Mohamed, S., Vedaldi, A.: Describing textures in the wild. In: IEEE Conference on Computer Vision and Pattern Recognition (CVPR) (2014)
8. Lowe, D.: Distinctive image features from scale-invariant keypoints. Int. J. Comput. Vis. **60**, 91–110 (2004)
9. Alexe, B., Deselaers, T., Ferrari, V.: Measuring the objectness of image windows. IEEE Trans. Pattern Anal. Mach. Intell. **34**(11), 2189–2202 (2012)
10. Bay, H., Tuytelaars, T., Van Gool, L.: SURF: speeded up robust features. In: Leonardis, A., Bischof, H., Pinz, A. (eds.) ECCV 2006, Part I. LNCS, vol. 3951, pp. 404–417. Springer, Heidelberg (2006)
11. Hou, X., Zhang, L.: Saliency detection: a spectral residual approach. In: IEEE Conference on Computer Vision and Pattern Recognition (CVPR), pp. 1–8 (2007)
12. Harel, J., Koch, C., Perona, P.: Graph-based visual saliency. In: Advances in Neural Information Processing Systems (NIPS) (2006)
13. Gao, D., Vasconcelos, N.: Bottom-up saliency is a discriminant process. In: IEEE International Conference on Computer Vision (ICCV) (2007)
14. Bruce, N., Tsotsos, J.: Saliency based on information maximization. In: Advances in Neural Information Processing Systems (NIPS) (2005)
15. Felzenszwalb, P.F., Girshick, R.B., McAllester, D., Ramanan, D.: Object detection with discriminatively trained part-based models. IEEE Trans. Pattern Anal. Mach. Intell. **32**, 1627–1645 (2010)
16. Dalal, N., Triggs, B.: Histograms of oriented gradients for human detection. In: IEEE Conference on Computer Vision and Pattern Recognition (CVPR) (2005)
17. Bosch, A., Zisserman, A., Munoz, X.: Representing shape with a spatial pyramid kernel. In: Proceedings of the 6th ACM International Conference on Image and Video Retrieval, pp. 401–408 (2007)
18. Leung, T., Malik, J.: Representing and recognizing the visual appearance of materials using three-dimensional textons. Int. J. Comput. Vis. **43**, 29–44 (2001)
19. Schmid, C.: Constructing models for content-based image retrieval. In: IEEE Conference on Computer Vision and Pattern Recognition (CVPR), vol. 2, p. II-39 (2001)

20. Varma, M., Zisserman, A.: A statistical approach to material classification using image patch exemplars. IEEE Trans. Pattern Anal. Mach. Intell. **31**, 2032–2047 (2009)
21. Guo, Z., Zhang, D.: A completed modeling of local binary pattern operator for texture classification. IEEE Trans. Image Process. **19**(6), 1657–1663 (2010)
22. Liao, S., Law, M.W., Chung, A.C.: Dominant local binary patterns for texture classification. IEEE Trans. Image Process. **18**(5), 1107–1118 (2009)
23. Sharan, L., Liu, C., Rosenholtz, R., Adelson, E.H.: Recognizing materials using perceptually inspired features. Int. J. Comput. Vis. **103**, 348–371 (2013)
24. Caputo, B., Hayman, E., Mallikarjuna, P.: Class-specific material categorisation. In: IEEE International Conference on Computer Vision (ICCV), vol. 2, pp. 1597–1604 (2005)
25. Caputo, B., Hayman, E., Fritz, M., Eklundh, J.O.: Classifying materials in the real world. Image Vis. Comput. **28**, 150–163 (2010)
26. Liu, C., Sharan, L., Adelson, E.H., Rosenholtz, R.: Exploring features in a bayesian framework for material recognition. In: IEEE Conference on Computer Vision and Pattern Recognition (CVPR), pp. 239–246 (2010)
27. Yamaguchi, K., Kiapour, M.H., Ortiz, L.E., Berg, T.L.: Parsing clothing in fashion photographs. In: IEEE Conference on Computer Vision and Pattern Recognition (CVPR), pp. 3570–3577 (2012)
28. Yamaguchi, K., Kiapour, M.H., Berg, T.L.: Paper doll parsing: retrieving similar styles to parse clothing items. In: IEEE International Conference on Computer Vision (ICCV), pp. 3519–3526 (2012)
29. Dong, J., Chen, Q., Xia, W., Huang, Z., Yan, S.: A deformable mixture parsing model with parselets. In: IEEE International Conference on Computer Vision (ICCV), pp. 3408–3415 (2013)
30. Kalantidis, Y., Kennedy, L., Li, L.J.: Getting the look: clothing recognition and segmentation for automatic product suggestions in everyday photos. In: Proceedings of the 3rd ACM conference on International conference on multimedia retrieval, pp. 105–112 (2013)
31. Hidayati, S.C., Cheng, W.H., Hua, K.L.: Clothing genre classification by exploiting the style elements. In: Proceedings of the 20th ACM International Conference on Multimedia, pp. 1137–1140. ACM (2012)
32. Liu, S., Feng, J., Song, Z., Zhang, T., Lu, H., Xu, C., Yan, S.: Hi, magic closet, tell me what to wear! In: Proceedings of the 20th ACM International Conference on Multimedia, pp. 619–628 (2012)
33. Blaschko, M.B., Hofmann, T.: Conformal multi-instance kernels. In: Workshop on Learning to Compare Examples (NIPS), pp. 1–6 (2006)
34. Gehler, P.V., Chapelle, O.: Deterministic annealing for multiple-instance learning. In: International Conference on Artificial Intelligence and Statistics, pp. 123–130 (2007)
35. Andrews, S., Tsochantaridis, I., Hofmann, T.: Support vector machines for multiple-instance learning. In: Advances in Neural Information Processing Systems (NIPS), pp. 561–568 (2002)
36. Perronnin, F., Sánchez, J., Mensink, T.: Improving the Fisher Kernel for large-scale image classification. In: Daniilidis, K., Maragos, P., Paragios, N. (eds.) ECCV 2010, Part IV. LNCS, vol. 6314, pp. 143–156. Springer, Heidelberg (2010)
37. Perronnin, F., Liu, Y., Sánchez, J., Poirier, H.: Large-scale image retrieval with compressed fisher vectors. In: IEEE Conference on Computer Vision and Pattern Recognition (CVPR), pp. 3384–3391 (2010)

Action Recognition from a Single Web Image Based on an Ensemble of Pose Experts

Peihao Zhang, Xiaoyang Tan[✉], and Xin Jin

Department of Computer Science and Technology,
Nanjing University of Aeronautics and Astronautics,
Nanjing 210016, China
x.tan@nuaa.edu.cn

Abstract. In this paper, we present a new method which estimates the pose of a human body and identifies its action from one single static image. This is a challenging task due to the high degrees of freedom of body poses and lack of any motion cues. Specifically, we build a pool of pose experts, each of which individually models a particular type of articulation for a group of human bodies with similar poses or semantics (actions). We investigate two ways to construct these pose experts and show that this method leads to improved pose estimation performance under difficult conditions. Furthermore, in contrast to previous wisdoms of combining the output of each pose expert for action recognition using such method as majority voting, we propose a flexible strategy which adaptively integrates them in a discriminative framework, allowing each pose expert to adjust their roles in action prediction according to their specificity when facing different action types. In particular, the spatial relationship between estimated part locations from each expert is encoded in a graph structure, capturing both the non-local and local spatial correlation of the body shape. Each graph is then treated as a separate group, on which an overall group sparse constraint is imposed to train the prediction model, with extra weight added according to the confidence of the corresponding expert. We show in our experiments on a challenging web data set with state of the art results that our method effectively improves the tolerance of our system to imperfect pose estimation.

1 Introduction

Human action recognition is an extremely important and active research field in computer vision [1–4]. Its purpose is to recognize what a person is doing or what the posture means. Human action recognition has many interesting and important applications, for example, surveillance, entertainment, human-computer interaction, image and video retrieval. Nowadays, most of the previous work in this area focused on recognizing human actions from videos, those work [5–7] mainly use motion cues and a lot of progress has been made in the recent years. However, compared with videos, human action recognition from static images is a relatively less-researched field. In fact, the analysis of human action in still images is very important. This can be very useful for image understanding

© Springer International Publishing Switzerland 2015
D. Cremers et al. (Eds.): ACCV 2014, Part I, LNCS 9003, pp. 477–493, 2015.
DOI: 10.1007/978-3-319-16865-4_31

and retrieval. Besides, it will not only help us to understand and analyze human actions under certain situations, but also can help us analyze and recognize human behaviors.

In this paper, we present a new method for recognizing human actions from still images. Our contribution is two-fold. First, we propose a global mixture of pose experts for more accurate articulation modeling. In contrast to a previously-proposed state of the art method [8] which uses a single pictorial tree with mixture of small, non-oriented parts to model the non-linear and non-convexity of the pose manifold of human being, we build a pool of pose experts, each of which individually models a particular type of articulation for a group of human bodies. We investigate two ways to construct the groups, one is based on the local shape statistics from pose annotations, and the other uses the semantic similarity related to action types. We show that both methods lead to improved pose estimation performance under difficult conditions. Furthermore, the estimated poses could be used for other tasks rather than action recognition, such as image retrieval by pose.

As our second contribution, we propose a flexible strategy which adaptively integrates the output of pose experts in a discriminative framework for action prediction (c.f., Fig. 1). In contrast to previous methods of combining the output of each pose expert using some relatively simple strategy such as majority voting, our method essentially allows each pose expert to adjust their roles in prediction according to their specificity when facing samples from different action types.

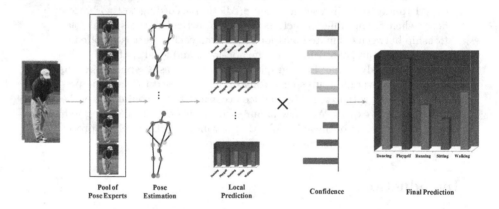

| Pool of Pose Experts | Pose Estimation | Local Prediction | Confidence | Final Prediction |

Fig. 1. The stages of our action prediction pipeline. For a test image shown in the leftmost, we use an ensemble of pose experts to extract pose cues from it, which are then respectively fed into the corresponding action predictor to evaluate its posterior probability distribution over action types. Finally, the conditional expectation is calculated for each action type over the pose experts involved, based on which the final decision is made. Technically, we use a discriminative framework with group sparse constraints to jointly train this series of action predictors (detailed in Sect. 3.2). This essentially allows each pose expert to play different roles in different action prediction tasks according to their specificity, and the strength of each experts is thus adaptively combined for the final action prediction.

To achieve this, we first use a graph structure to capture both the non-local and local spatial correlation of the body shape estimated by the pose expert. Each graph is then treated as a single unit, over which an overall group sparse constraint is imposed to train the prediction model, with extra weight added according to the confidence of the corresponding expert. We show in our experiments on a challenging web data set with state of the art results that our method effectively improves the tolerance of our system to imperfect pose estimation.

The rest of this paper is organized as follows. After a brief review of the related work in Sect. 2, we details our method in Sect. 3. Experimental results are given in Sect. 4. We conclude our paper in Sect. 5.

2 Related Work

The major challenges of action recognition from still images come from the variability of human visual appearances (possibly with highly cluttered background), many degrees of freedom in human body postures, and lack of motion cue. In this section we give a brief review on how to deal with these issues in the literature.

Particularly, these methods can be roughly categorized into two classes. The first type of methods are appearance-based, in which various invariant feature descriptors, such as SIFT, HOG [9], visual words [10], and so on, are used as cues for action recognition [1,10–12]. Despite many successes achieved by these methods, we argue that invariant feature sets are insufficient alone for this complicated task, since most of them can only provide partial invariance - some address this type of variations and others address that but not all; and even with these feature sets, lots of prototypes are still needed to cover the huge range of the variability exhibited in the pose space of human body, not to mention such a representation is usually with high dimension. To deal with these issues, some authors proposed to enhance the stability of feature sets using various context information (if available), such as human-object context [13–15] or group context [1,11,16], or using a multiple cues based approach to combine the strength of different features [2]. Recently, Wang et al. introduce a method which relies on more semantically meaningful features (i.e., pose-lets) and arrange them in a hierarchical manner to improve the invariance and discriminative power of the feature representation [3], and achieves the state of the art performance on a challenging web data set with still images [17].

Alternatively, one can decompose the task into two subsequent tasks by estimating the pose first and then recognizing the actions [9,15,18,19], due to the fact that the pose conveys a lot of information about the actions. These approaches can also be thought as a way to adopt a distributional representation (pose vector) as the feature sets and we call them pose-based methods. While the appearance-based methods enjoy the rich information extracted from the raw data, the pose-based ones take the advantages of more compact pose representation and higher degree of interpretableness for human beings (regarding the results of action recognition yielded).

However, it is worth mentioning that building the action classifier directly based on the output of pose estimator [18,19] could be dangerous due to the inherent uncertainty of the articulation modeling. To alleviate this issue, Yang et al. propose to couple the task of pose estimation with the goal of actions recognition such that more discriminative poses could be learnt [9]. This method proves to be very successful. However, in some real world situations, the boundary between two actions may be not so clear (e.g., running and walking), hence the supervision information injected through the action labels could be misleading.

If motion information is available, both of the above two types of representation could be extended to their 3D versions by modeling the input sequences as a tensor, as in dense trajectory [4,20], action bank [21], among others [22–24]. These methods are related to our method but is unfortunately beyond the scope of the current work. we note that there exist huge number of static images of human beings in the internet, and it is of interest to properly model them and infer their high-level semantics, e.g., their poses and actions.

3   The Proposed Method

The stages of our action prediction pipeline are shown in Fig. 1. In what follows, we give the details of two major components involved, i.e., the pose experts and the corresponding action prediction model.

3.1   Pose Experts

A Part-Based Method. In this work, we adopt a variant of part based model (PBM) as our pose expert. The basic idea of PBM [8,25,26] is to decompose the whole human body into many local parts (the feet, hands, arms, legs, torso, etc.), modeling them separately, and assembling them in such a way that the resulting configuration satisfying well the spatial constraints imposed by the exemplars. Mathematically, this is often equivalent to fit a tree structured model on the given image. One problem of PBM, however, is how to effectively characterize a large amount of poses in a single tree. Recently Yi Yang and Deva Ramanan [8,27] proposed a variant of PBM called flexible mixtures-of-parts (FMP), to address this issue, and successfully applied it for human pose estimation and human detection. Chen et al. [28] improve the model by incorporating the local context information in multiple scales, and achieve more accurate results.

The key idea behind FMP is to use mixture of small, non-oriented parts for articulation modeling and to learn the spatial constraints between these mixtures under a discriminative structural learning framework. Compared to the single modal Gaussian as adopted in many PBM models, the mixture structure effectively enhances the capability of PBM to represent human body with various poses. However, what the FMP learns is essentially still a tree model, which is limited in considering only the first order spatial relationship between two adjacent parts, thus ignoring the high order spatial constraints of human body. In other words, the FMP is a flexible model to impose the complex local compatibility on the pose space but somehow lacks non-local or global compatibility (e.g., the spatial regularity between one's left leg and his right leg, as usually exhibited in some type of actions).

To deal with this problem, we propose to group the pose space according to the desired global compatibility before articulation learning, with each group consisting of samples with similar poses or semantic meaning (e.g., actions). We then train for each group one pose estimator (called pose expert in this work) specific to that group, using the implementation of Chen et al. [28] (kindly provided by the authors). When testing (e.g., performing pose estimation for a never-seen image), we simply pick up the one output by the pose expert with highest confidence.

It is worthy mentioning that this idea of pose expert is related to that of poselet [29]. The major distinction between poselet and our method, however, is that the poselet groups parts of human body while we groups human bodies with similar poses. This different methodology leads to more broader difference when using them. For example, it is straightforward to apply our pose experts in the task of unsupervised human parsing, while a poselet model is more useful in detecting the parts of human body under different poses.

Grouping the Pose Space. The properties of the group have direct influence on the specificity of the pose expert trained on it. Here two methods are considered: one is based on some semantical similarity while the other is on pose similarity. For our task at hand, one straightforward way to measure the similarity between samples is their action types. Hence in the first method (called action-specific grouping), we group together those images with the same action type (i.e., walking, running, etc.), and train one pose expert for it. This is similar to [9], but the difference lies in that they have to perform a dynamic programming-based searching for the most likely latent pose for each test image, while we consider more pose candidates due to the inherent ambiguities of pose expert.

As another strategy, we consider a more generative way to construct the pose expert, by grouping the training samples in the pose space (hence called pose-specific grouping). For this we have to design a similarity metric which reliably measures the pose similarity between two pose vectors. The traditional Euclidean distance is not a good choice since the pose vectors may distribute in a rather non-linear way in the pose space and it does not take the spatial correlation between parts into consideration. To address this issue, we use shape context feature, first used in shape matching and object detection by Belongie [30], to capture such information.

In particular, consider the set of vectors originating from one part to all other parts on a pose. These vectors express both the local and non-local configuration information of the entire shape relative to the reference part, and this information is summarized by the shape context feature as a 2D histogram. Hence shape context feature sets could be used to represent well the internal structure of the parts of human pose. In our implementation, we calculate the 2D histogram for each part, vectorize it, and concatenate all these to get a representation for the pose of a human body. Usually this could lead to a vector with high dimension (e.g., over 6,000), and one can use PCA to condense it. With these in hand, we use the K-means algorithm with Mahalanobis distance as similarity measure to perform the grouping operation.

In either ways, we obtain several groups of poses with some degree of global compatibility preserved. We then use Chen et al.'s improved FMP model [28] to construct a pose expert for each group.

Human Parsing Using an Ensemble of Pose Experts. When the task of pose estimation is of interest by itself, we use a minimum error rate principle to regress for a test image the pose using the pre-trained ensemble of pose experts. This is done by simply picking up the one output by the pose expert with highest confidence as the estimation.

3.2   Action Recognition

Graph-Based Action Representation. The output of each pose expert is a tree with its each node corresponding to a part in a human body, we can simply vectorize this tree for action representation [8,27]. One limitation of this representation is that the non-local information between two non-adjacent parts is ignored, while it is well known that when training samples is few, preserving as rich information as possible is of importance for the subsequent classification task. Here we use an undirected complete graph structure, so that the spatial information regarding to any two body parts is explicitly encoded. This is similar to the shape context feature we used before when grouping the poses, and in fact the shape context feature can be interpreted as a more compact or discretized version of the complete graph.

Besides these first order features, we also incorporate a subset of second-order features by calculating the angle at the center part of an ordered triple parts. This kind of high order features is usually ignored in the previous work but is proven to be discriminative for some action types. For example, the angle formed by upper arm and lower arm in the action of walking is always bigger than that in a running action. As another example, the angle between upper leg and lower leg in playing golf would be always approximately equal to 180°.

More formally, assume that our training data set have been grouped into H clusters as described in Sect. 3.1, based on which we learn H pose expert, denoted as e_j. Then for a given image I, the output of the j-th expert is denoted as $R_j = e_j(I)$. Further assume that each human body has K body parts, and R_j is actually a vector with its component being the location $p_k = (x_k, y_k)$ of each part estimated by the expert, denoted as $R_j = (p_1, p_1, \ldots, p_K)$. With this, we construct a feature representation x^j for each pose expert j as follows:

$$x^j = (\psi_{1,2}, \psi_{1,3}, \ldots, \psi_{1,K}, \psi_{2,3}, \ldots, \psi_{K-1,K}, \theta_1, \theta_2, \ldots, \theta_{K'}) \tag{1}$$

where ψ and θ denotes respectively the first and second order features (i.e., angles mentioned before). In particular, the first order feature between any two parts m and n can be calculated as follows:

$$\psi_{m,n} = \varphi(I, p_m, p_n)$$

$$\varphi(I, p_m, p_n) = [dx\ dx^2\ dy\ dy^2]$$

where $dx = x_m - x_n$, $dx^2 = (x_m - x_n)^2$ and $dy = y_m - y_n$, $dy^2 = (y_m - y_n)^2$, accounting both the relative distance and the relative orientation between these two parts. This can also be understood as modeling the negative spring energy associated with pulling part i from a typical relative location with respect to part j. Hence given H pose experts, we have for each image I a feature representation x: $x = [x^1\ x^2 \dots x^H]$.

Combining Pose Experts via Group Sparse Model. One of the major challenges we face when identifying action type from the output of pose expert is the inherent ambiguity in articulation modeling. In other words, we cannot assume that the pose estimated by pose experts is perfect but in fact it is noisy and weak (in terms of performance). Hence it is risky to simply rely on the pose estimated by the pose expert with the highest score for action prediction. Instead, a better choice is to follow the Bayesian idea, i.e., taking all the output of pose experts in our pool into account.

Specifically, given a feature representation x, our goal is to estimate the maximum posterior probability of action a, i.e., $p(a|x)$. For this we train a series of action predictors corresponding to each pose expert in the pool and properly combine their responses for the final decision. Particularly, for a particular action type a, denote the parameter of the action predictor corresponding to the j-th pose expert as w^j. We jointly learn all the action predictors $w = \{w^1, w^2, ..., w^H\}$ by maximizing the following objective:

$$p(w|a, x^1, x^2, ..., x^H) \propto p(a|x^1, x^2, ..., x^H, w^1, w^2, ..., w^H) \prod_j p(w^j) \quad (2)$$

where the model parameter w is assumed to have multivariate independent and identical priors. We use the logistic regression to model $p(a|x, w)$ as,

$$p(a|x, w) = (1 + exp(-a(\sum_j (w^j)^T x^j + b)))^{-1} \quad (3)$$

and the prior of w^j is modeled as Laplace, whose energy is further scaled according the confidence of the corresponding pose expert (detailed below). Note that in the above formulation, although the behavior of each action predictor for a pose expert is independent by the prior assumption, they jointly make the final prediction by summarizing their responses before undergoing a nonlinear transformation (c.f., Eq. 3).

Now, assume that N training data points (a_i, x_i), $a_i \in \{+1, -1\}$ are available to us, we reach the following objective by Eq. 2,

$$\min_w \sum_{i=1}^N log(1 + exp(-a_i(\sum_j (w^j)^T x_i^j + b))) + \lambda \sum_{j=1}^H (\frac{1}{n_j} \sum_{i=1}^{n_j} S(I_i, e_j)) \|w^j\|_2 \quad (4)$$

where b is the bias shared by all the action predictors, and the scaling factor over the energy of laplace prior is defined to the average confidence of the corresponding pose expert, i.e.,

$$\alpha_j = \frac{1}{n_j} \sum_{i=1}^{n_j} S(I_i, e_j) \tag{5}$$

where n_j is the size of group j (c.f., Sect. 3.1), and $S(I, e_j)$ is the score or confidence of pose expert e_j for image I, which is known to us after the pose estimation stage.

Note that Eq. 4 imposes a critical constraint that the pool of action predictors should not contribute equally to the final prediction, and some of them will even be canceled with a probability related to the confidence of the corresponding pose expert. This effectively improves the robustness against ambiguity in articulation estimation. To solve Eq. 4, we use an efficient implementation of proximal methods [31]. After this, we can use these action predictors to perform action recognition in the test stage, as illustrated in Fig. 1.

4   Experiments

In this section, we report our experimental results concerning two series of experiments, i.e., human parsing (Sect. 4.1) and action recognition (Sect. 4.2).

4.1   Human Parsing Using an Ensemble of Pose Experts

We test our approach on two publicly available data set: the UIUC people data set [32] and the still web image data set collected by Ikizler-Cinbis et al. [17].

UIUC People Data Set. The UIUC people data set [32] contains 593 still images. Most of these images are about people playing various sports such as badminton, Frisbee, walking, jogging or standing, hence contains very aggressive pose and spatial variations (c.f., Fig. 2). We follow the commonly used evaluation protocols in this dataset with the standard data partitions (346 for training, 247 for testing). The original dataset has 14 parts location annotated on the human body in each image, but we use 26 parts model as in [8].

For performance evaluation, we use the Percentage of Correct Parts (PCP) metric [8,28]. A part is localized correctly only if both the distances of the endpoints from their respective ground truth endpoints are less than a fraction (usually set as 0.5) of the part length. With this, the percentage of correct parts can be calculated for each image and then be averaged across all images.

We compare with several related state-of-the-art approaches that do full-body parsing: the iterative parsing method [25], the improved pictorial structure [33], and the discriminative hierarchical part-based model [3], Poselet conditioned pictorial structures [34], the flexible mixture of parts model [8] and its improved version by Chen et al. [28]. Note that since the UIUC data set has no action

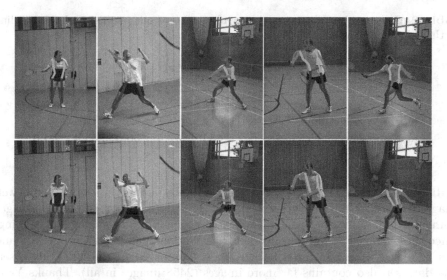

Fig. 2. Visualization of human parsing by the baseline method [28] (top row) and the proposed method (bottom row) on the UIUC people data set.

labels, we only built our pose experts according to the pose similarity (c.f., Sect. 3.1).

Table 1 and Fig. 2 give the results. It is clear from this table that our method based on an ensemble of pose-specific experts performs best among the compared ones. In particular, it improves the previous state-of-the-art performance [28] from 59.1 % to 63.4 %, and achieves better accuracy on most of key parts - notably, compared to [28], the proposed method significantly improves the localization accuracy of upper legs (from 64.2 % to 73.1 %) and upper arms (from 49.2 % to 50.2 %) (c.f., Fig. 2).

Table 1. Comparison of various part-based human parsing methods on the UIUC Peoples dataset.

Method	Torso	Head	Upper legs	Lower legs	Upper arms	Lower arms	Total
Ramanan [25]	44.1	30.8	9.5	25.3	11.1	25.5	21.8
Andriluka [33]	70.9	59.1	36.5	22.9	26.2	10.1	32.1
Wang [3]	86.6	68.8	56.3	50.2	30.8	20.3	47.0
Pishchulin [34]	**91.5**	85.0	66.8	54.7	38.3	23.9	54.4
Yang [8]	85.0	83.4	63.6	56.3	48.8	34.6	57.6
Chen [28]	87.9	**85.4**	64.2	57.5	49.2	**38.3**	59.1
Ours (pose-specific)	89.5	84.6	**73.1**	**63.8**	**50.2**	37.8	**63.4**

Table 2. Comparative human parsing performance of our method and the baseline method on the still web image data set.

Method	Torso	Head	Upper legs	Lower legs	Upper arms	Lower arms	Total
Baseline [28]	96.6	95.3	60.1	58.7	51.0	28.3	58.8
Ours (action-specific)	**97.7**	**96.1**	62.6	59.9	54.8	31.9	61.2
Ours (pose-specific)	97.6	95.2	**68.9**	**62.4**	**60.0**	**35.4**	**64.6**

Still Web Image Data Set. We also evaluate our method on the still web image data set by Ikizler-Cinbis et al. [17]. This data set consists of still images from 5 kinds of human action: dancing, sitting, playing golf, walking and running. Since those images are all downloaded from Web, human poses vary greatly and lots of images have cluttered backgrounds. Compared to the UIUC data set, this data set also contains far more images (2458 images in all). Thanks Yang et al. [9] for providing us their pose annotation with 14 joints on the human body on all the images in the data set. For evaluation, we follow Yang [9] and Wang [3] by partition 1/3 of the images from each kind of action for training, and the rest of the images are used for testing. Unfortunately, both authors do not perform human parsing experiments on this data set, and here we only compare our method with the baseline method [28].

Table 2 gives the result. It reveals that both grouping methods (action-specific and pose-specific) for pose experts construction lead to improved human parsing performance than the baseline algorithm, and the pose-specific grouping method works best as expected. It is worthy noting that an ensemble of action-specific pose experts still outperform the single-tree based model [28] - this is somewhat surprising since the grouping criteria is not originally designed for human parsing but for action recognition, but it can be partly explained by the conjecture that the top-level semantic information is beneficial to the task of pose estimation, as implied in Yang et al. [9]. Figure 3 illustrates some human parsing results yielded by the compared methods.

4.2 Action Recognition from a Single Web Image

Next we report our experiments on the task of action recognition from a single web image, based on the still web image data set described in Sect. 4.1. As stated before, our evaluation protocol follows the ones proposed by Yang [9] and Wang [3] , i.e., using 1/3 of the images from each kind of action for training, and the rest of the images for testing.

Effectiveness of the Proposed Method. To assess the effectiveness of the proposed method, we first designed several baseline algorithms by modifying one or some of its component, as follows,

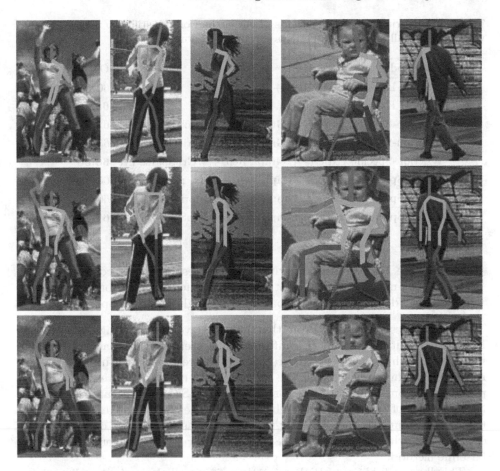

Fig. 3. Visualization of various methods for human parsing on the still web image data set. From top to bottom, each row shows the results yielded by the baseline model [28], our method with action-specific \ pose-specific experts, respectively.

- **Baseline algorithms:** We first learn a single tree-structured articulation model based on [28] from the training data. With the poses estimated by this model for the training set, we train a sparse logistic regression (LR) model as the action predictor. Two versions are implemented with different representation for action recognition, i.e., the tree-based representation and the graph-based representation (c.f., Sect. 3.2), as shown in the first two rows in Table 6;
- **Different grouping methods:** All the remaining variants use multiple pose experts, which are trained either in an action-specific way or in a pose specific way, as described in Sect. 3.1;
- **Different combining methods:** We test three kinds of ways to combine the output of pose experts for action prediction: (1) train a sparse logistic regression-based action predictor for each pose expert and combine their prediction by majority voting; (2) train the action predictors in the same as

Table 3. Performance (%) of variants of our method on the still web image data set, with both overall and average per-class accuracies reported.

Methods	Overall
Single Expert + Tree Rep. + Sparse LR	60.81
Single Expert + Graph Rep.+ Sparse LR	**63.79**
Action-Specific Experts + Graph Rep. + Max. resp	62.87
Action-Specific Experts + Graph Rep. + Majority Voting	63.10
Action-Specific Experts + Graph Rep. + wGrpSparse LR	**66.08**
Pose-Specific Experts + Graph Rep. + Max. resp	65.74
Pose-Specific Experts + Graph Rep. + Majority Voting	66.08
Pose-Specific Experts + Graph Rep. + wGrpSparse LR	**67.84**

previous one, but trust the one with maximum response when combining them (denoted as max. resp.); (3) jointly train those action predictors as described in Sect. 3.2, denoted as "wGrpSparse LR" (Weighted Group Sparse Logistic).

Table 3 gives the results. From this table we have the following observations: First, the results show that rich information is useful for more accurate action recognition - this can be seen by comparing the results shown in the first two rows - under the same settings, the method based on graph representation outperforms the one using tree-based representation. Secondly, it can be seen that the two types of action recognizers based on an ensemble of pose experts outperform the baselines. In fact, the best performer is based on a pool of pose-specific experts, achieving an accuracy of 68.84 % that is over 4.0 % higher than the best baseline method.

Thirdly, the table reveals that jointly training all the action predictors are effective in fusing the strength of each pose expert. By comparing the performance of jointly trained model with the ones trained independently (Max. resp. or Majority Voting), we find that the former consistently performs better than the later. To gain further understanding on this, we show for pose-specific experts-based method the energy of each action predictor assigned by the learner and the corresponding accuracy in Table 5 and Table 4, respectively. One can see from these two tables that different action predictors are good at predicting different type of actions while the energy assigned by the learner (Eq. 4) is proportion to this. For example, one can see from Table 4 that the 7-th action predictor is good at recognizing dancing and running, but not so good at playing golf and working. Accordingly, we see from the 7-th row of Table 5 that they receive large energy in both dancing and running, but will be excluded to make a prediction about playing golf and working.

Last but not least, it can be observed that the method based on the pose-specific experts work better than that based on the action-specific ones. This may be unexpected since pose-specific experts do not rely on any supervision information, while action-specific experts are trained deliberately for each type

Table 4. The action recognition accuracy (%) of each action predictor (each row), whose energy assigned by the learner is shown as one corresponding row in Table 5.

	dancing	playgolf	running	sitting	walking	mean
group 1	68.25	56.41	78.75	46.01	52.65	63.69
group 2	55.26	47.13	80.50	73.24	57.98	65.29
group 3	64.09	41.58	73.17	57.71	62.36	62.75
group 4	59.38	63.10	81.78	70.63	32.70	63.19
group 5	59.60	44.97	80.96	41.76	59.54	61.85
group 6	56.28	54.39	79.06	69.47	60.68	65.76
group 7	66.31	37.43	71.55	44.95	36.69	55.17
group 8	49.56	46.90	76.97	36.33	60.27	58.11

Table 5. The energy of each action predictor (each row, the group number is kept the same as the corresponding pose-specific expert) as a function of action type. These energy numbers are calculated as the l_2-norm of the corresponding weight vector w^j jointly learned by optimizing objective (4). The individual accuracy of these eight action predictors is shown in Table 4.

	Dancing	playgolf	running	sitting	Walking
group 1	1.9071	1.4831	1.0617	0.5722	0.6082
group 2	0.3056	0.7620	1.2251	1.3800	1.0011
group 3	1.0645	0.6213	0.8023	0.6384	1.0438
group 4	0.8377	1.6826	1.9567	1.7014	0.1466
group 5	0.9136	0.3988	1.0441	0.0000	1.4968
group 6	0.7858	1.6478	1.6883	0.9625	1.7677
group 7	1.9493	0.0000	0.7548	0.3556	0.0000
group 8	0.7763	0.5117	0.8766	0.0000	1.6639

of actions. Despite this, Table 2 shows that on average action-specific experts do not perform as well as pose-specific ones in the task of human parsing (61.2 % vs. 64.6 %) - this implies that a less accurate pose estimator may lead to a deteriorated overall performance for action prediction.

To further understand the behavior between the two types of experts, we detail their confusion matrix in Fig. 4(a) and Fig. 4(b), respectively. By comparing these, we find that about 24.0 % running actions are misclassified as walking by the approach based on pose-specific experts, while this number reduces to 20.0 % by the one based on action-specific experts. This indicates that injecting high-level semantic information into the articulation model is useful to reduce the ambiguity for action prediction. Actually, since the poses of walking and running are similar to each other in many cases, images with these two kinds of actions are highly possibly to be clustered into the same group.

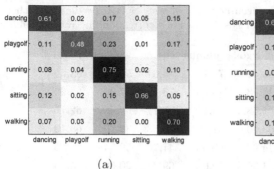 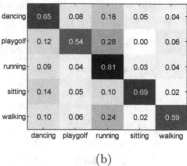

(a)   (b)

Fig. 4. Confusion matrix of the classification results on the still web image action dataset, based on (a) action-specific pose experts and (b) pose-specific experts. Horizontal rows are ground truths,and vertical columns are predictions.

Comparison with the State-of-the-art Methods. We compare our method with two state-of-the-art action recognition methods on still images, i.e., Yang [9] and Wang [3], and the results are given in Table 6. It can be seen from the table that our approach performs better than both methods. However, it should be noted that the accuracy numbers are not directly comparable since the training/testing data sets and features are not completely identical.

Table 6. Comparative performance (%) of our method and two state-of-the-art methods on the still web image data set.

Methods	Overall
Baseline	63.79
Yang [9]	61.07
Wang [3]	65.15
Ours (action-Specific)	**66.08**
Ours (pose-Specific)	**67.84**

5   Conclusions

In this paper, we present a new method for human parsing and action recognition from a single still image, which is a less-studied problem. We base our method on a pool of pose experts, and show how to construct these pose experts and how to flexibly combine the output of these experts for improved action recognition performance. Our experiments on a challenging data set with web images indicate that 1) compared to the single expert strategy, our multiple experts approach is more effective for both tasks when the training data are relatively few; 2) our modified group sparse logistic regression learner leads to better performance than the one that trains its module independently. The importance of rich information for action recognition is also highlighted. Our current search is focused on how to extend the proposed method to the situation when motion cues are available.

Acknowledgement. The authors want to thank the anonymous reviewers for their helpful comments and suggestions. This work was supported by the National Science Foundation of China (61073112, 61035003, 61373060), Jiangsu Science Foundation (BK2012793), Qing Lan Project, Research Fund for the Doctoral Program (RFDP) (20123218110033).

References

1. Sharma, G., Jurie, F., Schmid, C.: Expanded parts model for human attribute and action recognition in still images. In: 2013 IEEE Conference on Computer Vision and Pattern Recognition (CVPR), pp. 652–659. IEEE (2013)
2. Sener, F., Bas, C., Ikizler-Cinbis, N.: On Recognizing Actions in Still Images via Multiple Features. In: Fusiello, A., Murino, V., Cucchiara, R. (eds.) ECCV 2012 Ws/Demos, Part III. LNCS, vol. 7585, pp. 263–272. Springer, Heidelberg (2012)
3. Wang, Y., Tran, D., Liao, Z., Forsyth, D.: Discriminative hierarchical part-based models for human parsing and action recognition. J. Mach. Learn. Res. **13**, 3075–3102 (2012)
4. Wang, H., Kläser, A., Schmid, C., Liu, C.L.: Dense trajectories and motion boundary descriptors for action recognition. Int. J. Comput. Vis. **103**, 60–79 (2013)
5. Laptev, I., Marszalek, M., Schmid, C., Rozenfeld, B.: Learning realistic human actions from movies. In: 2008 IEEE Conference on Computer Vision and Pattern Recognition. CVPR 2008, pp. 1–8. IEEE (2008)
6. Niebles, J.C., Wang, H., Fei-Fei, L.: Unsupervised learning of human action categories using spatial-temporal words. Int. J. Comput. Vis. **79**, 299–318 (2008)
7. Schuldt, C., Laptev, I., Caputo, B.: Recognizing human actions: a local svm approach. In: 2004 Proceedings of the 17th International Conference on Pattern Recognition. ICPR 2004. vol. 3, pp. 32–36. IEEE (2004)
8. Yang, Y., Ramanan, D.: Articulated pose estimation with flexible mixtures-of-parts. In: 2011 IEEE Conference on Computer Vision and Pattern Recognition (CVPR), pp. 1385–1392. IEEE (2011)
9. Yang, W., Wang, Y., Mori, G.: Recognizing human actions from still images with latent poses. In: 2010 IEEE Conference on Computer Vision and Pattern Recognition (CVPR), pp. 2030–2037. IEEE (2010)
10. Delaitre, V., Laptev, I., Sivic, J.: Recognizing human actions in still images: a study of bag-of-features and part-based representations. In: The 2010 British Machine Vision Conference. vol. 2, pp. 1–11 (2010)
11. Maji, S., Bourdev, L., Malik, J.: Action recognition from a distributed representation of pose and appearance. In: 2011 IEEE Conference on Computer Vision and Pattern Recognition (CVPR), pp. 3177–3184. IEEE (2011)
12. Sharma, G., Jurie, F.: Learning discriminative spatial representation for image classification. In: Hoey, J., McKenna, S.J., Trucco, E., (eds.) The 2011 British Machine Vision Conference, pp. 1–11. BMVA Press (2011)

13. Desai, C., Ramanan, D., Fowlkes, C.: Discriminative models for static human-object interactions. In: 2010 IEEE Computer Society Conference on Computer Vision and Pattern Recognition Workshops (CVPRW), pp. 9–16. IEEE (2010)
14. Gupta, A., Kembhavi, A., Davis, L.S.: Observing human-object interactions: Using spatial and functional compatibility for recognition. IEEE Trans. Pattern Anal. Mach. Intell. **31**, 1775–1789 (2009)
15. Yao, B., Fei-Fei, L.: Modeling mutual context of object and human pose in human-object interaction activities. In: 2010 IEEE Conference on Computer Vision and Pattern Recognition (CVPR), pp. 17–24. IEEE (2010)
16. Lan, T., Wang, Y., Yang, W., Mori, G.: Beyond actions: Discriminative models for contextual group activities. NIPS. **4321**, 4322–4325 (2010)
17. Ikizler-Cinbis, N., Cinbis, R.G., Sclaroff, S.: Learning actions from the web. In: the IEEE 12th International Conference on Computer Vision (CVPR 2009), pp. 995–1002. IEEE (2009)
18. Sheikh, Y., Sheikh, M., Shah, M.: Exploring the space of a human action. In: The Tenth IEEE International Conference on Computer Vision (ICCV 2005). vol. 1, pp. 144–149. IEEE (2005)
19. Ramanan, D., Forsyth, D. A.: Automatic annotation of everyday movements. In: Advances in neural information processing systems (2003)
20. Jiang, Y.-G., Dai, Q., Xue, X., Liu, W., Ngo, C.-W.: Trajectory-Based Modeling of Human Actions with Motion Reference Points. In: Fitzgibbon, A., Lazebnik, S., Perona, P., Sato, Y., Schmid, C. (eds.) ECCV 2012, Part V. LNCS, vol. 7576, pp. 425–438. Springer, Heidelberg (2012)
21. Sadanand, S., Corso, J.J.: Action bank: a high-level representation of activity in video. In: 2012 IEEE Conference on Computer Vision and Pattern Recognition (CVPR), pp. 1234–1241. IEEE (2012)
22. Xia, L., Chen, C.C., Aggarwal, J.: View invariant human action recognition using histograms of 3d joints. In: 2012 IEEE Computer Society Conference on Computer Vision and Pattern Recognition Workshops (CVPRW), pp. 20–27. IEEE (2012)
23. Yuan, C., Li, X., Hu, W., Ling, H., Maybank, S.: 3D R transform on spatio-temporal interest points for action recognition. In: 2013 IEEE Conference on Computer Vision and Pattern Recognition (CVPR), pp. 724–730. IEEE (2013)
24. Zhu, Y., Chen, W., Guo, G.: Fusing spatiotemporal features and joints for 3d action recognition. In: 2013 IEEE Conference on Computer Vision and Pattern Recognition Workshops (CVPRW), pp. 486–491. IEEE (2013)
25. Ramanan, D.: Learning to parse images of articulated bodies. In: NIPS: The Twentieth Annual Conference on Neural Information Processing Systems, 4–7 December, 2006, Vancouver, Canada. vol. 19, pp. 1129–1136. MIT Press (2006)
26. Felzenszwalb, P.F., Huttenlocher, D.P.: Pictorial structures for object recognition. International Journal of Computer Vision **61**, 55–79 (2005)
27. Yang, Y., Ramanan, D.: Articulated human detection with flexible mixtures of parts. IEEE Trans. Pattern Anal. Mach. Intell. **35**, 2878–2890 (2013)
28. Chen, M., Tan, X.: Part-based pose estimation with local and non-local contextual information. IET Computer Vision, 1–12 (2014)
29. Bourdev, L., Malik, J.: Poselets: Body part detectors trained using 3d human pose annotations. In: 2009 IEEE 12th International Conference on Computer Vision, pp. 1365–1372. IEEE (2009)
30. Belongie, S., Malik, J., Puzicha, J.: Shape matching and object recognition using shape contexts. IEEE Trans. Pattern Anal. Mach. Intell. **24**, 509–522 (2002)
31. Liu, J., Ji, S., Ye, J.: SLEP: Sparse Learning with Efficient Projections. Arizona State University (2009)

32. Tran, D., Forsyth, D.: Improved Human Parsing with a Full Relational Model. In: Daniilidis, K., Maragos, P., Paragios, N. (eds.) ECCV 2010, Part IV. LNCS, vol. 6314, pp. 227–240. Springer, Heidelberg (2010)
33. Andriluka, M., Roth, S., Schiele, B.: Pictorial structures revisited: People detection and articulated pose estimation. In: 2009 IEEE Conference on Computer Vision and Pattern Recognition. CVPR 2009, pp. 1014–1021. IEEE (2009)
34. Pishchulin, L., Andriluka, M., Gehler, P., Schiele, B.: Poselet conditioned pictorial structures. In: 2013 IEEE Conference on Computer Vision and Pattern Recognition (CVPR), pp. 588–595. IEEE (2013)

Scene Text Recognition and Retrieval
for Large Lexicons

Udit Roy[1]([⊠]), Anand Mishra[1], Karteek Alahari[2], and C.V. Jawahar[1]

[1] CVIT, IIIT Hyderabad, Hyderabad, India
udit.roy@research.iiit.ac.in
[2] Inria, LEAR team, Inria Grenoble Rhône-Alpes, Laboratoire Jean Kuntzmann,
CNRS, Univ. Grenoble Alpes, Saint-Martin-d'Héres, France

Abstract. In this paper we propose a framework for recognition and retrieval tasks in the context of scene text images. In contrast to many of the recent works, we focus on the case where an image-specific list of words, known as the small lexicon setting, is unavailable. We present a conditional random field model defined on potential character locations and the interactions between them. Observing that the interaction potentials computed in the large lexicon setting are less effective than in the case of a small lexicon, we propose an iterative method, which alternates between finding the most likely solution and refining the interaction potentials. We evaluate our method on public datasets and show that it improves over baseline and state-of-the-art approaches. For example, we obtain nearly 15 % improvement in recognition accuracy and precision for our retrieval task over baseline methods on the IIIT-5K word dataset, with a large lexicon containing 0.5 million words.

1 Introduction

Text can play an important role in understanding street view images. In light of this, many attempts have been made to recognize scene text [1–6]. Scene text recognition is a challenging problem and its recent success is mostly limited to the *small lexicon setting*, where an image-specific lexicon containing the ground truth word is provided. Typically, these lexicons contain only 50 words [3]. This setting has many practical applications, but it does not scale well. As an example consider the scenario of assisting visually-impaired people in finding books by their titles in a library. Here the lexicon is populated with all the book titles. In this case, the small lexicon setting becomes less accurate as the lexicon sizes can range from a few thousands to a million. For instance, when lexicon size increases from 50 to 1000, the recognition accuracy drops by more than 10 % [6,7]. In other words, the general problem of scene text recognition, i.e., recognition with the help of a large lexicon (say a million dictionary words) is far from being solved. In this paper, we investigate this problem.

One way to address the task of recognizing scene text is to pose the problem in conditional random field (CRF) framework and obtain the maximum a posteriori (MAP) solution as proposed in [3,4,7–10]. In these frameworks,

© Springer International Publishing Switzerland 2015
D. Cremers et al. (Eds.): ACCV 2014, Part I, LNCS 9003, pp. 494–508, 2015.
DOI: 10.1007/978-3-319-16865-4_32

Word Image	Top-5 diverse solutions (ranked)
PITT	PITA, PASP, ENEP, **PITT**, AWAP
COM	AUM, NIM, **COM**, MUA, PLL
MONSTER	MINSTER, MINSHER, GRINNER, MINISTR, **MONSTER**
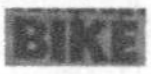 BIKE	BRKE, BNKE, **BIKE**, BAKE, BOKE
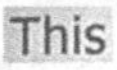 This	TOLS, TARS, **THIS**, TOHE, TALP

Fig. 1. Examples where the MAP solution is incorrect, as the pairwise priors become too generic when computed from large lexicons. The set of top-5 diverse solutions contains the correct result.

an energy function consisting of unary and pairwise potentials is defined, and the minimum of this function corresponds to the text contained in the word image. These methods demonstrated successful results in a small lexicon setting primarily due to the fact that the pairwise terms computed with this lexicon have a positive bias towards the ground truth word. However, when the pairwise terms are computed from large lexicons, they become too generic, and often in such cases the MAP solution does not correspond to the ground truth. Besides this, MAP solutions suffer from drawbacks, such as (i) approximation errors in inference, (ii) poor precision/recall for character detection, (iii) weak unary and pairwise potentials. Consider the word "PITT" shown in Fig. 1 as an example. The MAP solution for the word is "PITA", which is incorrect. Our approach addresses this problem by using the top-M solutions to ultimately find text that is most likely contained in the image.

We begin by generating a set of candidate words with M-best diverse solutions [11]. With these potential solutions, we refine the large lexicon by removing words from it with a large edit distance to any of the candidates, and then recompute the M-best diverse solutions. These two steps are repeated a few times, which ultimately results in set of words most likely to represent the word contained in the image. Then a desired solution can be picked using various means (e.g., using minimum edit distance based correction using a lexicon). We show significant performance gain for recognition tasks in the large lexicon setting using this framework. We also present an application of computing the top-M solutions, i.e., text to image retrieval, where the goal is to retrieve all the occurrences of the query text from a database of word images. We will show that our strategy of re-ranking the words with the refined lexicon improves the performance over baseline methods.

Related Work. The problem of cropped word recognition has been looked at in two broad settings: with an image-specific lexicon [3–6,10] and without the help of lexicon [1,7,8]. Approaches for scene text recognition typically follow a two-step process (i) A set of potential character locations are detected either by binarization [1,2] or sliding windows [3,4], (ii) Inference on CRF model [4,7], semi Markov model [1,8], finite automata [9] or beam search [2] in a graph (representing the character locations and their neighborhood relations) is performed.

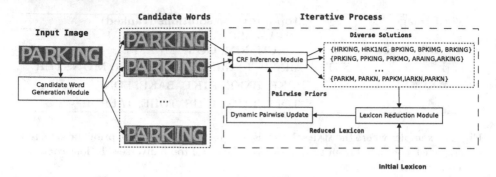

Fig. 2. Overview of the proposed framework. The input image is passed on to a multiple candidate word generation module which generates candidate words, each with a set of character regions and their corresponding unary potentials. With the help of an initial lexicon, pairwise priors are computed and diverse solutions are inferred from all the candidate words. These candidates are then used to reduce the lexicon. This process is repeated with the reduced lexicon until the lexicon is refined to a small size. The final solution is the word in the full lexicon closest to the diverse solutions computed in the last iteration.

These approaches work well especially in small lexicon settings, but suffer from two main drawbacks: (i) Obtaining a single set of true character windows in a word image in these methods is difficult, (ii) Pairwise information gets less influential as the lexicon size increases. We adopt a similar framework in this paper, but propose crucial changes to overcome the issues of previous approaches. First, we generate multiple word hypotheses and derive a set of candidate words likely to represent the word image. Second, we present a technique to prune the large lexicon based on edit distances between the candidate solutions and lexicon words. This proposed method allows us to significantly reduce the lexicon size and make the priors more specific to the image. Third, unlike prior works which yield a single solution, our method is also capable of yielding multiple solutions, and is applicable to the text-to-image retrieval task.

The remainder of the paper is organized as follows. In Sect. 2.1, we present CRF framework for word recognition. We utilize multiple segmentations of word images to obtain potential character locations in Sect. 2.2. We then present details of the inference method in Sect. 2.3. Our lexicon reduction and pairwise term update steps are described in Sect. 2.4. The two problem settings, i.e., recognition and retrieval, are then discussed Sect. 3. Section 4 describes the experiments and shows results on public datasets. Implementation details are also provided in this section. We then make concluding remarks in Sect. 5.

2   Proposed Method

We model the scene text recognition task as an inference problem on a CRF model, similar to [4], where unary potentials are computed from character classification scores and pairwise potentials from the lexicons. Small lexicon based pairwise potentials often help to recover from the errors made by character classification [12,13]. However, when the pairwise potentials are computed from large lexicons, they become too generic, and the overall model cannot cope with erroneous unary potentials. To overcome this issue, starting from a large lexicon recognition problem, we automatically refine the problem statement and convert it to a small lexicon inference task.

The framework has the following components, as shown in Fig. 2: (i) Candidate word generation module, where we generate multiple words with each word as a set of characters spanning over the image, (ii) CRF inference module, where each word is represented as a CRF and inferred to obtain diverse solutions, and (iii) Lexicon reduction module, where we prune the lexicon by removing distant words after re-ranking the lexicon with a novel group edit distance computed using the diverse solutions. It is accompanied by re-computation of pairwise potentials which become image specific as the lexicon size decreases. We use different stopping criteria for recognition and retrieval tasks as we alternatively reduce our lexicon and infer solutions.

2.1 CRF Framework

The CRF is defined over a set of random variables $x = \{x_i | i \subset \mathcal{V}\}$, where $\mathcal{V} = \{1, 2, ..., n\}$, denotes the set of n characters in a candidate word. Each random variable x_i denotes a potential character in the word, and can take a label from the label set $\mathcal{L}$ containing English characters and digits. The energy function, $E : \mathcal{L}^n \rightarrow \mathbb{R}$, corresponding to a candidate word can be typically written as the sum of unary and pairwise potentials:

$$E(x) = \sum_{i \in \mathcal{V}} E_i(x_i) + \sum_{(i,j) \in \mathcal{N}} E_{ij}(x_i, x_j), \tag{1}$$

where $\mathcal{N}$ represents the neigbourhood system defined over the candidate word. The set of potential characters is obtained by a segmentation procedure, discussed in Sect. 2.2.

Unary Potentials. The unary potential of a node is determined by the SVM confidence score. The unary term $E_i(x_i = c_j)$ represents the cost of a node x_i taking a character label c_j, and is defined as:

$$E_i(x_i = c_j) = 1 - p(c_j | x_i), \tag{2}$$

where $p(c_j | x_i)$ denotes the likelihood of character class c_j for node x_i.

Pairwise Potentials. The pairwise cost of two neighbouring nodes x_i and x_j taking a pair of character labels c_i and c_j is defined as,

$$E_{ij}(x_i, x_j) = \lambda_l(1 - p(c_i, c_j)), \tag{3}$$

where $p(c_i, c_j)$ is the bigram probability of the character pair c_i and c_j occurring together in the lexicon. The parameter λ_l determines the penalty for a character pair occurring in the lexicon. Similar to [4], we use node-specific prior, where the priors are computed independently for each edge from the bigrams in the lexicon that have the same relative position to that of the edge in the CRF. This enforces spatial constraints on prior computation, and are found to be more effective than the standard node prior [4].

2.2   Generating Candidate Words

Obtaining potential character locations with a high recall is desired for our approach. There are two popular methods for character extraction based on: (i) sliding window [4,7], (ii) binarization [1,2]. We follow the binarization based approach as it results in fewer potential character locations, in the form of connected components (CCs), than those generated by the sliding window based method. This avoids redundant character windows with similar size at a specific image location. Binarization based methods reduce the number of candidate windows with threshold parameters and by leveraging fast pruning techniques on the CCs. To ensure that all the characters are present in the candidate windows as CCs, we combine results with different thresholds. This significantly improves the character recall at the cost of generating some false windows that can be overcome in the latter steps.

To remove obvious false windows we use heuristics based on information such as character sizes, aspect ratio and spatial consistency, followed by a character specific non-maximal suppression. This step removes false positive windows occurring in the background or unwanted foreground text elements like text bounding boxes. We also detect other anomalous windows, like holes in characters and invalid windows present within the characters, by finding configurations where a smaller window is contained completely within a larger window, and then remove the smaller one.

After pruning, we get a set of potential character windows which are used to generate candidate words. We first build a graph by joining the potential character windows which are spatially consistent and likely to be adjacent characters. In other words, the windows are connected with an edge if (i) overlapping windows have an overlap less than a threshold, and (ii) non-overlapping windows are less than a threshold away. We remove a few edges connecting windows whose width or height ratio is not in a desired range, to ensure that only character-to-character links are preserved. Then we estimate the most probable words for further analysis as described in the following.

Selection of Candidate Words. Our objective is to find a set of probable candidate words from the directed graph described above. We define a candidate word as a set of character windows representing the text present in the image. We first find the most probable start and end character windows by selecting windows close to the left and right image boundaries. Representing these start and end windows as candidate start and end nodes, we find possible connected paths (i.e., candidate words) between all pairs of start and end nodes using a depth first all paths algorithm [14]. We reject candidate words which do not cover sufficient area over the word image. The shortlisted candidate words are represented as a CRF, inferred and re-ranked according to their minimum energy value which is normalized by the number of nodes in the CRF. The least energy candidate words are retained for the subsequent stage as the correct candidate words assuming they have nodes with better unary potentials.

2.3 Diversity Preserving Inference

Once the optimal candidate words are selected, we infer the text each of them contains by minimizing the energy (1). However, the minimum energy solution of the word may be at times incorrect due to poor unary or pairwise potentials. Hence, diverse solutions are preferred a over single solution. Inspired by [11], we obtain M-best solutions instead of one MAP solution. This is done for all the selected candidate words from the previous stage individually. We approach the problem of diversity preserving inference with a greedy algorithm. First, we obtain the MAP solution with TRW-S [15] and then, the next solution is defined as the lowest energy state with minimum similarity from the previously obtained solutions.

Rewriting the problem of optimizing the energy function (1) we obtain,

$$\min_{\mu} \sum_{i \in V} \sum_{s \in \mathcal{L}} \alpha_i(s)\mu_i(s) + \sum_{i,j \in \mathcal{N}} \sum_{s,t \in \mathcal{L}} \alpha_{ij}(s,t)\mu_{ij}(s,t), \qquad (4)$$

where $\alpha_i(s)$ is the unary potential and $\alpha_{ij}(s,t)$ is the pairwise potential. The terms $\mu_i(s)$ and $\mu_{ij}(s,t)$ are their corresponding binary indicator variables. This function (4) can be re-written with standard constraints on unary and pairwise potentials as well as the diversity constraint (to get the second best solution) in the form of function $\Delta(\hat{\mu}, \mu)$, where $\hat{\mu}$ is the best solution found after inferring with the diversity constraint as follows,

$$\min_{\mu} \sum_{i \in V} \sum_{s \in \mathcal{L}} \alpha_i(s)\mu_i(s) + \sum_{i,j \in \mathcal{N}} \sum_{s,t in \mathcal{L}} \alpha_{ij}(s,t)\mu_{ij}(s,t), \qquad (5)$$

$$\text{s.t.} \quad \sum_{s \in \mathcal{L}} \mu_i(s) = 1, \qquad (6)$$

$$\sum_{s \in \mathcal{L}} \mu_{ij}(s,t) = \mu_j(t), \quad \sum_{t \in \mathcal{L}} \mu_{ij}(s,t) = \mu_i(s), \qquad (7)$$

$$\Delta(\hat{\mu}, \mu) \geq k, \qquad (8)$$

$$\mu_i(s), \mu_{ij}(s,t) \in \{0,1\}. \qquad (9)$$

Here, (6) and (7) denote the constraints on unary and pairwise potentials. The constraint (8) is the diversity measure that has to be greater than a scalar k. The Langrangian relaxation of this optimization problem is formed by the dualizing the constraint (8), which yields,

$$\min_{\mu} \sum_{i \in \mathcal{V}} \sum_{s \in \mathcal{L}} \alpha_i(s) \mu_i(s) + \sum_{i,j \in \mathcal{N}} \sum_{s,t \in \mathcal{L}} \alpha_{ij}(s,t) \mu_{ij}(s,t) - \lambda(\Delta(\hat{\mu}, \mu) - k). \quad (10)$$

Using a dot product dissimilarity (Hamming distance) as our Δ function we obtain,

$$\min_{\mu} \sum_{i \in \mathcal{V}} \sum_{s \in \mathcal{L}} \alpha_i(s) \mu_i(s) + \sum_{i,j \in \mathcal{N}} \sum_{s,t \in \mathcal{L}} \alpha_{ij}(s,t) \mu_{ij}(s,t) - \lambda(-\hat{\mu} \cdot \mu - k), \quad (11)$$

which can be re-written as,

$$\min_{\mu} \sum_{i \in \mathcal{V}} \sum_{s \in \mathcal{L}} (\alpha_i(s) + \lambda \hat{\mu}_i(s)) \mu_i(s) + \sum_{i,j \in \mathcal{N}} \sum_{s,t \in \mathcal{L}} \alpha_{ij}(s,t) \mu_{ij}(s,t) + \lambda \cdot k. \quad (12)$$

In summary, only the unary potentials need to be modified by adding the original solution scaled by the diversity parameter λ. The TRW-S [15] algorithm can be utilized again to infer the second best solution.

2.4 Lexicon Reduction

Once the solutions are obtained from all the selected candidate words, they are used to reduce the large lexicon and compute pairwise potentials iteratively. We prefer to use the diverse solutions over the MAP solution as they maximize the chances of inferring the correct solution. Our first iteration involves shrinking the lexicon to a smaller size, i.e., 50. This is done by re-ranking the lexicon words using group edit distance (described below) to the solutions obtained, and retaining the top matches. This iteration reduces the lexicon size significantly and retains a small subset with a high recall of ground truth words. From the second iteration onwards, we use the new pairwise potentials (computed from the reduced lexicon) and re-infer the diverse solutions. Thereafter, we remove the word in the lexicon with maximum group edit distance from the diverse solutions. This lexicon reduction procedure is summarized in Algorithm 1.

Group Edit Distance. The standard way of re-ranking a lexicon using a single solution is by computing the edit distance between the solution and all the lexicon words. However in a multiple solution scenario, where diverse solutions from multiple words come into the picture, the correct inferred label is most likely to be present in the solution set. To be able to compute the edit distance between a solution set and lexicon, we find the minimum edit distance for each lexicon word from the solution set. This modification ensures that if the ground truth is very close to one of the diverse solutions, it will be ranked higher than others in the lexicon.

3   Recognition and Retrieval

The method described so far reduces the size of the lexicon by alternating between the two steps of estimating candidate words and refining the lexicon. We then use this lexicon for the recognition and retrieval tasks.

Input: Candidate words, Initial lexicon L_i, Reduced lexicon size r
Output: Reduced lexicon L_r
Initialization: $L_r = L_i$
while $size(L_r) > r$ **do**
> **1:** Perform inference on all the candidate words to obtain M diverse solutions (Sect. 2.3)
> **2:** Remove the lexicon word w with the maximum group edit distance from M diverse solutions
>
> $$L_r = L_r - \{w\}$$
>
> **3:** Compute new pairwise priors from the reduced lexicon

end

Algorithm 1. The lexicon reduction process alternates between removing words from the lexicon and re-computing the pairwise potentials.

Recognition. In the recognition task, our goal is to associate a text label to a given word image. The process begins by forming multiple candidate words using the graph construction described in Sect. 2.2. Candidate words are re-ranked and k optimal candidate words are retained. We reduce the lexicon (using the method in Sect. 2.4) to a size of 10 words and obtain diverse solutions with the newly computed pairwise potentials from this reduced lexicon. We now select a word from the original lexicon with the minimum group edit distance from the diverse solutions as our result.

Retrieval. In a retrieval task, our objective is to retrieve word images for a given text query word from a dataset. The traditional approach would be to reduce the lexicon for each word to size one (hereafter referred to as singleton lexicon), and search for the query word in the singleton lexicons of all the words in the dataset. However, since this approach is prone to failures in recognition, we relax the constraint of reducing the lexicon to size one, and instead reduce the lexicon to a very small size, say five words. This allows us to overcome recognition errors and retrieve word images where the ground truth in present in the reduced lexicon but not in the singleton lexicon. Word images with reduced lexicons having low similarity among their constituent words are further reduced to a singleton lexicon. We measure the similarity of words in the lexicon with a measure called average edit distance (AED) which is defined as,

$$\text{AED} = \frac{1}{P} \sum_{w_i, w_j \in L^P} ED(w_i, w_j), \tag{13}$$

where L^P is the lexicon with P words and $ED(w_i, w_j)$ is the edit distance between words w_i and w_j. A low AED implies that the reduced lexicon has similar words and hence, one more lexicon reduction iteration may result in arbitrary loss of ground truth from the reduced lexicon. On the other hand, in cases with high AED score, the words in the reduced lexicon are different from each other.

As a preprocessing step to our retrieval task, we prepare the dataset by reducing the lexicons for each word image to either a singleton or a reduced lexicon. The lexicon is reduced iteratively to a size n and the AED score is computed. If the score is found to be less than θ (i.e., showing high similarity among the words in the lexicon) we terminate the lexicon reduction process and associate the reduced lexicon of size n with the word image. We continue the process to get a singleton lexicon otherwise. For a given query word, we find all the word images in the dataset that have the query word in their respective singleton or reduced lexicons. All the selected images are then ranked using a combined score computed as the weighted sum of: (i) the lexicon size (one or n), and (ii) the position of the query word in the ranked lexicon. Note that in each iteration of the lexicon reduction process, the lexicon is ranked by group edit distance from the diverse solutions (Sect. 2.4). The intuition behind this combined score is that words retrieved from a small lexicon and words that rank better in the lexicon are more likely to be the correct retrieval, i.e., a low combined score. We give more weightage to the first term, as word images with smaller lexicons are more likely to retain the ground truth.

4 Experimental Analysis

4.1 Datasets

We used three public datasets, namely IIIT 5K-word dataset [7], ICDAR 2003 [16] and Street View Text (SVT) [17,18] in our evaluations.

IIIT 5K-word. The IIIT 5K-word dataset contains 5000 cropped word images from scene texts and born-digital images, harvested from Google image search engine. This is the largest dataset for natural image word spotting and recognition currently available. The dataset is partitioned into train (2000 word images) and test (3000 word images) sets. It also comes with a large lexicon of 0.5 million words. Further, each word is associated with two smaller lexicons, one containing 50 words (known as small lexicon), another with 1000 words (known as medium lexicon).

ICDAR 2003. The test dataset contains 890 cropped word images. They were released as a part of the robust reading competitions. We use small lexicons provided by [17] of size 50 for each image in this dataset.

SVT. The SVT dataset contains images taken from Google Street View. Since we focus on the word recognition task, we used the SVT-WORD dataset, which contains 647 word images and a 50-word sized lexicon for each image.

4.2 Multiple Candidate Word Generation

We binarize the image using Otsu's method [19] with ten thresholds equally spaced over the grayscale range. This provides a good set of potential character

Word Image	Iteration 1	Iteration 2	Iteration 3	Iteration 4
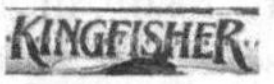 KINGFISHER	FGAIEESHER	FGAIERSHER	KINGFISHER	KINGFISHER
that	NHAI	AHAI	AHAI	THAT
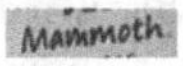 Mammoth	MAITOTA	MAITOTA	MACTOTH	MAMMOTH
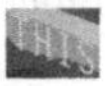	THTL	THEL	THEL	THIS

Fig. 3. Effect of the lexicon reduction technique on the inferred label. Here we show four iterations for each example. We observe that with stronger pairwise potentials the method recovers from the errors in the MAP solution.

locations, which are used to construct the graph (Sect. 2.2). The overlap, aspect ratio and width/height range parameters associated with the graph construction are chosen by cross-validating on an independent validation set. We add an edge between two overlapping windows if their X-axis projection intersection is less than 25 % of the left window width. If they are non-overlapping, they must be no farther than 50 % of the left window width. We remove edges with window width ratio or height ratio more than a factor of 4. For non-maximal suppression, we use 80 % overlap as our threshold. Once the graph is constructed, all candidate words are found (Sect. 2.2). We then re-rank them using their energy score (1) normalized by word length and select the top-10 candidate words for the lexicon reduction phase.

4.3 Diversity Preserving Inference

We train one-vs-all character classifiers with linear SVM for unary potentials, as described in [20], with dense HOG features [21] from character images. To obtain multiple CRF solutions we infer the top-5 diverse labels by modifying the unary potentials in each iteration (Sect. 2.3). The λ parameter in (12) is set by cross validation. We found $\lambda = 0.1$ to be an optimal value to moderate the influence of diversity. Note that with a small λ, the unary potentials will be modified by a very small amount in the next iteration, which will result in inferring the same solution. On the other hand, a large λ gives very diverse solutions, and in some cases words that are significantly different from each other.

4.4 Recognition

In our recognition experiment, we stop the lexicon reduction process when the reduced lexicon reaches a size of 10, and then find the nearest word in the original lexicon with minimum group edit distance from the most recently inferred solution set. We evaluate the performance of the system by checking if the nearest word is the ground truth or not.

For the large lexicon experiments, the group edit distance re-ranking becomes computationally expensive due to the lexicon size. To speed up the process, we represent each word by its character histogram and build a k-NN classifier.

Table 1. Word recognition accuracy comparison between various CRF and non-CRF methods. A word is said to be correctly recognized if the word nearest to result of a method in the lexicon is the ground truth. We compute top-5 diverse solutions and select one solution from the full lexicon with minimum group edit distance as the proposed method. We see that in the large and medium lexicon setting of IIIT 5K-word dataset, our method outperforms the existing ones. We also obtain similar performance as compared to the other CRF methods on small lexicons.

Method	IIIT 5K-word			ICDAR 03	SVT
	Large	Medium	Small	Small	Small
non-CRF based					
Wang et al. [3]	-	-	-	76.0	57.0
Bissacco et al. [2]	-	-	-	82.8	**90.3**
Alsharif et al. [22]	-	-	-	**93.1**	74.3
Goel et al. [5]	-	-	-	89.6	77.2
Rodriguez et al. [6]	-	57.4	**76.1**	-	-
CRF based					
Shi et al. [10]	-	-	-	87.4	73.5
Novikova et al. [9]	-	-	-	82.8	72.9
Mishra et al. [4]	-	-	-	81.7	73.2
Mishra et al. [7]	28.0	55.5	68.2	80.2	73.5
Our Method	**42.7**	**62.9**	71.6	85.5	76.4

Now, for a given solution set and a lexicon, we first find the top-100 nearest neighbours in the lexicon for each word in the solution set. We then consider the union of all top-100 nearest lexicon words to be the new lexicon and perform the group edit distance based re-ranking on it. This speeds up the process by around 200 times and reduces the computation time to less than a second.

Discussion. Figure 3 shows that lexicon reduction (and re-computation of priors using diverse solutions) corrects solutions in the first four iterations. We observe that the inferred label changes by one or more characters as the priors get stronger over iterations by assigning a lower pairwise cost to the bigrams from the ground truth.

Table 1 compares the performance of the proposed method with the state of the art over the three datasets. We see that our method outperforms the state of the art in the large lexicon setting. We obtain 14 % improvement over [7] because of stronger priors.[1] As a baseline, to evaluate the effectiveness of the diversity constraint, we searched for multiple candidate words using the

---

[1] It should also be noted that [7] follows an open vocabulary lexicon, i.e., it does not assume that the ground truth is present in the lexicon. We find that around 75 % of the ground truth words from the IIIT 5K-word dataset are present in the large lexicon by default. The rest of the ground truth words are language-specific and proper nouns like city and shop names.

Table 2. Top-1 precision for retrieval experiment on various datasets. We compare the results between two reduction methods, each with and without diverse solutions. The partial reduction method leaves some lexicons with around 5 words, while the full reduction method reduces all lexicons to size one. We see that our proposed method of partial reduction with diverse solutions works the best for the IIIT 5K-word dataset.

Method	IIIT 5K-word			ICDAR 03
	Large	Medium	Small	Small
Without diversity				
Full reduction	27.5	51.9	65.0	**81.7**
Partial reduction	35.1	35.6	60.7	76.9
With diversity				
Full reduction	23.1	52.0	65.0	78.9
Partial reduction	**42.1**	**59.0**	**66.5**	79.5

CRF energy without using the diversity constraint. For example, on the IIIT 5K-word dataset (with medium lexicon), this resulted in an accuracy of 55.6 without diversity compared to 62.9 (with diversity, shown in Table 1), when considering the top-5 candidate words.

For the small lexicon setting, non-CRF methods, like beam search on a graph in [2] perform well on the SVT dataset because of training the classifiers with millions of character images. This is around ten times larger than the amount of training data we use, and is unavailable to the public. The structured SVM formulation [6] shows a good performance on the small lexicon of IIIT 5K-word but deteriorates as the lexicon size increases. This is due to the model being incapable of effectively minimizing the distance between the label and image features in the embedded space for larger lexicons.

4.5   Retrieval

In this experiment we retrieve a word image for a given query word from the dataset. The dataset comprises of a singleton or a reduced lexicon for each image which is used for the task as described in Sect. 3. As our proposed method, we preprocess the dataset by reducing the lexicon to singleton if the AED value θ at the $5th$ (last) iteration is less than 3.5. We call this process the *partial reduction* method as it reduces the lexicon to size one only for some word images, and for the rest, the lexicon contains 5 words. As a baseline method, we also do a *full reduction*, reducing lexicons for all the word images to one corresponding word. Both, the proposed and the baseline methods, are performed with and without the diversity constraint, thus creating four different variations. The parameter θ that gives the best precision for the proposed method is selected after cross validation over an independent query set. For quantitative evaluation, we compute

Query	Retrieved Image	Reduced Lexicon: diversity + partial red.	Reduced Lexicon: diversity + full red.
BRADY	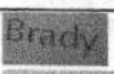	MY, BRADY, ANY, A	MY
SPACE	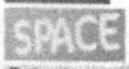	HOT, SPACE, LACEY, SALE	HOT
HAHN	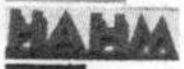	BUENA, HANDA, HAHN, PIPE	BUENA
DAILY		PEARL, MOUNTS, DAILY, NIKE	PEARL
TIMES	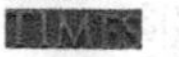	TIME, TIMES, WINE, MED	TIME
THREE	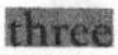	THE, THREE, THERE, USED	THE

Fig. 4. Cases where retrieval results are correct. The reduced lexicon from partial reduction method (partial red.) retains the ground truth word. The words in the reduced lexicon are similar to each other, and any further reduction could have resulted in loss of ground truth (Color figure online).

the precision of the first retrieved word image as the datasets do not have a significant number of repeating ground truth labels (i.e., word images with the same text).

We show quantitative results in Table 2, where we clearly see that partial reduction of lexicons with diversity outperforms full reduction without diversity on the IIIT 5K-word dataset. The diverse solutions improve the performance as they retain the ground truth in reduced lexicon after the lexicon reduction process in many cases. We also notice that on IIIT 5K-word dataset, the performance gap increases as the lexicon size increases, suggesting potential applicability to larger lexicon based query systems. Correct retrievals (in Fig. 4) show that a higher AED threshold based lexicon association has the ground truth in the reduced lexicon associated with it, as compared to its singleton lexicon. The method is less successful in cases (Fig. 5) where the ground truth is lost in the early stages of lexicon reduction leading to a reduced lexicon without the ground truth in it. This happens due to failure of the binarization method used to segment out the characters, which leads to abrupt short/long candidate word formation.

	Query	Retrieved Image	Reduced Lexicon
1	CLEAR	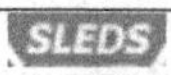	CLEAR
2	HOME	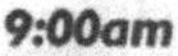	HOME, 900AM, 9080, 90
3	BAR		BAR
4	FOR	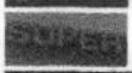	AND, ARTS, FOR, INN
5	311		311
6	JOIN	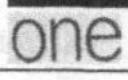	ONE, JOIN, OUT, OUR

Fig. 5. Failure cases for retrieval experiment with reduced lexicons after partial reduction. Some word images have reduced lexicons with no ground truth (rows 1, 3, 4, 5). Other cases have the ground truth word, but are retrieved for the wrong query word (rows 2, 6).

5   Summary

In this paper we proposed a novel framework for recognition and retrieval tasks in the large lexicon setting. We identify potential character locations and find words contained in the image. We reduce the large lexicon to a small image-specific lexicon. The lexicon reduction process alternates between recomputing priors and refining the lexicon. We evaluated our results on public datasets and show superior performance on large and medium lexicons for recognition and retrieval tasks.

Acknowledgements. This work was partially supported by the Ministry of Communications and Information Technology, Government of India, New Delhi. Anand Mishra was supported by Microsoft Corporation and Microsoft Research India under the Microsoft Research India PhD fellowship award.

References

1. Weinman, J., Butler, Z., Knoll, D., Feild, J.: Toward integrated scene text reading. TPAMI **36**, 375–387 (2014)
2. Bissacco, A., Cummins, M., Netzer, Y., Neven, H.: Photoocr: reading text in uncontrolled conditions. In: ICCV (2013)
3. Wang, K., Babenko, B., Belongie, S.: End-to-end scene text recognition. In: ICCV (2011)
4. Mishra, A., Alahari, K., Jawahar, C.V.: Top-down and bottom-up cues for scene text recognition. In: CVPR (2012)
5. Goel, V., Mishra, A., Alahari, K., Jawahar, C.V.: Whole is greater than sum of parts: recognizing scene text words. In: ICDAR (2013)
6. Rodriguez, J., Perronnin, F.: Label embedding for text recognition. In: BMVC (2013)
7. Mishra, A., Alahari, K., Jawahar, C.V.: Scene text recognition using higher order langauge priors. In: BMVC (2012)
8. Weinman, J.J., Learned-Miller, E., Hanson, A.R.: Scene text recognition using similarity and a lexicon with sparse belief propagation. TPAMI **31**, 1733–1746 (2009)
9. Novikova, T., Barinova, O., Kohli, P., Lempitsky, V.: Large-lexicon attribute-consistent text recognition in natural images. In: Fitzgibbon, A., Lazebnik, S., Perona, P., Sato, Y., Schmid, C. (eds.) ECCV 2012, Part VI. LNCS, vol. 7577, pp. 752–765. Springer, Heidelberg (2012)
10. Shi, C., Wang, C., Xiao, B., Zhang, Y., Gao, S., Zhang, Z.: Scene text recognition using part-based tree-structured character detection. In: CVPR (2013)
11. Batra, D., Yadollahpour, P., Guzman-Rivera, A., Shakhnarovich, G.: Diverse m-best solutions in markov random fields. In: Fitzgibbon, A., Lazebnik, S., Perona, P., Sato, Y., Schmid, C. (eds.) ECCV 2012, Part V. LNCS, vol. 7576, pp. 1–16. Springer, Heidelberg (2012)
12. Sheshadri, K., Divvala, S.K.: Exemplar driven character recognition in the wild. In: BMVC (2012)
13. Tian, S., Lu, S., Su, B., Tan, C.L.: Scene text recognition using co-occurrence of histogram of oriented gradients. In: ICDAR (2013)

14. Tarjan, R.: Depth-first search and linear graph algorithms. SIAM J. Comput. **1**, 146–160 (1972)
15. Kolmogorov, V.: Convergent tree-reweighted message passing for energy minimization. TPAMI **28**, 1568–1583 (2006)
16. ICDAR 2003 datasets. http://algoval.essex.ac.uk/icdar
17. Wang, K., Belongie, S.: Word spotting in the wild. In: Daniilidis, K., Maragos, P., Paragios, N. (eds.) ECCV 2010, Part I. LNCS, vol. 6311, pp. 591–604. Springer, Heidelberg (2010)
18. Street View Text dataset. http://vision.ucsd.edu/~kai/svt
19. Otsu, N.: A threshold selection method from gray-level histograms. IEEE Trans. Syst. Man Cybern. **9**, 62–66 (1979)
20. Mishra, A., Alahari, K., Jawahar, C.V.: Image retrieval using textual cues. In: ICCV (2013)
21. Dalal, N., Triggs, B.: Histograms of oriented gradients for human detection. In: CVPR (2005)
22. Alsharif, O., Pineau, J.: End-to-end text recognition with hybrid HMM maxout models. arXiv preprint arXiv:1310.1811 (2013)

Planar Structures from Line Correspondences in a Manhattan World

Chelhwon Kim[1]([✉]) and Roberto Manduchi[2]([✉])

[1] Electrical Engineering Department, University of California,
Santa Cruz, CA, USA
chkim@soe.ucsc.edu
[2] Computer Engineering Department, University of California,
Santa Cruz, CA, USA
manduchi@soe.ucsc.edu

Abstract. Traditional structure from motion is hard in indoor environments with only a few detectable point features. These environments, however, have other useful characteristics: they often contain severable visible lines, and their layout typically conforms to a Manhattan world geometry. We introduce a new algorithm to cluster visible lines in a Manhattan world, seen from two different viewpoints, into coplanar bundles. This algorithm is based on the notion of "characteristic line", which is an invariant of a set of parallel coplanar lines. Finding coplanar sets of lines becomes a problem of clustering characteristic lines, which can be accomplished using a modified mean shift procedure. The algorithm is computationally light and produces good results in real world situations.

1 Introduction

This paper addresses the problem of reconstructing the scene geometry from pictures taken from different viewpoints. Structure from motion (SFM) has a long history in computer vision [1,2], and SFM (or visual SLAM) algorithms have been ported on mobile phones [3,4]. Traditional SFM relies on the ability of detecting and matching across views a substantial number of point features. Unfortunately, robust point detection and matching in indoor environments can be challenging, as the density of detectable points (e.g. corners) may be low. At the same time, indoor environments are typically characterized by (1) the presence of multiple line segments (due to plane intersections and other linear structures), and (2) "Manhattan world" layouts, with a relatively small number of planes at mutually orthogonal orientations.

This paper introduces a new algorithm for the detection and localization of planar structures and relative camera pose in a Manhattan world, using line matches from two images taken from different viewpoints. As in previous approaches [5–7], the orientation (but not the position) of the two cameras with

Electronic supplementary material The online version of this chapter (doi:10. 1007/978-3-319-16865-4_33) contains supplementary material, which is available to authorized users.

© Springer International Publishing Switzerland 2015
D. Cremers et al. (Eds.): ACCV 2014, Part I, LNCS 9003, pp. 509–524, 2015.
DOI: 10.1007/978-3-319-16865-4_33

respect to the environment is computed using vanishing lines and inertial sensors (available in all new smartphones). The main novelty of our algorithm is in the criterion used to check whether groups of lines matched in the two images may be coplanar. Specifically, we introduce a new invariant feature ($\vec{n}$-*characteristic line*) of the image of a bundle of coplanar parallel lines, and show how this feature can be used to cluster visible lines into planar patches and to compute the relative camera pose. The algorithm has low complexity (quadratic in the number of matched line segments); implemented on an iPhone 5s, its average end-to-end execution time is of 0.28 s. Our algorithm fully exploits the strong constraints imposed by the Manhattan world hypothesis, and is able to produce good results even when very few lines are visible, as long as they are correctly matched across the two images.

2   Related Work

The standard approach to recovering scene structure and camera pose from multiple views is based on point feature matches across views [2]. When point features are scarce, line features can be used instead. Computation of 3-D line segments and camera pose from three images of a set of lines is possible using the trifocal tensor [2,8,9]. This approach follows three general steps: (1) trifocal tensor computation from triplets of line correspondences, producing the three camera matrices; (2) 3-D line computation via triangulation from line correspondences; (3) non-linear optimization for refinement. At least 13 triplets of line correspondences are necessary for computing the trifocal tensor [2]. Note that direct 3-D line computation requires at least three views because two views of 3-D lines in the scene do not impose enough constraints on camera displacements [9,10].

A few authors have attempted to recover structure and motion using line features from only two views (as in our contribution), under strong geometric priors such as the Manhattan world assumption. Košecka and Zhang [11] presented a method to extract dominant rectangular structures via line segments that are aligned to one of the principal vanishing points, thus recovering camera pose and planar surfaces. Elqursh and Elgammal [7] introduced an SFM algorithm based on line features from a man-made environment. Three line segments, two of which parallel to each other and orthogonal to the third one, are used to recover the relative camera rotation, and the camera translation is computed from any two intersections of two pairs of lines. This algorithm was shown to work even in the absence of dominant structures.

An alternative approach is to detect dominant planes and compute the induced homographies, from which the camera pose and planar geometry can be recovered [12–15]. Zhou et al. [16] presented a SFM system to compute structure and motion from one or more large planes in the scene. The system detects and tracks the scene plane using generalized RANSAC, and estimates the homographies induced by the scene plane across multiple views. The set of homographies are used to self-calibrate and recover the motion for all camera frames by solving a global optimization problem. Another possibility for planar surface recovery is to fit multiple instances of a plane to 3-D point cloud obtained by SFM using a robust estimation algorithm [17–19].

A more recent research direction looks to recover the spatial layout of an indoor scene from a single image [20–22]. Lee et al. [23] proposed a method based on an hypothesis-and-test framework. Layout hypotheses are generated by connecting line segments using geometric reasoning on the indoor environment, and verified to find the best fit to a map that expresses the local belief of region orientations computed from the line segments. Flint et al. [24] addressed the spatial layout estimation problem by integrating information from image features, stereo features, and 3-D point clouds in a MAP optimization problem, which is solved using dynamic programming. Ramalingam et al. [25] presented a method to detect junctions formed by line segments in three Manhattan orthogonal directions using a voting scheme. Possible cuboid layouts generated from the junctions are evaluated using an inference algorithm based on a conditional random field model. Tsai et al. [26] model an indoor environment as a ground plane and a set of wall planes; by analyzing ground-wall boundaries, a set of hypotheses of the local environment is generated. A Bayesian filtering framework is used to evaluate the hypotheses using information accumulated through motion.

3 The Characteristic Lines Method

3.1 Notation and Basic Concepts

By *Manhattan world* we mean an environment composed of planar surfaces, each of which is oriented along one of three *canonical* mutually orthogonal vectors[1] $(\vec{n}_1, \vec{n}_2, \vec{n}_3)$. In addition, we will assume that each line visible in the scene lies on a planar surface (possible at its edge) and is oriented along one of the three canonical vectors. Two pictures of the environment are taken by two different viewpoints (camera centers, $\vec{c}_1$ and $\vec{c}_2$) with *baseline* $\vec{t} = \vec{c}_1 - \vec{c}_2$. The rotation matrix representing the orientation of the frame of reference of the first camera with respect to the second one is denoted by $\mathbf{R}$. Previous work has shown how to reconstruct the orientation of a camera from a single picture of a Manhattan world, using the location of the three vanishing points of the visible lines [5]. This estimation can be made more robust by measuring the gravity vector using a 3-axis accelerometer, a sensor that is present in any modern smartphones [6]. We will assume that the intrinsic calibration matrices $\mathbf{K}_1$, $\mathbf{K}_2$ of the cameras have been obtained offline, and that the orientation of each cameras with respect to the canonical reference system $(\vec{n}_1, \vec{n}_2, \vec{n}_3)$ has been estimated using one of the methods mentioned above (and, consequently, that $\mathbf{R}$ is known). We will also assume that lines visible in both images have been correctly matched; the algorithm used in our implementation for line detection and matching is briefly discussed in Sect. 4.

---

[1] A vector is represented by an arrowed symbol ($\vec{n}$) when the frame of reference is immaterial, and by a boldface symbol ($\mathbf{n}$) when expressed in terms of a frame of reference.

A generic plane Π will be identified by the pair $(\vec{n}, d)$, where $\vec{n}$ is its orientation (unit-norm normal) and d is its signed offset with respect to the first camera ($d = \langle \vec{p} - \vec{c}_1, \vec{n} \rangle$, where $\vec{p}$ is a generic point on the plane, and $\langle \cdot, \cdot \rangle$ indicates inner product). A generic line $\mathcal{L}$ will be identified by its orientation $\vec{l}$ (unit-norm vector parallel to the line) and by the location of any point on the line. In a Manhattan world, surface planes and visible lines are oriented along one of the three canonical orientations.

It is well known that a plane $(\vec{n}, d)$ imaged by two cameras induces an homography $\mathbf{H}$ on the image points in the two cameras. Given a line $\mathcal{L}$ in the plane, the two homogeneous representations $\mathbf{L}_1$ and $\mathbf{L}_2$ of the image lines in the two camera are related to one another as by $\mathbf{L}_1 = \mathbf{H}^T \mathbf{L}_2$. The *lever vectors* $\vec{u}_1(\mathcal{L})$ and $\vec{u}_2(\mathcal{L})$ are unit-norm vectors orthogonal to the plane containing $\mathcal{L}$ and the optical center of camera 1 and camera 2, respectively (see Fig. 1, left panel). Expressed in terms of the associated camera reference frames, the lever vectors can be written as $\mathbf{u}_1 = \mathbf{K}_1^T \mathbf{L}_1$ and $\mathbf{u}_2 = \mathbf{K}_2^T \mathbf{L}_2$. The lever vectors are thus easily computed from the image of the line $\mathcal{L}$ in the two cameras. The following relation holds:

$$\mathbf{u}_1 = \mathbf{H}_c^T \mathbf{u}_2 \tag{1}$$

where $\mathbf{H}_c = \mathbf{K}_2^{-1} \mathbf{H} \mathbf{K}_1$ is the *calibrated homography matrix* induced by the plane, which can be decomposed [2] as

$$\mathbf{H}_c = \mathbf{R} + \mathbf{t}\mathbf{n}^T / d \tag{2}$$

In the above equation, the baseline $\mathbf{t}$ and plane normal $\mathbf{n}$ are expressed in terms of the reference frames defined at the second camera and at the first camera, respectively, and d is the distance between the plane and the first camera.

A set of lines will be termed $\vec{n}$-*coplanar* if the lines are all coplanar, and the common plane has orientation $\vec{n}$.

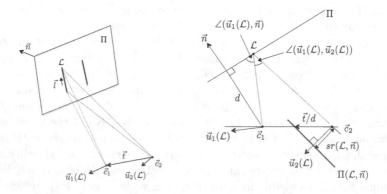

Fig. 1. Left: The two camera centers $\vec{c}_1$, $\vec{c}_2$ and the lever vectors $\vec{u}_1(\mathcal{L})$, $\vec{u}_2(\mathcal{L})$ for line $\mathcal{L}$. Right: Line $\mathcal{L}$ lies on the plane $\Pi \equiv (\vec{n}, d)$ (both line and plane orthogonal to this page). The thick blue line is the trace of the $\vec{n}$-characteristic plane $\Pi(\mathcal{L}, \vec{n})$ (also orthogonal to the page) (Color figure online).

3.2   Characteristic Planes

Given a line $\mathcal{L}$ and a vector $\vec{n}$, we define by *sin-ratio* $sr(\mathcal{L}, \vec{n})$ the following quantity:

$$sr(\mathcal{L}, \vec{n}) = \frac{\sin \angle(\vec{u}_1(\mathcal{L}), \vec{u}_2(\mathcal{L}))}{\sin \angle(\vec{u}_1(\mathcal{L}), \vec{n})} \tag{3}$$

where $\angle(\cdot, \cdot)$ indicates the signed angle between two vectors. Note that the numerator of (3) has magnitude equal to $\|(\mathbf{u}_1 \times \mathbf{R}^T \mathbf{u}_2)\|$, while the denominator has magnitude equal to $\|\mathbf{u}_1 \times \mathbf{n}\|$, where $\mathbf{n}$ is defined with respect to the first camera's reference frame. Hence, $sr(\mathcal{L}, \vec{n})$ can be computed from the two images of $\mathcal{L}$ and from $\mathbf{R}$ without knowledge of the baseline $\vec{t}$. The sin-ratio has an interesting property:

Proposition 1. If the line $\mathcal{L}$ lies on plane $(\vec{n}, d)$, then the projection $\langle \vec{t}/d, \vec{u}_2(\mathcal{L}) \rangle$ of $\vec{t}/d$ onto $\vec{u}_2(\mathcal{L})$ is equal to $sr(\mathcal{L}, \vec{n})$.

Proof. From (1) one derives

$$\mathbf{u}_1 \times \mathbf{H}_c^T \mathbf{u}_2 = 0 \tag{4}$$

Combining (4) with (2), one obtains

$$(\mathbf{R}^T \mathbf{u}_2) \times \mathbf{u}_1 = \mathbf{u}_1 \times \mathbf{n} \mathbf{u}_2^T \mathbf{t}/d \tag{5}$$

The vectors $(\mathbf{R}^T \mathbf{u}_2) \times \mathbf{u}_1$ and $\mathbf{u}_1 \times \mathbf{n}$ are both parallel to the line $\mathcal{L}$. The ratio of their magnitudes (multiplied by -1 if they have opposite orientation) is equal to the sin-ratio $sr(\mathcal{L}, \vec{n})$. This value is also equal to $\mathbf{u}_2^T \mathbf{t}/d = \langle \vec{u}_2(\mathcal{L}), \vec{t}/d \rangle$. ∎

This result may be restated as follows. Given a plane $(\vec{n}, d)$ and a line $\mathcal{L}$ on this plane, define by *characteristic plane* $\Pi(\mathcal{L}, \vec{n})$ the plane with normal equal to $\vec{u}_2(\mathcal{L})$ and offset with respect to the second camera center $\vec{c}_2$ equal to $sr(\mathcal{L}, \vec{n})$. Then, the "normalized" baseline vector $\vec{t}/d$ is guaranteed to lie on $\Pi(\mathcal{L}, \vec{n})$ (see Fig. 1, right panel). This constraint is at the basis of our *characteristic line* method, discussed in the next section. A parallel derivation of the characteristic plane and of its properties, based on algebraic manipulation, is presented in the Appendix.

3.3   Characteristic Lines and Coplanarity

Given a set of parallel lines $\{\mathcal{L}_i\}$, with common orientation $\vec{l}$, the associated characteristic planes $\{\Pi(\mathcal{L}_i, \vec{n})\}$ for a given unit norm vector $\vec{n}$ are all parallel to $\vec{l}$ by construction (since the lever vectors $\{\vec{u}_2(\mathcal{L}_i)\}$ are all coplanar and orthogonal to $\vec{l}$). Any two such planes intersect at a $\vec{n}$-*characteristic line* $\mathcal{L}^*$ oriented along $\vec{l}$. It may be interesting to study under which conditions *all* of the characteristic planes associated with $\{\mathcal{L}_i\}$ intersect at a common line, i.e., when the lines $\{\mathcal{L}_i\}$ *induce a $\vec{n}$-characteristic plane intersection at $\mathcal{L}^*$*.

Corollary 1. Let $\{\mathcal{L}_i\}$ be any number of parallel $\vec{n}$-coplanar lines. These lines induce a $\vec{n}$-characteristic plane intersection at $\mathcal{L}^*$, where the characteristic line $\mathcal{L}^*$ goes through $\vec{t}/d$, and d is the signed offset of the plane defined by the lines $\{\mathcal{L}_i\}$ to the first camera.

Proof. By definition of $\vec{n}$–coplanarity, all lines $\{\mathcal{L}_i\}$ lie on the plane $(\vec{n}, d)$. Hence, by Proposition 1, $\vec{t}/d$ is contained in all of the $\vec{n}$-characteristic planes defined by the lines. Since these planes are all parallel to the orientation of the lines $\{\mathcal{L}_i\}$, they must intersect at a single characteristic line containing $\vec{t}/d$.   ∎

Corollary 1 shows that a sufficient condition for a set of parallel lines to induce a $\vec{n}$-characteristic plane intersection is that they be $\vec{n}$-coplanar. The resulting characteristic line represents an *invariant* property of parallel, coplanar lines; importantly, it can be computed from the image lines, provided that the rotation **R** and the normal $\vec{n}$ of the plane are known. As discussed earlier in Sect. 3.1, this information can be easily obtained in a Manhattan world.

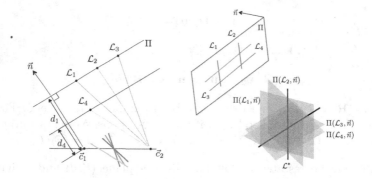

Fig. 2. Left: Lines $\mathcal{L}_1$, $\mathcal{L}_2$ and $\mathcal{L}_3$ (orthogonal to this page) are $\vec{n}$-coplanar. Their associated $\vec{n}$-characteristic planes all intersect at a characteristic line through the baseline (also orthogonal to this page). They also individually intersect with the $\vec{n}$-characteristic plane associated with line $\mathcal{L}_4$, parallel but not coplanar with the other lines, but these intersections are outside of the baseline. Right: The sets of parallel lines $(\mathcal{L}_1, \mathcal{L}_2)$ and $(\mathcal{L}_3, \mathcal{L}_4)$ are mutually orthogonal; all lines are $\vec{n}$-coplanar. The $\vec{n}$-characteristic line associated with $(\mathcal{L}_3, \mathcal{L}_4)$ intersects the $\vec{n}$-characteristic line associated with $(\mathcal{L}_1, \mathcal{L}_2)$, $\mathcal{L}^*$, at a point on the baseline.

Thus, for a given canonical orientation $\vec{n}$, one may test whether a group of parallel lines all belong to a plane oriented as $\vec{n}$ by observing whether the associated characteristic planes intersect at one line (see Fig. 2, left panel). In fact, one never needs to test many lines at once: the characteristic planes for multiple lines in a parallel bundle intersect at a single line if and only if the characteristic lines from pairwise plane intersection are identical. Hence, one needs only test two parallel lines at a time. This observation suggests the following algorithm to *cluster* parallel lines into coplanar groups for a given plane orientation $\vec{n}$:

1. For each pair of parallel lines, find the associated $\vec{n}$-characteristic line;
2. Find clusters of nearby characteristic lines. Each such cluster may signify the presence of a plane;
3. For all characteristic lines in a cluster, label the associated parallel lines $\{\mathcal{L}_i\}$ as belonging to the same plane $(\vec{n},d)$ for some d.

An example of application of this algorithm is shown in Fig. 3. Since all $\vec{n}$-characteristic lines for a given line orientation $\vec{l}$ are parallel to $\vec{l}$, in Fig. 3 we simply plot the intersections of these lines with a plane orthogonal to $\vec{l}$. To identify cluster centers, we run mean shift on these 2-D points.

A degenerate case occurs when the camera moves in the direction of $\vec{l}$. In this case, $\vec{u}_1 = \vec{u}_2$ and thus $sr(\mathcal{L}_i, \vec{n}) = 0$ for all lines $\mathcal{L}_i$, meaning that all $\vec{n}$-characteristic planes intersect at $\vec{c}_2$. This is consistent with the fact that the image of the lines does not change as the camera moves along $\vec{l}$.

Before closing this section, we note that from a set of coplanar parallel lines we cannot really say much about the baseline $\vec{t}$. As we will see next, multiple bundles of parallel lines allow us to also precisely compute $\vec{t}/d$.

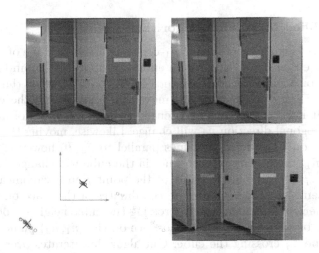

Fig. 3. Top row: Image pair with detected lines oriented along one canonical direction $(\vec{n}_1)$. Only lines that have been matched across images are shown. Bottom left: Traces of the $\vec{n}_2$- and $\vec{n}_3$-characteristic lines on a plane oriented as $\vec{n}_1$. The cluster centers, found by mean shift, are marked by a cross. Note that the cluster centers for the $\vec{n}_2$- and $\vec{n}_3$-characteristic lines are found separately. Characteristic line traces are shown by circles in dark blue color when associated with a cluster, by circles in pale blue color otherwise. Bottom right: The coplanar line sets defined by the characteristic line clusters. Each set drawn with a characteristic color (For line segments at the intersection of two planes, we used one color corresponding to one of the two planes) (Color figure online).

3.4 Multiple Line Orientations

In a Manhattan world, lines belonging to a plane orthogonal to a canonical orientation $\vec{n}_i$ must be oriented along one of the two other canonical orientations $(\vec{n}_j$

or $\vec{n}_k$), orthogonal to $\vec{n}_i$. For each such orientation, consider a bundle of coplanar parallel lines. These two line bundles induce an $\vec{n}_j$- and $\vec{n}_k$-characteristic line, respectively, where the first characteristic line contains $\vec{t}/d_j$ and the second one contains $\vec{t}/d_k$ (d_j and d_k being the offsets of the planes defined by the two line bundles to the first camera). If both bundles are coplanar, then obviously $d_j = d_k = d$, and the characteristic lines in both directions intersect at $\vec{t}/d$ (Fig. 2, right panel). This is a very interesting result: the intersection of characteristic lines induced by orthogonal coplanar lines directly provides the direction of camera translation. (Note again that this simple result is only possible in a Manhattan world, where the orientation of planes in the scene is known.)

The algorithm for testing coplanarity introduced in Sect. 3.3 can be easily modified to consider, for each canonical orientation $\vec{n}$, the two bundles of parallel lines in the two directions orthogonal to $\vec{n}$. This calls for an algorithm that can detect accumulation points of 3-D lines, defined as points in 3-D space that, within a cubic neighborhood, contain a high density of characteristic lines in both directions. For this purpose we propose a modified version of mean shift [27], described next.

3.5   A Modified Mean Shift Algorithm

Suppose we are looking for groups of $\vec{n}_1$-coplanar lines; each one of these lines is oriented along either $\vec{n}_2$ or $\vec{n}_3$. Given a cubic neighborhood around a point $\vec{p}$, it is convenient to consider the *traces* (intersections) of the lines on the cube's faces orthogonal to $\vec{n}_2$ and $\vec{n}_3$. Suppose to move the point $\vec{p}$ (and the cube around it) along $\vec{n}_2$; it is clear that only the density (within the cube) of lines oriented along the orthogonal direction $\vec{n}_3$ will change. Likewise, moving the point along $\vec{n}_3$ will change only the density of lines parallel to $\vec{n}_2$. If, however, the point is moved along $\vec{n}_1$, the density of both lines in the cube will change.

Let (p^1, p^2, p^3) be the coordinates of the point $\vec{p}$ in a canonically oriented reference system; let $(\mathcal{L}^1_{i,2}, \mathcal{L}^3_{i,2})$ be the coordinates of the trace on the $(\vec{n}_1, \vec{n}_3)$ plane of a generic $\vec{n}_2$-oriented line $\mathcal{L}_i$ crossing the cubic neighborhood of $\vec{p}$; and let $(\mathcal{L}^1_{j,3}, \mathcal{L}^2_{j,3})$ be the coordinates of the trace on the $(\vec{n}_1, \vec{n}_2)$ plane of a generic $\vec{n}_3$-oriented line $\mathcal{L}_j$ crossing the cube. Our algorithm iterates over a cycle of 3 steps, each requiring a 1-D (component-wise) mean shift update:

1. Implement a mean shift update of p^2 based on the measurements $\{\mathcal{L}^2_{j,3}\}$.
2. Implement a mean shift update of p^3 based on the measurements $\{\mathcal{L}^3_{i,2}\}$.
3. Implement a mean shift update of p^1 based on the measurements $\{\mathcal{L}^1_{i,2}\} \cup \{\mathcal{L}^1_{j,3}\}$.

At convergence, the point will be situated in a neighborhood with high density of lines in both directions. We also found it beneficial to assign a weight to each line (which is used in the mean shift updates) equal to the mean of a function $g(D)$ (with $g(D) = e^{-D/\sigma}$) of the line's distance D to each other line oriented in an orthogonal direction; this ensures that characteristic lines with a high density of neighbors in the orthogonal direction are given high weight. An example of application of this algorithm is shown in Fig. 4.

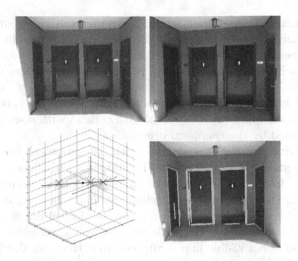

Fig. 4. Top row: Image pair with detected lines oriented along the three canonical directions (the color of each line identifies its orientation). Only lines that have been matched across images (including incorrect ones) are shown. Bottom left: Characteristic lines for the different orientations. The color of a characteristic line matches the color of the lines it represents. Clusters centers identified by the mean shift algorithm described in Sect. 3.5 are shown by black crosses. Characteristic lines not associated to a cluster are shown in pale color. The regressed baseline direction is represented by a black line through the origin (shown as a thick dot). Bottom right: The coplanar line sets defined by the characteristic line clusters (each set drawn with a characteristic color) (Color figure online).

3.6 Limitations

Corollary 1 provides a sufficient condition for characteristic plane intersection. This condition, however, is not necessary: there may exist groups of parallel, non-$\vec{n}$-coplanar lines (but still individually oriented orthogonally to $\vec{n}$) that induce a $\vec{n}$-characteristic plane intersection. This means that a cluster of characteristic lines could potentially be found even for non-coplanar lines.

In general, the occurrence of such "spurious" clusters is unlikely in a Manhattan world. For example, if two parallel lines are $\vec{n}$-coplanar, addition of a third, non-coplanar parallel line will *not* induce a characteristic plane intersection, as shown by the following corollary. (proof omitted for lack of space.)

Corollary 2. A bundle of parallel lines, two or more of which are $\vec{n}$-coplanar, induces a $\vec{n}$-characteristic plane intersection only if all lines in the bundle are $\vec{n}$-coplanar.

4 Implementation

We use the LSD (Line Segment Detector) algorithm [28] to find line segments. This algorithm works in linear time, and does not require any parameter tuning. A MSLD (Mean-Standard Deviation Line Descriptor) [29] feature vector is computed for each line; lines are matched based on a criterion that considers the Euclidean distance between feature vectors in a line match while ensuring that the angle between matched image lines in the two images is consistent across matches. For each image, the vanishing points of detected lines are computed. This information, together with data from the accelerometers (which measure the direction of gravity, assumed to be aligned to one of the canonical orientations), is used to compute the rotation of each camera with respect to the frame of reference defined by the canonical orientations.

Each image line segment is associated with one canonical direction. In addition, each line segment is rotated around its midpoint and aligned with the direction from the midpoint to the associated vanishing point. This pre-processing is particularly useful for short segments, whose estimated orientation can be noisy.

In addition to vanishing points, we compute the vanishing lines of planes in the canonical orientations. (In a Manhattan world, vanishing lines join the two vanishing points of visible lines.) Suppose that the vanishing line for planes orthogonal to $\vec{n}$ is visible in the image; since the image of a plane orthogonal to $\vec{n}$ cannot straddle the plane's vanishing line, when computing the $\vec{n}$-characteristic lines we can safely neglect to consider pairs of parallel lines whose images are on different sides of the vanishing line. This property, which is used extensively in the computation of structure from single images [23], helps reducing the risk of false positives.

We also implemented a simple procedure to remove characteristic lines from parallel line pairs that are unlikely to belong to the same planar surface. Given a pair of image segments from parallel lines (i.e. converging at one of the vanishing points), we compute the smallest quadrilateral Q, two sides of which are collinear with the line segments, and the remaining sides converge to one of the other vanishing points, such that all four segments endpoints are contained in the quadrilateral. This quadrilateral could be construed as the image of a rectangular planar surface, with edges parallel to the canonical directions. If this were in fact the case (i.e., if there existed a planar rectangular surface patch projecting onto the image quadrilateral), one would not expect to see a line orthogonal to the surface within the image of the surface. Accordingly, if a line aligned towards the third vanishing point crosses Q, the two line segments defining Q are assumed *not* to belong to the same planar patch, and the associated characteristic line is neglected. This simple procedure has given good results in our experiments, although it may lead to false negatives in more complex geometrical layouts.

As detailed in the previous sections, our algorithm searches for coplanar lines one canonical orientation at a time. All pairs of parallel lines that survive the tests discussed above generate characteristic lines, and 3-D clusters are found using our modified mean shift algorithm, seeded with multiple points chosen at the mid-point between nearby orthogonal characteristic line pairs. Each cluster represents a plane; the characteristic lines within each cluster identify coplanar 3-D lines. In some cases, the same line in space may be associated with two different characteristic lines, belonging to different clusters. This may be a legitimate situation for lines at the junction of two planes; otherwise, it represents an inconsistency. In order to reject outlier clusters, we exploit the property that clusters of characteristic lines defined by $\vec{n}$-coplanar lines must be collinear with the baseline vector $\vec{t}$ (Sect. 3.3). For each canonical orientation $\vec{n}_i$, we select the cluster of characteristic lines orthogonal to $\vec{n}_i$ with highest weight, where the weight of a cluster is equal to the sum of the weights of the characteristic lines it contains (with the characteristic line weights defined in Sect. 3.5). The selected cluster determines a tentative baseline direction $\vec{t}_i$. Among the remaining clusters, we only retain those that are at a distance to the line $\lambda\vec{t}_i$ closer than a threshold T. We repeat this for all canonical directions, obtaining up to three tentative baseline directions $\{\vec{t}_i\}$. Note that some canonical orientation may contain no characteristic lines, or the lines may not cluster. (In fact, in our experiments we never considered the vertical canonical orientation due to the general lack of line features on the floor and on the ceiling.) Finally, we linearly regress the direction of $\vec{t}$ from the vectors $\{\vec{t}_i\}$, and project the vectors $\{\vec{t}_i\}$ onto the resulting line to compute (up to a common scale) the distance of each plane to the first camera (and thus the location of the planes in space).

Our algorithm has been implemented on an iPhone 5s and tested in various scenarios. On images with resolution of 352×288, execution time is of 0.28 s on average, with 35 % of the computation due to line detection, 6 % to vanishing line detection, 7 % to line matching, and the remaining 52 % due to characteristic lines computation and clustering.

5 Experimental Evaluation

Quantitative comparative assessment of our algorithm was performed on a set of 10 image pairs. These image pairs were taken by hand, some with an iPhone 4 and some with an iPhone 5s. Examples can be seen in Fig. 5. The full set of images, with line detection and 3-D reconstruction, is provided in the Supplementary Material.

We devised an evaluation criterion based on a test for coplanarity of line triplets, that does not require ground truth measurements of relative camera pose (which are difficult to obtain without precisely calibrated instruments). This criterion requires manual evaluation of coplanarity of all line triplets seen in the image. In practice, we manually enumerated all planes in the scene and assigned each line to the one or two planes containing it. From this data, labeling of all line triplets as coplanar or not is trivial. Given three lines in space, one can test for their coplanarity using Plücker matrices [30]. More precisely, lines $(\mathcal{L}_1, \mathcal{L}_2, \mathcal{L}_3)$ are coplanar if $\mathbf{L}_1\mathbf{L}_2^*\mathbf{L}_3 = \mathbf{0}$, where $\mathbf{L}_1, \mathbf{L}_3$ are the Plücker L-matrices associated with $\mathcal{L}_1, \mathcal{L}_3$ and $\mathbf{L}_2^*$ is the Plücker L^*-matrix associated with $\mathcal{L}_2$ [30]. The ability of an algorithm to determine line coplanarity is critical for precise reconstruction of Manhattan environments; in addition, this criterion gives us an indirect assessment of the quality of pose estimation (as we expect that good pose estimation should result in good 3-D reconstruction and thus correct coplanarity assessment).

We compared our algorithm against two other techniques. The first is traditional structure from motion from point features *(SFM-P)*. We used the popular

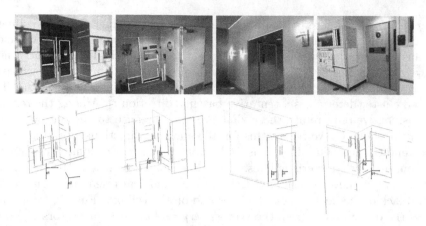

Fig. 5. Top row: Coplanar line sets produced by our algorithm for the image set considered in the evaluation. Only one image for each pair is shown. Different line sets are shown in different color. Note that some lines (especially those at a planar junction) may belong to more than one cluster (although they are displayed using only one color). All lines that have been matched (possibly incorrectly) across images are shown (by thick segments) and used for coplanarity estimation. The quadrilaterals $\mathcal{Q}$ shown by dotted lines represent potential planar patches. They contain all coplanar lines in a cluster, and are computed as described in Sect. 4. Bottom row: 3-D reconstruction of the visible line segments and camera center positions. Line segment are colored according to their orientation in space. The colored rectangles are the reconstructed planar patches corresponding to the quadrilateral $\mathcal{Q}$ shown with the same color as in the top row (Color figure online).

VisualSFM application [31], created and made freely available by Changchang Wu. The second technique is Elqursh and Elgammal's algorithm [7], which uses lines (rather than point features) in a pair of images to estimate the relative camera pose *(SFM-L)*. Once the motion parameters $(\mathbf{R}, \mathbf{t})$ are obtained with either algorithm, 3-D lines are reconstructed from matched image line pairs. To check for coplanarity of a triplet of lines (at least two of which are parallel), we compute the associated Plücker matrices $\mathbf{L}_1$, $\mathbf{L}_2^*$ and $\mathbf{L}_3$, each normalized to unit norm (largest singular value), and threshold the norm of $\mathbf{L}_1\mathbf{L}_2^*\mathbf{L}_3$. By varying this threshold, we obtain a precision/recall curve. This evaluation was conducted with and without the "corrective" pre-processing step, discussed in Sect. 4, that rotates each line segment to align it with the associated vanishing point.

When assessing our characteristic line algorithm, we considered two different approaches for determining line triplet coplanarity: (a) From the estimated relative camera pose $(\mathbf{R}, \mathbf{t})$, as discussed above *(SFM-CL)*; (b) From clusters of characteristic lines *(CL)*. In the second approach, we rely on the fact that each characteristic line cluster represents a set of $\vec{n}$-coplanar lines. If all three lines in a triplet are contained in one such set of $\vec{n}$-coplanar lines, they are classified as coplanar. For the *CL* approach, the precision/recall curve was replaced by the Pareto front [32] of precision/recall values computed by varying the following parameters: (1) the constant σ in the function $g(D)$ defined in Sect. 3.5;

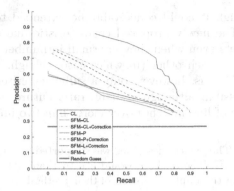

Fig. 6. Precision/recall curves for the algorithms considered (*SFM-P*, *SFM-L*, *SFM-CL*, *CL*) with and without the "correction" pre-processing step that aligns line segments with the associated vanishing point. (Note that the *CL* method is always computed with this correction.)

(2) the threshold T, defined in Sect. 4, used to select the inlier characteristic line clusters.

Note that line detection and matching across images was performed automatically as described in Sect. 4. In some cases, lines were incorrectly matched; in this situation, line triplets containing the incorrectly matched lines were removed from the evaluation set (although both correctly and incorrectly matched lines were fed to the algorithms).

The precision/recall curves for all methods (with and without line re-orientation pre-processing) are shown in Fig. 6. Note that for two of the 49 image pairs considered, the VisualSFM application could not find any reliable point features and thus did not produce any results. Those two images were removed from the set used for the construction of the precision/recall curves. Without the "correction" step, the curves for *SFM-P*, *SFM-L* and *SFM-CL* are fairly similar (with *SFM-P* showing higher precision than the other two for low recall). When the correction pre-processing step is implemented, *SFM-CL* produces better results than *SFM-L* and *SFM-P*. This suggests that our algorithm can reconstruct the relative camera pose as well as or better than the other methods. The curve for *CL*, which does not require explicit 3-D line reconstruction, shows a substantial improvement. This demonstrates the power of the proposed algorithm for planar surface modeling and reconstruction.

6   Conclusions

We have introduced a new algorithm for the explicit detection of coplanar line sets and for the estimation of the camera motion in a Manhattan world. The algorithm is simple, easy to implement, fast, and produces comparatively excellent experimental results in terms of detection of coplanar lines. The main drawback of this approach, of course, is that it doesn't work in non–Manhattan environments, although it could conceivably be extended to support multiple plane orientations. The newly proposed characteristic line criterion allows for the analysis of line sets even when they are small in number and even when the lines are all parallel to each other (in which case, though, the camera motion cannot be recovered). It is, however, only a sufficient criterion, meaning that false positives are possible, although arguably rare. Future work will extend this technique to the case of line matches over more than two images.

Acknowledgement. The project described was supported by Grant Number 1R21EY 021643-01 from NEI/NIH. The authors would like to thank Ali Elqursh and Ahmed Elgammal for providing the implementation of their method.

Appendix: Characteristic Planes Revisited

We present here a different derivation of the characteristic planes concept, obtained through algebraic manipulations. For simplicity's sake, we will restrict our attention to one canonical plane Π_i, assuming that both cameras are located on it. A 2-D reference system is centered at the first camera. In this 2-D world, each camera only sees an image line, and the cameras' relative pose is specified by the (unknown) 2-D vector $\mathbf{t}$ and the (known) 2-D rotation matrix $\mathbf{R}$. We'll assume that both cameras have identity calibration matrices. Consider a plane Π_j with (known) normal $\mathbf{n}_j$, orthogonal to Π_i. A line $\mathcal{L}$ in Π_j intersects Π_i at one point, $\mathbf{X}$. Note that, from the image of this point in the first camera and knowledge of the plane normal $\mathbf{n}_j$, one can recover $\mathbf{X}/d$, where d is the (unknown) distance of Π_j from the first camera. Let $\hat{\mathbf{x}}_2$ be the location of the projection of $\mathbf{X}$ in the second camera's (line) image, expressed in homogeneous coordinates. From Fig. 1 one easily sees that $\lambda\hat{\mathbf{x}}_2 = \mathbf{R}\mathbf{X} + \mathbf{t}$ for some λ, and thus

$$\mathbf{t}/d = \lambda\hat{\mathbf{x}}_2/d - \mathbf{R}\mathbf{X}/d = \lambda_2\hat{\mathbf{x}}_2 - (\mathbf{R}\mathbf{X})_\perp/d \tag{6}$$

for some λ_2, where $(\mathbf{R}\mathbf{X})_\perp = \mathbf{R}\mathbf{X} - (\hat{\mathbf{x}}_2^T\mathbf{R}\mathbf{X})\hat{\mathbf{x}}_2/(\hat{\mathbf{x}}_2^T\hat{\mathbf{x}}_2)$ is the component of $\mathbf{R}\mathbf{X}$ orthogonal to $\hat{\mathbf{x}}_2$. This imposes a linear constraint on $\mathbf{t}/d$. It is not difficult to see that $\hat{\mathbf{x}}_2$ is orthogonal to the lever vector $\vec{u}_2$ in Fig. 1, and that $\|(\mathbf{R}\mathbf{X})_\perp/d\|$ is equal to the modulus of the sin ratio for the line $\mathcal{L}$ seen by the two cameras. Hence, the linear constraint in (6) is simply an expression of the intersection of the characteristic plane $\Pi(\mathcal{L}, \vec{n}_j)$ with Π_i.

References

1. Harris, C.G., Pike, J.: 3D positional integration from image sequences. Image Vis. Comput. **6**, 87–90 (1988)
2. Hartley, R., Zisserman, A.: Multiple View Geometry in Computer Vision. Cambridge University Press, Cambridge (2000)
3. Arth, C., Klopschitz, M., Reitmayr, G., Schmalstieg, D.: Real-time self-localization from panoramic images on mobile devices. In: 10th IEEE International Symposium on Mixed and Augmented Reality (ISMAR), pp. 37–46 (2011)

4. Tanskanen, P., Kolev, K., Meier, L., Camposeco, F., Saurer, O., Pollefeys, M.: Live metric 3d reconstruction on mobile phones. In: IEEE International Conference on Computer Vision (ICCV), pp. 65–72 (2013)
5. Kosecká, J., Zhang, W.: Video compass. In: Heyden, A., Sparr, G., Nielsen, M., Johansen, P. (eds.) ECCV 2002, Part IV. LNCS, vol. 2353, pp. 476–490. Springer, Heidelberg (2002)
6. Hwangbo, M., Kanade, T.: Visual-inertial UAV attitude estimation using urban scene regularities. In: 2011 IEEE International Conference on Robotics and Automation (ICRA), pp. 2451–2458. IEEE (2011)
7. Elqursh, A., Elgammal, A.: Line-based relative pose estimation. In: 2011 IEEE Conference on Computer Vision and Pattern Recognition (CVPR), pp. 3049–3056 (2011)
8. Fitzgibbon, A.W., Zisserman, A.: Automatic camera recovery for closed or open image sequences. In: Burkhardt, H.-J., Neumann, B. (eds.) ECCV 1998. LNCS, vol. 1406, pp. 311–326. Springer, Heidelberg (1998)
9. Bartoli, A., Sturm, P.: Structure-from-motion using lines: representation, triangulation, and bundle adjustment. Comput. Vis. Image Underst. **100**, 416–441 (2005)
10. Navab, N., Faugeras, O.D.: The critical sets of lines for camera displacement estimation: a mixed euclidean-projective and constructive approach. Int. J. Comput. Vision **23**, 17–44 (1997)
11. Košecká, J., Zhang, W.: Extraction, matching, and pose recovery based on dominant rectangular structures. Comput. Vis. Image Underst. **100**, 274–293 (2005)
12. Vincent, E., Laganiére, R.: Detecting planar homographies in an image pair. In: Proceedings of the 2nd International Symposium on Image and Signal Processing and Analysis, ISPA 2001, pp. 182–187. IEEE (2001)
13. Sagüés, C., Murillo, A., Escudero, F., Guerrero, J.J.: From lines to epipoles through planes in two views. Pattern Recogn. **39**, 384–393 (2006)
14. Guerrero, J.J., Sagüés, C.: Robust line matching and estimate of homographies simultaneously. In: Perales, F.J., Campilho, A.C., Pérez, N., Sanfeliu, A. (eds.) IbPRIA 2003. LNCS, vol. 2652, pp. 297–307. Springer, Heidelberg (2003)
15. Montijano, E., Sagues, C.: Position-based navigation using multiple homographies. In: IEEE International Conference on Emerging Technologies and Factory Automation, ETFA 2008, pp. 994–1001. IEEE (2008)
16. Zhou, Z., Jin, H., Ma, Y.: Robust plane-based structure from motion. In: 2012 IEEE Conference on Computer Vision and Pattern Recognition (CVPR), pp. 1482–1489. IEEE (2012)
17. Zhou, Z., Jin, H., Ma, Y.: Plane-based content-preserving warps for video stabilization. In: Computer Vision and Pattern Recognition, CVPR 2013. IEEE (2013)
18. Toldo, R., Fusiello, A.: Robust multiple structures estimation with j-linkage. In: Forsyth, D., Torr, P., Zisserman, A. (eds.) ECCV 2008, Part I. LNCS, vol. 5302, pp. 537–547. Springer, Heidelberg (2008)
19. Sinha, S.N., Steedly, D., Szeliski, R.: Piecewise planar stereo for image-based rendering. In: ICCV, pp. 1881–1888. Citeseer (2009)
20. Hoiem, D., Efros, A.A., Hebert, M.: Recovering surface layout from an image. Int. J. Comput. Vis. **75**, 151–172 (2007)
21. Hedau, V., Hoiem, D., Forsyth, D.: Thinking inside the box: using appearance models and context based on room geometry. In: Daniilidis, K., Maragos, P., Paragios, N. (eds.) ECCV 2010, Part VI. LNCS, vol. 6316, pp. 224–237. Springer, Heidelberg (2010)

22. Delage, E., Lee, H., Ng, A.Y.: A dynamic bayesian network model for autonomous 3d reconstruction from a single indoor image. In: 2006 IEEE Computer Society Conference on Computer Vision and Pattern Recognition, vol. 2, pp. 2418–2428. IEEE (2006)

23. Lee, D.C., Hebert, M., Kanade, T.: Geometric reasoning for single image structure recovery. In: IEEE Conference on Computer Vision and Pattern Recognition, CVPR 2009, pp. 2136–2143. IEEE (2009)

24. Flint, A., Murray, D., Reid, I.: Manhattan scene understanding using monocular, stereo, and 3d features. In: 2011 IEEE International Conference on Computer Vision (ICCV), pp. 2228–2235. IEEE (2011)

25. Ramalingam, S., Pillai, J.K., Jain, A., Taguchi, Y.: Manhattan junction catalogue for spatial reasoning of indoor scenes. In: Computer Vision and Pattern Recognition, CVPR 2013. IEEE (2013)

26. Tsai, G., Kuipers, B.: Dynamic visual understanding of the local environment for an indoor navigating robot. In: 2012 IEEE/RSJ International Conference on Intelligent Robots and Systems (IROS), pp. 4695–4701. IEEE (2012)

27. Comaniciu, D., Meer, P.: Mean shift: a robust approach toward feature space analysis. IEEE Trans. Pattern Anal. Mach. Intell. **24**, 603–619 (2002)

28. Grompone von Gioi, R., Jakubowicz, J., Morel, J.M., Randall, G.: LSD: a line segment detector. Image Processing on Line 2012 (2012)

29. Wang, Z., Wu, F., Hu, Z.: Msld: a robust descriptor for line matching. Pattern Recogn. **42**, 941–953 (2009)

30. Ronda, J.I., Valdés, A., Gallego, G.: Line geometry and camera autocalibration. J. Math. Imaging Vis. **32**, 193–214 (2008)

31. Wu, C.: VisualSFM. http://ccwu.me/vsfm/ (last checked: 15 June 2014)

32. Boyd, S., Vandenberghe, L.: Convex Optimization. Cambridge University Press, Cambridge (2004)

LBP with Six Intersection Points: Reducing Redundant Information in LBP-TOP for Micro-expression Recognition

Yandan Wang[1]([⊠]), John See[2], Raphael C.-W. Phan[1], and Yee-Hui Oh[1]

[1] Faculty of Engineering,
Multimedia University (MMU), Cyberjaya, Malaysia
{yandvn,yeehui716}@gmail.com, raphael@mmu.edu.my
[2] Faculty of Computing and Informatics,
Multimedia University (MMU), Cyberjaya, Malaysia
johnsee@mmu.edu.my

Abstract. Facial micro-expression recognition is an upcoming area in computer vision research. Up until the recent emergence of the extensive CASMEII spontaneous micro-expression database, there were numerous obstacles faced in the elicitation and labeling of data involving facial micro-expressions. In this paper, we propose the Local Binary Patterns with Six Intersection Points (LBP-SIP) volumetric descriptor based on the three intersecting lines crossing over the center point. The proposed LBP-SIP reduces the redundancy in LBP-TOP patterns, providing a more compact and lightweight representation; leading to more efficient computational complexity. Furthermore, we also incorporated a Gaussian multi-resolution pyramid to our proposed approach by concatenating the patterns across all pyramid levels. Using an SVM classifier with leave-one-sample-out cross validation, we achieve the best recognition accuracy of 67.21 %, surpassing the baseline performance with further computational efficiency.

1 Introduction

Facial (macro-)expression recognition is a popular research area that has seen tremendous advancement in the past few decades. Indeed, macro-expression recognition research has reported accuracies of over 90 % for the six basic facial expressions (i.e. anger, disgust, surprise, fear, sadness and happiness).

In contrast, facial *micro-expression* recognition has recently seen more emphasis in the computer vision community, and addresses a more challenging research problem than its macro-expression counterpart.

A micro-expression is defined as a brief facial movement that reveals an emotion that a person tries to conceal [2]. Micro-expressions are distinctly different from macro-expressions in the aspect of its short duration and occurrence as a response towards a presented emotional stimuli. Its imperceptibility to the naked eyes is the primary motivation towards achieving machine detection and recognition of micro-expressions. There is also a notable lack of well-established

© Springer International Publishing Switzerland 2015
D. Cremers et al. (Eds.): ACCV 2014, Part I, LNCS 9003, pp. 525–537, 2015.
DOI: 10.1007/978-3-319-16865-4_34

databases due to difficulties in proper elicitation and labeling of micro-expression data. In current literature (and to our best knowledge), there are only two spontaneous micro-expression databases, i.e. SMIC [4] and CASME [10]/CASMEII [12] (both of these CASME variants can be seen as one as the former is a subset of the latter), while there are very few other works to date on automatic recognition of spontaneous micro-expressions.

Local Binary Patterns (LBP) is widely used in facial expression recognition [8] due to its ability to derive local statistical patterns that exhibit invariance towards illumination changes and simplicity in computation. In order to cope with dynamic textures and events across spatio-temporal dimensions, the classic LBP descriptor was extended to a volume-based LBP (VLBP) and LBP from three orthogonal planes (LBP-TOP) [14].

Among all the available work, Yan et al. [12] reported a baseline performance of up to 63.41 % accuracy for a 5-class classification task on their own CASMEII database, adopting LBP-TOP and SVM for feature extraction and classification respectively. The CASMEII has since superseded the original CASME database with the inclusion of more subjects and a higher sampling rate that is able to capture detailed facial muscle movements. While the LBP-TOP is an effective descriptor for dynamic textures, there are redundant pattern information within the overlapping orthogonal planes. This redundancy contributes to an increase in computational complexity, and also intuitively results in a less discriminative set of features.

In this paper, we propose Local Binary Pattern with Six Intersection Points (LBP-SIP), a computationally lightweight descriptor based on the LBP-TOP. In LBP-SIP, the unique distinct points that lie on the three intersecting lines of the three orthogonal planes are considered for computing the spatio-temporal patterns. The proposed descriptor is then incorporated in a multi-resolution Gaussian pyramid by concatenating the feature histograms of all four pyramid levels. Our proposed method is able to consistently match or outperform LBP-TOP in various aspects in addition to the computational efficiency it brings. Using SVM classifier with leave-one-sample-out cross validation, we obtain the best recognition accuracy of 67.21 %.

The rest of the paper is organized as follows: Sect. 2 reviews some recent methods in this area of research. Our proposed approach is presented in Sect. 4. Then we show our detailed experimental results in Sect. 5. Finally, the conclusion is given in Sect. 6.

2   Related Work

In dealing with dynamic textures that evolve over space-time dimensions, the LBP-TOP remains a popular choice of feature extraction for various applications such as texture recognition [13], face spoofing [1], gait and action recognition [3,5], and facial expression recognition [14,15].

Following its conception, several works were proposed to improve upon its effectiveness and robustness. Shan and Gritti [7] proposed to learn discriminative

LBP-Histogram bins which are able to provide a more compact yet discriminative representation for facial expressions. In the similar vein, Zhao et al. [15] extended the usage of LBP-TOP to multi-resolution space while utilizing AdaBoost to learn and select the most prominent expression-related features from different blocks and slices. To increase its robustness against view-based variations in texture, rotation-invariant descriptors [16] computed from the LBP-TOP features were proposed, to a good measure of success. Interestingly, the use of a multi-resolution pyramid of LBPs [6] was also found to be beneficial in extracting dominant structures in textures.

A majority of these methods are tailored towards texture recognition and *macro-expression* recognition, while very scant attention is given to address the challenging task of recognizing subtle facial *micro-expressions*. The use of LBP-TOP for feature description and SVM as classifier provides the baseline performance for the recently-proposed SMIC [4] and CASMEII [12] datasets, the latter obtaining a good accuracy rate of up to 63.41 %. As pointed out in [11], research in micro-expression recognition is still at an early stage with very few reported works to date. In a recent method, Wang et al. [9] proposed an efficient technique that uses discriminant tensor subspace for feature extraction and extreme learning machine (ELM) for classification. Experiments on the CASME micro-expression dataset showed some promising results (46.9 %, up from baseline of 41 % reported in [10]), especially when high-order tensors are applied.

In this paper, we improve the baseline performance in CASMEII by introducing an efficient and robust descriptor that trims the excess redundancy in feature patterns, resulting in a more compact and well-formed representation

3 LBP-Three Orthogonal Planes (LBP-TOP)

In this section, we describe the key idea of the LBP-TOP descriptor. Given a pixel c located at (x_c, y_c), its LBP code is computed as:

$$LBP_{P,R}(x_c, y_c) = \sum_{p=0}^{P-1} s(i_p - i_c) \times 2^P \qquad (1)$$

where

$$s(x) = \begin{cases} 1 \text{ if } x \geq 0, \\ 0 \text{ if } x < 0, \end{cases} \qquad (2)$$

i_c denotes the intensity of the central pixel c, P denotes the total number of neighbours of c parametrized by the radius of the neighbourhood R, while i_p indexed by p denotes the intensity of the neighbouring pixels. Then, the histogram of all r LBP patterns, $H_{LBP}(r)$ is computed for all pixels in an image, describing the LBP texture features of that image.

LBP-TOP computes the local spatio-temporal patterns based on LBP. More precisely, the LBP-TOP feature is constructed by the concatenation of LBP histograms on three orthogonal planes - XY, XT and YT respectively as shown in Fig. 1(a). The XT and YT planes contain the temporal transition information pertaining to the facial movement displacement e.g. how eyes, lips, muscle or eyebrows change over time. They are the stack of columns and rows of pixels respectively. In contrast, the XY plane (a frame itself) contains only spatial information which includes both expression and identity information of a face appearance.

However, by deeper inspection of the LBP-TOP formulation, we observe that not all the neighbour points on three othogonal planes respectively used to compute the LBP code (feature pattern) are distinctively different. In fact, when all three planes are considered in totality, some points are used more than once in the LBP-TOP computation of the center pixel, thus leading to redundant differencing and thresholding computations when the LBP codes are computed. Therefore, to compute more compactly while preserving the essential pattern information, we propose to uniquely compute the spatial and temporal two groups of neighbour points only in order to obtain the spatio-temporal LBP patterns. More precisely, we only consider the six distinct neighbour points on the three intersecting lines formed by the three orthogonal planes as shown in Fig. 1(b). The details of the proposed approach are elaborated in the next section.

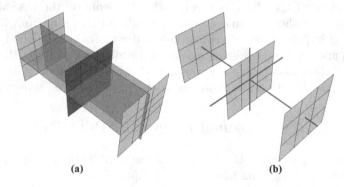

(a)   (b)

Fig. 1. (a) Three orthogonal planes in the LBP-TOP computation, and (b) Three intersecting lines crossing over the center pixel, formed by the three orthogonal planes, are considered to obtain the six distinct neighbour points surrounding the center point.

4 Proposed LBP-Six Intersection Points (LBP-SIP)

To further extend the LBP-TOP, we propose a more compact and efficient form while preserving much of robustness and the essential information that describes the dynamic textures. By closer examination of the neighbour points on all three orthogonal planes, the key property lies in the uniqueness of these neighbours.

Given a center pixel c in spatial location $(x_{c,t}, y_{c,t})$ at time t, its LBP-TOP feature can be denoted as $LBP - TOP_{P_{XY}, P_{XT}, P_{YT}, R_X, R_Y, R_T}(x_{c,t}, y_{c,t})$ with six parameters; the P parameters denote the number of neighbours in each of the planes, while the R parameters denote the radii in each of the axes. Three LBP histograms, one for each of the planes (XY, XY, YT) are concatenated to form the final LBP-TOP feature histogram, i.e. $H_{LBP-TOP} = H_{LBP,\pi}(\pi = XY, XT, YT)$.

In detail, the LBP-TOP neighbours of the pixel $(x_{c,t}, y_{c,t})$ are given as (without loss of generality, we consider only 4-neighbours for the proposal of this method):

- XY plane:
  $(x_{c,t}, y_{c,t} + R_Y), (x_{c,t} + R_X, y_{c,t}), (x_{c,t}, y_{c,t} - R_Y), (x_{c,t} - R_X, y_{c,t})$
- XT plane:
  $(x_{c,t} + R_X, y_{c,t}), (x_{c,(t+R_T)}, y_{c,(t+R_T)}), (x_{c,t} - R_X, y_{c,t}), (x_{c,(t-R_T)}, y_{c,(t-R_T)})$
- YT plane:
  $(x_{c,t}, y_{c,t} + R_Y), (x_{c,(t+R_T)}, y_{c,(t+R_T)}), (x_{c,t}, y_{c,t} - R_Y), (x_{c,(t-R_T)}, y_{c,(t-R_T)})$

Note that each neighbour pixel is used more than once in the computation of LBP-TOP, and that there are uniquely only 6 distinct neighbour points within the set of intersecting planes.

Building on this, we propose an LBP descriptor with reduced set of spatio-temporal neighbourhood points derived from the intersection of the three orthogonal planes. To better describe the method, consider the example in Fig. 2. In the original LBP-TOP computation, we compute for the central pixel C lying on the XY plane (in the middle frame) with 4 neighbour points considered on each plane that are the 4-neighbour points set $\{D, E, F, G\}$ for XY plane (middle frame), $\{E, A, G, B\}$ for XT plane (red plane), and $\{D, A, F, B\}$ for YT plane (blue plane). Observing that from these three point sets, every point is used twice to compute the resulting pattern.

Therefore, we propose to reduce the computational complexity by discarding the redundant *intersection points*. From Fig. 2, we can clearly see that the three orthogonal planes produce three intersecting lines (AB, DF, EG), all crossing over the center point C. Regardless of the radius between the center point and the original neighbour points, there are only six unique neighbour points on the intersection lines surrounding the center point—the six intersection points. Concisely from this example,

$$XY \cap XT \cap YT = \{A, B, D, E, F, G\} \tag{3}$$

Intuitively, these 6 unique neighbour points carry enough information to describe the spatio-temporal textures that center upon point C. Geometrically, we can view the new neighbour point set in two groups representing both spatial and temporal texture information. Firstly, we regard points $\{D, E, G, F\}$ as the spatial neighbour set while the two end points $\{A, B\}$ along the temporal axis (that is on the intersection line of the XT and YT planes) make up the temporal neighbour set. As such, the final feature histogram consists of two concatenated histograms of length $2^4 + 2^2 = 20$.

In contrast, the three orthogonal planes of the LBP-TOP produce a concatenated feature histogram of length $2^4 \times 3 = 48$, more than two times that of the proposed LBP-SIP. In terms of computational complexity, this results in a much compact feature length (or dimension). This is much desirable as high-dimensional feature spaces often suffer from the curse of dimensionality whereby the represented data becomes increasingly sparse, affecting classification ability.

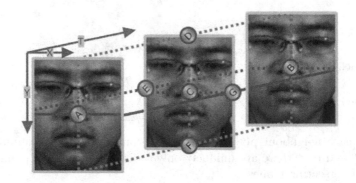

Fig. 2. The three orthogonal planes (XY, XT, YT) shown in different colors, and the intersecting points that are the neighbour points of point C shared by all three planes (A, B, D, E, F, G) (Color figure online).

Consistent with the previously described methods, we formally denote the proposed descriptor as: $LBP - SIP_{P_{XY},R_X,R_Y,R_T}(x_{c,t}, y_{c,t})$ where P_{XY} is fixed to 4, leaving only the radii parameters free. Good values for R_X, R_Y and R_T have been reported in [12] by empirical means.

5   Experiments

In this section, we present our experimental results. Firstly, We describe the dataset we used for our experiments in Sect. 5.1. In Sect. 5.3, we compare the performance of the proposed LBP-SIP with LBP-TOP through a multi-resolution Gaussian pyramid to examine the robustness of the methods across scale. In Sect. 5.4, we further demonstrate the robustness of the intuitive spatial and temporal neighbour point grouping exemplified in our proposed method. Finally, the complexity of both LBP-TOP and LBP-SIP methods are analyzed in Sect. 5.5.

5.1   Dataset

Experiments were conducted on two recently-proposed datasets—SMIC [4] and CASMEII [12]. We intensively test our proposed method on the CASMEII dataset, since it is the more comprehensive dataset between the two. In addition, we also substantiate our proposed idea by testing on the SMIC dataset for the basic case without using Gaussian pyramids (see Sect. 5.2).

SMIC [4] consists of both micro and macro expression videos. In this paper, we focus on the micro-expression only. A high speed (HS) camera (PixeLINK

PL-B774U, 640 × 480) of 100 fps was used to record the short duration of micro-expressions. 20 participants (164 videos) participated in the recording experiment. Only 3 micro-expression classes (positive, surprise and negative) are provided.

CASMEII [12] is the most extensive spontaneous micro-expression dataset to date, and it is publicly made available by the Chinese Academy of Science (CAS). Due to the lack of samples in some expression classes, the CAS team suggested a baseline experimental setup of 5 expression classes (Happiness, Disgust, Surprise, Repression, Tense) with a total of 247 different spontaneous micro-expression videos used for experiment. The micro-expression samples were recorded with high-speed camera (at 200 *fps*) from 26 participants with higher face resolution of around 280 × 340 pixels (original resolution). These samples were selected from nearly 3,000 elicited facial movements with their onset and offset frames coded. The Action Units (AU) and emotions are also properly marked and labelled according to the FACS coding system. The selection procedure was implemented as some samples are too subtle to be coded or labelled by the naked eye. This enforces the nature of micro-expressions and the obvious difficulties in creating a micro-expression database.

In our experiments, we strive to achieve consistency with the baseline work [12]. The smaller version of the cropped faces are used without frame size (X-Y dimension) normalization and video length (T dimension) normalization. This is possible as the descriptors tested (LBP-TOP, LBP-SIP) can accommodate different spatial and temporal scales. We also employ the same number of classes used. The details of the experimental results are shown in the following subsections.

5.2   Baseline Comparison: LBP-SIP vs LBP-TOP

We test our proposed LBP-SIP against LBP-TOP on both CASMEII and SMIC databases. We use 5 × 5 block partition and set the radii to $\{R_X, R_Y, R_T\} = \{1, 1, 4\}$, corresponding to the best results in [12]. Table 1 shows the results. From the results shown in Table 1, the LBP-SIP is clearly superior on all accounts.

On an Intel Core i7 machine with 8GB RAM, the average feature extraction time per video on CASMEII dataset for LBP-TOP is 18.289 s, while ours took 15.888 s. The recognition time for LBP-TOP is 0.584 s per video while ours took 0.208 s per video (an improvement of ≈2.8 times).

Table 1. Comparison of LBP-TOP and LBP-SIP on the CASMEII and SMIC datasets using SVM and RBF kernels for SVM

	CASMEII		SMIC	
	LBP-TOP (%)	LBP-SIP (%)	LBP-TOP (%)	LBP-SIP (%)
Linear	62.75	63.56	60.98	64.02
RBF	65.99	66.40	60.98	62.80

5.3   LBP-SIP vs LBP-TOP on a Gaussian Pyramid

From previous works, Zhao et al. [14] conducted intensive experiments on LBP-TOP for facial expression recognition, recommending that the neighbourhood radii takes the values $\{R_X, R_Y, R_T\} = \{1, 1, 2\}$. Meanwhile, Yan et al. [12] empirically showed that the best values applied to facial micro-expression recognition are $\{R_X, R_Y, R_T\} = \{1, 1, 4\}$ though the result is not significantly better than with $\{1, 1, 2\}$. Hence, for ease of comparison with the best known works, we consider both settings in this experiment.

We use a Gaussian pyramid to downsample every single image frame into 4 levels, where level 0 denotes the original size of image. Let the original frame resolution be $w \times h$ (width and height), and pyramid level be l which ranges from 0 to 3 for our case (as shown in Fig. 3). Applying Gaussian low pass filtering, which is a smoothing process at each level l results in a frame resolution of $(w \times h)/2^l$. In other words, the image size at each level will be half that of the previous level.

To better visualize the effect on different levels of the multi-resolution Gaussian pyramid, we normalize the processed images to the size of 163×134, as shown in the second row of Fig. 3. The third row shows the LBP coding at different resolution levels of the pyramid.

We use 5×5 blocks partition to compute the LBP-TOP and LBP-SIP feature histograms. Due to different pre-processing applied (e.g. image sequence normalization), our accuracy rate for LBP-TOP appears to be slightly different from the reported baseline [12]. As such, we maintain the same pre-processing for all our experiments on both LBP-TOP (as our baseline) and LBP-SIP to ensure comparisons can be made under fair conditions. We then follow through the rest of the recognition process using the SVM classifier with leave-one-sample-out cross validation.

Tables 2 and 3 show the performance of LBP-TOP and LBP-SIP using features derived from the different levels of the Gaussian pyramid as well as the concatenated features of all levels, with the temporal radius R_T of 2 and 4 respectively. In Table 2, in the linear case, we can see that LBP-TOP outperforms LBP-SIP at some levels, while at some other levels LBP-SIP slightly outperforms LBP-TOP. There is little difference between the two. On the other hand, LBP-SIP always outperforms LBP-TOP when the nonlinear RBF kernel is applied.

The performance results shown in Table 3 where $R_T = 4$ can be better visualized in Figs. 4(a) and (b), showing the linear and RBF kernel respectively. In Fig. 4(a), it is obvious that the performance of LBP-SIP (marked with triangular points) on the Linear kernel is almost consistently above or superposing the LBP-TOP line (marked with circular points) through all individual pyramid levels and the concatenated levels.

Overall, it may seemed that there is no significant difference between LBP-TOP and LBP-SIP in terms of accuracy (except when the RBF kernel is used), but the increase in computational efficiency and robustness in high dimensionality (concatenated feature) are promising advantages for practical purposes.

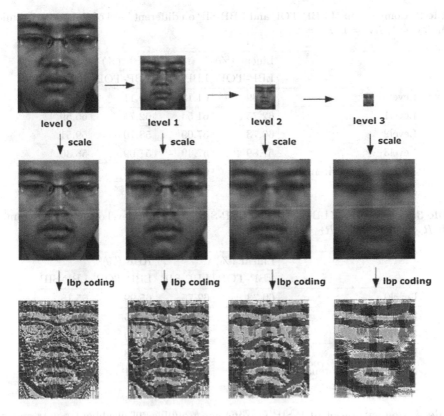

level 0   level 1   level 2   level 3

Fig. 3. LBP coding at different levels of a Gaussian pyramid

5.4   Spatial and Temporal Grouping of Neighbour Points

We further demonstrate the intuitiveness of considering a group of 4 intersecting points as the spatial LBP pattern on XY plane and the 2 remaining intersecting points as the temporal LBP pattern (XY+2), as compared to the two other possible grouping permutations that can arise from the 6 unique neighbour points. Two other combination of groupings are tested out: spatial grouping on XT plane and two points along the Y dimension (XT+2), and spatial grouping on YT plane and two points along the X dimension (YT+2). An illustration of how the six unique neighbour points can be grouped is shown in Fig. 5. For simplicity, we compare the recognition performance of the different neighbour groupings with $R_T = 4$ (since it was shown earlier to be better temporal radius).

Table 4 clearly shows that irrespective of the choice of kernels used, the XY+2 grouping outperforms the XT+2 and YT+2 groupings in most of the evaluated cases. We observe that the spatial and temporal grouping of neighbour points on the XY+2 setting is more robust across different levels of the Gaussian pyramid. The XY+2 grouping is also the most intuitive considering that the spatial

Table 2. Comparison of LBP-TOP and LBP-SIP on different level of Gaussion pyramid with $R_X = 1$, $R_Y = 1$, $R_T = 2$

	Linear (%)		RBF (%)	
	LBP-TOP	LBP-SIP	LBP-TOP	LBP-SIP
Level0	57.89	61.13	59.11	63.16
Level1	62.75	61.54	62.75	65.59
Level2	60.73	57.09	58.70	59.51
Level3	57.89	57.49	57.09	58.30
All levels (concatenated)	65.59	63.97	64.78	64.78

Table 3. Comparison of LBP-TOP and LBP-SIP on different level of Gaussion pyramid with $R_X = 1$, $R_Y = 1$, $R_T = 4$

	Linear (%)		RBF (%)	
	LBP-TOP	LBP-SIP	LBP-TOP	LBP-SIP
Level0	60.73	62.75	65.99	65.18
Level1	61.94	62.75	62.75	65.59
Level2	65.99	65.18	66.40	67.21
Level3	63.16	63.16	64.78	62.75
All levels (concatenated)	66.80	67.21	67.61	67.21

Table 4. Comparison of LBP-SIP for different groupings of neighbour points on different level of Gaussion pyramid with $R_X = 1$, $R_Y = 1$, $R_T = 4$

	Linear (%)			RBF (%)		
	XY+2	XT+2	YT+2	XY+2	XT+2	YT+2
Level0	62.75	61.94	60.73	65.18	61.13	63.56
Level1	62.75	60.73	61.13	65.59	63.97	64.37
Level2	65.78	57.49	67.20	67.21	62.75	66.40
Level3	63.16	62.35	57.89	62.75	61.94	61.13
All levels (concatenated)	67.21	65.59	66.40	67.21	66.40	65.18

pattern that resides on the XY plane is akin to a classic LBP pattern while the temporal pattern straddles across the T axis.

5.5   Complexity of LBP-TOP vs LBP-SIP

LBP-TOP. For each video sample, the use of 4 neighbour points on each of the 3 othogonal planes result in $4 \times 3 \times w \times h \times l$ number of computations where $w \times h$ is the spatial resolution of the image (frame) and l is the length of the video

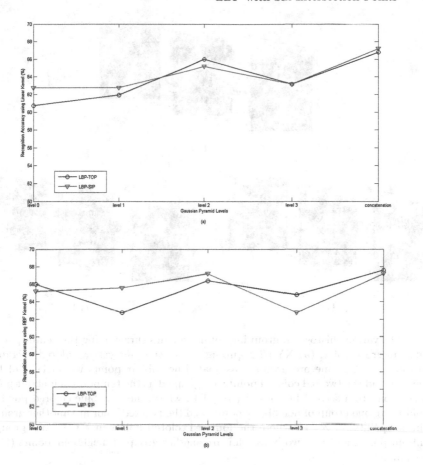

Fig. 4. The comparison between LBP-TOP and LBP-SIP using SVM linear in (a) and RBF kernel in (b) with $R_T = 4$

(i.e. number of frames). The length of the entire concatenated feature histogram is $2^4 \times 3 \times (5 \times 5) = 1200$ dimensions, where $2^4 \times 3$ is the dimensionality of feature in a single block partition with three othogonal planes while 5×5 gives the number of block partitions applied (to the XY plane).

LBP-SIP. In the proposed LBP-SIP approach, there are only 6 unique points derived from the three intersecting lines formed by the three orthogonal planes. We separate these neighbour points into two groups; namely a spatial LBP group that consists of 4 points along the spatial XY plane, and a temporal LBP group containing the remaining 2 points along the T axis. This results in $(4 + 2) \times w \times h \times l$ computations, which is half the number of computations required for the LBP-TOP. Furthermore, the dimensionality is reduced by 2.4 times from the LBP-TOP approach to a compact size of $(2^4 + 2^2) \times (5 \times 5) = 500$ dimensions, which is sufficient to represent the essential spatio-temporal patterns while maintaining a competitive performance.

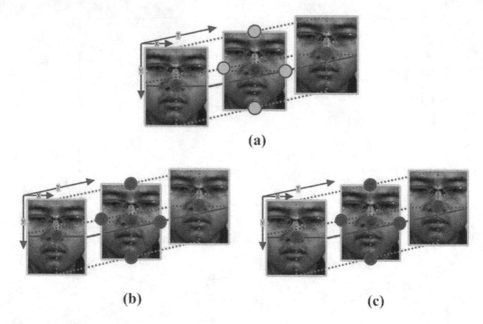

Fig. 5. The various histogram groupings of neighbours surrounding the center point c, denoted in green color: (a) XY+2 grouping, where the four yellow colored neighbour points in the XY plane are grouped as spatial neighbour points to correspond to a histogram, and the two red colored points are grouped as the temporal neighbour points to correspond to a second histogram (b) YT+2 where the four blue colored points in YT plane are one group of neighbour points and the two red color are another group of neighbour points (c) XT+2 where the four red colored points in XT are one group of neighbour points and the two blue color are another group of neighbour points (Color figure online)

6   Conclusion

In this paper, we propose LBP-SIP as a more compact and efficient formulation over LBP-TOP. Instead of considering all three othogonal planes which contain redundant points, we propose a reduced set of unique spatio-temporal neighbour points derived from the intersecting lines of the three orthogonal planes. LBP-SIP is then computed through a multi-resolution Gaussian pyramid by concatenating feature patterns from every level to improve on the task of facial micro-expression recognition. In various experiments conducted on the recently proposed CASMEII database, the LBP-SIP has consistently matched or outperformed the LBP-TOP in accuracy terms while exhibiting stability and robustness in high feature dimensionality. Most noteworthy here is its computational efficiency and a clear reduction in the length of feature histogram without deterioration in performance.

Acknowledgement. We thank the Chinese Academy of Sciences for access to the CASMEII micro-expression database and Su-Jing Wang for providing more details on their CASMEII work [12]. We also thank the anonymous reviewers for their constructive comments. This research work is funded by the TM Grant under project UbeAware.

References

1. de Freitas Pereira, T., Anjos, A., De Martino, J.M., Marcel, S.: *LBP − TOP* based countermeasure against face spoofing attacks. In: Park, J.-I., Kim, J. (eds.) ACCV Workshops 2012, Part I. LNCS, vol. 7728, pp. 121–132. Springer, Heidelberg (2013)
2. Ekman, P.: Lie catching and microexpressions. In: Martin, C.W. (ed.) The Philosophy of Deception, pp. 118–133. Oxford University Press, Oxford (2009)
3. Kellokumpu, V., Zhao, G., Li, S.Z., Pietikäinen, M.: Dynamic texture based gait recognition. In: Tistarelli, M., Nixon, M.S. (eds.) ICB 2009. LNCS, vol. 5558, pp. 1000–1009. Springer, Heidelberg (2009)
4. Li, X., Pfister, T., Huang, X., Zhao, G., Pietikainen, M.: A spontaneous microexpression database: inducement, collection and baseline. In: 10th IEEE International Conference and Workshops on Automatic Face and Gesture Recognition (FG), pp. 1–6 (2013)
5. Mattivi, R., Shao, L.: Human action recognition using LBP-TOP as sparse spatio-temporal feature descriptor. In: Jiang, X., Petkov, N. (eds.) CAIP 2009. LNCS, vol. 5702, pp. 740–747. Springer, Heidelberg (2009)
6. Qian, X., Hua, X.S., Chen, P., Ke, L.: PLBP: an effective local binary patterns texture descriptor with pyramid representation. Pattern Recogn. **44**(10), 2502–2515 (2011)
7. Shan, C., Gritti, T.: Learning discriminative LBP-histogram bins for facial expression recognition. In: BMVC, pp. 1–10 (2008)
8. Shan, C., Gong, S., McOwan, P.W.: Facial expression recognition based on local binary patterns: a comprehensive study. Image Vis. Comput. **27**(6), 803–816 (2009)
9. Wang, S.J., Chen, H.L., Yan, W.J., Chen, Y.H., Fu, X.: Face recognition and micro-expression recognition based on discriminant tensor subspace analysis plus extreme learning machine. Neural Process. Lett. **39**(1), 25–43 (2014)
10. Yan, W.J., Wu, Q., Liu, Y.J., Wang, S.J., Fu, X.: CASME database: a dataset of spontaneous micro-expressions collected from neutralized faces. In: 10th IEEE International Conference and Workshops on Automatic Face and Gesture Recognition (FG), pp. 1–7 (2013)
11. Yan, W.J., Wang, S.J., Liu, Y.J., Wu, Q., Fu, X.: For micro-expression recognition: database and suggestions. Neurocomputing **136**, 82–87 (2014)
12. Yan, W.J., Li, X., Wang, S.J., Zhao, G., Liu, Y.J., Chen, Y.H., Fu, X.: CASME II: an improved spontaneous micro-expression database and the baseline evaluation. PloS One **9**(1), e86041 (2014)
13. Zhao, G., Pietikainen, M.: Local binary pattern descriptors for dynamic texture recognition. In: 18th International Conference on Pattern Recognition (ICPR), vol. 2, pp. 211–214. IEEE (2006)
14. Zhao, G., Pietikainen, M.: Dynamic texture recognition using local binary patterns with an application to facial expressions. IEEE Trans. Pattern Anal. Mach. Intell. **29**(6), 915–928 (2007)
15. Zhao, G., Pietikainen, M.: Boosted multi-resolution spatiotemporal descriptors for facial expression recognition. Pattern Recogn. Lett. **30**(12), 1117–1127 (2009)
16. Zhao, G., Ahonen, T., Matas, J., Pietikainen, M.: Rotation-invariant image and video description with local binary pattern features. IEEE Trans. Image Process. **21**(4), 1465–1477 (2012)

Deep Convolutional Neural Networks for Efficient Pose Estimation in Gesture Videos

Tomas Pfister[1]([✉]), Karen Simonyan[1],
James Charles[2], and Andrew Zisserman[1]

[1] Visual Geometry Group, Department of Engineering Science,
University of Oxford, Oxford, UK
tp@robots.ox.ac.uk
[2] Computer Vision Group, School of Computing,
University of Leeds, Leeds, UK

Abstract. Our objective is to efficiently and accurately estimate the upper body pose of humans in gesture videos. To this end, we build on the recent successful applications of deep convolutional neural networks (ConvNets). Our novelties are: (i) our method is the first to our knowledge to use ConvNets for estimating human pose in videos; (ii) a new network that exploits temporal information from multiple frames, leading to better performance; (iii) showing that pre-segmenting the foreground of the video improves performance; and (iv) demonstrating that even without foreground segmentations, the network learns to abstract away from the background and can estimate the pose even in the presence of a complex, varying background.

We evaluate our method on the BBC TV Signing dataset and show that our pose predictions are significantly better, and an order of magnitude faster to compute, than the state of the art [3].

1 Introduction

The goal of this work is to track the 2D human upper body pose over long gesture videos. As a case study, we experiment on a dataset of sign language gestures, which contains high variation in pose and body shape in videos over an hour in length. The foreground appearance in these videos is very varied (as shown in Fig. 3), with highly varying clothing, self-occlusion, self-shadowing, motion blur due to the speed of the gesturing, and in particular a changing background (due to the person being superimposed over a moving video, as shown in Fig. 2).

We build upon recent work in video upper body pose estimation. Buehler *et al.* [2] proposed a generative model capable of tracking a person's upper body continuously for hours, but required manual annotation of 64 frames per video, and was computationally expensive. Charles *et al.* later used this generative model to train a faster and more reliable pose estimator [3,4,15] using a random

---

Electronic supplementary material The online version of this chapter (doi:10.1007/978-3-319-16865-4_35) contains supplementary material, which is available to authorized users. Videos can also be accessed at http://www.springerimages.com/videos/978-3-319-16864-7.

© Springer International Publishing Switzerland 2015
D. Cremers et al. (Eds.): ACCV 2014, Part I, LNCS 9003, pp. 538–552, 2015.
DOI: 10.1007/978-3-319-16865-4_35

forest. However, their method relied on a hand-tuned foreground segmentation algorithm for preprocessing the videos, without which their method performed poorly. The segmentation method had to be manually tuned for each different type of video, and failed on certain videos with unusual body shapes, unusual absolute positions of persons in the video, or similar foreground and background colours. Further, the extensive preprocessing was computationally expensive, reducing the speed of the method to near-realtime. In our method (pictured in Fig. 1) we solve these issues by exploiting recent advances in deep convolutional neural networks (ConvNets) to accurately predict the pose without the need for foreground segmentation, and in real-time (100fps on a single GPU). Further, we show that our method implicitly learns constraints about the human kinematic chain, resulting in significantly better constrained pose estimates (*i.e.*, significantly smoother pose tracks with fewer serious prediction errors) than in previous work.

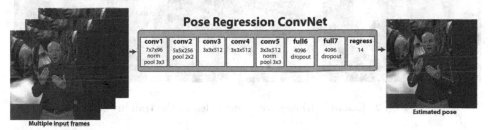

Fig. 1. Method overview. Given a set of input frames, the convolutional neural network regresses the positions of the head, shoulder, elbows and wrists.

Many recent works have demonstrated the power of ConvNets in a wide variety of vision tasks – object classification and detection [7,13,17,23], face recognition [20], text recognition [1,8,9], video action recognition [12,18] and many more [6,14,16]. These networks comprise several layers of non-linear feature extractors and are therefore said to be 'deep' (in contrast to classic methods that are 'shallow'). Very recent works have also explored the use of ConvNets for estimating the human pose. Toshev and Szegedy [22] proposed to use a cascade of ConvNets to improve precision over a single network in unconstrained 2D pose estimation. Very recently, Tompson *et al.* [10,21] proposed a hybrid architecture combining a ConvNet with a Markov Random Field-based spatial model. In this work we demonstrate that in gesture videos, a more computationally efficient conventional ConvNet alone outperforms previous work.

We evaluate our method on the BBC TV Signing dataset [3]. Our method achieves significantly better constrained pose estimates than the state of the art [3], without the need for hand-tuned foreground segmentation algorithms, and with over an order of magnitude faster computation speed.

2   Pose Estimation with ConvNets

In this paper we treat the task of estimating the pose as a regression problem. As the regressor we use a convolutional neural network, which consists of several stacked layers of convolutions and non-linearities. The input to the network is a set of RGB video frames, and the outputs of the last layer are the (x, y) coordinates of the upper-body joints.

We base our network architecture on that of Sermanet *et al.* [17] which has achieved excellent results on ImageNet Challenge 2013 object classification and localisation tasks. The network is shown in Fig. 1. Our network differs from Sermanet *et al.* in that we use multiple input frames and video-specific information to significantly improve generalisation performance, and we modify training time augmentation to better suit the task of pose estimation. We note that applying the ConvNets to a new problem domain (gesture videos) is all but straightforward, and requires taking into account many domain specifics.

We next give an overview of the architecture, followed by a discussion on the aspects in which our method differs from previous methods.

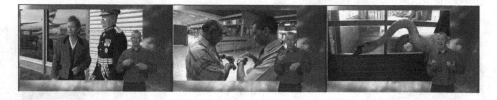

Fig. 2. Example frames from one video in the training set.

2.1 Architecture Overview

Figure 1 shows the network architecture. It consists of five convolutional layers followed by three fully connected layers. A selection of convolutional layers are followed by pooling and local response normalisation layers, and the fully connected layers are regularised by dropout [13]. All hidden weight layers use a rectification activation function (RELU).

A generic ConvNet architecture is used due to its outstanding performance in image recognition tasks. In the experiments we show that using this generic architecture, along with a few important changes, we outperform previous work on a challenging video gesture pose dataset.

2.2 Pose Regression

Regression Layer. Our network is trained for regressing the location of the human upper-body joints. Instead of the softmax loss layer, found in the image classification ConvNets [13], we employ an l_2 loss layer, which penalises the l_2 distance between the pose predictions and ground truth. Since the absolute image coordinates of the people vary across videos, we first normalise the training set with regards to a bounding box. The bounding boxes are estimated using a face detector: the estimated face bounding boxes are scaled by a fixed scaler (learnt from the training data such that joints in all training frames are contained within the bounding boxes). In the image domain, we crop out the bounding box, and rescale it to a fixed height. In the human joint domain, we rescale accordingly,

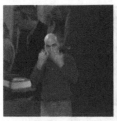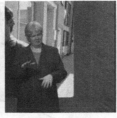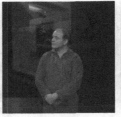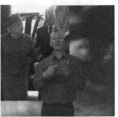

(a) Motion blur   (b) Similar foreground   (c) Self-occluding hands   (d) Faces in background
                         & background colour

Fig. 3. Challenges in the BBC TV Signing dataset. (a) Motion blur removes much of the edges of the hand; (b) similar foreground & background colours render colour information less informative; (c) self-occluding hands makes the assignment of left/right hand ambiguous; (d) faces in the background renders face detection-based bounding box detection difficult.

and in addition re-normalise the labels to the range $[0, 1]$. We found hyperparameter optimisation difficult without $[0, 1]$-normalised joints – in particular, the last fully-connected (regression) layer would require a different learning rate from other layers in order to converge.

We denote $(x, \mathbf{y})$ as a training example, where $\mathbf{y}$ stands for the coordinates of the k joints in the image x. Given normalised training data $N = (x, \mathbf{y})$ and a ConvNet regressor ψ, the training objective becomes the task of estimating the network weights λ:

$$\arg\min_{\lambda} \sum_{(x,\mathbf{y}) \in N} \sum_{i=1}^{k} \|\mathbf{y}_i - \phi(x, \lambda)\|^2 \tag{1}$$

The ConvNet weights are optimised using backpropagation using the open-source Caffe framework [11].

Multiple Input Frames. To exploit the temporal information available in videos, our network is trained on multiple video frames. This is in contrast to CNN pose estimators in previous work, which typically operate on a single frame. This is done by inserting multiple frames (or their difference images) into the data layer colour channels. So for example, a network with three input frames contains 9 colour channels in its data layer. The network is then retrained from scratch. In practice, for the training of such a network to converge, input RGB values need to be rescaled by the number of input frames to preserve the dynamic range of the hyperparameters.

Video-Specific Learning. Pose estimation in long videos comes with its own challenges. Here we discuss how we overcome them.

The major difference to general RGB image pose estimation is that videos generally contain several frames of the same person, as depicted in Fig. 2. Further, in the gesture communication scenario in particular, the person stands

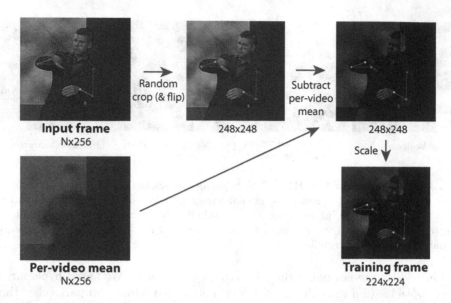

Fig. 4. Per-video mean and training augmentation. At training time, the training data is augmented with random crops and flips. A per-video mean is computed from a subset of frames to provide some invariance to different background colours. The per-video mean is obtained once per video, and can be computed on-the-fly in online pose estimation scenarios.

against a partially static background. We exploit this for an additional pre-processing step in our learning.

In particular, when training a generic network on videos without this preprocessing step, we noticed that the network would overfit to the static background behind the person. To alleviate this overfitting, we compute the mean image μ_V over 2,000 sampled frames for each video V in our training and testing datasets and subtract the video-specific mean from each input image: $x = x - \mu_V$ for frame x of video V. As shown in Fig. 4, this removes the video-specific static background and yields an input representation for the ConvNet that generalises much better across different videos.

This method differs from previous static image ConvNets, which generally compute a mean image over the full dataset, and subtract the same mean from each input frame.

We note that this preprocessing can also be applied to test scenarios where there is no access to the full video. In those scenarios, the mean image can be computed over a small set of frames before the test frame. In practice we did not find this to cause a significant drop in prediction accuracy.

Training Augmentation. Works on classification ConvNets commonly find that applying data augmentation (in the form of flips and crops) at training time increases performance [13]. In the classification tasks each image is typically associated with a single class; however, in our regression setting each image is associated with multiple target values dependent on the position of objects (body parts) in the image. We found that the level of data augmentation in the classification nets was too substantial for a regression task like ours.

Chatfield *et al.* [5] randomly crop (and randomly horizontally flip) a 224×224 subimage out of an image that has been resized so its smallest dimension is 256. This adds robustness to the absolute position of the object and improves generalisation in object recognition. However, when the input images are human bounding boxes, this crop is too substantial, and frequently crops off a part of the human body. One solution would be to scrap augmentation altogether. However, in experiments we found adding a small amount of invariance (as follows) to be helpful. We resize each input bounding box to height 256, randomly crop and flip a 248×248 image from it and update the joint positions accordingly. This results in each body part always being present in the image.

3 Implementation Details

Training. The training procedure is an adaptation of that of Krizhevsky *et al.* [13]. The network weights are learnt using mini-batch stochastic gradient descent with momentum set to 0.9. Each iteration samples 256 training frames randomly across the training videos and uses them as a mini-batch. The input frames are rescaled to height 256. A 248×248 sub-image (of the $N \times 256$ input image) is randomly cropped, randomly horizontally flipped and RGB jittered, and resized to 224×224. When re-training the ConvNet from scratch, the learning rate is set to 10^{-2}, and decreased to 10^{-3} at 80 K iterations, to 10^{-4} after 90 K iterations and stopped at 110 K iterations. In the experiments in which we pretrain the weights on ImageNet ILSVRC-2012, learning rates are similarly decreased at 50 K and 60K, and training is stopped at 70 K iterations.

Testing. At test time, we crop the centre 248×248 of the input image, resize to 224×224 and feed forward through the network to obtain human joint location predictions. Test augmentation (*e.g.* computing the mean/median of predictions for 10 random image crops and flips, as done in classification ConvNet works) did not yield improved results over using the centre crop only.

Training Time. Training was performed on a single NVIDIA GTX Titan GPU using a modified version of the Caffe framework [11]. Training the network from scratch took 3 days, while fine-tuning took 2 days.

Pretraining on ImageNet. In the evaluation section we also evaluate a setting where we pretrain the weights on ImageNet ILSVRC-2012 (rather than starting training from scratch), and fine-tune the weights on the new dataset. For those experiments, we use the publicly available "CNN-S" net provided by the authors of [5], which achieves 13.1 % top-5 error on the ILSVRC-2012 test set.

4 Datasets

Experiments in this work are conducted on BBC sign language TV broadcasts. In addition to providing benchmarks on the original dataset, we also show experiments on an extended version of the dataset with an order of magnitude more training data.

Original BBC TV sign language broadcast dataset. This dataset consists of 20 TV broadcast videos overlaid with a person interpreting what is being spoken into British Sign Language (BSL) (see Fig. 5). The videos, each between 0.5 h–1.5 h in length, contain content from a variety of TV programmes. All frames of the videos have been automatically assigned joint locations (which we use as ground truth for training) using a slow (and semi-automatic) but reliable tracker by Buehler *et al.* [2]. The full set of 20 videos are split into three disjoint sets: 13 videos for training, 2 for validation, 5 for testing. The test set videos contain different people wearing different clothing from those in the training and validation sets. 1,000 annotated frames (200 per video) of the test set have been manually annotated for evaluation purposes.

Extended BBC TV sign language broadcast dataset. This dataset contains 72 additional training videos, which are used to evaluate the benefits of additional training data. This dataset is combined with the original BBC TV dataset to yield a total of 92 videos (85 training, 2 validation and 5 testing). The frames of the new 72 videos are automatically assigned joint locations (used for ground truth in training) using the tracker of Charles *et al.* [3].

Foreground segmentations for both of these datasets are obtained automatically (but with some parameter tuning) using the co-segmentation algorithm of Charles *et al.* [3]. The output of the segmentation algorithm is an estimate of the person's silhouette (which can be noisy).

5 Evaluation

Experiments are conducted on the two BBC TV sign language datasets. We first present comparisons to alternative network architectures and preprocessing methods. We follow this by a comparison to the state of the art [3], both in terms of accuracy and computational performance.

5.1 Evaluation Protocol and Details

Evaluation Protocol. In all pose estimation experiments we compare the estimated joints against frames with manual ground truth. We present results as graphs that plot accuracy vs distance from ground truth in pixels. A joint is deemed correctly located if it is within a set distance of d pixels from a marked joint centre in ground truth. Unless otherwise stated, the experiments use $d = 6$. Figure 5(top-left) shows the image scale.

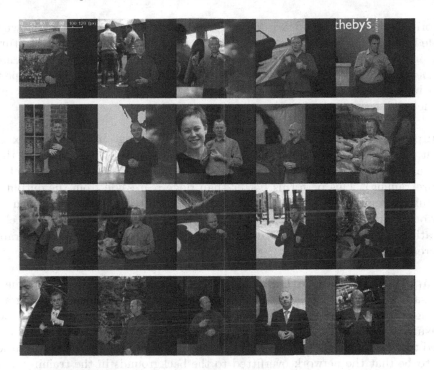

Fig. 5. Original BBC TV sign language dataset. The first three rows show the training and validation videos, and the last row shows the test videos. The upper-left figure gives a pixel scale.

Experimental Details. All frames of the videos are used for training (with each frame randomly augmented as detailed above). The frames are randomly shuffled prior to training to present maximally varying input data to the network.

The hyperparameters (early stopping and weights for combining multiple nets, see below) are estimated using the validation set.

5.2   Evaluation of Components

Table 1 shows comparisons to ConvNets with different number of input frames, input representations, levels of preprocessing and pretraining. We next discuss each of these results in detail.

Comparing Ridge Regression from ImageNet Fully Connected Layer Features. ConvNets trained on ImageNet have been shown to generalise extremely well to a wide variety of classification tasks [5,16,23]. Often the state of the art can be achieved by simply using the output from one of the fully connected layers as a feature. Here we investigate the performance of this approach for pose estimation.

In the first experiment, we extract features from the last fully connected layers of a network trained on ImageNet (a 4096 dimensional feature) applied to the original BBC TV broadcast dataset, and learn a ridge regressor. As shown in Table 1(row 1), this performs surprisingly poorly. This implies that these features that are extremely powerful for various real-world image classification tasks may not be quite as powerful when it comes to predicting precise locations of parts with high appearance variation in an image. One reason for this is likely that the network learns some location invariance.

Comparing to ImageNet Pretraining/Fine-Tuning. In the second experiment, we first pretrain network weights on ImageNet ILSVRC-2012, and then fine-tune them on the BBC TV sign language dataset (Sect. 3 provides details on pretraining). This performs better than ridge regression from the output of the fully connected layers, but still does not match the performance when the network is trained from scratch. This indicates that the two tasks (image classification and pose estimation) are sufficiently different to require considerably different weights.

Comparison to Using a Different Mean Image. In the third experiment, as a sanity check, we investigate using a single mean image for all training and testing. When using the standard ImageNet mean image, the average evaluation measure drops from 72.0 % to 57.6 %. The drop is caused by nearly completely failed tracking in some test videos. When investigating further, the reason turned out to be that the network overfitted to the backgrounds in the training data, and did not generalise to videos with different static backgrounds (as is the case for some of the test videos). This motivated the idea to use a per-video mean image, which removes the static background and so prevents the network from overfitting to it.

Comparison to a Smaller ConvNet. In the fourth experiment, we turn to comparing our method to a smaller (and slightly faster) network (set up with same architecture as the "CNN-M" network in Chatfield et al. [5] – i.e., same depth as our other network, "CNN-S", but with fewer parameters). This performs slightly worse than the larger network used in this work (60.4 % vs 72.0 %). This hints at that even deeper and larger networks could yield improved performance [19].

Comparison to No Training Augmentation. In the fifth experiment we test different levels of training augmentation. As shown in Table 1(row 3), training augmentation yields a small improvement over no training augmentation (using the centre crop of the image only), thanks to the added slight invariance in absolute position of the body inside the bounding box.

Comparisons with Different Training Sets. In the sixth experiment we compare results when training either on the original, or extended, training dataset. The network trained on the extended dataset performs worse on shoulders (87.7 % vs 89.1 %), but better on wrists (53.0 % vs 47.1 %) and elbows

Table 1. Evaluation of different architectures. The evaluation measure is the percentage of predictions within 6 pixels from ground truth. 'Scratch/Last only/FT all' refer to training from scratch/training the last layer from scratch (keeping the rest of the ImNet-pretrained network fixed)/finetuning all layers of an ImNet-pretrained network; 'Aug' to training time augmentation; 'Multi' to using multiple input frames; and 'Seg' to using an input representation with the foreground pre-segmented.

Training	Aug	Multi	Seg	Head	Wrists	Elbows	Shoulders	Average
Last only	✓			15.4	5.8	8.4	18.3	12.0
FT all	✓			95.6	44.0	53.6	80.8	68.5
Scratch				94.3	52.1	51.9	87.9	71.5
Scratch	✓			95.9	47.1	56.0	89.1	72.0
Scratch	✓	✓		95.6	50.1	58.1	89.5	73.3
Scratch	✓		✓	96.1	58.0	66.8	91.2	78.0

(56.4 % vs 56.0 %), and slightly better on average (72.6 % vs 72.0 %). We hypothesise the better wrist performance is due to the network seeing a larger variety of poses, whereas the worse shoulder performance is due to less precise ground truth shoulder locations in the extended dataset.

Comparison to Multi-frame Net. In the seventh experiment we test the improvement from using multiple input frames. Table 1(row 5) shows a consistent performance improvement over wrists, elbows and shoulders, with a particularly noticeable improvement in wrist predictions. The head predictions are slightly worse, likely because the head is fairly stationary and hence does not benefit from the additional temporal information. Qualitatively, when visualising the predictions, the wrists are better localised and the output looks better smoothed.

The multi-frame network has two parameters: the number of input frames n (how many frames are used as input for each pose estimate) and the temporal spacing t between the input frames (time between each of the n input frames). In a parameter optimisation experiments we searched over $n = \{1, 3, 5\}$ and $t = \{1, 2, 3, 5, 8, 10, 15, 25\}$ on the validation set. $n = 3$ and $t = 1$ (three input frames with one-frame time spacing) were selected as the optimal parameters. We also explored using difference images (subtracting the current frame from the additional input frames), however this did not improve performance.

Weighted Combination of Nets. In the eighth experiment, we demonstrate a further improvement in performance by combining predictions from the two best-performing nets so far (with training augmentation that were trained from scratch – one single-frame and the other multi-frame). We define the prediction of each joint y_i as

$$y_i = \alpha_i C_1(x) + (1 - \alpha_i) C_2(x) \tag{2}$$

where $C_l(x)$ are the predictions of the two nets for input image x. The parameter α_i is learnt separately for each joint i on the validation set.

This combination yields the best performance of all the nets without foreground segmentations: 74.2 % (vs 72.0 % and 73.3 % for the single-frame and multi-frame nets respectively).

Comparison to Foreground-Segmented Input Representation. In the ninth experiment we test our approach with the input representation of Charles *et al.*, who pre-segment the foreground of the input frames using an algorithm with some manually tuned parameters, and black out the background. As shown in Table 1(row 6), even though our method does not require foreground segmentations, it does benefit from using them. On the downside, using them would require manual tuning of segmentation parameters and significantly slow down the runtime (from 100fps to around 5fps).

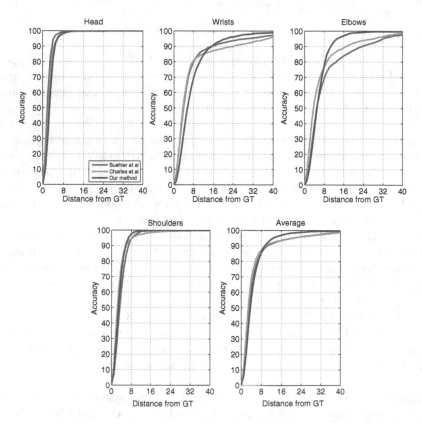

Fig. 6. Comparison to previous work. Comparison of pose estimation accuracy of the best-performing ConvNet versus the methods of Charles *et al.* [3] and Buehler *et al.* [2] (all trained and tested on the original dataset). Our method achieves much better constrained poses than previous work, without requiring any additional manual annotation (while [2] need per-video manual labelling, and [3] need manual tuning for the parameters of the foreground segmentation algorithm). Plots show accuracy per joint type (average over left and right body parts) as the allowed distance from manual ground truth is increased.

5.3   Comparison to Previous Work

Figure 6 presents a comparison of our method to previous work. Our method results on average in much better constrained poses and a significantly higher area under the curve, without requiring any of the video-specific manual segmentation algorithm tuning [3] or manual annotation [2] in previous work. We hypothesise that the better constrained poses are due to the ConvNet learning constraints for what poses a human body can perform (*i.e.*, the constraints of the human kinematic chain). While our method doesn't require any manual annotation (unlike previous work), our results in fact improve further if the input includes the foreground segmentations (as used in Charles *et al.*) – this is shown in Table 1.

Further, the ConvNet rarely predicts incorrect joint positions in the background (which is in contrast to previous work on this dataset, which reports 'catching the background' as the main challenge when not using a foreground segmentation algorithm [3] – Fig. 9 shows examples of corrected frames). We conjecture that this is due to the high capacity of the model, which enables it to essentially learn a foreground segmentation and ignore any pixels in the background.

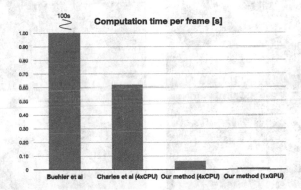

Fig. 7. Computation time. Comparison of computation times versus the methods of Charles *et al.* [3] and Buehler *et al.* [2]. Note that the reliable semi-automatic method of Buehler *et al.* is far off the scale as computing a pose for a single frame takes around 100s. Our method outperforms previous methods by over an order of magnitude using the same hardware. Using a single GPU instead of 4 CPUs increases speed by another order of magnitude.

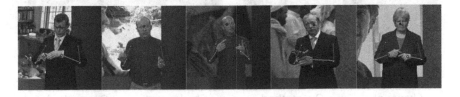

Fig. 8. Example pose estimates on the test set.

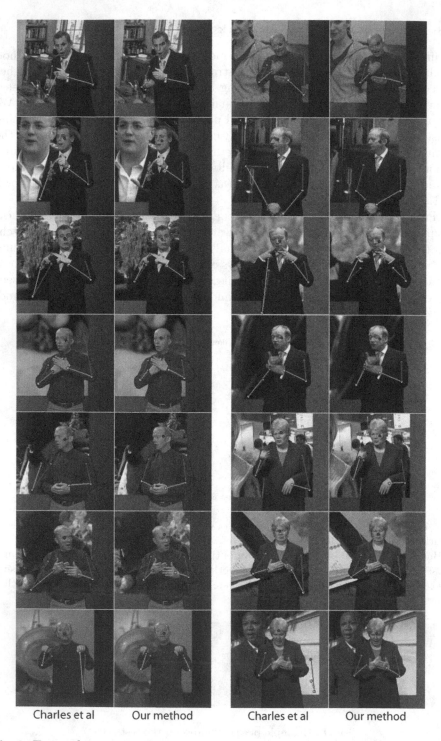

Charles et al   Our method   Charles et al   Our method

Fig. 9. Example test set frames comparing our estimates versus previous work [3]. The pose estimates of our method are much better localised.

In practice, this 'more constrained' estimation output manifests itself as significantly fewer serious prediction errors, and as much smoother pose tracks.

We achieve on average very similar pose estimates to previous work within the range of 0 − 8 pixels from ground truth, and outperform from 8 pixels onwards. On elbows this marked improvement is clear from 8 pixels onwards, and for wrists from 14 pixels onwards. The performance on shoulders and head predictions is very similar to previous methods. The performance in the near range on wrists is slightly poorer, which we attribute to the lower resolution of our network (selected due to computational limitations) which makes accurate learning of the highly varying wrist positions more challenging. However, this is more than compensated for by (1) significantly better constrained predictions (see examples in Figs. 8 and 9), (2) not needing a foreground segmentation algorithm that needs to be tuned manually, and (3) an order of magnitude faster prediction speed.

5.4 Computation Time

Figure 7 shows a comparison of our method's computation time to previous work. The computation times are measured on a 2.4 GHz Intel i7 Quad Core CPU. We improve by an order of magnitude over previous methods using the same hardware. If we instead predict with a single GPU, performance increases by yet another order of magnitude. Note that the timing of our method assumes a cropped bounding box around the person. Our current method for computing this takes 0.06 s on the CPU or 0.01 on the GPU using OpenCV's face detector. Even when taking these costs into account, our method is still over 5x faster on the CPU and 30x faster on the GPU.

6 Conclusion and Future Work

We have presented a ConvNet pose estimation method for gesture videos. The method produces much better constrained poses than previous work on the gesture dataset, is much faster and does not require a manually tuned foreground segmentation algorithm.

In the future we plan to investigate various avenues of improvement, including alternative ways of integrating temporal information from the videos into our networks, and training on significantly larger datasets.

Acknowledgements. We are grateful to Sophia Pfister for discussions. Financial support was provided by Osk. Huttunen Foundation and EPSRC grant EP/I012001/1.

References

1. Alsharif, O., Pineau, J.: End-to-end text recognition with hybrid HMM maxout models. In: ICLR (2014)
2. Buehler, P., Everingham, M., Huttenlocher, D.P., Zisserman, A.: Upper body detection and tracking in extended signing sequences. IJCV **95**(2), 180–197 (2011)

3. Charles, J., Pfister, T., Everingham, M., Zisserman, A.: Automatic and efficient human pose estimation for sign language videos. IJCV **110**, 70–90 (2014)
4. Charles, J., Pfister, T., Magee, D., Hogg, D., Zisserman, A.: Domain adaptation for upper body pose tracking in signed TV broadcasts. In: Proceedings of the BMVC (2013)
5. Chatfield, K., Simonyan, K., Vedaldi, A., Zisserman, A.: Return of the devil in the details: delving deep into convolutional nets. In: BMVC (2014)
6. Donahue, J., Jia, Y., Vinyals, O., Hoffman, J., Zhang, N., Tzeng, E., Darrell, T.: Decaf: a deep convolutional activation feature for generic visual recognition. In: ICML (2014)
7. Girshick, R., Donahue, J., Darrell, T., Malik, J.: Rich feature hierarchies for accurate object detection and semantic segmentation. In: Proceedings of the CVPR (2014)
8. Goodfellow, I.J., Bulatov, Y., Ibarz, J., Arnoud, S., Shet, V.: Multi-digit number recognition from street view imagery using deep convolutional neural networks. In: ICLR (2014)
9. Jaderberg, M., Simonyan, K., Vedaldi, A., Zisserman, A.: Synthetic data and artificial neural networks for natural scene text recognition. arXiv preprint arXiv:1406.2227 (2014)
10. Jain, A., Tompson, J., Andriluka, M., Taylor, G., Bregler, C.: Learning human pose estimation features with convolutional networks. In: ICLR (2014)
11. Jia, Y.: Caffe: an open source convolutional architecture for fast feature embedding (2013). http://caffe.berkeleyvision.org/
12. Karpathy, A., Toderici, G., Shetty, S., Leung, T., Sukthankar, R., Fei-Fei, L.: Large-scale video classification with convolutional neural networks. In: Proceedings of the CVPR (2014)
13. Krizhevsky, A., Sutskever, I., Hinton, G.: Imagenet classification with deep convolutional neural networks. In: NIPS (2012)
14. Osadchy, M., LeCun, Y., Miller, M.: Synergistic face detection and pose estimation with energy-based models. JMLR **8**, 1197–1215 (2007)
15. Pfister, T., Charles, J., Everingham, M., Zisserman, A.: Automatic and efficient long term arm and hand tracking for continuous sign language TV broadcasts. In: Proceedings of the BMVC (2012)
16. Razavian, S., Azizpour, H., Sullivan, J., Carlsson, S.: CNN features off-the-shelf: an astounding baseline for recognition. In: CVPR Workshops (2014)
17. Sermanet, P., Eigen, D., Zhang, X., Mathieu, M., Fergus, R., LeCun, Y.: Overfeat: integrated recognition, localization and detection using convolutional networks. In: ICLR (2014)
18. Simonyan, K., Zisserman, A.: Two-stream convolutional networks for action recognition in videos. In: NIPS (2014)
19. Simonyan, K., Zisserman, A.: Very deep convolutional networks for large-scale image recognition. arXiv preprint arXiv:1409.1556 (2014)
20. Taigman, Y., Yang, M., Ranzato, M., Wolf, L.: Deepface: Closing the gap to human-level performance in face verification. In: Proceedings of the CVPR (2014)
21. Tompson, J., Jain, A., LeCun, Y., Bregler, C.: Joint training of a convolutional network and a graphical model for human pose estimation. In: NIPS (2014)
22. Toshev, A., Szegedy, C.: DeepPose: human pose estimation via deep neural networks. In: CVPR (2014)
23. Zeiler, M.D., Fergus, R.: Visualizing and understanding convolutional networks. In: Fleet, D., Pajdla, T., Schiele, B., Tuytelaars, T. (eds.) ECCV 2014, Part I. LNCS, vol. 8689, pp. 818–833. Springer, Heidelberg (2014)

Robust Edge Aware Descriptor for Image Matching

Rouzbeh Maani$^{(\boxtimes)}$, Sanjay Kalra, and Yee-Hong Yang

Department of Computing Science, University of Alberta, Edmonton, Canada
rmaani@ualberta.ca

Abstract. This paper presents a method called Robust Edge Aware Descriptor (READ) to compute local gradient information. The proposed method measures the similarity of the underlying structure to an edge using the 1D Fourier transform on a set of points located on a circle around a pixel. It is shown that the magnitude and the phase of READ can well represent the magnitude and orientation of the local gradients and present robustness to imaging effects and artifacts. In addition, the proposed method can be efficiently implemented by kernels. Next, we define a robust region descriptor for image matching using the READ gradient operator. The presented descriptor uses a novel approach to define support regions by rotation and anisotropical scaling of the original regions. The experimental results on the Oxford dataset and on additional datasets with more challenging imaging effects such as motion blur and non-uniform illumination changes show the superiority and robustness of the proposed descriptor to the state-of-the-art descriptors.

1 Introduction

Local feature detection and description are among the most important tasks in computer vision. The extracted descriptors are used in a variety of applications such as object recognition and image matching, motion tracking, facial expression recognition, and human action recognition. The whole process can be divided into two major tasks: region detection, and region description. The goal of the first task is to detect regions that are invariant to a class of transformations such as rotation, change of scale, and change of viewpoint. The detected regions are then described by a feature vector. An ideal region descriptor should not only be invariant to geometric transformations but also be robust to imaging effects such as blurriness, noise, distortions, and illumination changes [1].

This paper focuses on the second task, region description. Local gradients are commonly used by the state-of-the-art methods. Although local gradient information is very powerful, it is susceptible to imaging effects such as noise, illumination changes, and blurriness. The first contribution of this paper is a

---

Electronic supplementary material The online version of this chapter (doi:10.1007/978-3-319-16865-4_36) contains supplementary material, which is available to authorized users.

© Springer International Publishing Switzerland 2015
D. Cremers et al. (Eds.): ACCV 2014, Part I, LNCS 9003, pp. 553–568, 2015.
DOI: 10.1007/978-3-319-16865-4_36

novel method to compute local edge information. The proposed READ method is similar to local gradients but is computed in a novel way. It provides both magnitude and orientational information at each pixel, and is robust to imaging effects. Similar to using gradients, the proposed READ method can be used in basic image processing operations such as edge detection, segmentation, and texture analysis. In particular, due to its robustness, READ is useful in conditions where undesirable imaging effects are unavoidable (e.g., noise in magnetic resonance images or blurriness in underwater imaging). The second contribution of this paper is the kernel implementation of the proposed READ method. The presented implementation makes the method fast for practical use. The third contribution of this paper is a novel method for determining support regions around the regions detected by affine detectors. First, it is shown that in theory the support regions can be scaled (with different scaling factors along the eigenvectors of the elliptical affine region) and rotated. Then, through experiments it is demonstrated that this method of support region definition can improve the results compared to the simple method of isotropic scaling of the original regions detected by affine detectors which is suggested in [2]. The advantages of the new descriptor are first explored in common geometric transformations, and then in more challenging imaging effects such as motion blur, non-uniform illumination changes with moving shadows, and images with different levels and types of noise. Although they are very important, these challenging effects are less noted in the evaluation of the previous descriptors.

2   Related Works

There are two main steps in finding corresponding points in two images. In the first step, interest points (regions) are found in the images. Ideal points should be highly discriminative and robustly detectable under different imaging conditions and geometric transformations. Some examples of detection methods include Difference of Gaussian (DoG) [3], Harris-Affine [4], and Hessian-Affine [5]. A review and comparison of region detection methods can be found in [5,6].

Many detectors provide circular or elliptical regions with different sizes around the detected points for point description. The size of the detected region is determined by the detected scale of the region. By transforming the detected regions (elliptical and circular) to a circular region of a fixed radius, the regions are normalized into a canonical form. As a result, an affine transformation is reduced to a rotation, and an affine invariance on the original image can be obtained by rotation invariance on the canonical region [5]. Hence, region descriptors usually define rotation invariant features to provide descriptors that are invariant to local affine geometric transformations.

One of the most popular descriptors is the Scale Invariant Feature Transform (SIFT) [3]. The main information used in SIFT is the magnitude and orientation of local gradients accumulated in subregions. SIFT is later extended in the Gradient Location and Orientation Histogram (GLOH) method [1]. Mikolajczyk and Schmid [1] demonstrate that SIFT and GLOH outperform other descriptors obtained using shape context, steerable filters, spin images, differential invariants, complex filters, and moment invariants. Some other descriptors include the Center-Symmetric Local Binary Pattern (CS-LBP) [7], the shape of MSER [8], the Local Intensity Order Pattern (LIOP) [9], and KAZE [10].

DAISY is a successful method recently proposed by Tola et al. [11]. Similar to SIFT, DAISY uses the magnitude and orientation of local gradients; however, the weighted sum of gradient orientation is replaced by the convolution of the gradient in specific directions with several Gaussian filters. Recently, it has been shown that the intensity ordinal information is more useful than the fixed location bins used by many descriptors such as SIFT and DAISY. The idea has been used by several descriptors such as LIOP [9], MROGH, and MRRID [2,12].

A new promising approach is in developing "binary" descriptors such as BRIEF [13], Brisk [14], ORB [15], Freak [16], and BinBoost [17] for real-time applications. A comparative evaluation of these descriptors is presented in [18]. The recent paper by Miksik and Mikolajczyk [19] also compares some of these methods in the accuracy and speed trade-offs suggesting that binary descriptors provide comparable precision/recall results with SIFT and outperform in speed. On the other hand this paper reports that LIOP, MRRID, MROGH are slower but outperform SIFT and other binary descriptors.

3   Robust Edge Aware Descriptor

Considering neighbors on a circle (or multiple circles) around a pixel is a popular approach in rotation invariant methods. The values of the circular neighbors are usually encoded in two ways: (1) by applying a threshold (e.g., the center pixel's intensity) similar to the LBP [20] and its variants, (2) by transforming the values into frequency components as suggested by some texture classification methods [21–25]. It is argued that applying a threshold by the LBP-based methods compromises some important information and demonstrated that the latter approach outperforms the first one [24]. The 1D Discrete Fourier Transform (DFT) of the neighbor's intensity values is defined as

$$F(n) = \sum_{k=1}^{P} f(k)e^{\frac{-2\pi i(k-1)(n-1)}{P}}, (n = 1, \ldots, P), \tag{1}$$

where $F(n)$ consists of P complex numbers, known as the frequency components. Since $f(k)$ consists of real numbers, the frequency components of $F(n)$ are conjugate symmetric about the DC component. That is, the 2nd and the Pth components (similarly the 3rd and the $(P-1)^{th}$, and so on) have the same magnitude but opposite phase. A recent work [23] shows that the low frequency components ($F(1)$, $F(2)$, and $F(P)$) comprise more than 90 % of the $f(k)$ signal in some well known texture datasets, and therefore can well represent the texture around a pixel. Inspired by this work, we demonstrate that the *second frequency component* (or equivalently the Pth component) can be used to robustly compute the edge information. To better explain the edge detection ability of $F(2)$, we need to show the characteristics of function $f(k)$ when it is around an edge.

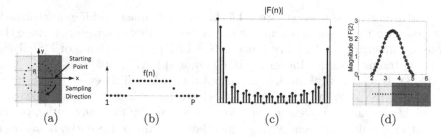

Fig. 1. Using READ operator to compute local edge. (a) P sample are located on radius of R around a pixel. (b) The function of samples have a rectangular shape. (c) The DFT of a rectangular shape function is a sinc. The highest values of the sinc function are at $n = 1$ and $n = \{2, P\}$. (d) $|F(2)|$ as a function of the distance of the center of the sampling circle from the edge.

We define an edge as the line separating a dark region from a bright region as shown in Fig. 1(a). In this example, we traverse the circular samples in the clockwise direction. We start from a dark region, cross the edge and go into the bright region, cross the edge again, and come back to the starting point in the dark region. Using this circular sampling method, the function of an edge can be characterized as a rectangular shape function as shown in Fig. 1(b). For simplicity, assume that the rectangular function has a value of one in the bright region. The DFT of the rectangular shape function with width M (using Eq. 1) is a sinc shape function of the following form:

$$F(n)_{rect} = \frac{sin(\frac{\pi(n-1)M}{P})}{sin(\frac{\pi(n-1)}{P})} \times e^{-\frac{i\pi(n-1)(M-1)}{P}}. \tag{2}$$

It can be easily observed that the magnitude of this sinc shape function, $|\frac{sin(\pi(n-1)M/P)}{sin(\pi(n-1)/P)}|$, has the maximum value at $n = 1$ and then at $n = \{2, P\}$ (Fig. 1(c)). As a result, an edge manifests itself with maximum values in $F(1)$, $F(2)$, and $F(P)$. It is noteworthy that among these three components, $F(1)$ represents the average intensity (known as DC component), which gives information if the pixel is located in a dark or bright region, while $F(2)$ (or $F(P)$) is more sensitive to the actual edge information around the pixel. Another possible interpretation of $F(2)$ is that it approximates a rectangular shape function better than the other components. To better demonstrate the edge detection ability we plot $|F(2)|$ as a function of the distance of the center of the circle from the edge for the given example shown in Fig. 1(d). In this example, we choose points between pixels 2 and 5 with an increment of 0.1 pixels. The magnitude of $F(2)$ is shown for each point in Fig. 1(d). As one can see, $|F(2)|$ reaches its maximum value at location 3.5 which is the exact point separating the dark region from the bright region. Now, we formally define READ by setting $n = 2$ in Eq. 1:

$$READ = \sum_{k=1}^{P} f(k)e^{\frac{-2\pi i(k-1)}{P}}. \tag{3}$$

Equation 3 gives a complex number; hence, it can be further decomposed into real and imaginary parts:

$$Re(READ) = \sum_{k=1}^{P} f(k)cos(\frac{2\pi(k-1)}{P}), \tag{4}$$

$$Im(READ) = -\sum_{k=1}^{P} f(k)sin(\frac{2\pi(k-1)}{P}). \tag{5}$$

The magnitude and the phase of READ can be simply computed from the real and imaginary parts. The magnitude of READ represents the amount of rectangular shape function (i.e., the strength of an edge), while the phase indicates the starting location of the rectangular shape function (i.e., the edge orientation). One may note that the exact value of the phase depends on the neighbor ordering strategy. We start from the x axis and traverse the neighbors in the clockwise direction as shown in Fig. 1(a). Using this protocol will result in the same orientation value computed by the conventional gradient orientation formula.

The rectangular shape function of $f(n)$ (which characterizes an edge) is comparable to the *uniform* patterns in the LBP method which represent edges of varying positive and negative curvatures [20]. However, the uniform patterns are acquired by applying a threshold which makes the patterns sensitive to noise, while in READ, an edge appears as a low frequency component ($F(2)$) which is less affected by noise. Similar to the LBP, the READ can be acquired using different R and P. Figure 2 compares the gradient calculation of the READ operator with that of the central difference ($\Delta_h f(x) = f(x+h/2) - f(x-h/2)$) on a synthetic and a real image. READ is computed with setting ($P = 8, R = 1$) and $h = 1$ pixel in the central difference method. To make a fair visual comparison, the magnitude of the gradients are normalized in the range [0 1].

As one can observe the magnitude of the READ is zero in flat regions, while it is maximized on pixels located on an edge. However, this change is gradual in contrast to the central difference (this was also demonstrated in Fig. 1(d)). The phase of READ faithfully represents the orientation of the local edge. One may consider the orientational values around the circle in the synthetic image. The color map in the bottom right of the phase image shows the color representing a given angle. Similarly the change in phase is smoother than that of the central difference. The second row of Fig. 2 compares edge characterization on a real image. It can be observed that the outputs of the two methods look very similar both in magnitude of the detected edges and in their orientations. However, one may note that the READ is more sensitive to finding faint edges. For example, the edges in the background on the upper left side and above the hat are more clear in the magnitude of READ compared to that of the local gradients.

3.1   Properties of READ

READ has several advantages that make it favorable for computer vision and image processing applications. The first advantage is its robustness to noise.

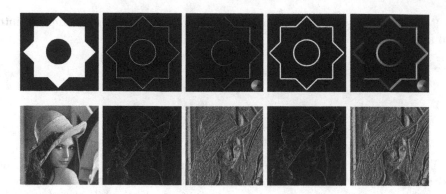

Fig. 2. Computing gradient on a synthetic (first row) and a real image (second row). The first column is the original image. The 2nd and 3rd columns are the magnitude and orientation of gradient computed by the central difference. The 4th and 5th columns are the magnitude and orientation of gradient computed by READ.

The reason is that noise appears in high frequency components. However, READ is defined based on a low frequency component, $F(2)$, which is not sensitive to noise. This property will be further demonstrated in Sect. 4. The next property of READ is its invariance to linear changes of illumination. One can simply observe that any linear change of illumination linearly changes the magnitude of function $f(k)$. This effect, however, does not change the phase of READ. To keep the magnitude of READ invariant to linear illumination changes, the image intensity is normalized to have zero mean and unit standard deviation. Finally, READ is robust to blur effect. The reason is that the blur effect mainly dampens the high frequency components and the low frequencies are less affected. These properties are further explored in Sect. 4.

3.2   Efficient Implementation

Speed is one important factor for descriptors. As a result a good descriptor should also have a reasonable runtime. In this regard, we present an efficient implementation for the READ operator. The idea is to define kernels to represent Eqs. 4 and 5 and finding the gradients by convolution of the defined kernels with the image. For a radius of R, the kernel has a size of $N \times N$ where $N = 2R + 1$. There are two factors to compute in the kernel as defined in Eqs. 4, 5: the value of the samples, $f(k)$, and the cos/sin coefficients. Since, the location of the samples are known for a specific R and P, both factors could be found easily.

The value of each sample is found using bilinear interpolation from its four nearest neighbors if it is not exactly located on a pixel. To compute the value of $f(k)$ we consider a $P \times N^2$ matrix. The kth row of the matrix represents the kth sample and each column represents the weight of each element in the kernel for the bilinear interpolation (we order the elements of the kernel in a $1 \times N^2$ row vector). We call this matrix B representing the bilinear weights of the kernel.

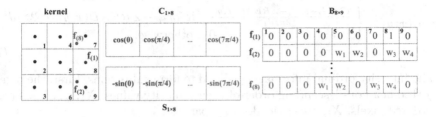

Fig. 3. Construction of matrix B, C, and S for $R = 1$ and $P = 8$ setting. The kernel size is 3×3. Samples are either located on a pixel ($f(1)$) or between pixels ($f(2)$, $f(8)$). In the latter case, we need bilinear interpolation to compute the value of the sample.

Now, we consider two $1 \times P$ row vectors called C and S to represent the *cos* and $-sin$ weights in Eqs. 4 and 5. Figure 3 illustrates the construction of B, C, and S for $R = 1$, $P = 8$ setting. The two kernels representing the equations can be simply computed by matrix multiplication $G_x = CB$ and $G_y = SB$. To use the kernel in the convolution operation we reshape G_x and G_y from $1 \times N^2$ to $N \times N$ matrices and reflect the values around the center of the matrix.

3.3   Region Descriptor

In this section we present a region descriptor for an arbitrary affine region detector. The orientation and magnitude of the underlying structure can be found by READ. However, although the magnitude of READ is rotation invariant, the phase of READ changes by rotation. Assume that the phase of READ at an arbitrary point x is α. When a rotation by $\theta°$ occurs, the phase will change to $\alpha' = \alpha + \theta$. Rotation invariance can be obtained by decomposing the phase of READ (i.e., α, α') into two components: a constant part related to the underlying structure (β) and a variable part related to the location of the point (γ, γ') as shown in Fig. 4. This approach is sim-

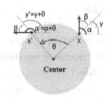

Fig. 4. Rotation invariant phase information.

ilar to the local rotation invariant coordinate system used by some descriptors such as MROGH [12], RIFT [26], and RIFF [27]. Instead of considering a new coordinate system, this can be easily done in READ by just subtracting the angle of the location of the point from the phase of READ computed in the regular coordinate system (i.e., $\beta = \gamma - \alpha = \gamma' - \alpha'$) which makes the computation fast.

By considering d orientational bins centering at ori_i, $(1 \leq i \leq d)$, the phase of READ is linearly assigned to the two closest orientational bins:

$$ori_i = (2\pi/d) \times (i - 1). \qquad (6)$$

$$Bin_i(x,y) = \begin{cases} \frac{(2\pi/d) - |ori_i - \angle READ(x,y)|}{(2\pi/d)} & , \text{ if } |ori_i - \angle READ(x,y)| < 2\pi/d \\ 0 & , \text{ otherwise.} \end{cases}$$

(7)

The intensity ordinal information is used to form subregions. First, the pixels are sorted in a non-descending order of their intensity values, $X_1, \ldots, X_n$. Then, the ordered pixels, X_i, are divided into k partitions,

$$Pr(p) = \{X_i | X_{\lceil n(p-1)/k+1 \rceil} \leq X_i \leq X_{\lceil np/k \rceil}\},$$

(8)

where $\lceil \rceil$ denotes the ceiling operator. The orientational histograms in each partition, $Pr(p)$, is accumulated and weighted with the average magnitude of the READ in that partition,

$$Hist(p,i) = \sum_{\forall(x,y) \in Pr(p)} Bin_i(x,y).\mu_{READ}(p),$$

(9)

where $Bin_i(x,y)$ is computed by Eq. 7 and $\mu_{READ}(p)$ by

$$\mu_{READ}(p) = \frac{1}{|Pr(p)|} \sum_{\forall(x,y) \in Pr(p)} |READ(x,y)|,$$

(10)

where $|Pr(p)|$ denotes the number of pixels in partition p. The final descriptor is a $d \times k$ feature vector constructed by concatenating the orientational histograms in all subregions.

Some descriptors (e.g., MROGH, MRRID) use support regions defined as the scaled version of the original detected region to improve their performance. Here, a novel and more flexible support region definition is presented. We suggest that the support region can be obtained by rotating and scaling with different scaling factors along the eigenvectors of the elliptical affine region (anisotropic scaling).

Using vector notation, a point X_L in an ellipse satisfies $X_L^T M_L X_L = 0$ in the homogeneous representation, where M_L is a symmetric matrix. As shown by Mikolajczyk and Schmid [4], when two elliptical regions $X_L^T M_L X_L = 0$ and $X_R^T M_R X_R = 0$ are corresponding, their canonical regions, $X_{Lc} = M_L^{1/2} X_L$ and $X_{Rc} = M_R^{1/2} X_R$, are related by a rotation:

$$\begin{aligned} X_{Rc} &= R(\alpha) X_{Lc} \\ \Rightarrow X_R &= M_R^{-1/2} R(\alpha) M_L^{1/2} X_L. \end{aligned}$$

(11)

Since M_L (and similarly M_R) is a symmetric matrix, it can be decomposed as $M_L = \Sigma_L \Lambda_L \Sigma_L^T$, where Σ_L is the orthogonal eigenvector matrix, and Λ_L the diagonal eigenvalue matrix. We define the transformation H for the scale matrix $S = \begin{bmatrix} s_1 & 0 \\ 0 & s_2 \end{bmatrix}$:

$$H = \Sigma_L S^{-1} \Sigma_L^T,$$

(12)

Lemma 1. *Transformation H maps $X_L^T M_L X_L = 0$ into a new ellipse, the eigenvectors of which are the same as the old ellipse but the eigenvalues are scaled by the $(s_1)^2$ and $(s_2)^2$ factors.*

Proof. If the ellipse $X_L^T M_L X_L = 0$ undergoes the H transformation, the new ellipse is defined as $X_L'^T M_L' X_L' = 0$, where $X_L' = H X_L$ and $M_L' = H^{-T} M_L H^{-1}$. Substituting $M_L = \Sigma_L \Lambda_L \Sigma_L^T$ in the M_L' equation will results in:

$$M_L' = (\Sigma_L S^{-1} \Sigma_L^T)^{-T} \Sigma_L \Lambda_L \Sigma_L^T (\Sigma_L S^{-1} \Sigma_L^T)^{-1} \tag{13}$$

After a few steps of reduction this equation results in $M_L' = \Sigma_L S \Lambda_L S^T \Sigma_L^T$. Considering the new eigenvalue matrix, $\Lambda_L' = S \Lambda_L S^T$, results in $M_L' = \Sigma_L \Lambda_L' \Sigma_L^T$ which is claimed in Lemma 1. ⊓

Before presenting the theorem we present the following equations (used in the proofs). Assume that S and D are diagonal and Q is orthogonal, then it is easy to show:

$$(Q D Q^T)^{1/2} = Q D^{1/2} Q^T = Q D^{1/2} Q^{-1}, \text{ and} \tag{14}$$

$$(Q S D S^T Q^T)^{1/2} = Q D^{1/2} S^T Q^T = Q D^{1/2} S Q^T. \tag{15}$$

Theorem 1. *Assume that the original ellipses defined by M_L and M_R undergo the H_L and H_R transformations, $X_L' = R \Sigma_L S^{-1} \Sigma_L^T X_L$, and $X_R' = R \Sigma_R S^{-1} \Sigma_R^T X_R$, where R is an arbitrary rotation matrix. The canonical regions of X_L' and X_R' are related by a rotation.*

Proof. We need to show that Eq. 11 holds for X_L' and X_R' with the new elliptical regions defined by M_L' and M_R'. We start by multiplying Eq. 11 with H_R

$$
\begin{aligned}
H_R X_R &= H_R M_R^{-1/2} R(\alpha) M_L^{1/2} X_L \\
&= H_R M_R^{-1/2} R(\alpha) M_L^{1/2} H_L^{-1} H_L X_L \\
&= (R \Sigma_R S^{-1} \Sigma_R^T)(\Sigma_R \Lambda_R^{-1/2} \Sigma_R^T) R(\alpha)(\Sigma_L \Lambda_L^{1/2} \Sigma_L^T)(\Sigma_L^{-T} S \Sigma_L^{-1} R^{-1}) H_L X_L \\
&= (R \Sigma_R S^{-1} \Lambda_R^{-1/2} \Sigma_R^T R^{-1}) R R(\alpha) R^{-1} (R \Sigma_L \Lambda_L^{1/2} S \Sigma_L^{-1} R^{-1}) H_L X_L \\
&= (H_R^{-T} M_R H_R^{-1})^{-1/2} R R(\alpha) R^{-1} (H_L^{-T} M_L H_L^{-1})^{1/2} H_L X_L. \\
\Rightarrow X_R' &= M_R'^{-1/2} R(\gamma) M_L'^{1/2} X_L'.
\end{aligned}
$$
$$\tag{16}$$
□

Figure 5 illustrates the concept. The original regions detected by an affine detector (yellow) are related by rotation. The red regions are anisotropically scaled and rotated version of the original regions detected by affine detectors (yellow). It can be observed that the red regions are related by rotation as well. This idea can be considered as a generalized form of support regions suggested in MROGH in which R in the H transformation is an identity matrix and $s_1 = s_2$ in the S matrix. Nonetheless, this generalized form gives more flexibility to choose the support regions.

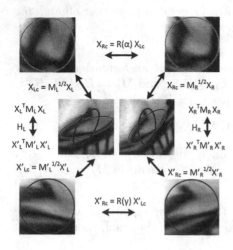

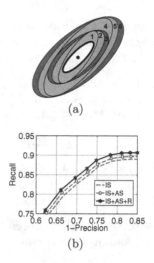

(a)

(b)

Fig. 5. Using new support regions (red) as anisotropically scaled and rotated version of the original regions detected by affine detectors (yellow). The new red regions are related by rotation (color figure online).

Fig. 6. (a) Support regions. (b) Comparing different support region strategies: IS, and its combination with AS, and R.

4   Experimental Results

4.1   Gradient Calculator Robustness

In the first experiment, we examine the robustness of the READ operator for gradient calculation for different imaging effects and artifacts. We compare the *READ* gradient operator with the central difference, the first order derivative of Gaussian (i.e., $\Delta f(x) = f(x) * \Delta_G(\sigma)$, where $*$ is convolution and $\Delta_G(\sigma) = \frac{-2x}{\sqrt{2\pi}\sigma^3}e^{-\frac{x^2}{2\sigma^2}}$), and Sobel. Central difference is an old operator which is still used by some descriptors (e.g., MROGH). First order derivative of Gaussian is used in the Canny edge detector (a popular edge detector) and Sobel is a known gradient operator. For the experiments we use Flower, Foliage, Fruit, Winter, and Man Made datasets from the McGill color image collections[1]. This includes 821 color images which are converted to the gray scale format. For the noise experiments, two types of noise are added: Gaussian noise with a specific standard deviation ($\sigma = 1, 1.5, \ldots, 3$) and the Salt & Pepper noise with different noise densities ($density = 0.05, 0.10, \ldots, 0.35$). For the blur effect experiment, the images are smoothed with a Gaussian kernel (i.e., $K(x, y) = e^{-\frac{x^2+y^2}{2\sigma^2}}$) with a window size of $W \times W$ ($W = (1.5 \times \sigma + .5) \times 2 + 1$). The experiment is performed for

---

[1] http://tabby.vision.mcgill.ca/html/welcome.html.

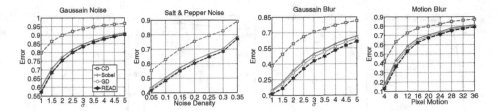

Fig. 7. The robustness of Central Difference (CD), Gaussian Derivative (GD), Sobel, and READ for different imaging effects.

$\sigma = 1, 1.5, \ldots, 3$. Finally, the motion blur effect is generated by Matlab using distances of 4 to 36 pixels with a step size of 4 pixels. To make the result of the methods comparable, the gradient vector at pixels ($G_i = [g_x, g_y]^T$) is normalized in each image I:

$$G_i = \frac{G_i}{\sum_{\forall G_i \in I} |G_i|}. \tag{17}$$

Then we measure the normalized error:

$$Err = \frac{1}{N} \sum_{i=1}^{N} \frac{|G_i^{cor} - G_i^{orig}|}{|G_i^{orig}|}, \tag{18}$$

where G_i^{cor} and G_i^{orig} are the gradient vectors in the corrupted and the original image, and N the number of pixels in the image. To avoid instability due to small values in the denominator, the vectors with small magnitudes ($|G_i^{orig}| < 10^{-6}$) are excluded. Figure 7 compares the normalized error of the compared methods. In the noise conditions (both Gaussian and Salt & Pepper) the proposed READ operator and the first order derivative of Gaussian are equally the most robust methods. However, in blur conditions (Motion and Gaussian) the READ operator outperforms the other methods. The central difference is the most sensitive method in all experiments.

4.2 Tuning Parameters

The next experiment is performed to find the best tuning parameters for the gradient scale, rotation, and scaling factors of the supporting regions. A total of 50 image pairs with different transformations (mainly rotation and zoom) are used[2]. Six regions are considered (Fig. 6(a)). All regions undergo isotropic scaling (IS) by a factor of 1.5 from the previous region, regions 1–3 undergo anisotropic scaling (AS) in the direction of eigenvectors of the elliptic region, regions 1 and 4 and regions 3 and 6 are rotated by $\theta°$ and $-\theta°$. The best gradient scale is searched for $R = 1, 2, 3, 4, 5$ with corresponsing $P = 6, 8, 10, 12, 14$. The best s_1 and s_2 are searched in the range $[0.7, 1.3]$ in steps of 0.05, and the best rotation

---

[2] Images downloaded from http://lear.inrialpes.fr/people/mikolajczyk/.

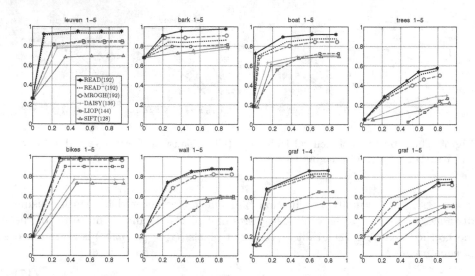

Fig. 8. The performance of the descriptors. The $READ^-$ is our descriptor with no anisotropic scaling or rotation of support regions. The y axis is recall and the x axis is 1-precision.

angle from the range $[0, 25]°$ with a step of $5°$, respectively. One may note that other configurations are also possible, and similar to DAISY the best parameters can be learned systematically [28]. Nonetheless, this specific configuration is sufficient to show the capability of the new descriptor. The best configuration is found to be $R = 4$, $P = 12$, $s_1 = 0.75$, $s_2 = 1.25$, and $\theta = 20°$. Figure 6(b) compares the configuration with only isotropic scaling (IS), and its combinations with anisotropic scaling (AS) and rotation (R). As one can see, the suggested strategy to define support region improves the performance of the descriptor.

4.3 Oxford Dataset

To evaluate the performance of the proposed descriptor we follow the evaluation protocol described by Mikolajczyk and Schmid [1] using the standard Oxford dataset[3]. The dataset includes image sets to evaluate different geometric transformations and imaging effects. The first image in each set is considered as a reference image and the other images are acquired under the designated change. A match is considered correct if the overlap error in the image area covered by two corresponding regions is less than 50 % of the union of the regions and the recall/1-precision is reported.

We compare our method to SIFT (as the baseline), DAISY, and LIOP and MROGH which have the highest performance according to the recent descriptor comparison study by Miksik and Mikolajczyk [19]. Figure 8 shows the performence of the descriptors. Two versions of our method are shown: (1) using

---

[3] Available at http://www.robots.ox.ac.uk/vgg/research/affine/.

only isotropic scaling for support regions ($READ^-$), and (2) adding anisotropic scaling and rotation to the previous version ($READ$). As one can see, the proposed method outperforms the other methods in all cases including illumination change (leuven), rotation and zoom (bark, boat), blur effect (trees, bikes), and view point change (wall, graf). An interesting case is the "1–5" pair in the graf dataset in which adding anisotropic scaling and rotation degrades the performance. This case shows that the performance of rotated and anisotropically scaled support regions relies on the accuracy of the affine region detector. The regions detected by the Hessian-affine detector is not very precise on the graf dataset due to the textureless nature of the scene. Therefore, due to a large viewpoint change, a small inaccuracy produces a large error when we use rotation and anisotropic scaling to define the support regions. Without using rotation or scaling ($READ^-$), however, we can get a much better result for this special case. Nevertheless, if the viewpoint change is smaller (e.g., less than 40° as shown in "1–4" pair in graf) or if the scene has some texture to help better detection (e.g., the wall), anisotropic scaling and rotation improve the result as shown in the other cases. With the exception of leuven, the MROGH is the second best method. In general, all the examined descriptors perform better than SIFT. The average runtime to compute the descriptors on a PC with an Intel quad core 2.60 GHz CPU with 16GB RAM running Windows 7 Professional is 2.4 ms for READ, 3.1 ms for MROGH, 2.1 ms for LIOP, 1.9 ms for DAISY, and 1.0 ms for SIFT. Therefore, our method not only outperforms MROGH but also is quite faster.

4.4   Noise

To evaluate the performance of the descriptors in the presence of noise, the "1–5" image pairs of the Oxford dataset and two types of noise (i.e., Gaussian and the salt & pepper, SP) are considered. The Gassian noise with different Signal to Noise Ratio (SNR), and SP noise with different noise density are added to the "5" image while the reference image "1" is unchanged. We compute the area under the curve (AUC) for the recall/1-precision graphs for the original (AUC^{orig}) and the noisy (AUC^{noise}) conditions. The AUC drop ratio (($AUC^{orig} - AUC^{noise})/AUC^{orig}$) is shown in Fig. 9. As one can see, the READ method is the most robust one in all levels of both types of noise. In some levels of noise $READ^-$ is slightly more robust than READ. After READ, the next robust methods are MROGH, and DAISY. SIFT and LIOP are the most sensitive methods in the Gaussian and SP noise, respectively.

4.5   Motion Blur

Motion blur is one of the common and challenging problems in many computer vision applications. In spite of its importance, and to the best of our knowledge, the effect of motion blur on the performance of descriptors have not been explored. To do so, we apply the motion blur effect function in MATLAB to our images and generate and add motion blur effect with distances of 4 to 16 pixels

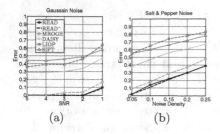

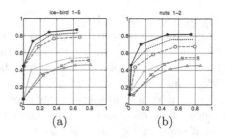

Fig. 9. The AUC drop ratio in different levels of noise for (a) Gaussian noise, (b) salt & pepper noise.

Fig. 10. Performence of descriptors on (a) motion blur, (b) non-uniform illumination change. The y axis is recall and the x axis is 1-precision.

with a step of 4. Figure 10(a) shows the performance of the descriptors for the "1–5" pair (16 pixels distance). One can see that the READ descriptor notably outperforms the other methods.

4.6 Non-uniform Illumination

Non-uniform illumination and shadows are among the most challenging effects. To evaluate the performance of the descriptors we use the "1–2" image pairs from the nuts dataset[4]. As can be seen in Fig. 10(b), the READ descriptor remarkably outperforms the other methods with about 14 % higher maximum recall than the second best method.

5   Conclusions

In this paper we propose a new gradient operator called READ which is robust to imaging effects. A kernel implementation of the READ is presented which makes the computation efficient. We demonstrate the ability of READ by defining a region descriptor and comparing it with other state-of-the-art descriptors. This paper presents a novel method to define support regions for the regions detected by an affine detector. The experimental results show that the READ descriptor outperforms the state-of-the-art descriptors such as SIFT, LIOP, DAISY, and MROGH in ordinary geometric transformations and common imaging effects. Additional experiments on noise, motion blur, and non-uniform illumination change further demonstrate the robustness and superior performance of the proposed method. The proposed READ gradient calculator can be used in other image processing and computer vision applications such as segmentation, texture classification, object recognition, and in applications that need robust gradient estimation.

---

[4] Accessible at http://lear.inrialpes.fr/people/mikolajczyk/Database/.

References

1. Mikolajczyk, K., Schmid, C.: A performance evaluation of local descriptors. IEEE Trans. Pattern Anal. Machine Intell. **27**, 1615–1630 (2005)
2. Fan, B., Wu, F., Hu, Z.: Rotationally invariant descriptors using intensity order pooling. IEEE Trans. Pattern Anal. Machine Intell. **34**, 2031–2045 (2012)
3. Lowe, D.: Distinctive image features from scale-invariant keypoints. Intl. J. Comput. Vis. **60**, 91–110 (2004)
4. Mikolajczyk, K., Schmid, C.: Scale & affine invariant interest point detectors. Intl. J. Comput. Vis. **60**, 63–86 (2004)
5. Mikolajczyk, K., Tuytelaars, T., Schmid, C.: A comparison of affine region detectors. Intl. J. Comput. Vis. **65**, 43–72 (2005)
6. Tuytelaars, T., Mikolajczyk, K.: Local invariant feature detectors: a survey. Found. Trends Comput. Graph. Vis. **3**, 177–280 (2008)
7. Heikkilä, M., Pietikäinen, M., Schmid, C.: Description of interest regions with local binary patterns. Pattern Recogn. **42**, 425–436 (2009)
8. Forssen, P., Lowe, D.: Shape descriptors for maximally stable extremal regions. In: International Conference on Computer Vision, ICCV, pp. 1–8 (2007)
9. Wang, Z., Fan, B., Wu, F.: Local intensity order pattern for feature description. In: International Conference on Computer Vision, ICCV, pp. 603–610 (2011)
10. Alcantarilla, P.F., Bartoli, A., Davison, A.J.: KAZE features. In: Fitzgibbon, A., Lazebnik, S., Perona, P., Sato, Y., Schmid, C. (eds.) ECCV 2012, Part VI. LNCS, vol. 7577, pp. 214–227. Springer, Heidelberg (2012)
11. Tola, E., Lepetit, V., Fua, P.: Daisy: An efficient dense descriptor applied to wide-baseline stereo. IEEE Trans. Pattern Anal. Machine Intell. **32**, 815–830 (2010)
12. Fan, B., Wu, F., Hu, Z.: Aggregating gradient distributions into intensity orders: A novel local image descriptor. In: IEEE Conference on Computer Vision and Pattern Recognition, CVPR, pp. 2377–2384 (2011)
13. Calonder, M., Lepetit, V., Strecha, C., Fua, P.: BRIEF: binary robust independent elementary features. In: Daniilidis, K., Maragos, P., Paragios, N. (eds.) ECCV 2010, Part IV. LNCS, vol. 6314, pp. 778–792. Springer, Heidelberg (2010)
14. Leutenegger, S., Chli, M., Siegwart, R.Y.: Brisk: Binary robust invariant scalable keypoints. In: International Conference on Computer Vision, ICCV, pp. 2548–2555 (2011)
15. Rublee, E., Rabaud, V., Konolige, K., Bradski, G.: Orb: an efficient alternative to sift or surf. In: International Conference on Computer Vision, ICCV, pp. 2564–2571 (2011)
16. Alahi, A., Ortiz, R., Vandergheynst, P.: Freak: Fast retina keypoint. In: IEEE Conference on Computer Vision and Pattern Recognition, CVPR, pp. 510–517 (2012)
17. Trzcinski, T., Christoudias, M., Fua, P., Lepetit, V.: Boosting binary keypoint descriptors. In: IEEE Conference on Computer Vision and Pattern Recognition, CVPR, pp. 2874–2881 (2013)
18. Heinly, J., Dunn, E., Frahm, J.-M.: Comparative evaluation of binary features. In: Fitzgibbon, A., Lazebnik, S., Perona, P., Sato, Y., Schmid, C. (eds.) ECCV 2012, Part II. LNCS, vol. 7573, pp. 759–773. Springer, Heidelberg (2012)
19. Miksik, O., Mikolajczyk, K.: Evaluation of local detectors and descriptors for fast feature matching. In: International Conference on Pattern Recognition, ICPR, pp. 2681–2684 (2012)

20. Ojala, T., Pietikäinen, M., Mäenpää, T.: Multiresolution gray-scale and rotation invariant texture classification with local binary patterns. IEEE Trans. Pattern Anal. Machine Intell. **24**, 971–987 (2002)
21. Arof, H., Deravi, F.: Circular neighbourhood and 1-d dft features for texture classification and segmentation. IEE Proc. Vis. Image Signal Process. **145**, 167–172 (1998)
22. Liao, S., Chung, A.: A new subspace learning method in fourier domain for texture classification. In: International Conference on Image Processing, ICIP, pp. 4589–4592 (2010)
23. Maani, R., Kalra, S., Yang, Y.: Rotation invariant local frequency descriptors for texture classification. IEEE Trans. Image Process. **22**, 2409–2419 (2013)
24. Maani, R., Kalra, S., Yang, Y.H.: Noise robust rotation invariant features for texture classification. Pattern Recogn. **46**, 2103–2116 (2013)
25. Maani, R., Kalra, S., Yang, Y.: Robust volumetric texture classification of magnetic resonance images of the brain using local frequency descriptor. IEEE Trans. Image Process. **23**, 4625–4636 (2014)
26. Lazebnik, S., Schmid, C., Ponce, J.: A sparse texture representation using local affine regions. IEEE Trans. Pattern Anal. Machine Intell. **27**, 1265–1278 (2005)
27. Takacs, G., Chandrasekhar, V., Tsai, S.S., Chen, D., Grzeszczuk, R., Girod, B.: Fast computation of rotation-invariant image features by an approximate radial gradient transform. IEEE Trans. Image Process. **22**, 2970–2982 (2013)
28. Winder, S., Hua, G., Brown, M.: Picking the best daisy. In: IEEE Conference on Computer Vision and Pattern Recognition, CVPR, pp. 178–185 (2009)

Robust Binary Feature Using the Intensity Order

Yukyung Choi, Chaehoon Park, Joon-Young Lee, and In So Kweon$^{(\boxtimes)}$

Robotics and Computer Vision Laboratory, KAIST, Daejeon, Korea
iskweon77@kaist.ac.kr

Abstract. Binary features have received much attention with regard to memory and computational efficiency with the emerging demands in the mobile and embedded vision systems fields. In this context, we present a robust binary feature using the intensity order. By analyzing feature regions, we devise a simple but effective strategy to detect keypoints. We adopt an ordinal description and encode the intensity order into a binary descriptor with proper binarization. As a result, our method obtains high repeatability and shows better performance with regard to feature matching with much less storage usage than other conventional features. We evaluate the performance of the proposed binary feature with various experiments, demonstrate its efficiency in terms of storage and computation time, and show its robustness under various geometric and photometric transformations.

1 Introduction

Finding correspondences between images is a fundamental step in many computer vision methods, such as object recognition, image retrieval, and wide-baseline stereo. The key component of a correspondence search is to extract invariant image features, and many computer vision researchers have focused on extracting invariant image features based on their importance.

The main concerns with regard to invariant features are localization accuracy, invariance to geometric and photometric deformations, and distinctiveness to be correctly matched against a large number of features. SIFT [1] and SURF [2] are known as the best known and most widely used methods among all various image features. They find scale-invariant distinctive image regions and represent local regions using feature vectors which are invariant to rotation and illumination changes. The discriminative power of SIFT and SURF has been validated in many computer vision techniques, and variants of these methods are widely used for robust image representation.

Two other important factors pertaining to invariant features are time and space efficiency levels when detecting, matching, and storing features. Recently,

Electronic supplementary material The online version of this chapter (doi:10.1007/978-3-319-16865-4_37) contains supplementary material, which is available to authorized users.

Y. Choi and C. Park—The first and the second authors provided equal contributions to this work.

© Springer International Publishing Switzerland 2015
D. Cremers et al. (Eds.): ACCV 2014, Part I, LNCS 9003, pp. 569–584, 2015.
DOI: 10.1007/978-3-319-16865-4_37

demand has increased for such efficient image features, as mobile and embedded vision systems are emerging for visual searches [3] and for direct 2D to 3D matching [4, 5]. Also, for mobile visual search applications, the amount of data sent over the network needs to be as small as possible so as to reduce latency and lower costs. Several binary features, such as BRIEF [6], ORB [7], BRISK [8] have been developed to describe local image regions with small binary strings which can be matched much faster with the Hamming distance compared to SIFT. However, despite the effort and advances in this area, SIFT has remained the best option for various deformation tasks apart from non-geometric transforms [9].

In this paper, we aim to extract binary features with a method that can achieve matching performance levels comparable to those of SIFT and SURF with even less storage than that required for existing binary features. We apply FAST-like binary tests [10] to reject non-feature regions quickly and present an efficient approximation of the Determinant of the Hessian for robust feature detection with high repeatability. Motivated by earlier work [11], we employ ordinal descriptions of local image measurements for robust representations of feature regions. The ordinal description encodes the rank order of each measurement and is therefore invariant to monotonic deformations of the measurements. Also, an ordinal description is insensitive to moderate rank-order errors, thus enabling the quantization of descriptions into small-sized binary descriptors without a noticeable degradation in the performance. Experimental results show that our feature outperforms other state-of-the-art binary features with fewer dimensional descriptors in terms of repeatability and matching performance.

2   Related Work

2.1   Feature Detection

The first stage of image feature extraction is to detect interest points, which are known as keypoints. Many feature extractors detect blobs or corners as keypoints because they can be repeatedly detected despite the presence of various geometric and photometric deformations. SIFT [1] convolves images with Gaussian filters at different scales and approximates the Laplacian of the Gaussian using the Difference of Gaussians (DoG) method. SIFT then detects blob-like areas as keypoints by taking the maxima and minima of the Difference of Gaussians (DoG). Scale invariance is obtained from the scale of DoG. Instead of using DoG, SURF [2] uses an approximated Determinant of Hessian measure via box filters which are implemented efficiently using an integral image. Harris corner [12] is the best known corner detector; it uses the second moment matrix, also known as the auto-correlation matrix. Harris-Affine [13] introduces a multi-scale version of Harris corner. FAST [10, 14] is one of the fastest keypoint detectors. FAST is considered as a modification of SUSAN [15], demonstrating that a simple segment test is enough to detect corner-like areas. AGAST [16] improves FAST with an adaptive and generic accelerated segment test. CensurE [17] introduces a scale-invariant center-surround detector. A simplified center-surround filter with an integral image is used for efficiency, and non-features are removed by a Harris measure. FRIF [18] is a fast approximated LoG (FALoG) detector based on the Harris matrix. FALoG can be quickly computed by means of factorization with an integral image while preserving the properties of LoG. BRISK [8] and ORB [7] use multi-scale FAST for scale-invariance and efficiency. Inspired by SURF and FAST, we use a simple sampling pattern to measure and classify features and non-features.

2.2 Feature Description

A descriptor encodes the local image information around a keypoint. It is used to distinguish keypoints under various transformations. SIFT descriptor describes a local image patch using a gradient histogram. It quantizes gradient orientations and accumulates gradient magnitudes into an orientation histogram with eight bins over 4×4 sub-regions. The form of the SURF descriptor is similar to that of the SIFT descriptor. Instead of quantizing gradient orientations, the SURF descriptor computes a histogram with four bins, dx, dy, $|dx|$, and $|dy|$. There are many SIFT variants, such as GLOH and DAISY. GLOH [19] uses a polar arrangement of sub-regions and DAISY [20] uses a flower-like spatial division for dense descriptions.

Because gradient-based descriptors can only deal with linear deformations, rank-order-based methods have been proposed to handle more general non-linear deformations. Rank-order-based methods such as SIFT-Rank [11] and LUCID [21] encode *relative* order information rather than raw values such as the gradient and intensity. Wang et al. [22] propose a Local Intensity Order Pattern (LIOP) to encode the local ordinal information and create a histogram of the LIOP for each ordinal sub-region. Motivated by these methods, we introduce a new binary descriptor using ordinal information.

In the computer-vision community, recent progress has shown that a simple brightness comparison test is a good choice when attempting to generate a robust binary descriptor. BRIEF [6] presents a binary feature using an intensity difference test and demonstrates a high recognition rate with low computational complexity during the feature construction and matching processes, though it is not designed to be rotationally invariant. BRISK [8] is a combination of the scale-normalized FAST keypoint detector and the BRISK descriptor. BRISK divides point pairs into two groups: long-distance pairs and short-distance pairs. It calculates the characteristic pattern direction using long-distance pairs and computes the descriptor using intensity comparisons of short-distance pairs after rotation- and scale-normalization. ORB [7] demonstrates that the steered BRIEF loses discriminancy from rotation-normalization and introduces rBRIEF, which uses a learning strategy to recover from the loss of variance in steered BRIEF. The rBRIEF method demonstrates variance and correlation improvements over the steered BRIEF. Inspired by the human visual system, FREAK [23] uses the learning strategy of ORB with a DAISY-like sampling pattern [20]. For our feature description, we apply a similar sampling pattern with BRISK, but we generate a binary string using a different strategy based on the rank order.

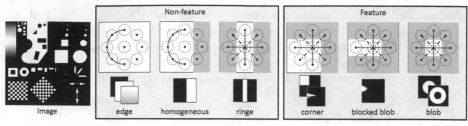

(a) Abstractive representation of six classes of local image region

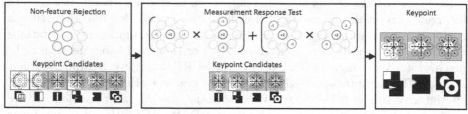

(b) Pipeline for keypoint detection

Fig. 1. The proposed feature detection algorithm.

3   Keypoint Detector

For fast keypoint detection, previous binary features [6–8] adopt the FAST detector [10] with modifications such as the scale-space feature and/or a Harris filter to obtain additional scale and rotation invariances. While these methods obtain very fast detection results, they have relatively low repeatability levels compared to SIFT and SURF, as will be shown in Sect. 5.1. Repeatability is one of the most important properties of a keypoint detector for localization accuracy.

We introduce a new keypoint detection algorithm in an effort to improve the repeatability. We apply a FAST-like binary comparison test and propose a keypoint measure to balance computational efficiency and repeatability performance.

We initially analyze the tendencies of image patches and categorize these into six types, *homogeneous*, *edge*, *ridge*, *corner*, *blob*, and *blocked blob*. Abstractive representations of the six types of local image regions are given in Fig. 1(a). For repeatable keypoint detection robust to image deformations, we detect corner and blob regions as keypoints and reject homogeneous, edge, and ridge regions as non-features. Therefore, we consider the *homogeneous*, *edge*, and *ridge* types as non-feature regions and the *corner*, *blob*, and *blocked blob* types as feature regions.

The overall pipeline for our keypoint detection is depicted in Fig. 1(b). For a given local image patch, we compute the differences between the intensities of a center and surrounding points and assign the *similar* label when the difference is under a certain threshold, assigning the *dissimilar* label otherwise. If more than five surrounding points have *similar* labels, the region is classified as a non-feature region because the *homogeneous* and *edge* types apply in this case. Classification between other categories also may be possible with additional rule-based comparison tests. However, we use another measure for classification in this case instead of adding more rules for robust and repeatable keypoint detections.

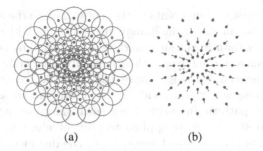

(a)   (b)

Fig. 2. Sample pattern of our descriptor with N = 80 points. (a) The blue dots indicate sampling points, the red circles show the radii corresponding to the standard deviation of a box kernel that is used to smooth intensity values around sampling points. (b) The red lines denote the predefined local directional vector at each sampling point and those are used for estimating dominant orientation (Color figure online).

When we compute the difference between intensity levels on a central and a surrounding point, large differences arise along a single axis in *ridge*-type regions. For *corner*- and *blob*-type regions, large differences arise along two perpendicular directions $(+, \times)$. We use this characteristic as a keypoint measure and formulate an equation to have high response values for features and low response values for non-features. The proposed keypoint measure μ is defined as

$$\mu - (2I_C - I_L - I_R)(2I_C - I_T - I_B) + (2I_C - I_{TL} - I_{BR})(2I_C - I_{TR} - I_{BL}), \quad (1)$$

where $I_{C,L,R,T,B}$ represents the intensities of the center, left, right, top, and bottom locations. This measure can be seen as an approximation of the Determinant of Hessian (DoH). Here, $(2I_C - I_L - I_R)$ denotes the second-order partial derivatives in the x direction and $(2I_C - I_T - I_B)$ denotes second-order partial derivatives in the y direction. Similarly, $(2I_C - I_{TL} - I_{BR})$ and $(2I_C - I_{TR} - I_{BL})$ represent the second-order partial derivative in the xy direction. The keypoint measure μ has a large response on corner or blob regions; therefore, we finally classify locations as keypoints when there are large keypoint responses.

In practice, we construct a scale-space for scale invariance and sample intensities from one center and eight surrounding points. The surrounding points are centrally symmetric and equidistant from the center point, as depicted in Fig. 1.

4   Descriptor

In this section, we present a new binary descriptor using the intensity order. Given a keypoint location with a scale, we extract pattern intensities from a sampling pattern and determine the dominant orientation for rotation invariance. Then, we establish the rank order of the pattern intensities and binarize it to produce a binary descriptor.

4.1   Sampling Pattern

To generate the descriptor, we use a sampling pattern, as shown in Fig. 2(a). As in previous methods, we sample intensities from a spatial division of the polar form. We assign more sampling points to the center than to the surrounding areas according to the retina model of the human visual system, which has a higher cell density at the center than in the surrounding areas [23]. The central part is less affected than the surrounding areas when there are geometric transformations; therefore, it is beneficial to assign more points to the center. The sampling pattern consists of one center point and 79 surrounding points around the center.

We sample the pattern intensity from each sampling point with spatial smoothing. Spatial smoothing is applied to prevent aliasing, and the scale of the smoothing region is determined according to the distances between adjacent sampling points. In Fig. 2(a), the blue dots indicate the sampling points and the red circles represent the radius corresponding to the standard deviation of the smoothing kernels.

4.2   Dominant Orientation

For rotation invariance, we estimate the dominant orientation of a keypoint and construct a descriptor vector along the dominant orientation. The dominant orientation is determined by the weighted average of the local directional vectors. Each local directional vector is oriented toward the center point from a sampling point, and its magnitude set such that it is inversely proportional to the distance from the sampling points and to the center point. Figure 2(b) shows the local directional vectors. The red lines show the directions of the local vectors, and the lengths of these lines indicate the magnitudes of the vectors.

The weight of each local directional vector is assigned as the difference between its pattern intensity and the median of the pattern intensities. With the pattern intensities and predefined local directional vectors, the dominant orientation θ of a keypoint is computed as

$$\theta = \arctan \sum_{i=1}^{N} |I_i - M| \frac{dy_i}{dx_i} \quad \text{s.t.} \quad M = \operatorname*{median}_{i \in \{1,...,N\}} (I_i), \tag{2}$$

where N is the total number of sampling points, I_i represents an ith pattern intensity, M is the median of pattern intensities, and (dx, dy) indicates a local directional vector.

4.3   Binary Descriptor

We employ an ordinal description of pattern intensities. The ordinal description for an invariant feature was introduced in earlier work [11]. It describes each measurement using its rank order with sorted measurement values. Employing the ordinal description technique is shown to have strong discriminative power and to be invariant to monotonic deformations of embedding measurements. While the ordinal description has good invariance characteristics for many deformations, it is not designed for use with binary descriptors. The binary descriptor is of greater

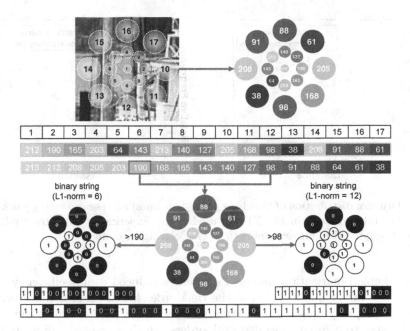

Fig. 3. The overall process of our binary description, which is explained in Sect. 4.3.

importance due to its compact storage size and fast matching performance. To take advantage of both approaches, we present an ordinal binary descriptor.

After determining the dominant orientation, we obtain a measurement vector by tracing the pattern intensities aligned with the dominant orientation. Then, we transform the measurement vector into a rank-order vector by computing the rank of each element value in the measurement vector. Our descriptor is formed by binarizing the rank-order vector. The binarization process is performed by means of a binary comparison test of a certain threshold rank. Our binary descriptor D with the binary comparison test is denoted as

$$D = \sum_{j=1}^{k}\sum_{i=1}^{N} 2^{N(j-1)} 2^{i-1} b_i, \quad \text{s.t.} \quad b_i = \begin{cases} 1, & r_i \geq T_j \\ 0, & otherwise, \end{cases} \quad (3)$$

where N is the total number of sampling points, k is the number of threshold values, T_j represents a jth threshold rank, and r_i denotes the ith element of the rank-order vector. Given N and k, we determine the threshold rank T as

$$T_j = \frac{j}{k+1} N, \quad \text{s.t.} \quad j \in \{1, ..., k\}. \quad (4)$$

We set the number of threshold values k to 2 throughout the paper; therefore, our descriptor becomes a 160-dimensional binary descriptor with 80 sampling points. The overall process of our binary description is illustrated in Fig. 3.

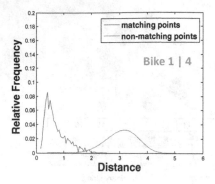 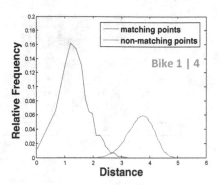

Fig. 4. Distance distribution of matching pairs (blue lines) and non-matching pairs (red lines). The Bikes dataset in Fig. 5 (c) is used in this experiment. (a) Intensity-based ordinal descriptor (b) Our descriptor ($k = 2$) (Color figure online).

Our simple binarization process experiences reduced coding efficiency compared to the direct quantization of the rank order into 2^k ranks. However, the important property of our binarization process is that we can utilize the Hamming distance to compare encoded rank orders, which is one order of magnitude faster than the Euclidean distance.

Ordinal descriptions are insensitive to moderate rank-order errors, which enables us to quantize rank-order descriptions into binary descriptors without a noticeable degradation in the performance. Figure 4 shows a comparison of an intensity-based ordinal descriptor and our quantized binary descriptor. For this experiment, the intensity-based ordinal descriptor directly employs the rank orders as a descriptor, while our descriptor uses the binarized version of the intensity-based ordinal descriptor according to Eq. 3 with $k = 2$. The distributions of the two descriptors are very similar, indicating that our descriptor retains the discriminative power of the intensity-based ordinal descriptor even after binarization with $k = 2$.

Also, as illustrated in Sect. 5, we achieve good performance only with two threshold values, which shows that the reduction in the coding efficiency is very small while the gain in the computational efficiency is considerable.

4.4 Comparison to Other Descriptors

Our descriptor is closely related to ordinal descriptors [11, 21, 22] and binary descriptors [6–8, 23] based on a brightness comparison test. For clarity, we present a description of the similarities and the differences between the proposed method and two category descriptors.

Ordinal Descriptor. The SIFT-Rank and the proposed descriptor are similar in terms of their use of ordinal information to take advantage of ordinal descriptions which are invariant to any monotonic transformations of the raw measurements. SIFT-Rank encodes ordinal information from raw SIFT descriptor values and the proposed descriptor utilizes the rank of the pattern intensities to describe a keypoint. The difference between the two methods is as follows. SIFT-Rank utilizes post-processing of the gradient-based SIFT descriptor and is therefore not designed to improve the time and storage efficiency. Also, SIFT-Rank uses a rank-order vector as a descriptor directly; thus, it may require specialized matching metrics. On the other hand, the proposed descriptor is an independent descriptor that uses the rank of the pattern intensities. It is also a binary descriptor with an elaborate binarization method. This allows the proposed descriptor to have very efficient time performance with low memory usage.

Binary Descriptor. The similarity between existing binary descriptors and the proposed descriptor is the use of a brightness comparison test to binarize a descriptor. The difference between them lies in the method used to select point pairs for the binary test. In existing binary descriptors, those point pairs are fixed to all keypoints. BRIEF chooses point pairs randomly or it depends on a certain distribution. BRISK uses the distance between point pairs as a condition and selects some from all possible point pairs. ORB selects point pairs according to decreases in correlations and increases in the degree of variation. Instead of predetermining point pairs for the binary test, our method implicitly selects point pairs based on an analysis of the pattern intensity distribution.

In the next section, it will be shown through experiments that our method shows better or comparable results relative to those of existing methods with fewer bits.

5   Experiments

To validate the performance of the proposed feature detector and descriptor, we conduct experiments using publicly available evaluation toolkits and datasets. First, we give a brief description of the experimental configuration, after which we present the experimental results pertaining to the detector and descriptor evaluations. In this evaluation, we mainly compare our method to methods that proposed both a detector and a descriptor simultaneously.

Evaluation toolkits and Dataset. Our method was mainly tested using the evaluation toolkits proposed by Mikolajczyk *et al.* [24], Mikolajczyk and Schmid [19], and the OpenCV-Features-Comparison toolkits (CVT)[1]. The evaluation codes are available on the authors' webpage. With the evaluation toolkits, we perform the evaluations using the dataset used in earlier studies [19,24]. There are eight datasets with different geometric and photometric transformations. These transformations include brightness changes (Leuven), JPEG compression (UBC), blur (bikes and tress), zoom and rotation (bark and boat), and view-point changes (graffiti and wall). Each set consists of six images with gradually increasing levels of transformation. The dataset provides homographies between the first and the other images, and the homographies are used to estimate ground-truth matches. Figure 5 shows sample images of the dataset.

---

[1] http://computer-vision-talks.com/2011/08/feature-descriptor-comparison-report/.

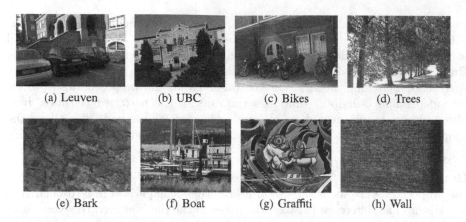

(a) Leuven   (b) UBC   (c) Bikes   (d) Trees

(e) Bark   (f) Boat   (g) Graffiti   (h) Wall

Fig. 5. Example images of Mikolajczyk and Schmid's dataset used for evaluation: brightness (Leuven), JPEG compression (UBC), blur (Bikes, Trees), zoom and rotation (Bark, Boat), viewpoint change (Graffiti, Wall).

Experimental Settings. We compare our method to the state-of-the-art keypoint detectors and descriptors of SIFT, SURF, STAR, ORB, and BRISK. STAR uses only a keypoint detector while the other methods use both detectors and descriptors. All of the compared methods are implemented in OpenCV 2.4.5, and we use the library with default parameters, except for ORB. For ORB, we set the number of features adaptively to have it extract the same number of features used by our method. We present more detailed information about each method in Table 1.

5.1   Repeatability Performance

Mikolajczyk *et al.* [24] proposed the concept of *repeatability* to evaluate the performance levels of keypoint detectors. Repeatability measures how much the keypoints detected from two images overlap the same regions. It is a desirable property for invariant local features, as a high degree of repeatability refers to the robustness of a keypoint detector under various transformations.

We evaluate the performance of the detectors according to a method used in earlier work [24]. Figure 6 shows the evaluation results pertaining to the repeatability of each detector under various transformations. SURF shows high repeatability over all images. For binary features, BRISK has relatively low repeatability and ORB has different appearances depending on the dataset. Both binary features commonly have low repeatability for scale changes, as they are based on multi-scale FAST, which is oriented for fast keypoint detections. The proposed method demonstrates repeatability performance similar to that of SURF because both methods detect keypoints using approximated DoH measures.

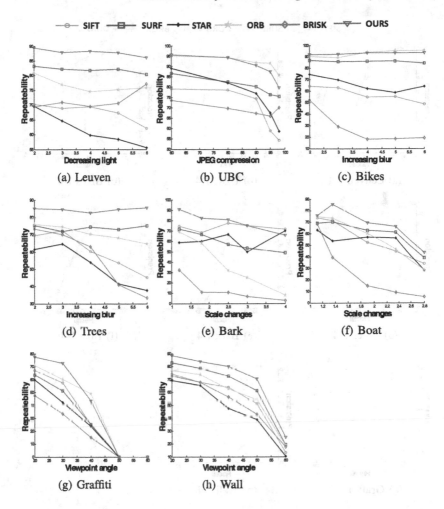

Fig. 6. Repeatability of keypoint detection.

5.2   Matching Performance

We evaluate the matching performance using Mikolajczyk and Schmids evaluation toolkit [19] and the CVT toolkit. Their evaluation toolkit [19] is publicly
available and evaluates descriptors by means of a precision-recall approach. The
CVT toolkit evaluates the performances of descriptors using synthetically transformed images. This evaluation tool provides brightness, blur, rotation, and scale
changes as the transformations.

Precision-Recall. Figure 7 shows the evaluation results using the aforementioned descriptor evaluation toolkit [19]. Both the SIFT and the proposed methods outperform the other methods in general. Specifically, SIFT outperforms
other methods in terms of scale and rotation transformations, and our method

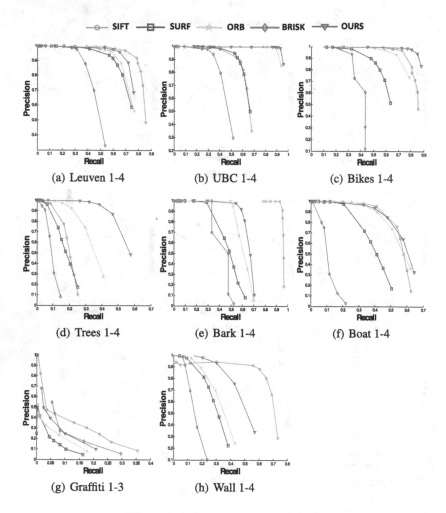

Fig. 7. Precision-recall performance.

shows good performance with transformations of brightness changes, blurring, and JPEG images.

CVT Toolkit. As the second matching experiment, the CVT evaluation toolkit is used and the degree of transformation is finely adjusted for the evaluation. Figure 8 shows the performance with each level of transformation. SIFT generally shows good performance, as shown in the previous precision-recall test. SURF shows matching performance that follows SIFT. ORB shows relatively strong performance compared to BRISK; however, both methods do not perform as well as SURF or SIFT. Our method specifically shows robustness to brightness changes and Gaussian blurring. Our method approaches state-of-the-art performance levels with relatively few bits.

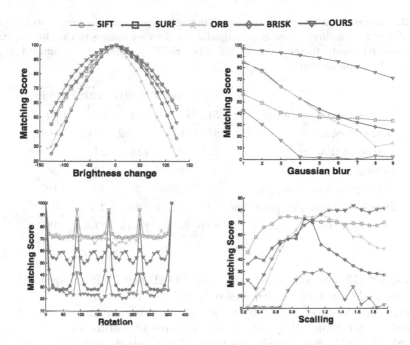

Fig. 8. Matching performance under four kinds of transformations (Brightness change, Gaussian blur, Rotation and Scaling)

Table 1. Feature detectors used for evaluation. Information about each feature detector is summarized.

	SIFT	SURF	ORB	BRISK	Ours
Non-feature removal	edge	-	FAST	FAST	FAST-variant
Detector measure	DoG	DoH	Harris	FAST	DoH-variant
Sampling pattern	grid	grid	polar	polar	polar
Dimensions	128	64	256	256	160
Storage/dimension	4bytes	4bytes	1bit	1bit	1bit
Feature information	gradient	gradient	intensity	intensity	order of intensity

5.3   Storage and Time

All experiments are performed using an Intel i7 3.4 GHz processor without multi-core parallelism. Table 2 summarizes the computation time and storage amounts for feature extractions, descriptions, and matching using the Boat dataset. To measure the computation time, we run 100 trials for each task and average them after dropping the best 10 % and worst 10 % of the results. For matching, we use a brute-force method.

The storage of the proposed descriptor is the lowest among the compared methods. SIFT and SURF are 128- and 64-dimensional floating descriptors

Table 2. Computation time and storage. The table represents storage, feature detection, and description time. Time is measured using the first images in the Boat dataset. SIFT shows relatively faster than SURF since SIFT is delicately optimized in the OpenCV 2.4.5 implementation.

	SIFT	SURF	ORB	BRISK	Ours
Storage/keypoint [bytes]	512	256	64	64	20
# of keypoints	8802	6752	5682	2442	5682
Detection time [ms]	221	278	19	27	67
Description time [ms]	506	961	16	12	38
Total extraction time [ms]	727	1239	35	43	105
Description time/keypoint [ns]	57.5	142.3	2.8	4.9	6.7
Total time/keypoint [ns]	82.6	183.5	6.16	17.6	18.4

which require 512 and 256 bytes, respectively. ORB and BRISK require 64 bytes (512 bits), while our method requires only 20 bytes (160 bits).

Though our method is not fully optimized, it is nonetheless one order of magnitude faster than SIFT and SURF in terms of feature extraction and is comparable to ORB and BRISK in a trade-off between detection time efficiency and the repeatability gain. Distance computation times between the descriptors are directly influenced by the descriptor length; therefore, the use of a short descriptor has advantages in terms of the matching time and the amount of required storage. Also, because our descriptor is a binary descriptor consisting of 0s and 1s, we can use a bitwise XOR operator to compare two descriptors with the Hamming distance, which is much more efficient than the Euclidean distance.

6   Conclusions

In this paper, we presented a robust binary feature using the intensity order. We achieved better detection results than other binary features in terms of repeatability. For robust feature descriptions, we employ an ordinal description which is invariant to monotonic transformations. We also presented a binarization method which encodes the intensity order into a binary descriptor, which enables us to take advantage of better storage and computational efficiency. We evaluated the proposed binary feature with various experiments and demonstrated that our feature shows performance analogous to that of SIFT and that it outperforms other binary features under various transformations with much less storage use for feature descriptions.

Acknowledgement. We would like to thank Jungho Kim and Jiyoung Jung for their support. This work was supported by the National Research Foundation of Korea(NRF) grant funded by the Korea government (No. 2010-0028680).

References

1. Lowe, D.G.: Distinctive image features from scale-invariant keypoints. Int. J. Comput. Vis. (IJCV) **60**, 91–110 (2004)
2. Bay, H., Ess, A., Tuytelaars, T., Van Gool, L.: Speeded-up robust features (surf). Comput. Vis. Image Underst. (CVIU) **110**, 346–359 (2008)
3. Chandrasekhar, V., Takacs, G., Chen, D.M., Tsai, S.S., Reznik, Y.A., Grzeszczuk, R., Girod, B.: Compressed histogram of gradients: A low-bitrate descriptor. Int. J. Comput. Vis. (IJCV) **96**, 384–399 (2012)
4. Sattler, T., Leibe, B., Kobbelt, L.: Fast image-based localization using direct 2d-to-3d matching. In: Proceedings of International Conference on Computer Vision (ICCV), pp. 667–674 (2011)
5. Li, Y., Snavely, N., Huttenlocher, D., Fua, P.: Worldwide pose estimation using 3D point clouds. In: Fitzgibbon, A., Lazebnik, S., Perona, P., Sato, Y., Schmid, C. (eds.) ECCV 2012, Part I. LNCS, vol. 7572, pp. 15–29. Springer, Heidelberg (2012)
6. Calonder, M., Lepetit, V., Strecha, C., Fua, P.: BRIEF: binary robust independent elementary features. In: Daniilidis, K., Maragos, P., Paragios, N. (eds.) ECCV 2010, Part IV. LNCS, vol. 6314, pp. 778–792. Springer, Heidelberg (2010)
7. Rublee, E., Rabaud, V., Konolige, K., Bradski, G.R.: Orb: An efficient alternative to sift or surf. In: Proceedings of International Conference on Computer Vision (ICCV), pp. 2564–2571 (2011)
8. Leutenegger, S., Chli, M., Siegwart, R.: Brisk: Binary robust invariant scalable keypoints. In: Proceedings of International Conference on Computer Vision (ICCV), pp. 2548–2555 (2011)
9. Heinly, J., Dunn, E., Frahm, J.-M.: Comparative evaluation of binary features. In: Fitzgibbon, A., Lazebnik, S., Perona, P., Sato, Y., Schmid, C. (eds.) ECCV 2012, Part II. LNCS, vol. 7573, pp. 759–773. Springer, Heidelberg (2012)
10. Rosten, E., Porter, R., Drummond, T.: Faster and better: A machine learning approach to corner detection. IEEE Trans. Pattern Anal. Mach. Intell. (PAMI) **32**, 105–119 (2010)
11. Toews, M., Wells III, W.: Sift-rank: Ordinal description for invariant feature correspondence. In: Proceedings of IEEE Conference on Computer Vision and Pattern Recognition (CVPR), pp. 172–177 (2009)
12. Harris, C., Stephens, M.: A combined corner and edge detection. In: Proceedings of the Fourth Alvey Vision Conference, pp. 147–151 (1988)
13. Mikolajczyk, K., Schmid, C.: Scale and affine invariant interest point detectors. Int. J. Comput. Vis. (IJCV) **60**, 63–86 (2004)
14. Rosten, E., Drummond, T.: Machine learning for high-speed corner detection. In: Leonardis, A., Bischof, H., Pinz, A. (eds.) ECCV 2006, Part I. LNCS, vol. 3951, pp. 430–443. Springer, Heidelberg (2006)
15. Smith, S.M., Brady, J.M.: SUSAN-a new approach to low level image processing. Int. J. Comput. Vis. (IJCV) **23**, 45–78 (1997)
16. Mair, E., Hager, G.D., Burschka, D., Suppa, M., Hirzinger, G.: Adaptive and generic corner detection based on the accelerated segment test. In: Daniilidis, K., Maragos, P., Paragios, N. (eds.) ECCV 2010, Part II. LNCS, vol. 6312, pp. 183–196. Springer, Heidelberg (2010)
17. Agrawal, M., Konolige, K., Blas, M.R.: CenSurE: center surround extremas for realtime feature detection and matching. In: Forsyth, D., Torr, P., Zisserman, A. (eds.) ECCV 2008, Part IV. LNCS, vol. 5305, pp. 102–115. Springer, Heidelberg (2008)

18. Wang, Z., Fan, B., Wu, F.: Frif:fast robust invariant feature. In: Proceedings of British Machine Vision Conference (BMVC) (2013)
19. Mikolajczyk, K., Schmid, C.: A performance evaluation of local descriptors. IEEE Trans. Pattern Anal. Mach. Intell. (PAMI) **27**, 1615–1630 (2005)
20. Tola, E., Lepetit, V., Fua, P.: Daisy: An efficient dense descriptor applied to wide-baseline stereo. IEEE Trans. Pattern Anal. Mach. Intell. (PAMI) **32**, 815–830 (2010)
21. Ziegler, A., Christiansen, E.M., Kriegman, D.J., Belongie, S.J.: Locally uniform comparison image descriptor. In: Neural Information Processing Systems (NIPS), pp. 1–9 (2012)
22. Wang, Z., Fan, B., Wu, F.: Local intensity order pattern for feature description. In: Proceedings of International Conference on Computer Vision (ICCV), pp. 603–610 (2011)
23. Alahi, A., Ortiz, R., Vandergheynst, P.: Freak: Fast retina keypoint. In: Proceedings of IEEE Conference on Computer Vision and Pattern Recognition (CVPR), pp. 510–517 (2012)
24. Mikolajczyk, K., Tuytelaars, T., Schmid, C., Zisserman, A., Matas, J., Schaffalitzky, F., Kadir, T., Gool, L.V.: A comparison of affine region detectors. Int. J. Comput. Vis. (IJCV) **65**, 43–72 (2005)

Minimal Solution for Computing Pairs of Lines in Non-central Cameras

Jesus Bermudez-Cameo[1]($\boxtimes$), João P. Barreto[2], Gonzalo Lopez-Nicolas[1], and Jose J. Guerrero[1]

[1] Instituto de Investigación en Ingeniería de Aragón,
Universidad de Zaragoza, Zaragoza, Spain
{bermudez,gonlopez,josechu.guerrero}@unizar.es
[2] Institute of Systems and Robotics,
University of Coimbra, 3030 Coimbra, Portugal
jpbar@deec.uc.pt

Abstract. In non-central cameras, the complete geometry of a 3D line is mapped to each corresponding projection, therefore each line can be theoretically recovered from a single view. However, the solution of this problem is ill-conditioned due to the lack of effective baseline between rays. This limitation prevents from a practical implementation of the approach if lines are not close to the visual system. In this paper, we exploit additional geometric constraints to improve the results of line reconstruction from single images in non-central systems. In particular, we obtain the minimal solution for the case of a pair of intersecting orthogonal lines and for the case of a pair of parallel lines considering three rays from each line. The proposal has been evaluated with simulations and tested with real images.

1 Introduction

In any central camera the projection surface of a 3D line is a plane. Any line contained in this plane is projected on the same line-image, and therefore two of the four degrees of freedom (DOF) of the 3D line are lost in the projection. By contrast, in certain non-central cameras (non-central implies that the projecting rays do not intersect in a common point) the projection surface of a line is a ruled surface composed by skew rays (except in certain degenerate cases). Through this surface there exist a unique mapping between a 3D line and its projection on the image (line-image) which can be exploited to recover the geometry of the 3D line from a single image. In particular, four generic rays[1] corresponding to four points on a line projection provide four independent constraints allowing to compute the complete geometry of the 3D line [1]. In practice, this is an

---

Electronic supplementary material The online version of this chapter (doi:10.1007/978-3-319-16865-4_38) contains supplementary material, which is available to authorized users.

[1] Four lines are generic if no two of them are coplanar, no three of them are coconical or cocylindrical, and the four are not cohyperbolic, i.e. do not lie on the same ruled quadric surface.

© Springer International Publishing Switzerland 2015
D. Cremers et al. (Eds.): ACCV 2014, Part I, LNCS 9003, pp. 585–597, 2015.
DOI: 10.1007/978-3-319-16865-4_38

ill-posed problem and the geometry of the 3D line can be only recovered if the relative depth of the line with respect to the system dimensions is low enough for guaranteeing effective baseline between rays.

In this paper we exploit the structure of the scene reducing the number of DOFs of the sought solution. In central systems with conventional cameras this idea is used for inferring layouts from line projections which only provide two independent constraints [2,3] for each line-image. In the case of non-central systems we propose to solve the four DOFs of each line using the redundant independent constraints provided by line projections by imposing geometric constraints between pairs of lines. The proposed geometric constraints are: orthogonal intersection between lines and parallelism between lines reducing to six the number of rays needed for a minimal solution of a pair of lines.

1.1 Previous Work

The basis for computing the geometry of the 3D line from a single line projection (line-image) is that given four generic lines there exist only two lines intersecting them [4,5]. In [1] this reasoning is introduced for application in computer graphics. In [6,7] this approach is exploited to compute 3D lines from 4 rays in non-central systems comparing the linear approach with different computation methods and considering the degeneracies and singular configurations. In [8] the approach is used with spherical catadioptric mirrors, and in addition two non-central systems are used for reconstruction. Work in [9] extends the approach to planar curves. To improve the accuracy in reconstruction some simplifications have been proposed: considering only horizontal lines [10,11] or exploiting cross-ratio properties [12]. In [13] the degeneracies caused by the revolution symmetry are avoided using an off-axis system. More recently in [14] the approach is particularized to the case of conical mirrors allowing to compute both the 3D line and the mirror geometry from a single line projection.

1.2 Contributions

In this paper we present the minimal solution for computing a junction composed by two orthogonal intersecting lines and for computing two parallel lines in non-central systems. This allows to obtain the complete geometry of these pairs of lines from three rays belonging to each line in a calibrated non-central system. The interest of this result can be in robust extraction methods based on minimal sets like RANSAC or in the improvement of the reconstruction accuracy in line fitting. The approach has been implemented for spherical catadioptric systems, using the projection model described in [15]. The proposal has been evaluated in simulation, and tested with real images.

2 Recovering a 3D Line from Four Skew Generic Rays

In this section we present the background, geometric concepts and notation used for computing a 3D line from four generic rays. The description used for lines are the Plücker coordinates based on Grassmann algebra.

2.1 Plücker Coordinates of a Line

The Plücker coordinates of a 3D line is a $\mathbb{P}^5$ representation of a line obtained from the null space of any pair of points $X = \left(x_0, \mathbf{x}^\mathsf{T}\right)^\mathsf{T}$, and $Y = \left(y_0, \mathbf{y}^\mathsf{T}\right)^\mathsf{T}$ belonging to the line. The description of a Plücker line from the coordinates of the defining points are $\mathbf{L} = \left(\mathbf{l}^\mathsf{T}, \bar{\mathbf{l}}^\mathsf{T}\right)^\mathsf{T}$ where $\mathbf{l} \in \mathbb{R}^3$, $\mathbf{l} = x_0\mathbf{y} - y_0\mathbf{x}$ and $\bar{\mathbf{l}} \in \mathbb{R}^3$, $\bar{\mathbf{l}} = \mathbf{x} \times \mathbf{y}$ (depending on the author the order and the sign of the elements can differ, here we follow the standard in [16]).

Notice that not all the elements of the $\mathbb{P}^5$ space correspond to 3D lines. The points of $\mathbb{P}^5$ corresponding to lines in $\mathbb{P}^3$ must hold $\mathbf{l}^\mathsf{T}\bar{\mathbf{l}} = 0$ which is known as Plücker identity. This identity is a quadratic constraint which defines a two dimensional subspace in $\mathbb{P}^5$ called the Klein quadric M_2^4 [16]. Plücker representation has a geometric interpretation in Euclidean geometry. Vector $\mathbf{l}$ represents the direction of $\mathbf{L}$ (see Fig. 1(a)) and $\bar{\mathbf{l}}$ is the moment vector which can be seen as the normal to a plane passing through the 3D line and the origin of the reference system. The Plücker identity expresses the orthogonality of $\mathbf{l}$ and $\bar{\mathbf{l}}$ given that the direction vector must be contained in the plane defined by $\bar{\mathbf{l}}$. $\mathbf{L}$ is an homogeneous vector but when normalizing respect to $\mathbf{l}$, $|\bar{\mathbf{l}}|$ is the minimum distance from the origin to the 3D line. Therefore, when normalizing respect to $\bar{\mathbf{l}}$, $|\mathbf{l}|$ is the inverse of that distance.

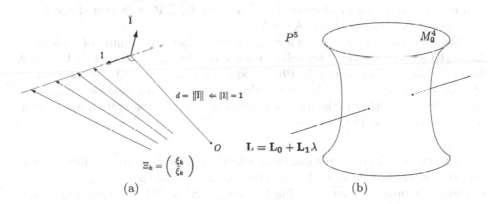

Fig. 1. (a) Plücker description for lines and line projection. (b) One dimensional subspace in $\mathbb{P}^5$ and Klein Quadric.

2.2 Intersection of Rays with a 3D Line

The constraint resulting of the intersection of a 3D line with a projection ray can be expressed linearly by the side operator which defines the signed distance between two lines $\mathbf{L} = \left(\mathbf{l}^\mathsf{T}, \bar{\mathbf{l}}^\mathsf{T}\right)^\mathsf{T}$ and $\mathbf{M} = \left(\mathbf{m}^\mathsf{T}, \bar{\mathbf{m}}^\mathsf{T}\right)^\mathsf{T}$. It is described as

$$side\,(\mathbf{L}, \mathbf{M}) = \mathbf{L}^\mathsf{T}\mathsf{W}\mathbf{M} = \mathbf{l}^\mathsf{T}\bar{\mathbf{m}} + \bar{\mathbf{l}}^\mathsf{T}\mathbf{m} \tag{1}$$

where $\mathsf{W} = \begin{pmatrix} 0_{3\times3} & I_{3\times3} \\ I_{3\times3} & 0_{3\times3} \end{pmatrix}$.

If the Plücker representation of both skew lines is normalized with the direction vector then this distance is metric in $\mathbb{R}^3$. The sign of this distance depends on the *side* where a line is located with respect to the other (clockwise or counterclockwise). The intersection between two lines is given by the constraint $\mathbf{L}^\mathsf{T}\mathsf{W}\mathbf{M} = 0$. Notice that the self-operation ($side\,(\mathbf{L}, \mathbf{L}) = 0$) becomes the Plücker identity.

A 3D line has four degrees of freedom (DOF), as consequence at least four independent constraints are needed to solve the corresponding equations system. In non-central systems, four projection rays provide four independent constraints when they are generic (Fig. 1(a)). Notice that in a central system the four equations are not independent given that the four rays are coplanar.

However, given that Plücker coordinates set (without taking into account the Plücker identity) is an over-parametrized description of a line, the solution of a system of four homogeneous equations in $\mathbb{P}^5$ is a one dimensional subspace of $\mathbb{P}^5$. The solution of these equations system can be expressed as a singular value decomposition problem in which A is the collection of constraints such that $\mathsf{A}\mathbf{L} = \mathbf{0}$ with $\mathsf{A}_i = \left(\bar{\boldsymbol{\xi}}_i^\mathsf{T}, \boldsymbol{\xi}_i^\mathsf{T}\right)$ where A_i is the ith row of A, in order that it can be written as the product of three matrices, U, Σ,V, such that U and V are orthogonal, Σ is diagonal and $\mathsf{A} = \mathsf{U}\Sigma\mathsf{V}^\mathsf{T}$.

The null space of this system is spanned by the last two columns of V (denoted $\mathbf{L}_0$ and $\mathbf{L}_1$ respectively). The null-space can be parametrized by $\mathbf{L} = \mathbf{L}_0 + \mathbf{L}_1\lambda$ (see Fig. 1(b)) and imposing the Plücker identity we can compute the intersection of this subspace with the Klein Quadric obtaining two solutions: One is the sought line, the other is the axis of revolution of the visual system if it is axial or an arbitrary line in other case.

Degeneracies. There are some cases where the four rays are not independent and the system is degenerated. When the camera is axial the defining rays can be coplanar forming a Planar Viewing Surface (PVS) [7]. These degenerated cases are: the Axial-PVS case when the line is coplanar with the axis of symmetry and the Horizontal-PVS case when all the projecting rays lie in an horizontal plane. If the projection surface of the line is a ruled surface defined by only three rays this surface is called a regulus and the system is also under-determined.

3   Orthogonal Junction of Two Lines

In this section we present the minimal solution for a junction of two orthogonal intersecting lines in non-central systems. Computing a junction composed by two orthogonal intersecting lines is a problem with 6 degrees of freedom (DOF). Four DOFs for one of the 3D lines, other for the depth of the line intersection and the 6th DOF for the angle defining the direction of the orthogonal line.

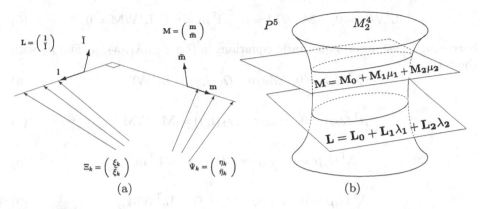

Fig. 2. (a) Orthogonal junction of two lines. (b) Two dimensional subspaces in $\mathbb{P}^5$ and Klein Quadric.

Given the lines $\mathbf{L} = \left(\mathbf{l}^\mathsf{T}, \bar{\mathbf{l}}^\mathsf{T}\right)^\mathsf{T}$, $\mathbf{M} = \left(\mathbf{m}^\mathsf{T}, \bar{\mathbf{m}}^\mathsf{T}\right)^\mathsf{T}$ and considering three generic rays $\boldsymbol{\Xi}_k$ intersecting the line $\mathbf{L}$ and three generic rays $\boldsymbol{\Psi}_k$ intersecting $\mathbf{M}$ (see Fig. 2(a)), the corresponding null spaces of the under determined linear systems

$$\boldsymbol{\Xi}_k^\mathsf{T}\mathsf{W}\mathbf{L} = 0 \quad , \quad \boldsymbol{\Psi}_k^\mathsf{T}\mathsf{W}\mathbf{M} = 0 \tag{2}$$

are two subspaces of dimension 2 in $\mathbb{P}^5$. These subspaces are not contained in the Klein quadric and intersect the Klein quadric in two one-dimensional curves (see Fig. 2(b)). A parametrized description of these 2-dimensional subspaces can be obtained by solving the null space of these systems with a singular value decomposition algorithm.

Taking as example the case of $\mathbf{L}$ and $\boldsymbol{\Xi}_k = \left(\boldsymbol{\xi}_k^\mathsf{T}, \bar{\boldsymbol{\xi}}_k^\mathsf{T}\right)^\mathsf{T}$: the matrix $\mathsf{A} = \begin{bmatrix} \bar{\boldsymbol{\xi}}_1 \ \bar{\boldsymbol{\xi}}_2 \ \bar{\boldsymbol{\xi}}_3 \\ \boldsymbol{\xi}_1 \ \boldsymbol{\xi}_2 \ \boldsymbol{\xi}_3 \end{bmatrix}^\mathsf{T}$ can be written as the product of the three matrices, $\mathsf{A} = \mathsf{U}\boldsymbol{\Sigma}\mathsf{V}^\mathsf{T}$ and the null space is spanned by the three last columns of matrix V denoted as $\mathbf{L}_0$, $\mathbf{L}_1$ and $\mathbf{L}_2$ parametrizing it with $L : \mathbb{P}^2 \mapsto \mathbb{P}^5$ defined as

$$\mathbf{L} = \mathbf{L}_0 + \mathbf{L}_1\lambda_1 + \mathbf{L}_2\lambda_2 \sim \mathsf{L}_m\boldsymbol{\lambda} \tag{3}$$

where $\mathsf{L}_m = \begin{bmatrix} \mathbf{L}_0 \ \mathbf{L}_1 \ \mathbf{L}_2 \end{bmatrix}$ and $\boldsymbol{\lambda} \in \mathbb{P}^2$ with $\boldsymbol{\lambda} = \left(\tilde{\lambda}_0, \tilde{\lambda}_1, \tilde{\lambda}_2\right)^\mathsf{T} \sim (1, \lambda_1, \lambda_2)^\mathsf{T}$.

Analogously, for $\mathbf{M}$ we parametrize the null space with

$$\mathbf{M} = \mathbf{M}_0 + \mathbf{M}_1\lambda_1 + \mathbf{M}_2\lambda_2 \sim \mathsf{M}_m\boldsymbol{\mu} \tag{4}$$

where $\mathsf{M}_m = \begin{bmatrix} \mathbf{M}_0 \ \mathbf{M}_1 \ \mathbf{M}_2 \end{bmatrix}$ and $\boldsymbol{\mu} \in \mathbb{P}^2$ with $\boldsymbol{\mu} = (\tilde{\mu}_0, \tilde{\mu}_1, \tilde{\mu}_2)^\mathsf{T} \sim (1, \mu_1, \mu_2)^\mathsf{T}$.

To obtain the four parameters λ_1, λ_2, μ_1 and μ_2 we need four additional independent constraints. These constraints are the condition of belonging at the Klein quadric for both lines, the perpendicularity between them and the intersection between them. These constraints are explicitly defined by

$$\mathbf{L}^{\mathsf{T}}\mathbf{WL} = 0, \quad \mathbf{M}^{\mathsf{T}}\mathbf{WM} = 0, \quad \mathbf{1}^{\mathsf{T}}\mathbf{m} = 0, \quad \mathbf{L}^{\mathsf{T}}\mathbf{WM} = 0 \tag{5}$$

becoming a system of 4 quadratic equations in terms of λ_1, λ_2, μ_1 and μ_2 with the form

$$\boldsymbol{\lambda}^{\mathsf{T}}\Omega_1\boldsymbol{\lambda} = 0 \quad \text{where} \quad \Omega_1(i,j) = \mathbf{L}_i^{\mathsf{T}}\mathbf{WL}_j \tag{6}$$

$$\boldsymbol{\mu}^{\mathsf{T}}\Omega_2\boldsymbol{\mu} = 0 \quad \text{where} \quad \Omega_2(i,j) = \mathbf{M}_i^{\mathsf{T}}\mathbf{WM}_j \tag{7}$$

$$\boldsymbol{\lambda}^{\mathsf{T}}\Omega_3\boldsymbol{\mu} = 0 \quad \text{where} \quad \Omega_3(i,j) = \mathbf{1}_i^{\mathsf{T}}\mathbf{m}_j \tag{8}$$

$$\boldsymbol{\lambda}^{\mathsf{T}}\Omega_4\boldsymbol{\mu} = 0 \quad \text{where} \quad \Omega_4(i,j) = \mathbf{L}_i^{\mathsf{T}}\mathbf{WM}_j. \tag{9}$$

This system can be manipulated to reduce the number of dimensions but increasing the degree of equations. Given the Eqs. (8) and (9), imagine the $\mathbb{P}^2$ space of $\boldsymbol{\lambda}$ and the lines depending on $\boldsymbol{\mu}$:

$$\mathbf{U} = \Omega_3\boldsymbol{\mu} \quad , \quad \mathbf{V} = \Omega_4\boldsymbol{\mu} \tag{10}$$

Solving these equations for $\boldsymbol{\lambda}$

$$\begin{bmatrix} \mathbf{U}^{\mathsf{T}} \\ \mathbf{V}^{\mathsf{T}} \end{bmatrix}\boldsymbol{\lambda} = 0 \tag{11}$$

we obtain an explicit linear morphism

$$\boldsymbol{\lambda} = \mathsf{C}\hat{\boldsymbol{\mu}} \tag{12}$$

where $\hat{\boldsymbol{\mu}} = \left(\tilde{\mu}_0^2, \tilde{\mu}_0\tilde{\mu}_1, \tilde{\mu}_0\tilde{\mu}_2, \tilde{\mu}_1^2, \tilde{\mu}_1\tilde{\mu}_2, \tilde{\mu}_2^2\right)^{\mathsf{T}} \sim \left(1, \mu_1, \mu_2, \mu_1^2, \mu_1\mu_2, \mu_2^2\right)^{\mathsf{T}}$ and $\mathsf{C}_{3\times 6}$ is computed analytically.

Substituting $\boldsymbol{\lambda}$ in Eq. (6) we have a system of two equations with two unknowns, the first is a quartic expression and the second a quadratic equation.

$$\hat{\boldsymbol{\mu}}^{\mathsf{T}}\mathsf{C}^{\mathsf{T}}\Omega_1\mathsf{C}\hat{\boldsymbol{\mu}} = 0 \tag{13}$$

$$\boldsymbol{\mu}^{\mathsf{T}}\Omega_2\boldsymbol{\mu} = 0 \tag{14}$$

Substituting (14) in (13) we obtain a single polynomial equation with one unknown of degree 8 which can be solved for μ_1.

$$\sum_{i=0}^{8} c_i\mu_1^i = 0 \tag{15}$$

From the fundamental theorem of algebra we know that the number of solutions of this polynomial is 8. Using Eq. (14) we obtain 2 solutions of μ_2 from each solution for μ_1. One solution of (λ_1, λ_2) is obtained from each solution (μ_1, μ_2) (12), therefore the maximum number of solutions is 16. However, the majority of them are removed considering only real solutions, compatible with the equations and coherent with the orientation of the defining rays. Usually only 2 solutions remain.

4   Two Parallel Lines

In this section we present the minimal solution for computing the geometry of two parallel lines in non-central systems. Computing two parallel lines is a problem with 6 DOFs: in this particular case two DOFs for the common direction and two additional DOFs for each line. From three generic rays $\boldsymbol{\Xi}_k$ intersecting a line $\mathbf{L}$ and three generic rays $\boldsymbol{\Psi}_k$ intersecting a line $\mathbf{M}$ we compute the two dimensional subspaces (see Fig. 2(b)),

$$\mathbf{L} = \mathbf{L}_0 + \mathbf{L}_1\lambda_1 + \mathbf{L}_2\lambda_2 \sim \mathsf{L}_m\boldsymbol{\lambda} \tag{16}$$
$$\mathbf{M} = \mathbf{M}_0 + \mathbf{M}_1\lambda_1 + \mathbf{M}_2\lambda_2 \sim \mathsf{M}_m\boldsymbol{\mu} \tag{17}$$

To obtain the four parameters λ_1, λ_2, μ_1 and μ_2 we need four additional constraints. First two are the constraint for each line of being in the Klein quadric or being a line,

$$\mathbf{L}^\mathsf{T}\mathbf{W}\mathbf{L} = 0, \tag{18}$$

$$\mathbf{M}^\mathsf{T}\mathbf{W}\mathbf{M} = 0 . \tag{19}$$

The constraint of being parallels can be expressed as follows,

$$\mathbf{l} = (\mathbf{l}_0 + \mathbf{l}_1\lambda_1 + \mathbf{l}_2\lambda_2) - K(\mathbf{m}_0 + \mathbf{m}_1\mu_1 + \mathbf{m}_2\mu_2) , \tag{20}$$

which means three equations involving an additional unknown K. From (20) it is possible to compute $\boldsymbol{\mu}$ in terms of $\boldsymbol{\lambda}$ obtaining the linear mapping between $\boldsymbol{\mu}$ and $\boldsymbol{\lambda}$

$$\boldsymbol{\mu} = (\mathbf{m}_0, \mathbf{m}_1, \mathbf{m}_2)^{-1} (\mathbf{l}_0, \mathbf{l}_1, \mathbf{l}_2) \boldsymbol{\lambda}. \tag{21}$$

Substituting $\boldsymbol{\mu}$ in Eq. (19) we obtain two quadratic equations (18) and (19) depending on $\boldsymbol{\lambda}$, which can be considered as the intersection between two conics in $\mathbb{P}^2$ having four solutions.

5   Simulations

In this section we evaluate the proposed method performing simulations of the line fitting process. As reference method we take the approach of Teller et al. [1] which is denoted as unconstrained linear method.

We consider two different cases: orthogonal junctions and parallel lines. In both cases, a collection of 100 pairs of lines are randomly generated. The length of the lines is 20 m. In the case of a junction, the intersection between each pair of lines is located in a cube of side 4 m(see Fig. 3(a)). In the case of parallel lines, two points are randomly located in a cube of side 4 m and then the orientation on the line is randomly computed (see Fig. 3(a)). These lines are projected on an spherical-mirror-based image [15]. The catadioptric system is composed of a spherical mirror with radius of 1.2 m and a perspective camera located at 1.8 m from the center of the sphere. The resolution of the simulated camera is 1024 × 768.

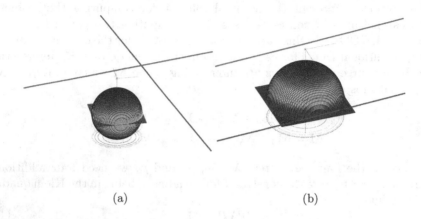

(a)   (b)

Fig. 3. Lines configuration example. (a) Junction. (b) Parallel.

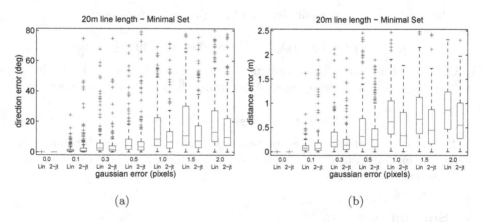

(a)   (b)

Fig. 4. Lines estimation using the minimal set of points comparing the linear approach (Lin) and junction approach (2-jt): (a) Direction error (deg) (b) Distance error (m)

Gaussian noise of a given σ is added to the projected points. The value of σ variates from 0.1 to 2. Then 3D lines are computed from its projection in a single image using the linear Teller approach and using our proposal. For each value of σ we compute 100 pairs of lines. The 100 pairs of lines are the same for each value of σ.

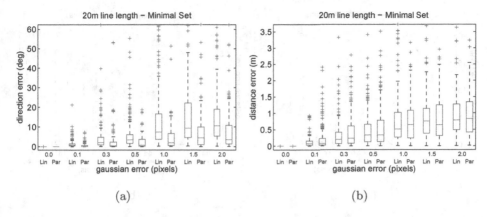

(a)   (b)

Fig. 5. Lines estimation using the minimal set of points comparing the linear approach (Lin) and parallel lines approach (Par): (a) Direction error (deg) (b) Distance error (m)

The first simulation, is a comparison between the unconstrained linear approach and our proposals (junction in Fig. 4 and parallel lines in Fig. 5) considering the minimal set of defining points. The length of the lines in this setup is 20m. The linear approach is computed from 8 points (4 for each line) and the proposal (junction or parallel) is computed from 6 points (3 for each line). The 6 points used for the proposal is a subset of the 8 points used for the unconstrained linear approach to avoid biasing. When using orthogonal junctions we take care of not using the intersection between lines which is a degenerated configuration with only 5 independent constraints.

The second simulation (see Figs. 6 and 7), is a comparison between the linear approach and our proposal considering more than the minimal set of points in the fitting. Considering more points (200 points), we obtain a least square fitting of the null spaces of dimension two in $\mathbb{P}^5$ described by L_m and M_m. In this case the number of points is the same for both linear and our proposal.

From the results we conclude that there is an improvement in the accuracy of the extracted lines. As expected, the improvement is more evident in the direction of the extracted line than in depth.

6   Experiments with Real Images

A reconstruction has been carried out to evaluate the performance of the method using a catadioptric system composed by a spherical mirror seen by a conventional camera with resolution 1280×1024 pixels.

6.1   Calibration of the Non-central System

First, the perspective camera has been independently calibrated. As the spherical catadioptric system is always axial the extrinsic parameters to calibrate are the tilt in the orientation of the camera, the radius of the sphere r_{sph} and the

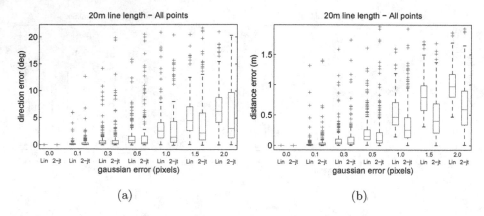

(a)   (b)

Fig. 6. Lines estimation using all points comparing the linear approach (Lin) and junction approach (2-jt): (a) Direction error (deg) in 20 m length lines. (b) Distance error (m) in 20 m length lines.

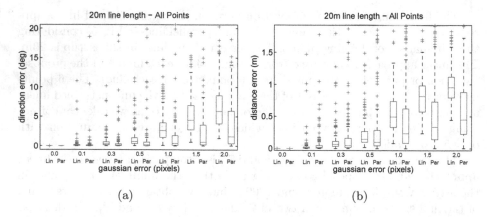

(a)   (b)

Fig. 7. Lines estimation of parallel lines using all points comparing the linear approach (Lin) and parallel lines approach (Par): (a) Direction error (deg) in 20 m length lines. (b) Distance error (m) in 20 m length lines.

distance from the center of the sphere to the perspective camera d. Notice that in spherical catadioptric systems d and r_{sph} are coupled in the line projection. Therefore, only $d_{rel} = \frac{d}{r_{sph}}$ can be recovered from a single line-image (Figs. 6 and 7).

In this case we have computed the tilt in the orientation and the relative distance d_{rel} from the contour projection of the sphere which is a conic in the image plane of the perspective camera and also using the projection of the camera reflection on the image which is related with the direction of the center of the sphere. The radius of the sphere has been estimated from a 3D reconstruction of the mirror obtained from a RGB-D device. This metric can be finally refined using projections of patterns with a known dimension like in the calibration method presented in [17].

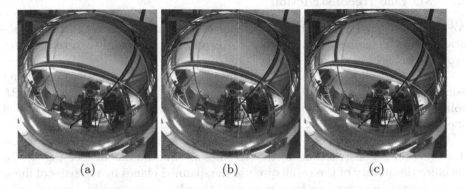

(a)   (b)   (c)

Fig. 8. Lines projection after fitting: (a) Linear. (b) junction. (c) Parallel.

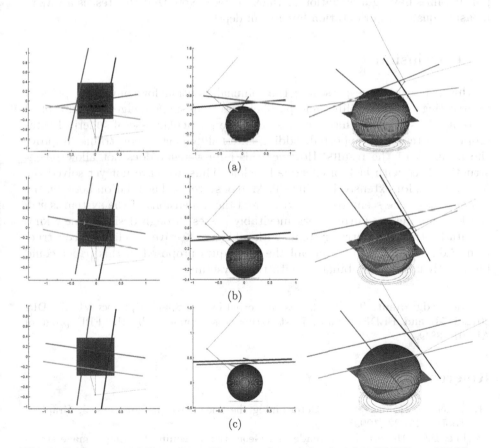

(a)

(b)

(c)

Fig. 9. Reconstructed lines from 15 points, from left to right: XY-View, YZ-View, Orthographic-View (a) Teller's method, (b) junction proposal. (c) Parallel proposal

6.2   3D Line Reconstruction

We have performed a reconstruction of four lines forming a rectangle. This disposition allows us to first reconstruct two different junctions and then reconstruct two different sets of parallel lines.

In Fig. 8 we show the forward projection of these four lines after the fitting using the junction. In Fig. 9 we show the reconstructions of these lines from 15 points using the Tellers linear method, our junction approach and our parallel lines approach.

As we can see in Fig. 8, line projections are very similar in the three cases. However, the reconstructions of the 3D lines are quite different (see Fig. 9). To measure the quality of the results we use the spanned planes by the pairs of lines. In the case of junctions we have compared the planes spanned by the two pairs of intersecting orthogonal lines. Both planes have a deviation of 9.72 degrees. In the case of parallel lines we compare the planes spanned by the two pairs of parallel lines having a deviation of 15.69 degrees. Note that this test is a way to measure quality in orientation but not in depth.

7   Conclusion

In this paper we have presented the minimal solution for computing pairs of intersecting orthogonal lines and parallel lines from single images in non-central systems. This proposal has been tested in the particular case of spherical catadioptric systems. As expected, adding external geometric constraints improve the accuracy of the results. However this improvement does not allow reconstructing lines with lack of effective baseline. Thus, we have not yet solved the impediments for extensively using this kind of systems. The relation between the dimensions of the scene to reconstruct and the dimensions of the system is still too low in practice. Future work inevitably passes through designing new kind of catadioptric or dioptric systems with a bigger effective baseline by construction. Additionally, notice that all the techniques proposed in this paper could be directly used in combination with these systems.

Acknowledgement. This work was supported by the Spanish project VINEA DPI 2012-31781 and FEDER funds. First author was supported by the FPU program AP2010-3849.

References

1. Teller, S., Hohmeyer, M.: Determining the lines through four lines. J. Graphics Tools **4**, 11–22 (1999)
2. Lee, D.C., Hebert, M., Kanade, T.: Geometric reasoning for single image structure recovery. In: IEEE Conference on Computer Vision and Pattern Recognition (CVPR 2009), pp. 2136–2143 (2009)

3. Ramalingam, S., Brand, M.: Lifting 3D manhattan lines from a single image. In: IEEE International Conference on Computer Vision (ICCV 2013), pp. 497–504 (2013)
4. Semple, J.G., Kneebone, G.T.: Algebraic Projective Geometry. Oxford University Press, USA (1998)
5. Griffiths, P., Harris, J.: Principles of Algebraic Geometry, vol. 52. Wiley, New York (2011)
6. Caglioti, V., Gasparini, S.: On the localization of straight lines in 3D space from single 2D images. In: IEEE Computer Society Conference on Computer Vision and Pattern Recognition (CVPR 2005), vol. 1, pp. 1129–1134 (2005)
7. Gasparini, S., Caglioti, V.: Line localization from single catadioptric images. Int. J. Comput. Vis. **94**, 361–374 (2011)
8. Lanman, D., Wachs, M., Taubin, G., Cukierman, F.: Reconstructing a 3D line from a single catadioptric image. In: Third International Symposium on 3D Data Processing, Visualization, and Transmission (3DPVT 2006), pp. 89–96 (2006)
9. Swaminathan, R., Wu, A., Dong, H., et al.: Depth from distortions. In: The 8th Workshop on Omnidirectional Vision, Camera Networks and Non-classical Cameras (OMNIVIS 2008) (2008)
10. Pinciroli, C., Bonarini, A., Matteucci, M.: Robust detection of 3D scene horizontal and vertical lines in conical catadioptric sensors. In: The 6th Workshop on Omnidirectional Vision (OMNIVIS 2005) (2005)
11. Chen, W., Cheng, I., Xiong, Z., Basu, A., Zhang, M.: A 2-point algorithm for 3D reconstruction of horizontal lines from a single omni-directional image. Pattern Recognit. Lett. **32**, 524–531 (2011)
12. Perdigoto, L., Araujo, H.: Reconstruction of 3D lines from a single axial catadioptric image using cross-ratio. In: 21th International Conference on Pattern Recognition (ICPR 2012), pp. 057–800 (2012)
13. Caglioti, V., Taddei, P., Boracchi, G., Gasparini, S., Giusti, A.: Single-image calibration of off-axis catadioptric cameras using lines. In: International Conference on Computer Vision (ICCV 2007), pp. 1–6 (2007)
14. Bermudez-Cameo, J., Lopez-Nicolas, G., Guerrero, J.J.: Line-images in cone mirror catadioptric systems. In: 22nd International Conference on Pattern Recognition (ICPR 2014) (2014)
15. Agrawal, A., Taguchi, Y., Ramalingam, S.: Analytical forward projection for axial non-central dioptric and catadioptric cameras. In: European Conference on Computer Vision (ECCV 2010), pp. 129–143 (2010)
16. Pottmann, H., Wallner, J.: Computational Line Geometry. Springer, Heidelberg (2001)
17. Agrawal, A., Ramalingam, S.: Single image calibration of multi-axial imaging systems. In: IEEE Computer Society Conference on Computer Vision and Pattern Recognition (CVPR 2013), pp. 1399–1406 (2013)

Asymmetric Feature Representation for Object Recognition in Client Server System

Yuji Yamauchi[1]([⊠]), Mitsuru Ambai[2], Ikuro Sato[2], Yuichi Yoshida[2],
Hironobu Fujiyoshi[1], and Takayoshi Yamashita[1]

[1] Chubu University, Kasugai, Japan
yuu@vision.cs.chubu.ac.jp
[2] Denso IT Laboratory, Inc., Tokyo, Japan

Abstract. This paper proposes asymmetric feature representation and
efficient fitting feature spaces for object recognition in client server system. We focus on the fact that the server-side has more sufficient memory and computation power compared to the client-side. Although local
descriptors must be compressed on the client-side due to the narrow
bandwidth of the Internet, feature vector compression on the server-side
is not always necessary. Therefore, we propose asymmetric feature representation for descriptor matching. Our method is characterized by the
following three factors. The first is asymmetric feature representation
between client- and server-side. Although the binary hashing function
causes quantization errors due to the computation of the sgn function ($\cdot$),
which binarizes a real value into $\{1, -1\}$, such errors only occur on the
client-side. As a result, performance degradation is suppressed while the
volume of data traffic is reduced. The second is scale optimization to
fit two different feature spaces. The third is fast implementation of distance computation based on real-vector decomposition. We can compute
efficiently the squared Euclidean distance between the binary code and
the real vector. Experimental results revealed that the proposed method
helps reduce data traffic while maintaining the object retrieval performance of a client server system.

1 Introduction

Advances in object recognition technology and mobile device technology have
enabled the realization of object recognition applications operating in partner-
ship with client server systems. In such applications, a user captures the image
of an object with a mobile device and the image or features computed from
the image are then sent to a server. On the server, the image is recognized
from its features and meta-information about the image is returned to the user.
Many such systems operate using local descriptors [1–3], as typified by scale-
invariant feature transform (SIFT) [4], which delivers excellent performance in
object recognition.

In practice, extracting local descriptors on a client-side and then sending
them to a server is problematic, since the data size of local descriptors is too

© Springer International Publishing Switzerland 2015
D. Cremers et al. (Eds.): ACCV 2014, Part I, LNCS 9003, pp. 598–612, 2015.
DOI: 10.1007/978-3-319-16865-4_39

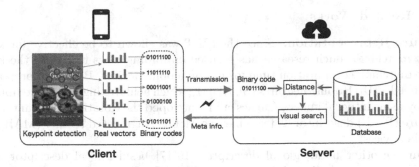

Fig. 1. Our system framework in client server system.

large to transfer through the Internet. For example, the SIFT descriptors is a 128-dimensional vector that consumes 128 bytes when represented as a 1-byte unsigned integer array. Since an image has anywhere from a few hundred to a few thousand SIFT descriptors, the total memory consumption reaches a few hundred KBytes per image. This has created a need to reduce the volume of data traffic sent from the client to the server in consideration of network load.

Chandrasekhar et al. suggested that the volume of data traffic can be reduced by having the client send compressed local descriptors instead of compressed images [5]. Memory-efficient descriptors have been proposed that represent a feature as a binary code, a sequence of binary values $\{-1, 1\}^1$, that can be compactly stored in main memory. BRIEF [7] and its extensions [8–10] generate a binary code by using L pixel pairs chosen from inside a nearby region around a keypoint, which produces an L bits binary sequence. One drawback to these methods is that they produce relatively longer binary codes with lengths ranging from 256 to 512 bits.

While these approaches directly compute a binary code by comparing pixel intensities around a keypoint, binary hashing [6,11–15] converts a local descriptor represented as a real vector into a much shorter binary code by using a hashing function. In general, binary representation degrades matching performance along with decreasing bit length. Generating a short yet informative feature description remains an open problem.

We focus on the fact that the server-side has more sufficient memory and computation power compared to the client-side. Figure 1 shows the our framework of object recognition in client server system. Although local descriptors must be compressed on the client-side due to the narrow bandwidth of the Internet, feature vector compression on the server-side is not always necessary. Therefore, we propose asymmetric feature representation for descriptor matching. Our method consisted of three factors. The first is asymmetric feature representation between client- and server-side. The second is scale optimization to fit two different feature spaces. The third is fast implementation of distance computation based on real-vector decomposition.

---

1 In this paper, as with [6], a binary code is expressed by $\{-1, 1\}$ instead of $\{0, 1\}$ in order to simplify the mathematical expressions.

1.1 Related Works

Feature Representation. Since the SIFT was shown to be effective for keypoint matching, much research has focused on finding ways to reduce the keypoint matching computation time for use on mobile devices. Bay et al. proposed the Speeded-Up Robust Features (SURF) [1], which achieves high-speed computation by using integral images. Takacs et al. developed the Rotation-Invariant, Fast Feature (RIFF) descriptor [2] for achieving Mobile Augmented Reality (MAR) on mobile devices.

On the other hand, global descriptor [16,17] besides local descriptor also have been proposed. Global descriptor such as VLAD [17], computational cost-large because it requires further computation after extracting local descriptor. Furthermore, the approach based on global descriptor, there is a disadvantage that the adoption of the strategy of improving performance by re-ranking using location information of the keypoints is difficult [18]. Therefore, we adopt a local descriptor at client for transmitting to server, as shown in Fig. 1.

These local descriptors require much memory, in order to represent as a high-dimensional real vector. Several methods in which local descriptors are extracted as binary code have been proposed for overcoming these problems [7–10]. These approaches generate binary code on the basis of the relation between the intensity of two pixels around each keypoint. One drawback to these methods is that they produce relatively longer binary codes with lengths ranging from 256 to 512 bits.

While these approaches directly compute a binary code by comparing pixel intensities around a keypoint, binary hashing [6,11–15] converts a local descriptor represented as a real vector into a much shorter binary code by using a hashing function. In this approach, a feature vector $\mathbf{x} \in \mathbb{R}^D$ is mapped into short binary code $\mathbf{b} \in \{-1, 1\}^L$ by using a binary hashing function $\mathbf{b} = \mathrm{sgn}(f(\mathbf{W}^T\mathbf{x}))$, where D is a dimension, L is the bit length of the binary code, and $\mathbf{W} \in \mathbb{R}^{D \times L}$ is a weight matrix. Weight matrix $\mathbf{W}$ and function $f(\cdot)^2$ characterize each binary hashing. The simplest method proposed is random projection (RP) [11]. $f(\cdot)$ is an identity function, and the elements in $\mathbf{W}$ are sampled from a normal distribution in random projection. The Very Sparse Random Projections (VSRP) [12] was developed to speed up the calculation. It does this by limiting each element in $\mathbf{W}$ to $\{-1, 0, 1\}$. The very supervised sparse hashing (VSSH) [13] improves performance by introducing the concept of learning to VSRP. The VSSH has been proposed that learns each element of $\mathbf{W}$. Spectral hashing (SH) [14] uses principal directions of training data for $\mathbf{W}$ and applies a cosine-like function for $f(\cdot)$. The iterative quantization (ITQ) [6] defines $\mathbf{W} = \mathbf{W}_{PCA}\mathbf{R}$, where $\mathbf{W}_{PCA}$ is obtained by principal component analysis, and rotation matrix $\mathbf{R}$ is optimized to minimize the quantization error before and after binary code conversion. In general, binary representation degrades matching performance along with decreasing bit length L. Generating a short yet informative feature description remains an open problem.

---

² In many cases [6,11–13,15,19], $f(\cdot)$ is an identity function.

Domain Adaptation. Domain adaptation is often used for fitting two or more feature spaces. Domain adaptation aims to learn classifier using a large number of samples in the source domain and a small number of samples or classifier in target domain. In order to achieve this, integrating feature spaces [20], adaptation of classifier [21,22], and fitting two feature spaces [23–25] have been proposed. The proposed method is related to domain adaptation for fitting two feature spaces.

Saenko et. al proposed a method for learning metric using Information-Theoretic Metric Learning (ITML)[26] to form a feature space in consideration of relationships between different domains [23]. High accuracy object recognition is achieved by using of k-Nearest Neighbor on the learned feature space. In addition, it is extended to non-linear mapping to apply the kernel method [25]. Geng et al. proposed Domain Adaptation Metric Learning (DAML) which learned a metric in reproducing kernel Hilbert space [24]. A common point of these methods is to learn a metric while considering the relations of a domains and the target categories.

The proposed method is also related to methods for fitting two feature spaces. However, a local descriptor of the same domain is represented by two feature spaces in the proposed method. The proposed method transforms the local descriptor $\mathbf{x} \in \mathbb{R}^D$ to short real vector $\mathbf{y} \in \mathbb{R}^L$, and it is transformed binary code $\mathbf{b} \in \{-1,1\}^L$ by sgn ($\cdot$) function. We obtain binary code and real vector from a same local descriptor. Since this is our specific problem, method to solve it has not been proposed.

1.2   Overview of Our Approach

In this paper, we focus on the fact that the server-side has more sufficient memory and computation power compared to the client-side. Although local descriptors must be compressed on the client-side due to the narrow bandwidth of the Internet, feature vector compression on the server-side is not always necessary. Therefore, we propose asymmetric feature representation for descriptor matching. Our method is characterized by the following three factors.

1. *Asymmetric feature representation*
   In our approach, local descriptors are computed on the client-side and converted into short binary codes, and the server stores local descriptors as real vectors. Although the binary hashing function causes quantization errors due to the computation of the sgn function ($\cdot$), which binarizes a real value into $\{1, -1\}$, such errors only occur on the client-side. As a result, performance degradation is suppressed while the volume of data traffic is reduced.
2. *Defining distances between binary codes and real vectors*
   Since the feature space of the real vectors is different from that of the binary codes, they cannot be directly compared. We propose a simple method to scale one feature space to fit the other feature space that enables the computation of distances between such asymmetrically represented features.
3. *Fast implementation for computing distances*
   It has already been reported that by decomposing a real vector into a few scholar weight factors and a few binary basis vectors, the Euclidean distance

between the binary code and the real vector can be computed extremely quickly [27]. We propose a decomposition method based on alternative optimization strategies that can approximate the real vector with fewer basis vectors than [27].

2 Asymmetric Representation and Distance

This section describes asymmetric feature representation and defining distances between binary codes and real vectors.

2.1 Euclidean Distance Between Binary Code and Real Vector

The binary hashing consists of two steps. First, an input vector $\mathbf{x} \in \mathbb{R}^{D3}$ is converted into a short real vector $\mathbf{y} \in \mathbb{R}^L$ by

$$\mathbf{y} = f(\mathbf{W}^{\mathrm{T}}\mathbf{x}). \tag{1}$$

Second, a binary code $\mathbf{b} \in \{-1, 1\}^L$ is computed by

$$\mathbf{b} = \mathrm{sgn}(f(\mathbf{W}^{\mathrm{T}}\mathbf{x})). \tag{2}$$

In our framework, any conventional binary hashing method is available for use. The $f(\cdot)$ and the $\mathbf{W} \in \mathbb{R}^{D \times L}$ follow the definitions of conventional binary hashing methods.

As shown in [6], the sgn($\cdot$) function used in the binary hashing can cause quantization errors that may degrade matching performance. Therefore, in our approach, while local descriptors computed on the client-side are converted into short binary codes $\mathbf{b}$, the server stores local descriptors as real vectors $\mathbf{y}$. As a result, since quantization errors only occur on the client-side, performance degradation is suppressed while the volume of data traffic is reduced. However, since each feature space is different, they cannot be directly compared.

2.2 Optimization of Adjustment Matrix

Since two feature spaces are different, it is necessary to fit the other feature space that enables the computation of distances between such asymmetrically represented features. An approach using the domain adaptation [23–25] introduced the metric learning for fitting feature spaces in different domains. These methods proposed introducing metric learning to form a feature space in consideration of relationships between different domains. However, a local descriptor of the same domain is represented by two feature spaces in the proposed method. We obtain binary code and real vector from a same local descriptor. Therefore, in order to minimize the error between real vectors and binary codes, we optimize the objective function as follows :

$$J(\mathbf{Q}) = ||\mathbf{B} - \mathbf{Q}\mathbf{Y}||_F^2, \tag{3}$$

---

[3] Before the local features are converted, they are mean-centered by using an average descriptor which is computed from training samples.

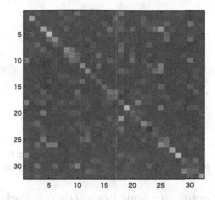

Fig. 2. Visualization of adjustment matrix ($L = 32$ bits). The red color means a high value (Color figure online).

Table 1. Euclidean norm and scale factor in each binary hashing method.

Binary hashing	Average Euclidean norm	Scale factor
Binry code	5.66	—
RP [11]	4.22	1.09
VSRP [12]	1.32	3.41
SH [14]	2.46	1.86
ITQ [6]	0.65	6.17

where $\mathbf{B} \in \{-1, 1\}^{L \times N}$ is a matrix of binary code corresponding to N keypoints obtained from training images. The matrix of real vectors $\mathbf{Y} \in \mathbb{R}^{L \times N}$ is similar. $\mathbf{Q} \in \mathbb{R}^{L \times L}$ is a adjustment matrix for fitting the two feature spaces. Two feature spaces can be fitted using optimized adjustment matrix.

Figure 2 shows example of visualization of optimized adjustment matrix. The adjustment matrix is very similar to the diagonal matrix, and diagonal elements have high value. This means that the optimized adjustment matrix can be replaced as a scalar matrix. Furthermore, the size of the adjustment matrix $\mathbf{Q}$ is a square of the bit length L of the binary code. If the bit length is greater, there is a possibility that the matrix becomes over-fit to the training samples. Therefore, we fit two feature spaces by more simpler way.

2.3   Optimization of Scale Factor

We propose a simple method to scale one feature space to fit the other feature space and enable the computation of distances between such asymmetrically represented features. We introduce the optimization of scale factor α to absorb the scale difference between feature spaces. Optimization is done using a cost function:

$$J(\alpha) = ||\mathbf{B} - \alpha \mathbf{Y}||_F^2, \tag{4}$$

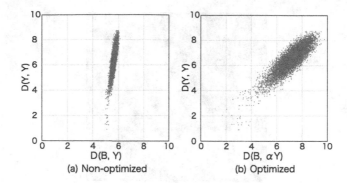

Fig. 3. Effect of optimizing scale factor. $D(\cdot, \cdot)$ is Euclidean distance.

where $\mathbf{B} \in \{-1, 1\}^{L \times N}$ is a matrix of binary code $\mathbf{b}$ corresponding to N key-points obtained from training images. The matrix of real vectors $\mathbf{Y} \in \mathbb{R}^{L \times N}$ is a matrix of real vector $\mathbf{y}$.

The Euclidean norms of binary code and real vectors when L is set to 32 are shown in Table 1 for several binary hashing methods. The Euclidean norm of a binary code $\mathbf{b}$ is a constant value $\sqrt{L}$ because the elements of the binary code only take two integer values $\{-1, 1\}$. In contrast, the Euclidean norm of a real vector depends on the binary hashing method. This difference may significantly degrade matching performance. Table 1 shows the optimized scale factors for each binary hashing method. The smaller the Euclidean norm of the real vector, the larger the scale factor becomes. The effect of the optimization of the scale factor is shown in Fig. 3. We used the ITQ binary hashing method. Without optimization (Fig. 3(a)), the distribution of the Euclidean distance between the binary code and real vectors was biased compared with the distribution of the Euclidean distance between real vectors. This is because the Euclidean norm of a real vector is very small compared to that of a binary code. With optimization (Fig. 3(b)), the Euclidean distances were about the same. For brevity purposes, $\mathbf{y}_\alpha = \alpha \mathbf{y}$ is used hereafter.

3   Fast Computation of Euclidean Distance by Introducing Decomposition Method

This section describes fast computation of Euclidean distance by introducing decomposition method.

3.1   Real Vector Decomposition

In this section, we consider the efficient computation of squared Euclidean distance between the binary code $\mathbf{b}$ and the real vector $\mathbf{y}_\alpha$. This computation can be expanded as

$$d(\mathbf{b}, \mathbf{y}_\alpha) = \|\mathbf{b} - \mathbf{y}_\alpha\|_2^2$$
$$= \mathbf{b}^{\mathrm{T}}\mathbf{b} - 2\mathbf{b}^{\mathrm{T}}\mathbf{y}_\alpha + \mathbf{y}_\alpha^{\mathrm{T}}\mathbf{y}_\alpha. \tag{5}$$

The first term of Eq. (5) is the dot product between binary codes in the client. This becomes a constant value because all of the elements in $\mathbf{b}$ take only two values $\{1, -1\}$. The third term is the dot product between real vectors stored in the server that can be calculated in advance. The problem here is computing the second term: it cannot be calculated in advance, so it requires a large number of floating-point computations.

To overcome this problem, Hare et al. [27] proposed decomposing the real vector $\mathbf{y}_\alpha$ into k weight factors and k binary basis vectors as

$$\mathbf{y}_\alpha \approx \mathbf{Mc}, \tag{6}$$

where $\mathbf{c} = (c_1, c_2, \cdots, c_k)^\mathrm{T} \in \mathbb{R}^k$ is the weight factor and $\mathbf{M} = \{\mathbf{m}_1, \mathbf{m}_2, \cdots, \mathbf{m}_k\} \in \{-1, 1\}^{L \times k}$ is the binary matrix composed of k binary basis vectors $\mathbf{m}_i \in \{-1, 1\}^k$.

Letting Eq. (6) into the second term of Eq. (5), we obtain

$$\mathbf{b}^\mathrm{T}\mathbf{y}_\alpha \approx \mathbf{b}^\mathrm{T}\mathbf{Mc}$$
$$= \sum_{i=1}^{k} c_i \mathbf{b}^\mathrm{T}\mathbf{m}_i. \tag{7}$$

The computations $\mathbf{b}^\mathrm{T}\mathbf{m}_i$ that appeared in Eq. (7) are extremely fast because this is equivalent to computing the Hamming distance between $\mathbf{b}$ and $\mathbf{m}_i$, as

$$\mathbf{b}^\mathrm{T}\mathbf{m}_i = L - 2\mathrm{HammingDistance}(\mathbf{b}, \mathbf{m}_i) \tag{8}$$

Since the Hamming distance can be computed efficiently using a bitwise XOR followed by a bit-count, Eq. (7) can also be computed very fast.

Introducing the decomposition method provides one more advantage. The server only has to store $\mathbf{c}$, $\mathbf{M}$, and $\mathbf{y}_\alpha^\mathrm{T}\mathbf{y}_\alpha$ instead of $\mathbf{y}_\alpha$. This reduces memory usage in the server substantially.

3.2   Decomposition Algorithms

The rest of this section discusses the decomposition algorithms used to obtain $\mathbf{M}$ and $\mathbf{c}$. Hare et al. [27] proposed a greedy algorithm that sequentially determines pairs of c_i and $\mathbf{m}_i$ one after another. In contrast to this, we propose a decomposition method based on an alternative optimization strategy that can approximate $\mathbf{y}_\alpha$ with fewer weights c_i and basis vectors $\mathbf{m}_i$ than Hare's greedy optimization.

In our approach, $\mathbf{M}$ and $\mathbf{c}$ are determined by minimizing the following cost function:

$$J(\mathbf{c}, \mathbf{M}) = \|\mathbf{y}_\alpha - \mathbf{Mc}\|_2^2. \tag{9}$$

Our decomposition algorithm is shown in **Algorithm 1**. Since it is difficult to optimize $\mathbf{M}$ and $\mathbf{c}$ at the same time, we do so alternately. If the basis vector $\mathbf{M}$ is fixed, the weight factor $\mathbf{c}$ can be optimized by using the least squares method.

Algorithm 1. Decomposition.

for $i = 1 : I$ do
   Set **c** and **M** to random values.
   for $j = 1 : \infty$ do
      (1) Minimize $J(\mathbf{c}, \mathbf{M})$ by fixing **M** and updating **c**.
         This optimization can be done by least squares method.
      (2) Minimize $J(\mathbf{c}, \mathbf{M})$ by fixing **c** and updating **M**.
         This optimization can be done by exhaustive search.
      (3) Exit loop if converged.
   end for
end for
Select the best **c** and **M** that minimize $J(\mathbf{c}, \mathbf{M})$.

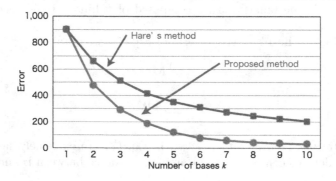

Fig. 4. Comparison of the proposed method with Hare's method [27].

In contrast, if **c** is fixed, the basis vector **M** can be optimized by exhaustive search. Thanks to the constraint that the binary basis vector **M** only takes two integer values $\{1, -1\}$, the i th row in the matrix **M** takes 2^k combinations. Therefore, all of the 2^k combinations can be exhaustively tested if k is small enough. We initialize **M** and **c** by random values and alternately update them until convergence. To avoid falling to a local minimum, several different initial values are tested.

In contrast to Hare's method, our method determines k pairs of c_i and $\mathbf{m}_i$ simultaneously. Therefore, the difference between the two methods appears in the approximate performance. It is obvious from Fig. 4 that our method can approximate $\mathbf{y}_\alpha$ using fewer basis vectors $\mathbf{m}_i$ than Hare's method.

4   Experiments

We evaluated the performance of the asymmetric feature representation proposed in this paper by testing to find corresponding points between two images.

4.1   Datasets for Evaluating Keypoint Matching

We evaluate the proposed method on two datasets of the IEEE Spectrum magazine dataset and Mikolajczyk's dataset [3].

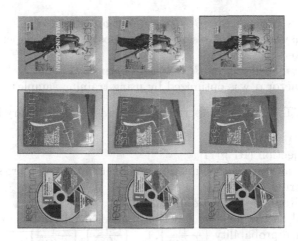

Fig. 5. Example images in dataset.

IEEE Spectrum Magazine Dataset. We prepared seven issues of the IEEE Spectrum magazine and captured them from six viewpoints. Example images from some various viewpoints are shown in Fig. 5. Let I_j^i denote an image in the database, with the number of where i is the magazine index ($1 \leq i \leq 7$), and j is the viewpoint index ($1 \leq j \leq 6$). Assuming that the magazines are planar, we prepared a homography matrix $\mathbf{H}_{1 \rightarrow j}^i$ between I_1^i and I_j^i in advance, which gives ground truth correspondences between the image pairs. We used $I_j^1 \sim I_j^3$ for training to compute the weight matrix $\mathbf{W}$, and used $I_j^4 \sim I_j^7$ for testing.

Keypoint matching performance can be evaluated by using the image pairs I_1^i, I_j^i, and their homography matrix $\mathbf{H}_{1 \rightarrow j}^i$. For each keypoint obtained from the I_1^i, the first and second nearest neighbors were searched from the keypoints extracted from the I_j^i. Let d_1 and d_2 denote the distances to the first and second nearest neighbors, respectively. If the ratio of the distances d_1/d_2 was less than a pre-defined threshold T, the query keypoint in I_1^i and the first nearest neighbor in I_j^i were regarded as corresponding points. If the first nearest neighbor was located within $\sqrt{(1+1)}$ pixels from the true location derived from $\mathbf{H}_{1 \rightarrow j}^i$, such keypoint pair is regarded as inlier. We computed the average number of matches over test image pairs and the rate of correct matching.

Mikolajczyk's Dataset. We evaluate the proposed method using the standard dataset [3] for keypoint matching. Mikolajczyk's dataset is captured at eight places from six viewpoints. We use images from four viewpoints for training to compute weight matrix $\mathbf{W}$, and used the remaining images for testing.

4.2   Comparing Symmetric and Asymmetric Representation

We compared three kinds of feature representation:

- *Binary code vs. Binary code: BC-BC*
  This is conventional symmetric representation.

– *Binary code vs. Real vector: BC-RV without optimizing* α
This is the asymmetric representation proposed in this paper. The scaling factor α is fixed to 1.
– *Binary code vs. Real vector: BC-RV with optimizing* α
The scaling factor α was optimized by using training samples.

We used SIFT [4] as local descriptors, and we test four binary hashing functions as follow:

– Random Projection (RP) [11]
$f(\cdot)$ was used as the identity function, and elements in $\mathbf{W}$ were sampled from a normal distribution.
– Very Sparse Random Projection (VSRP) [12]
$f(\cdot)$ was used as the identity function, and elements in $\mathbf{W}$ were limited to $\{-1, 0, 1\}$, with probability $\{\frac{1}{2\sqrt{(D)}}\}, 1 - \{\frac{1}{\sqrt{(D)}}\}, \{\frac{1}{2\sqrt{(D)}}\}$.
– Spectral Hashing (SH) [14]
Basis vectors obtained by principal component analysis were used as $\mathbf{W}$, and $f(\cdot)$ was used as an eigenfunction.
– Iterative Quantization (ITQ) [6]
ITQ was used to define $\mathbf{W} = \mathbf{W}_{PCA}\mathbf{R}$, $\mathbf{W}_{PCA}$ was obtained by principal component analysis, and rotation matrix $\mathbf{R}$ was optimized to minimize the quantization error before and after binary code conversion.

The results are shown in Fig. 6. The asymmetric representation with optimizing α clearly outperformed the conventional symmetric representation when the shorter binary codes were used. This means that the proposed method can improve matching performance when short binary codes are used to reduce network traffic. The scaling factor α played an important role when ITQ and VSRP were used as the binary hashing function. In the case of ITQ and VSRP, the average Euclidean norm of binary codes in the client-side significantly differed from that of real vectors in the server-side, as shown in Table 1. This means that the scaling factor α absorbed such difference and contributed to improving the matching performance.

4.3   Effect of Decomposition

We evaluated the effect of decomposition in terms of matching rate, computational time, and memory usage. In this experiment, random projections were used as binary hashing methods. Bit length L was set to 32.

Matching Performance. The results of a comparison between our decomposition algorithm and Hare's method [27] are shown in Fig. 7. When the number of basis vectors k was set to 1, there was little difference between our algorithm and Hare's method. However, when $k > 1$, the performance of the proposed method was higher. While Hare's method needed four basis vectors to sufficiently approximate the original real vector $\mathbf{y}_\alpha$, our algorithm only required three, which helped reduce the memory usage and computational time of matching.

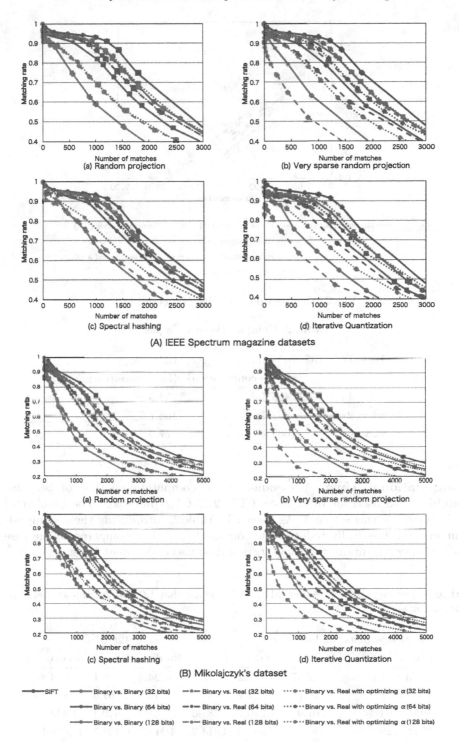

(a) Random projection

(b) Very sparse random projection

(c) Spectral hashing

(d) Iterative Quantization

(A) IEEE Spectrum magazine datasets

(a) Random projection

(b) Very sparse random projection

(c) Spectral hashing

(d) Iterative Quantization

(B) Mikolajczyk's dataset

SIFT
Binary vs. Binary (32 bits)
Binary vs. Real (32 bits)
Binary vs. Real with optimizing α (32 bits)
Binary vs. Binary (64 bits)
Binary vs. Real (64 bits)
Binary vs. Real with optimizing α (64 bits)
Binary vs. Binary (128 bits)
Binary vs. Real (128 bits)
Binary vs. Real with optimizing α (128 bits)

Fig. 6. Comparison with state-of-the-art methods.

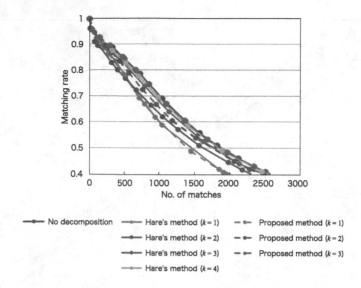

Fig. 7. Comparison with Hare's method [27]

Table 2. Computational time [ns].

Bits	BC - BC	BC - RV (No Decomposition)	BC - RV (Decomposition)
32	14.2	433.5	54.5
64	27.6	852.3	105.7
128	61.9	1683.2	177.5

Computational Time. We evaluated the computational time of keypoint matching. We used an Intel Xeon CPU 2.27-GHz processor. The number of basis vectors k was set to 3. As shown in Table 2, introducing the decomposition method drastically reduced the computational time compared to the case without decomposition: the computation time was eight times faster.

Table 3. Memory usage in server [MB]. (We assume that 1,000 keypoints are detected from an image.)

No. of keypoints (No. of images)	32 bits		64 bits		128 bits	
	Dec	No dec	Dec	No dec	Dec	No dec
0.1 M (0.1 K)	2.67	12.2	3.8	24.4	6.1	48.8
1 M (1 K)	26.7	122.1	38.1	244.1	61.0	488.3
10 M (10 K)	267.0	1,220.7	381.5	2,441.4	610.4	4,882.8
100 M (100 K)	2,670.3	12,207.0	3,814.7	24,414.1	6,103.5	48,828.1

Memory Usage. We compared memory usage with and without decomposing y_α. The number of basis vectors k was set to 3. Table 3 shows the results. One example shows that if the server stores 100,000 images and the length of the binary code is set to 32 bits, memory usage is reduced to about 21 %.

5   Conclusion

In this paper, we proposed asymmetric feature representation for matching local descriptors. Experimental results revealed that the proposed method helps reduce data traffic while maintaining the object retrieval performance of a client server system. Our method consisted of three factors. The first was asymmetric feature representation between client- and server-side. The second was scale optimization to fit two different feature spaces. The third was fast implementation of distance computation based on real-vector decomposition.

The range of application is not limited to object retrieval. We believe our method can be used not only for computer vision applications but also for similar applications such as speech recognition systems.

References

1. Bay, H., Ess, A., Tuytelaars, T., Van Gool, L.: Speeded-up robust features (surf). Comput. Vis. Image Underst. **110**, 346–359 (2008)
2. Takacs, G., Chandrasekhar, V., Tsai, S., Chen, D., Grzeszczuk, R., Girod, B.: Unified real-time tracking and recognition with rotation-invariant fast features. In: IEEE Computer Society Conference on Computer Vision and Pattern Recognition (2010)
3. Mikolajczyk, K., Schmid, C.: A performance evaluation of local descriptors. IEEE Trans. Pattern Anal. Mach. Intell. **27**, 1615–1630 (2005)
4. Lowe, D.G.: Distinctive image features from scale-invariant keypoints. Int. J. Comput. Vis. **60**, 91–110 (2004)
5. Chandrasekhar, V., Takacs, G., Reznik, Y., Grzeszczuk, R., Girod, B.: Compressed histogram of gradients: A low-bitrate descriptor. Int. J. Comput. Vis. **96**(3), 384–399 (2011)
6. Gong, Y., Lazebnik, S.: Iterative quantization : A procrustean approach to learning binary codes. In: IEEE Computer Society Conference on Computer Vision and Pattern Recognition (2011)
7. Calonder, M., Lepetit, V., Ozuysal, M., Trzcinski, T., Strecha, C., Fua, P.: BRIEF: Computing a local binary descriptor very fast. IEEE Trans. Pattern Anal. Mach. Intell. **34**, 1281–1298 (2012)
8. Leutenegger, S., Chli, M., Siegwart, R.: BRISK: Binary robust invariant scalable keypoints. In: IEEE International Conference on Computer Vision (2011)
9. Rublee, E., Rabaud, V., Konolige, K., Bradski, G.: ORB: An efficient alternative to SIFT or SURF. In: IEEE International Conference on Computer Vision (2011)
10. Alahi, A., Ortiz, R., Vandergheynst, P.: FREAK: Fast retina keypoint. In: IEEE Computer Society Conference on Computer Vision and Pattern Recognition (2012)
11. Achlioptas, D.: Database-friendly random projections: Johnson-Lindenstrauss with binary coins. J. Comput. Syst. Sci. **66**, 671–687 (2003)

12. Li, P., Hastie, T.J., Church, K.W.: Very Sparse Random Projections. In: International Conference on Knowledge Discovery and Data Mining (2006)
13. Ambai, M., Yoshida, Y.: CARD: Compact and real-time descriptors. In: IEEE International Conference on Computer Vision, pp. 97–104 (2011)
14. Weiss, Y., Torralba, A., Fergus, R.: Spectral hashing. In: Neural Information Processing Systems, pp. 1753–1760 (2008)
15. Heo, J.P., Lee, Y., He, J., Chang, S.F., Yoon, S.E.: Spherical hashing. In: IEEE Computer Society Conference on Computer Vision and Pattern Recognition (2012)
16. Csurka, G., Dance, C.R., Fan, L., Willamowski, J., Bray, C.: Visual categorization with bags of keypoints. In: Workshop on Statistical Learning in Computer Vision, in conjunction European Conference on Computer Vision (2004)
17. Jégou, H., Douze, M., Schmid, C., Pérez, P.: Aggregating local descriptors into a compact image representation. In: IEEE Computer Society Conference on Computer Vision and Pattern Recognition, pp. 3304–3311 (2010)
18. Philbin, J., Chum, O., Isard, M., Sivic, J., Zisserman, A.: Object retrieval with large vocabularies and fast spatial matching. In: IEEE Computer Society Conference on Computer Vision and Pattern Recognition (2007)
19. Weiss, Y., Fergus, R., Torralba, A.: Multidimensional spectral hashing. In: Fitzgibbon, A., Lazebnik, S., Perona, P., Sato, Y., Schmid, C. (eds.) ECCV 2012, Part V. LNCS, vol. 7576, pp. 340–353. Springer, Heidelberg (2012)
20. Daume III, H.: Frustratingly easy domain adaptation. In: Annual Meeting of the Association of Computational Linguistics, pp. 256–263 (2007)
21. Duan, L., Tsang, I.W., Xu, D., Chua, T.S.: Domain adaptation from multiple sources via auxiliary classifiers. In: Annual International Conference on Machine Learning, pp. 289–296 (2009)
22. Yang, J., Yan, R., Hauptmann, A.G.: Cross-domain video concept detection using adaptive svms. In: International Conference on Multimedia, pp. 188–197 (2007)
23. Saenko, K., Kulis, B., Fritz, M., Darrell, T.: Adapting visual category models to new domains. In: Daniilidis, K., Maragos, P., Paragios, N. (eds.) ECCV 2010, Part IV. LNCS, vol. 6314, pp. 213–226. Springer, Heidelberg (2010)
24. Geng, B., Tao, D., Xu, C.: Daml : Domain adaptation metric learning. IEEE Trans. Image Process. **20**, 2980–2989 (2011)
25. Kulis, B., Saenko, K., Darrell, T.: What you saw is not what you get: Domain adaptation using asymmetric kernel transforms. In: IEEE Computer Society Conference on Computer Vision and Pattern Recognition, pp. 1785–1792 (2011)
26. Davis, J.V., Kulis, B., Jain, P., Sra, S., Dhillon, I.S.: Information-theoretic metric learning. In: International Conference on Machine Learning, pp. 209–216 (2007)
27. Hare, S., Saffari, A., Torr, P.H.S.: Efficient online structured output learning for keypoint-based object tracking. In: IEEE Computer Society Conference on Computer Vision and Pattern Recognition, pp. 1894–1901 (2012)

Leveraging High Level Visual Information for Matching Images and Captions

Fei Yan[✉] and Krystian Mikolajczyk

Centre for Vision, Speech and Signal Processing,
University of Surrey, Guildford, Surrey GU2 7XH, UK
{f.yan,k.mikolajczyk}@surrey.ac.uk

Abstract. In this paper we investigate the problem of matching images and captions. We exploit the kernel canonical correlation analysis (KCCA) to learn a similarity between images and texts. We then propose methods to build improved visual and text kernels. The visual kernels are based on visual classifiers that use responses of a deep convolutional neural network as features, and the text kernel improves the Bag-of-Words (BoW) representation by learning a vision based lexical similarity between words. We consider two application scenarios, one where only an external image set weakly related to the evaluation dataset is available for training the visual classifiers, and one where visual data closely related to the evaluation set can be used. We evaluate our visual and text kernels on a large and publicly available benchmark, where we show that our proposed methods substantially improve upon the state-of-the-art.

1 Introduction

The explosive growth of visual and textual data on the web and in personal collections demands effective methods for image and video search, visual content description and text-to-image generation. Owing to recent advances in computer vision (CV), natural language processing (NLP) and machine learning (ML), integrated modelling of vision and language is finding more and more applications, e.g. face recognition from caption-based supervision [1], text-to-image coreference [2], and zero-shot visual learning using purely textural description [3]. In particular, generating natural language description for image and video has attracted much interest in both CV and NLP communities [4–16].

One of the main issues with the work in [4–16], however, is the lack of automatic and objective evaluation metric. In [17] the problem of generating natural language description for a given image is relaxed to one of ranking a set of human-written captions, by assuming the set contains the original (human-written) caption of the image. Hodosh et al. [17] builds a dataset (dubbed Flickr8K) of image and caption pairs, and employs the kernel canonical correlation analysis (KCCA) [18,19] to learn a latent space in which a similarity measure between an image and a caption is defined. KCCA requires two kernels to be built, one for the images and the other for the captions. Hodosh et al. [17] fixes the image kernel to a relatively simple one that uses only low level and mid-level visual

© Springer International Publishing Switzerland 2015
D. Cremers et al. (Eds.): ACCV 2014, Part I, LNCS 9003, pp. 613–627, 2015.
DOI: 10.1007/978-3-319-16865-4_40

information such as colour, texture and SIFT descriptors, and demonstrates that text kernels that exploit lexical similarities and high-order co-occurrence information outperform the basic Bag-of-Word (BoW) text kernel.

In this paper, we build on the results from [17], and propose an approach that significantly improves the performance of image-to-text annotation and text-to-image retrieval. In particular we consider the scenario where there is no image data for training visual classifiers for synsets in the application domain at hand. Our contributions can be summaries as follows:

- Our approach makes use of additional visual classifiers for synsets different than those contained in the evaluation data. We show that the combination of the basic BoW text kernel and a high level image kernel based on the probabilities given by visual classifiers outperforms the best combination in [17] in most evaluation metrics (Sect. 5.1);
- We demonstrate that visual classifiers trained for synsets included in the evaluation dataset improve the retrieval scores by a factor of two compared to the best method in [17] (Sect. 5.2);
- Finally, in contrast to lexical similarities computed using text corpora, we propose to use the high level visual information to learn a lexical similarity, and show that the BoW text kernel enriched with such lexical similarity further boosts the performance (Sect. 6).

The remainder of this paper is organised as follows: in Sect. 2 we brief review existing work on description generation for image and video. In particular, we present the dataset and experimental setup introduced in [17], which we compare our approaches to. The BoW text kernel used in our studies is presented in Sect. 3, followed by an introduction in Sect. 4 to our visual recognition pipeline that is based on a deep convolutional neural network (CNN). In Sect. 5, the performance of high level visual kernels built using external and internal sets of synsets is presented respectively, with analysis and discussions. In Sect. 6, we propose a vision based lexical similarity to model partial matches in the text representation, and compare it to language based lexical similarities. Finally, Sect. 7 concludes the paper.

2   Related Work

Generating natural language description for image and video has become a popular research topic in recent years. Among existing work on this topic, the goal in [4] is automatic caption generation for a given news image with an associated news article. A good caption for such an image is often only loosely related to the content of the image. The setting of this work is therefore different from that in [5–12], where the objective is to generate a caption that describes what is depicted in the image.

In [5], a dataset with 1 million image-caption pairs is leveraged, and the caption of the image in the dataset that is visually most similar to the given image is transferred as its caption. However, even with 1 million images, it is unrealistic to expect that every possible query image with various objects and actions can be represented and found in such dataset. In contrast to this caption transfer approach, the work in [6–12] adopts the conventional content selection and surface realisation approach. Starting from the output of visual processing engines e.g. object classifiers, object detectors and attribute classifiers, image content that will be described is selected in the form of tuples such as subject-action-object triplets, object-preposition-object triplets, and object-action-preposition-scene triplets quadruplet. A surface realiser is then employed to produce captions as constrained by the lexicon and grammar.

While [6] focuses on the investigation of surface realisation techniques, the work in [7–12] differs primarily in the way the tuples of image content are generated. In [7,8], structured output learning techniques i.e. structured support vector machine (S-SVM) and conditional random field (CRF) are employed to learn the mapping from the output of visual processing engines to the tuples. In [11] the tuples for the test image are a weighted collection of those for the training examples, and the weights are learnt from training image-caption pairs. In [12] content selection and planning is formulated as an integer linear program (ILP). Finally, [9,10] employ language corpora to learn word co-occurrence statistics and use the statistics to filter and enrich the output of visual processing engines. While [9] uses a hidden Markov model (HMM) to determine the quadruplet of image content, [10] generates syntactic trees to encode what the visual engines see.

In parallel to image captioning, automatic video description is also receiving increasing attention [13–16]. Although details differ, [13–16] operate within the same paradigm of content selection and surface realisation. Compared to image description, typically video description systems additionally employ spatio-temporal methods for action recognition.

2.1 Image Description as a Ranking Task

The approaches discussed above can produce human-like description for image and video. However, [17] argues that these approaches lack automatic and objective evaluation methods. On the one hand, although automatic evaluation metrics such as BLEU [20] and ROUGE [21] are useful for measuring the fluency of the generated text [22], it is shown in [17] that they are not reliable metrics for how accurately a caption describes an image. On the other hand, human judgements can be quite reliable but are expensive and time-consuming to collect. To address this issue, [17] builds a dataset of image-caption pairs, and formulates the image captioning problem as one of ranking a set of available human-written captions.

The Flickr8K dataset. The authors of [17] collected 8000 images from the Flickr.com website, which focused on people or animal performing actions. Using a crowdsourcing service, five captions were generated by different annotators for each image. The annotators were asked to describe the actors, objects, scenes and activities that were shown in the image, i.e., information that could be obtained

Table 1. Two example image-caption pairs in the Flickr8K dataset.

- A cat standing on carpet is interested in a piece of string in the air nearby wood flooring.
- A white and brown cat bats at a frayed string dangling in front of him.
- Cat playing with a dangling string.
- Cat standing to play with string.
- The white and black cat pawed at the piece of fabric.

- A couple of several people sitting on a ledge overlooking the beach.
- A group of people sit on a wall at the beach.
- A group of teens sit on a wall by a beach.
- Crowd of people at the beach.
- Several young people sitting on a rail above a crowded beach.

from the image alone. Two examples of image-caption pairs are illustrated in Table 1. The dataset is split into predefined training, validation, and test sets with 6000, 1000, and 1000 pairs respectively. The five captions are pooled into one for the training set, and in the validation and test sets only caption 2 is used. Each image-caption pair therefore can be thought of as consisting of one image and one caption.

Kernel canonical correlation analysis (KCCA). Given m samples of two sets of variables $\{\mathbf{x}_i\}_{i=1}^m$ and $\{\mathbf{y}_i\}_{i=1}^m$ where $\mathbf{x}_i \in \mathcal{R}^{d_x}$ and $\mathbf{y}_i \in \mathcal{R}^{d_y}$. Canonical correlation analysis (CCA) [23] finds a projection for each set such that in the projected common space the linear correlation of the samples is maximised. CCA can be kernelised by implicitly embedding $\mathbf{x}_i$ and $\mathbf{y}_i$ into feature spaces through kernel functions $k_x(\mathbf{x}_i, \mathbf{x}_j)$ and $k_y(\mathbf{y}_i, \mathbf{y}_j)$ [18,19]. The resulting kernel CCA (KCCA) finds the two projections by solving:

$$\underset{\alpha,\beta}{\operatorname{argmax}} \frac{\alpha^T K_x K_y \beta}{\sqrt{(\alpha^T K_x^2 \alpha + \kappa \alpha^T K_x \alpha)(\beta^T K_y^2 \beta + \kappa \beta^T K_y \beta)}} \tag{1}$$

where K_x and K_y are the $m \times m$ training kernel matrices with $K_x[i,j] = k_x(\mathbf{x}_i, \mathbf{x}_j)$ and $K_y[i,j] = k_y(\mathbf{y}_i, \mathbf{y}_j)$, and κ is a regularisation parameter. Let l be the number of test examples, and K_x' and K_y' be the $m \times l$ test kernel matrices. The similarity measure between test image i' and test caption j' is defined as the cosine of the angle between the two projected points in the learnt common space:

$$\operatorname{Sim}(\mathbf{x}_{i'}, \mathbf{y}_{j'}) = \cos(\alpha^T K_x'[:, i'], \beta^T K_y'[:, j']) \tag{2}$$

or the linear correlation between them:

$$\operatorname{Sim}(\mathbf{x}_{i'}, \mathbf{y}_{j'}) = \operatorname{corr}(\alpha^T K_x'[:, i'], \beta^T K_y'[:, j']) \tag{3}$$

where $K'_x[:, i']$ denotes the i'^{th} column of K'_x, and $K'_y[:, j']$ denotes the j'^{th} column of K'_y.

Evaluation metrics. Given an image kernel and a text kernel, [17] learns the common space using KCCA. For each test image, the 1000 captions in the test set are ranked according to their similarity to the image using Eq. (2). This ranked list allows to define metrics that measure how well images and captions are matched in the learnt common space. Hodosh et al. [17] proposes to use the recall of the caption originally paired with the image at positions 1, 5, 10 of the ranked list (R@1, R@5, R@10), and the median rank (MR) of this original gold caption for all test images.

Formulating caption generation as a ranking task allows different approaches to be compared in an automatic, efficient and objective fashion. Moreover, such a framework can be trivially extended to perform the symmetric task of image retrieval using captions. We therefore employ the KCCA approach for both image-to-text annotation and text-to-image retrieval. We use the metrics R@1, R@5, R@10 and MR to measure the performance of our kernels on both annotation and retrieval tasks, and compare with that in [17].

3   Bag-of-Words (BoW) Text Kernel

In this section, we introduce the text kernel K_y used in our study. First, all captions are processed using the linguistic analyser of [24]. This analyser performs tokenisation, lemmatisation, part-of-speech (POS) tagging and word-sense disambiguation. There are 5768 unique lemmatised words in the training captions. We build a $d_y = 5768$ dimensional bag-of-words (BoW) representation for each caption, with the rth dimension:

$$y^r = t^r \log \frac{D}{d^r + 1} \tag{4}$$

where t^r is the term frequency (TF) of the rth lemmatised word i.e. the number it appears in the caption, d^r is document frequency of the lemmatised word i.e. the number of training captions where it appears, and D is the total number of training captions. We adopt the linear correlation as the kernel function:

$$k_y(\mathbf{y}_i, \mathbf{y}_j) = \text{corr}(\mathbf{y}_i, \mathbf{y}_j) \tag{5}$$

and denote the resulting kernel $BoW5'$, where "5" indicates that for the training set the five captions are pooled into one, and the prime symbol indicates that $BoW5'$ is a close variant of the $BoW5$ kernel used in [17] with the following differences: (1) $BoW5'$ adopts the linear correlation as kernel function while $BoW5$ adopts the cosine; (2) $BoW5'$ uses the standard inverse document frequency (IDF) weight while $BoW5$ uses a square-rooted version which is found to perform better in [17]; (3) stop words are kept when building $BoW5'$ while they are removed in $BoW5$.

Table 2. Statistics of the sets of synsets involved in our work. Visual classifiers are trained for the two sets in boldface.

Synset set	# of synsets	# of images
{ILSVRC12}	1000	1,281,169
{Caption}	3335	-
{ImageNet}	21841	-
{ILSVRC12} ∩ {ImageNet}	999	-
{ILSVRC12} ∩ {Caption}	197	-
{Caption} ∩ {ImageNet}	1372	1,571,576

The word-sense disambiguation component of the linguistic analyser also maps each token to a WordNet synset. We denote by {Caption} the set of 3335 synsets that correspond to tokens in the captions labelled as nouns by the POS tagger. In the following, we train visual classifiers for a subset of {Caption}, and use the output of the classifiers to build a high level visual kernel.

4   Building High Level Visual Kernels with Deep Learning

Following the success of deep convolutional neural network (CNN) [25] in the ImageNet large scale visual recognition challenge 2012 (ILSVRC12) [26], deep learning [27,28] has become the de-facto approach for large scale visual recognition. Moreover, it has recently been shown in [29] that features extracted from the activations of a deep CNN trained in a fully supervised fashion can be re-purposed to novel generic tasks that differ significantly from the original task.

Inspired by [29], we extract such activations as features for novel visual recognition tasks. More specifically, we train binary classifiers for two sets of WordNet synsets: the first set, denoted {ILSVRC12}, is the synsets in the ILSVRC12 challenge; and the second set, denoted {Caption} ∩ {ImageNet}, is the intersection of the 3335 noun synsets in the captions of Flickr8K and the 21841 synsets in the 2011 Fall release of the ImageNet [30]. Statistics of the sets involved are summarised in Table 2.

For each of the two sets, we extract activations of a pre-trained CNN model as features for images in the synsets. Similarly, features are also extracted for the images in Flickr8K. The pre-trained CNN model is a reference implementation of the structure proposed in [25] with minor modifications, and is made publicly available through the Caffe project [31]. It is shown in [29] that the activations of layer six of the CNN perform the best for novel tasks. Our study on a toy example with ten ImageNet synsets however suggests that the activations of layer seven have a small edge.

Again for each of the two sets, once the 4096 dimensional activations of layer seven are extracted, we train binary support vector machines (SVMs) using the LIBSVM toolbox [32] for each synset, with 5000 images randomly sampled from

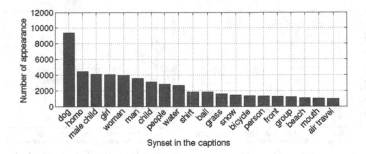

Fig. 1. The top 20 most frequently appearing synsets in Flickr8K. X-axis: the first word/phrase in the WordNet definition of a synset; Y-axis: number of appearances in the $8000 \times 5 = 40000$ original captions (before pooling for training set).

all synsets as negative examples. The trained SVMs are used to predict the probabilities of the presence of the n synsets in the Flickr8K images.

Let $\mathbf{x}$ be the $d_x = n$ dimensional representation of an image, where its tth element x^t is the probability that synset t is present in the image, as given by the tth SVM. We again use the linear correlation as kernel function:

$$k_x(\mathbf{x}_i, \mathbf{x}_j) = \text{corr}(\mathbf{x}_i, \mathbf{x}_j) \tag{6}$$

Compared to the visual kernel in [17] which uses only low and mid-level visual information such as colour, texture and SIFT descriptors, our kernel encodes high level visual information in terms of presence of objects, actions, and scenes.

5 Evaluation of High Level Visual Kernels

In this section, we evaluate the high level visual kernels in conjunction with the $BoW5'$ text kernel under the KCCA framework, and provide analysis and discussions on the results. To enable a fair comparison, we follow [17] and find 15 best performing models on the validation set by tuning the KCCA regularisation parameter κ and the dimensionality d of the learnt common space. The final rank on the test set is obtained by aggregating the ranks given by the 15 sets of optimal parameters. In the following, we consider two scenarios: when visual classifiers are leant for sysnets that are external to the Flickr8K dataset i.e. synsets in {ILSVRC12} (Sect. 5.1); and when they are learnt for synsets from the captions of Flickr8K i.e. synsets in {Caption} ∩ {ImageNet} (Sect. 5.2).

5.1 Learning for Synsets in {ILSVRC12}

To build the Flickr8K dataset, images were collected from six Flickr groups: *strangers!*, *Wild-Child*, *Dogs in Action*, *Outdoor Activities*, *Action Photography*, and *Flickr-Social*. As a result, the images tend to depict people or animals (mainly dogs) performing some action. The top 20 most frequently appearing

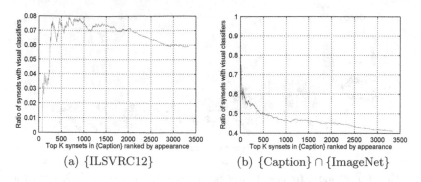

(a) {ILSVRC12}   (b) {Caption} ∩ {ImageNet}

Fig. 2. Ratio of top K synsets in {Caption} ranked by appearances that have visual classifiers. (a): when learning for synsets in {ILSVRC12}; (b): when learning for synsets in {Caption} ∩ {ImageNet}.

Table 3. Performance of high level visual kernel learnt on {ILSVRC12}, *ILS*.

Image	Text	Image annotation				Image retrieval			
		R@1	R@5	R@10	MR	R@1	R@5	R@10	MR
Pyr	*BoW5*	6.2	17.1	24.3	58.0	5.8	16.7	23.6	60.0
Pyr	*TagRank*	6.0	17.0	23.8	56.0	5.4	17.4	24.3	52.5
Pyr	*Tri5*	7.1	17.2	23.7	53.0	6.0	17.8	26.2	55.0
Pyr	*Tri5Sem*	**8.3**	21.6	30.3	34.0	**7.6**	20.7	30.1	38.0
ILS	*BoW5'*	7.5	**21.8**	**33.3**	**26.0**	6.6	**24.6**	**34.7**	**26.0**

synsets in the set {Caption} are shown in Fig. 1, where we can see that synset *dog, domestic dog, Canis familiaris* (WordNet ID n02084071) appears in more than 9000 captions out of the original 40000, twice more than synset *homo, man, human being, human* (WordNet ID n02472293). Note that to avoid clutter, in Fig. 1 as well as in the rest of this paper, we use the first word of the WordNet definition to refer to a synset, e.g., we use *dog* instead of *dog, domestic dog, Canis familiaris* for synset n02084071.

{ILSVRC12} provides training images for synsets external to Flickr8K and has a very small intersection with {Caption}. According to Table 2, the two sets have 197 common elements. More details are presented Fig. 2(a), which shows the ratio of the top K synsets in {Caption} that have visual classifiers (i.e. also in {ILSVRC12}). The first synset with a visual classifier appears at $K = 83$, and the fraction of Flickr8K noun synsets with visual classifiers is lower than 8 %. The low level of overlapping between {ILSVRC12} and {Caption} fits our application scenario where little directly related training data is available.

In Table 3 we present the performance of our high level visual kernel *ILS* that is built by visual classifiers for the synsets in {ILSVRC12}. For comparison we also include the performance of the methods reported in [17], where *Pyr* denotes the visual kernel in [17] that uses only low and mid-level visual information,

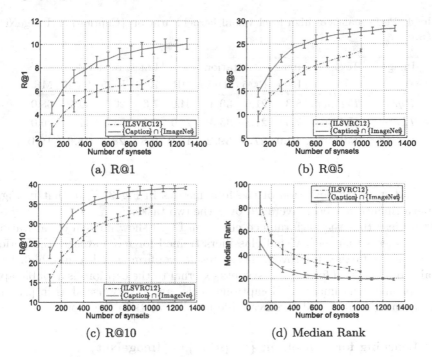

Fig. 3. Mean and standard deviation of performance averaged over "annotation" and "retrieval" tasks as functions of the number of random synsets.

TagRank, *Tri5* and *Tri5Sem* are sophisticated text kernels that use high-order word statistics and lexical similarities. Table 3 shows the recalls R@1, R@5, R@10 and the median rank on both annotation and retrieval tasks.

The results in Table 3 demonstrate that *ILS* performs well despite the small overlap between {ILSVRC12} and {Caption}. When the basic text kernels *BoW5* or *BoW5′* are used, *ILS* outperforms *Pyr* by large margins in all metrics and on both tasks. For example, with the same *Pyr* visual kernel, the text kernels *TagRank* and *Tri5* that exploit high-order word statistics reduce the median rank of *BoW5* from 58 to 56 and 53 respectively, while *ILS* takes it to 26. This suggests that compared to noisy low level visual representation, better alignment can be found between high level visual information and captions.

When compared to the best combination in [17] *Pyr/Tri5Sem*, where *Tri5 Sem* encodes both third-order word co-occurrence statistics and lexical similarities learnt from several external corpora, the *ILS/BoW5′* combination still leads in most metrics. Interestingly, while *Tri5Sem* seems better at finding the exact gold item as indicted by the higher R@1 scores, *ILS* can bring good matches to the query overall, leading to better R@5, R@10 and median rank scores.

We also randomly sample 100–900 synsets at a step size of 100 and build visual kernels using only the predicted probabilities from the corresponding SVMs. For each sample size we repeat the experiment 15 times, and report the

Table 4. Performance of high level visual kernel learnt on {Caption} ∩ {ImageNet}, *CapIma*.

Image	Text	Image annotation				Image retrieval			
		R@1	R@5	R@10	MR	R@1	R@5	R@10	MR
Pyr	*Tri5Sem*	8.3	21.6	30.3	34.0	7.6	20.7	30.1	38.0
ILS	*BoW5'*	7.5	21.8	33.3	26.0	6.6	24.6	34.7	26.0
CapIma	*BoW5'*	**10.0**	**27.3**	**39.2**	**19.0**	**9.8**	**28.8**	**38.6**	**19.0**

mean and standard deviation of the four metrics in Fig. 3. Note that in Fig. 3 the performance has been averaged over the two tasks.

It is clear that the performance curves in Fig. 3 show no sign of saturation, which suggests that with visual classifiers trained for more sysnets the performance can be further improved. These results confirm that learning high level visual representation for a set of sysnets external to the captions is a viable approach for matching images and captions. This can be very useful as in practice training images are not always available for all synsets in the captions.

5.2　Learning for Synsets in {Caption} ∩ {ImageNet}

In the second scenario, we learn for synsets that are actually in the captions. To obtain training images we use the intersection of {Caption} and {ImageNet}. The resulting set {Caption} ∩ {ImageNet} has 1372 synsets with image data available for training visual classifiers.

Figure 2(b) plots the ratio of the top K synsets in {Caption} that have visual classifiers. Compared to Fig. 2(a) the ratio here is much higher. For example, out of 10, 50, and 100 top ranked synsets, 7, 31, and 57 respectively have corresponding visual classifiers. Overall, 1372 synsets out of the total 3335 have visual classifiers.

In Table 4 we report the performance of the visual kernel *CapIma* that is built using {Caption}∩{ImageNet}. For convenience we also repeat the results of *Pyr/BoW*5 and *ILS/BoW*5' from Table 3. Table 4 shows that *CapIma/BoW*5' combination outperforms the other two by large margins in all metrics and on both tasks. For example, its median rank (19.0) almost halves that of *Pyr/BoW*5 (36.0), which is the best reported in [17]. The significant edge of *CapIma/BoW*5' over *ILS/BoW*5' demonstrates the advantage of learning the visual appearance of the objects, scenes and actions that are actually mentioned in the captions, rather than learn the context.

Figure 3 plots the performance when using varying numbers of randomly sampled synsets to build visual kernels, where for each number the averaged result for 15 random sets is reported. It gives a flavour of the performance that can be expected when training images are available only for limited number of synsets. For instance, when only 250 synsets have visual classifiers, the R@10 score is approximately 30, which is similar to that of *Pyr/Tri5Sem*.

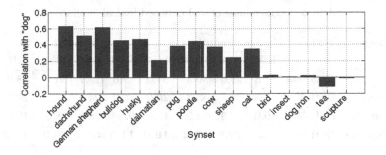

Fig. 4. Visual correlation with *dog* synset.

6 . Vision Based Lexical Similarity

One of the key problems with the basic $BoW5/BoW5'$ text kernels is that they require exact match of words, and cannot account for the fact that the same entity can be described in different words. In [17] three lexical similarity measures are leant on text corpora. These similarities capture semantic relatedness, hence allow partial matches between words. The $Tri5Sem$ text kernel is then built by combining the lexical similarities, and is shown to be the best performing text kernel.

In contrast to the linguistics based similarities, we propose a vision based lexical similarity measure. This measure exploits the high level visual information encoded in the output of the visual classifiers. Recall that x^t in the representation of an image is the prediction of the visual classifier corresponding to the tth synset. Let $\mathbf{x}^t \in \mathcal{R}^m$ and $\mathbf{x}^{t'} \in \mathcal{R}^m$ be predictions of the presence of synsets t and t' for all training images in Flickr8K. The linear correlation $c(t, t') = \text{corr}(\mathbf{x}^t, \mathbf{x}^{t'}) \in [-1, 1]$ can be thought of as a visually informed lexical similarity between synsets t and t'.

Figure 4 plots the correlations between the *dog* synset and another 16 synsets. The figure shows that all breeds of dog have high positive correlations with *dog*. The correlations between the three mammals *cow*, *sheep*, *cat* and *dog* are also high, although in general not as high as the dog breeds. On the other hand, *bird*, *insect*, and the semantically unrelated ones all correlate poorly with *dog*. This demonstrates the potential advantages of the vision based lexical similarity.

The Lin similarity [33] used in [17] exploits the hypernym/hyponym relations in WordNet. As a result, synsets that have close relations but are not visually similar may have high similarity, for example, *dog* and *bird*, *swimming* and *football*. This particularly poses a problem when alignment between image and text is sought. Our vision based similarity measure, on the the hand, tackles the very problem. Moreover, the vision based similarity is not confused by the presence of words in semantically unrelated sysnets, e.g. *dog* in *dog iron*, which are visually dissimilar.

Recall that the word-sense disambiguation component of the linguistic analyser of [24] establishes correspondences between the lemmatised words and

Table 5. Performance of vision based lexical similarity.

Image	Text	Image annotation				Image retrieval			
		R@1	R@5	R@10	MR	R@1	R@5	R@10	MR
Pyr	$Tri5Sem$	8.3	21.6	30.3	34.0	7.6	20.7	30.1	38.0
ILS	$BoW5'$	7.5	21.8	33.3	26.0	6.6	24.6	34.7	26.0
$CapIma$	$BoW5'$	10.0	27.3	39.2	19.0	9.8	28.8	38.6	19.0
$CapIma$	$BoW5'_V$	**11.1**	**29.8**	**42.2**	**16.0**	**11.2**	**30.7**	**40.9**	**15.0**

synsets. We consider the case where visual classifiers are trained for synsets in {Caption} ∩ {ImageNet}. Let syn(r) be the synset ID in {Caption} ∩ {ImageNet} that corresponds to the rth word in the dictionary of 5768 unique words. The rth dimension of the BoW representation with vision based similarity incorporated, is then:

$$y^r = \left(t^r + \gamma \sum_{s \in \{S\} \backslash r} t^s c\big(\text{syn}(r), \text{syn}(s)\big) \right) \log \frac{D}{d^r + 1} \tag{7}$$

where $\{S\}$ is the set of word IDs in the dictionary whose corresponding sysnets have visual classifiers, t^s is the term frequency of the sth word in the dictionary, and $\gamma \in [0, 1]$ is a parameter that is learnt on the validation set. When γ is set to 0, Eq. (7) reduces to the standard BoW representation in Eq. (4). Otherwise, the additional term accounts for partial matches between words: not only the rth word activates the rth bin of the BoW representation, other words also contribute an amount determined by the visual similarity between them and the rth word.

We denote by $BoW5'_V$ the text kernel using vision based lexical similarity and report its performance in Table 5, where for comparison we repeat the content of Table 4. The $CapIma/BoW5'_V$ combination outperforms the previous best $CapIma/BoW5'$ in all metrics, reducing the median rank from 19.0 to 15.5. This clearly indicates the advantage of exploiting vision based lexical similarity.

The $Tri5Sem$ kernel in [17] combines several linguistics based lexical similarities trained on both internal (captions) and external corpora. Among them, the alignment based similarity takes advantage of the fact that each image in Flickr8K is associated with five independently written captions. Our vision based similarity does not rely on this and is therefore more general. Moreover, note that ideally we would like to compute the visual similarity between every pair of noun synsets, or even ever pair of sysnets, in the captions. In practice, however, we are constrained by available training images, and as a result we have pairwise similarity only for 1372 synsets. The potentials of the vision based lexical similarity are therefore not fully realised.

Finally, the five top ranked and the gold captions/images for three random test examples on both tasks are shown in Tables 6 and 7, where the best kernels $CapIma/BoW5'_V$ are used.

Table 6. Query image, the five top ranked captions retrieved (from top to bottom), and the gold caption (in boldface). In the three random examples the rank of the gold caption is 9, 5, and 11 respectively.

- A boy in a park playing with two orange balls.
- little girls in swimsuits are laughing
- A boy in a bathing suit stands in water.
- A dark man in a white and green feathered mask with green jewelry and pants.
- A child wearing swim goggles.
- ...
- **A man and a woman in festive costumes dancing.**

- A black dog in water.
- A child slides down a slide and into the water.
- A boy is diving through the air into a swimming pool.
- a person doing the backstroke in a swimming pool
- **a brown and white dog swimming towards some in the pool**

- A basketball player wearing a black and white uniform dribbles the ball.
- A boy with red shorts is holding a basketball in a basketball court.
- A basketball player dribbles the ball while another blocks him and an official looks on.
- Several basketball players are grabbing for the ball during a game.
- A basketball game
- ...
- **A player from the white and green highschool team dribbles down court defended by a player from the other team.**

Table 7. Query caption, the five top ranked images retrieved (from left to right), and the gold image (in column 6). In the three random examples the rank of the gold image is 22, 16, and 810 respectively.

The dogs are in the snow in front of a fence.

A hiker ascends a snowy hill.

Three boys in a building under construction.

7   Conclusions

We have presented an approach for matching images and captions based on KCCA. Our visual kernels encode high level visual information resulting from state-of-the-art image recognition, leading to a significant improvement compared to low level visual representation in [17]. We successfully make use of additional annotated data with very few labels directly related to the test images, and we quantify the gain in performance when the visual classifiers are trained for directly related synsets. We have also proposed to exploit responses of visual classifiers to compute a lexical similarity between words. We evaluated the proposed approaches on a large and publicly available dataset, and showed that our methods substantially improved the state-of-the-art performance.

Acknowledgement. This work has been supported by EU Chist-Era EPSRC EP/ K01904X/1 Visual Sense project.

References

1. Guillaumin, M., Mensink, T., Verbeek, J., Schmid, C.: Face recognition from caption-based supervision. IJCV **96**(1), 64–82 (2012)
2. Kong, C., Lin, D., Bansal, M., Urtasun, R., Fidler, S.: What are you talking about? text-to-image coreference. In: CVPR (2014)
3. Elhoseiny, M., Saleh, B., Elgammal, A.: Write a classifier: zero-shot learning using purely textural description. In: ICCV (2013)
4. Feng, Y., Lapata, M.: Automatic caption generation for news images. PAMI **35**(4), 797–812 (2013)
5. Ordonez, V., Kulkarni, G., Berg, T.: Im2text: describing images using 1 million captioned photographs. In: NIPS (2011)
6. Li, S., Kulkarni, G., Berg, T., Berg, A., Choi, Y.: Composing simple image descriptions using web-scale n-grams. In: CoNLL (2011)
7. Farhadi, A., Hejrati, M., Sadeghi, M.A., Young, P., Rashtchian, C., Hockenmaier, J., Forsyth, D.: Every picture tells a story: generating sentences from images. In: Daniilidis, K., Maragos, P., Paragios, N. (eds.) ECCV 2010, Part IV. LNCS, vol. 6314, pp. 15–29. Springer, Heidelberg (2010)
8. Kulkarni, G., Premraj, V., Dhar, S., Li, S., Choi, Y., Berg, A., Berg, T.: Baby talk: understanding and generating simple image descriptions. In: CVPR (2011)
9. Yang, Y., Teo, C., Daumé III, H.D., Aloimonos, Y.: Corpus-guided sentence generation of natural images. In: EMNLP (2011)
10. Mitchell, M., Han, X., Dodge, J., Mensch, A., Goyal, A., Berg, A., Yamaguchi, K., Berg, T., Stratos, K., Daume, H.: Midge: generating image descriptions from computer vision detections. In: EACL (2012)
11. Gupta, A., Verma, Y., Jawahar, C.: Choosing linguistics over vision to describe images. In: AAAI Conference on Artificial Intelligence (2012)
12. Kuznetsova, P., Ordonez, V., Berg, A., Berg, T., Choi, Y.: Collective generation of natural image descriptions. In: ACL (2012)
13. Krishnamoorthy, N., Malkarnenkar, G., Mooney, R., Saenko, K., Guadarrama, S.: Generating natural-language video descriptions using text-mined knowledge. In: AAAI Conference on Artificial Intelligence (2013)

14. Das, P., Xu, C., Doell, R., Corso, J.: A thousand frames in just a few words: lingual description of videos through latent topic and sparse object stitching. In: CVPR (2013)
15. Guadarrama, S., Krishnamoorthy, N., Malkarnenkar, G., Venugopalan, S., Mooney, R., Darrell, T., Saenko, K.: Youtube2text: recognizing and describing arbitrary activities using semantic hierarchies and zero-shot recognition. In: ICCV (2013)
16. Rohrbach, M., Qiu, W., Titov, I., Thater, S., Pinkal, M., Schiele, B.: Translating video content to natural language descriptions. In: ICCV (2013)
17. Hodosh, M., Young, P., Hockenmaier, J.: Framing image description as a ranking task: data, models and evaluation metrics. J. Artif. Intell. Res. **47**, 853–899 (2013)
18. Bach, F., Jordan, M.: Kernel independent component analysis. JMLR **3**, 1–48 (2002)
19. Hardoon, D., Szedmak, S., Shawe-Taylor, J.: Canonical correlation analysis: an overview with application to learning methods. Neural Comput. **16**(12), 2639–2664 (2004)
20. Papineni, K., Roukos, S., Ward, T., Zhu, W.: BLEU: a method for automatic evaluation of machine translation. In: ACL (2002)
21. Lin, C.: ROUGE: a package for automatic evaluation of summaries. In: Workshop on Text Summarization Branches Out (2004)
22. Reiter, E., Belz, A.: An investigation into the validity of some metrics for automatically evaluating natural lanugage generation systems. Comput. Linguist. **35**(4), 338–529 (2009)
23. Hotelling, H.: Relations between two sets of variates. Biometrika **28**(3/4), 321–377 (1936)
24. Padro, L., Stanivlosky, E.: Freeling 3.0: towards wider multilinguality. In: Language Resources and Evaluation Conference (2012)
25. Krizhevsky, A., Sutskever, I., Hinton, G.: ImageNet classification with deep convolutional neural networks. In: NIPS (2012)
26. Deng, J., Berg, A., Satheesh, S., Su, H., Khosla, A., Feifei, L.: ImageNet large scale visual recognition challenge (ILSVRC) 2012 (2012). http://image-net.org/challenges/LSVRC/2012/
27. LeCun, Y., Boser, B., Denker, J., Henerson, D., Howard, R., Hubbard, W., Jackel, L.: Backpropagation applied to handwritten zip code recognition. Neural Comput. **1**(4), 541–551 (1989)
28. Hinton, G., Salakhutdinov, R.: Reducing the dimensionality of data with neural networks. Science **313**, 504–507 (2006)
29. Donahue, J., Jia, Y., Vinyals, O., Hoffman, J., Zhang, N., Tzeng, E., Darrell, T.: DeCAF: a deep convolutional activation feature for generic visual recognition (2013). arXiv:1310.1531 [cs.CV]
30. Deng, J., Dong, W., Socher, R., Li, L., Li, K., Fei-Fei, L.: Imagenet: a large scale hierarchical image database. In: CVPR (2009)
31. Jia, Y.: Caffe: an open source convolutional architecture for fast feature embedding (2013). http://caffe.berkeleyvision.org
32. Chang, C., Lin, C.: LIBSVM: a library for support vector machines. ACM Trans. Intell. Syst. Technol. **2**(3), 1–27 (2011). http://www.csie.ntu.edu.tw/cjlin/libsvm
33. Lin, D.: An information-theoretic definition on similarity. In: ICML (1998)

Efficient Feature Coding Based on Auto-encoder Network for Image Classification

Guo-Sen Xie[✉], Xu-Yao Zhang, and Cheng-Lin Liu

National Laboratory of Pattern Recognition, Institute of Automation,
Chinese Academy of Sciences, Beijing 100190, China
{guosen.xie,xyz,liucl}@nlpr.ia.ac.cn

Abstract. Local descriptor coding is one crucial step in traditional Bag of Words (BoW) framework for image categorization. However, the slow coding speed of previous methods is one limitation for applications in large scale problems. Recently, neural network based models have been widely applied in various classification tasks. Using neural network models for descriptor coding is straightforward and efficient due to their fast forward propagation. In this paper, we propose to use the Auto-Encoder (AE) network as a local descriptor coding block, and further embed AE network in the BoW framework for the purpose of image classification. To make the hidden activities of AE network to be both selective and sparse, we add an efficient and effective regularization term into the learning process of AE network, which can promote sparsity of the hidden layer for each input descriptor as well as the selectivity for each hidden node. By incorporating the AE network coding with the BoW framework, we can achieve better results and faster speeds than other state-of-the-art feature coding methods on Caltech101, Scene15 and UIUC 8-Sports databases.

1 Introduction

Image classification is one basic and challenging vision task which aims at classifying images into correct categories. The original Bag of Words (BoW) model is derived from the document retrieval field, and has been successfully applied to image classification [1] with state-of-the-art performance [2–5]. An unified framework of BoW model consists of several steps including (a) local feature (e.g., SIFT, HOG, SURF, etc.) extraction [6–8], (b) dictionary learning and feature coding, (c) pooling (Max, Average, and Sum) of the coded features [2–4], and (d) classifier learning (e.g., one-vs-all SVMs). To incorporate spatial information into the BoW framework, Lazebnik et al. [9] proposed the spatial pyramid matching (SPM) model to improve the performance which is usually denoted as BoW+SPM.

Local descriptor coding is an essential step in the BoW framework, which has drawn great attention in recent years. Given the codebook (dictionary), descriptor coding can be seen as the process of activating a small number of codewords (based on the coding process of the descriptor), which can then generate a coding

© Springer International Publishing Switzerland 2015
D. Cremers et al. (Eds.): ACCV 2014, Part I, LNCS 9003, pp. 628–642, 2015.
DOI: 10.1007/978-3-319-16865-4_41

vector with the same size (dimension) of the codebook [10]. One class of local descriptor coding methods is the reconstruction based model, which is usually designed to minimize the norm (distance) of the descriptors and a linear combination of codewords (defined as reconstruction error), along with constraints on the coding vectors. For example, besides the reconstruction term, sparse coding (SC) [2] adds sparsity constraint on the coding vectors, and locality-constrained linear coding (LLC) [3] incorporates local neighborhood based constraints. Moreover, voting based coding [1,4,11] can also be viewed as reconstruction based models with some special constraints on the coding vector.

The optimization formulations of the above models are all based on minimization of the reconstruction error and subjection to various kinds of constraints on the final coding vectors. However, they deal with different descriptors independently. To further improve the performance, Gao et al. [12] proposed the Laplacian sparse coding (LaSC) which incorporates Laplacian constraints of the descriptors into the sparse coding model. Another class of models considering the relationships of descriptors are based on the context information of descriptors [13–15].

Recently, the development of deep neural networks (DNNs) has triggered many interests of using neural network (NN) models for automatical feature learning in image classification, e.g., the convolutional neural network (CNN) [16] and the restricted Boltzmann machines (RBM) [17] models. The learned weights of the neural networks can also be viewed as the codebook when compared with traditional coding methods. One obvious advantage of NN based feature learning is the fast speed of descriptor coding after learning the weights. Goh et al. [18] proposed a feature learning model based on regularized RBM. The regularizer used there can guarantee the sparsity of hidden activates for each input descriptor, and meanwhile the selectivity of one hidden node for a batch of input descriptors. Sohn et al. [19] also advocated complex sparse convolutional RBM for feature learning.

Considering the slow learning process of CNN and complex contrastive divergence (CD) [20] algorithm used in the RBM training process, in this paper, we explore to use another neural network for local descriptor learning, namely the Auto-Encoder (AE) network [21]. The training of AE network is based on an efficient accessible back propagation (BP) algorithm [22], and we also use an improved version of regularizer proposed by [18] to constrain the learning process of AE network. It is obvious that the regularized AE network is also in the class of reconstruction based coding method. Compared with traditional BoW models as mentioned above, the selectivity of hidden node in the AE network can be explained as one kind of context constraint derived from one batch descriptors, which can bring superior performance for image classification.

The contributions of this paper are: (1) Integrating AE network based feature learning into BoW+SPM framework (Fig. 1) which is both efficient and effective. To the best of our knowledge, this is the first trial to integrate AE network into BoW framework. (2) Incorporating the improved regularizer proposed by [18] into the AE network learning process. (3) Extensive experiments on Caltech101, Scene15, and UIUC 8-Sports demonstrate the effectiveness of the proposed method.

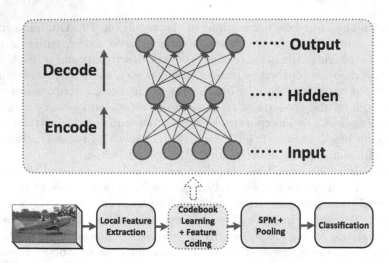

Fig. 1. The hybrid BoW+SPM framework, based on regularized AE network learning for local descriptor coding. After learning the weights and biases of the AE network, the hidden activates are coding vectors of descriptors.

The rest of this paper is organized as follows: The related work about descriptor coding are presented in Sect. 2. The proposed regularized AE network is detailed in Sect. 3. Experimental results, influence of parameter settings and comparison of coding speed are presented in Sect. 4. Section 5 concludes this paper and discusses the future works.

2   Related Work

Descriptor coding methods can be roughly classified into five categories [10]: (i) Voting based methods, e.g., hard assignment coding (HAC) [1], soft assignment coding (SAC) [11] and local soft assignment coding (LSAC) [4]. (ii) Reconstruction based methods, e.g., sparse coding (SC) [2], local coordinate coding (LCC) [23], locality-constrained linear coding (LLC) [3], and so on. (iii) Salient coding (SaC) [5] and group salient coding (GSC) [24]. (iv) Fisher coding [25,26]. (v) Local tangent coding, e.g., super vector coding [27].

Let $X = [x_1, x_2, \cdots, x_n] \in \mathbb{R}^{d \times N}$ be N d−dimensional local features extracted from an image. $B = [b_1, b_2, \cdots, b_M] \in \mathbb{R}^{d \times M}$ denotes the codebook which is usually obtained by k-means algorithm. And $V = [v_1, v_2, \cdots, v_M] \in \mathbb{R}^{M \times N}$ is the coding matrix of these N features, here v_i is the coding vector of x_i, with $i = 1, 2, \cdots, N$. Notations denoted above are used in the whole paper.

The initial BoW model was proposed by [1], where hard assignment was taken to quantize the local descriptors. HAC records the number of local descriptors assigned to each codeword in the codebook B, thus obtaining one M dimensional coding vector for these descriptors. The assignment criteria for descriptor x_i is:

$$v_{i,j} = \begin{cases} 1, & \text{if } j = \arg\min_k \|x_i - b_k\|_2^2, \\ 0, & \text{else.} \end{cases} \quad (1)$$

Different to HAC, SAC [11] assigns weighted value to all codewords of the codebook for each descriptor. An improved version of SAC is localized SAC (LSAC) [4] which only assigns value to neighbor codewords of the descriptor. When the size M of the codebook is large, the searching of neighbor codewords is time consuming. The performances of HAC, SAC and LSAC are all relative poor when compared with other more complicated models.

Besides the reconstruction error, SC [2] was proposed to add another sparse constraint onto the coding vector v. SC can be formulated as an optimization problem:

$$v^* = \arg\min_v \|x - Bv\|_2^2 + \lambda\|v\|_1, \quad (2)$$

where λ controls the tradeoff of the reconstruction and sparsity. We can get the best coding v^* of descriptor x through optimizing Eq. (2). Then LCC [28] was proposed to add locality constraint instead of sparse constraint. Though, the performances of SC and LCC are better than voting based coding, the optimization of them are both time consuming. To speed up, LLC was proposed by [3], which is formulated as follow:

$$v^* = \arg\min_v \|x - Bv\|_2^2 + \lambda\|dist \odot v\|_2, \quad (3)$$

where $\odot$ denotes element-wise product and $dist = [\exp(\|x - b_1\|_2/\delta), \exp(\|x - b_2\|_2/\delta), \cdots, \exp(\|x - b_M\|_2/\delta)]^T \in \mathbb{R}^M$. In Eq. (3), LLC incorporates locality constraint by L2-norm of element-wise product.

To consider the saliency of codewords, salient coding was proposed by [5], wherein relative proximity is used to represent the salient response of the codewords. Given K nearest neighbor codewords of one descriptor, salient coding utilizes the difference between the nearest codeword and the rest $K-1$ neighbor codewords to represent saliency. Recently, group saliency coding (GSC) [24] was also proposed to utilize all the saliency responses of a group of codewords, where the final coding vector of a descriptor on one codeword is the maximum value of all responses under different group sizes [10].

3   Auto-Encoder (AE) Network Based Descriptor Coding

In this paper, the descriptor coding process is based on Auto-Encoder (AE) network [21]. The AE network consists of an encoder process of descriptors and an decoder process of hidden outputs (Fig. 1). The objective is to minimize the reconstruction error and the activate functions of the hidden layer are usually nonlinear, (e.g., sigmoid and tangent), therefore, AE network is a reconstruction based and nonlinear coding process. To further improve the descriptor coding performance, we also add a regularization term in the learning process to guarantee both sparsity and selectivity of the AE network.

3.1   Auto-Encoder Network

We use the notations denoted in Sect. 2 for convenience. The number of nodes for both the input and output layer are d, which is the same as the descriptor dimension. In the BoW framework, we have M codewords in the codebook B, therefore, we also set the number of hidden nodes in the AE network as M, which means the coded vectors of AE network and other BoW models have the same discrete dimensionality (M can be set as 1024, 2048, etc.).

Let $W^{(1)} \in \mathbb{R}^{d \times M}, b^{(1)} \in \mathbb{R}^{M}$ be the weight and bias of the input-hidden layer, $W^{(2)} \in \mathbb{R}^{M \times d}, b^{(2)} \in \mathbb{R}^{d}$ be the weight and bias of the hidden-output layer. Figure 1 shows the architecture of the AE network. Suppose we have extracted N descriptors: $X = [x_1, x_2, \cdots, x_N] \in \mathbb{R}^{d \times N}$ from the training images around N interesting points (by dense sampling or interesting points detection). Then the formulation of AE network is:

$$\arg \min_{\Theta} \mathcal{L} = \frac{1}{2N} \sum_{t=1}^{N} \|x_t - h(x_t)\|_2^2 + \frac{\lambda_1}{2}(\|W^{(1)}\|_F^2 + \|W^{(2)}\|_F^2), \qquad (4)$$

where $\Theta = \{W^{(i)}, b^{(i)} | i = 1, 2\}$ and λ_1 controls the elements of the weights to be small, which can avoid over-fitting. The $h(x_t)$ is the reconstruction of x_t which is defined as

$$h(x_t) = \sigma(W^{(2)^\top} \sigma(W^{(1)^\top} x_t + b^{(1)}) + b^{(2)}), \qquad (5)$$

where $\sigma(x) = \frac{1}{1+e^{-x}}$ is the sigmoid activate function. Then Eq. (4) is optimized by batch gradient decent (BGD) based on BP algorithm [22].

3.2   Sparsity and Selectivity Regularizer with Random Distortion

In the striate complex cells, the selectivity is the response distribution of a neuron across a set of stimuli, and sparsity is the response distribution of several neurons to one single stimulus [29]. In the AE network, each hidden node can be viewed as a neuron and each descriptor can be viewed as a stimuli. To make the AE network to be both sparse and selective, i.e., the output hidden activate vector of one input descriptor is sparse, and the activate vector of one hidden node for the batch descriptors is selective, we should regularize our AE network learning process with sparsity and selectivity just the same as the striate complex cells [29].

To facilitate the next steps of pooling and classification in the hybrid BoW framework (Fig. 1), Goh et al. [18] have proposed one regularizer into the learning process of RBM. In this paper, we also incorporate this regularizer into the AE network. To further improve the performance, we also add random distortion into the constructing of the regularization term.

Let $X_{batch} = [x_1, x_2, \cdots, x_K] \in \mathbb{R}^{d \times K}$ be one batch descriptors during the AE network training, $H = [\sigma(W^{(1)^\top} x_1 + b^{(1)}), \sigma(W^{(1)^\top} x_2 + b^{(1)}), \cdots, \sigma(W^{(1)^\top} x_K + b^{(1)})] \in \mathbb{R}^{M \times K}$ be the forward activates matrix of X_{batch}. The sparsity and selectivity of the hidden activates can be introduced by forcing $\gamma(W^{(1)}, b^{(1)}) = \|H - P\|_F^2 \to 0$ during the AE network learning process, where $P \in \mathbb{R}^{M \times K}$ is

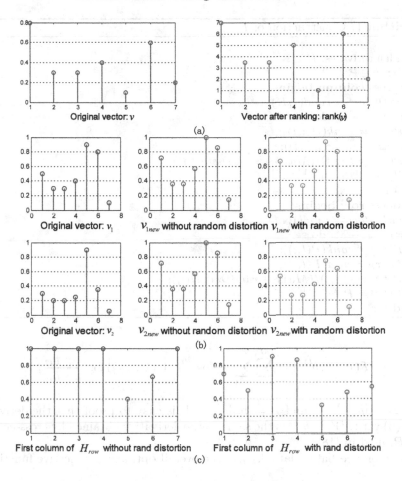

Fig. 2. (a) v and its corresponding rank(v), here $v =$[0.8 0.3 0.3 0.4 0.1 0.6 0.2], rank(v)=[7 3.5 3.5 5 1 6 2]. (b) v_i, $(i-1,2)$ and their normalized ranking vectors, without and with random distortion. It can be seen that $v_{1new} = v_{2new}$ when no distortion added, $v_{1new} \neq v_{2new}$ when distortion added. (c) H_{row} is the matrix obtained by row ranking of H, without or with random distortion. Left: first column of H_{row} without distortion. Right: first column of H_{row} with distortion. It's obvious we get better H_{row} with distortion added.

a matrix constructed based on H forcing both sparsity and selectivity. Then the gradient updating of $W^{(1)}, b^{(1)}$ is modified by adding the increments of $\gamma(W^{(1)}, b^{(1)})$ w.r.t. its parameters during the regularized AE network learning process.

In practice, many choices of penalty satisfying $H \rightarrow P$ can be taken. In order to embed the derivative calculation into the residual error during the back propagation [30], we use another penalty, i.e., KL divergence of H and P instead of the F-norm of them. The KL divergence of H and P is:

Algorithm 1. Construction of P
___
Input:
    Hidden activates: $H \in \mathbb{R}^{M \times K}$, μ_1, μ_2
Output: $P \in \mathbb{R}^{M \times K}$
1: **Process column begins:**
2: $randDistort = rand(1, K)$.
3: **for** t = 1 → K **do**
4:     $P(:, t) = rank(H(:, t))$;
5:     $Max_P = max(P(:, t))$;
6:     $P(:, t) = P(:, t)/(Max_P + randDistort(t))$;
7:     $P(:, t) = P(:, t)^{1-1/\mu_1}$;
8: **end for**
9: **Process row begins:**
10: $randDistort = rand(1, M)$.
11: **for** t = 1 → M **do**
12:    $P(t, :) = rank(P(t, :))$;
13:    $Max_P = max(P(t, :))$;
14:    $P(t, :) = P(t, :)/(Max_P + randDistort(t))$;
15:    $P(t, :) = P(t, :)^{1-1/\mu_2}$;
16: **end for**
___

$$T(W^{(1)}, b^{(1)}) = \sum_{i=1}^{M} \sum_{j=1}^{K} p_{ij} \log \frac{p_{ij}}{h_{ij}} + (1 - p_{ij}) \log \frac{1 - p_{ij}}{1 - h_{ij}}, \tag{6}$$

where $H = [h_{ij}]^{M \times K}$ and $P = [p_{ij}]^{M \times K}$. It is easy to proof that the derivative of Eq. (6) w.r.t. $W^{(1)}, b^{(1)}$ is the same as the derivative obtained by cross-entropy of H, P, used in [18].

Based on the batch data X_{batch}, the overall optimizing objective function is

$$\mathcal{L} = \frac{1}{2K} \sum_{t=1}^{K} \|x_t - h(x_t)\|_2^2 + \frac{\lambda_1}{2}(\|W^{(1)}\|_F^2 + \|W^{(2)}\|_F^2) + \lambda_2 T(W^{(1)}, b^{(1)}), \tag{7}$$

where λ_2 controls the tradeoff between sparsity, selectivity and the reconstruction.

Construction of Sparse and Selective Matrix P, based on H. In this Subsection, we present the construction of P.

Based on the initial algorithm in [18], we propose to add random distortion after getting the rank score of the column or row of H. Denote ν as one column or row of H, the distorted and normalized new vector ν_{new} is:

$$\nu_{new} = rank(\nu)/(max(\nu) + \tau * rand), \tag{8}$$

where τ controls the extent of random distortion, $\tau = 1$ in all our experiments. And rank(ν) returns the ranks of the values in ν. If any values in ν are equal, rank(ν) returns their average rank (Fig. 2(a)).

Adding random number into Eq. (8) can enhance the robustness of ν_{new}. On the one hand, when two different vectors ν_1, ν_2 have the same ranking results: $\nu_{1new} = \nu_{2new}$, adding random number can make them also different (Fig. 2(b)), which is more reasonable for afterward processing. On the other hand, after obtaining the ranked matrix H_{row} by ranking all rows of H by Eq. (8), equal value elements will occur in some columns, that is confused for afterward max-pooling operation (Fig. 2(c)). Adding random number in generating H_{row} can avoid this problem.

After ν_{new} is obtained, another step, transforming it into a long-tailed vector is carried out as follow:

$$\nu_{last} = \nu_{new}^{(1-1/\mu)}, \tag{9}$$

where μ controls the shape of the long-tailed vector. Inspired by [18,23], we first carry out column ranking of H, then row ranking. Complete constructing procedure of P is listed in Algorithm 1.

3.3 The Hybrid Algorithm of AE Network with Sparse and Selective Regularization

In this Subsection, we summary the modified BP algorithm used to train the regularized AE network. BP algorithm [22] is usually run on batch data. Based on notations in the above Sections, the batch mode gradient descending procedure on $X_{batch} = [x_1, x_2, \cdots, x_K] \in \mathbb{R}^{d \times K}$ is listed in Algorithm 2. The $\odot$ and $\oslash$ denote element-wise product and division of matrices respectively.

Based on Algorithm 2, we can train the regularized AE network to cover all training data for several iterative epoches. After $(W^{(i)}, b^{(i)}), i = 1, 2$ have been learned, we can use them to do forward propagation to code all local descriptors, e.g., given descriptor $x_i \in \mathbb{R}^d$, its coding vector is

$$v_i = \text{sigmoid}(W^{(1)^T} * x_i + b^{(1)}) \in \mathbb{R}^M.$$

After coding the local descriptors by our trained AE network, $1 \times 1, 2 \times 2, 4 \times 4$ spatial partitions (SPM) [9] are adopted to incorporate spatial information. Then, max pooling on each sub-regions are adopted. By concatenating all the pooled sub-region vectors, we get the final image representations, which are fed into the linear SVM [31] (one-vs-rest) to train classifier.[1]

4   Experiments

In this Section, we first present the experimental settings in Subsect. 4.1. Then Subsect. 4.2 gives classification accuracy and illustrates the impact of different hidden node size on three datasets. Subsection 4.3 shows the impact of μ_1, μ_2 and λ_2. Subsection 4.4 compares the speed of the proposed methods with several other coding methods.

---

[1] We utilized lib-linear toolkit [32] in this paper for SVM training.

Algorithm 2. One batch Learning of Regularized AE Network

Input:

Batch data: $X_{batch} \in \mathbb{R}^{d \times K}$

$\lambda_1 = 0.0001, \lambda_2, \mu_1, \mu_2, hiddenNodes = M$

$momentum = 0.05, learnRate = 1, layer = 3$

Output: $(W^{(i)}, b^{(i)}), i = 1, 2$

1: **Forward propagation:**
2: $H^{(1)} = X_{batch}$;
3: **for** t = 2 → layer **do**
4:     $H^{(t)} = sigmoid(repmat(b^{(t-1)}, 1, K) + W^{(t-1)^T} * H^{(t-1)})$;
5: **end for**
6: Calculate P based on $H^{(2)} \in \mathbb{R}^{M \times K}$
7: **Back propagation:**
8: $D^{(layer)} = -(X_{batch} - H^{(3)}) \odot H^{(3)} \odot (1 - H^{(3)})$;
9: **for** t = layer − 1 → 2 **do**
10:     $SparsitySelectivity = \lambda_2 * ((1 - P) \oslash (1 - H^{(t)}) - P \oslash H^{(t)})$;
11:     $D^{(t)} = (W^{(t)} * D^{(t+1)} + SparsitySelectivity) \odot H^{(t)} \odot (1 - H^{(t)})$;
12: **end for**
13: **for** t = 1 → layer-1 **do**
14:     $DW^{(t)} = H^{(t)} * D^{(t+1)^T}/K$;
15:     $Db^{(t)} = sum(D^{(t+1)}, 2)/K$;
16: **end for**
17: **Gradient updating** :
18: **for** t = 1 → layer-1 **do**
19:     $vW^{(t)} = momentum * vW^{(t)} + learnRate * (DW^{(t)} + \lambda_1 * W^{(t)})$;
20:     $vb^{(t)} = momentum * vb^{(t)} + learnRate * Db^{(t)}$;
21:     $W^{(t)} = W^{(t)} - vW^{(t)}$;
22:     $b^{(t)} = b^{(t)} - vb^{(t)}$;
23: **end for**

4.1 Experimental Settings

In this paper, three datasets, i.e., Caltech101 [33], Scene15 [9], and UIUC 8-sports [34] are used to validate the proposed model. Images in Caltech101 and Scene15 datasets are resized to be no larger than 300 in height or width, and images in UIUC 8-sports no larger than 400. In all our experiments, single scale (16×16) 128-dim SIFT [6] are densely extracted from all images. The step sizes of extracting SIFT for Caltech101, Scene15 and UIUC 8-sports datasets are 6 pixels, 8 pixels and 4 pixels respectively. 20 k descriptors are used for regularized AE network learning in three datasets.

As for training-test set partition, we randomly select 30 training images per category for training, the rest for testing for Caltech101 dataset. For Scene15 dataset, we follow the partition manner in [9], i.e., randomly select 100 images per category for training, the rest for testing. For UIUC 8-sports dataset [34], 70 training images and 60 test images are randomly chosen from each category. The final result is the mean accuracy and standard deviations, which is based on 5 times experiments with different random partition of the training and test set.

Table 1. Classification rate (%) comparison on Caltech101, Scene15 and 8-Sports datasets.

Algorithms	Caltech101(30train)	Scene15	8-Sports
Hard Assignment [9]	64.60±0.80	81.40±0.50	–
Soft Assignment [4]	72.56±0.65	81.09±0.43	82.04±2.37
Local Soft Assignment [4]	74.21±0.81	82.70±0.39	82.29±1.84
ScSPM [2,12]	73.20±0.50	80.30±0.90	82.74±1.46
LLC [3,4]	73.40	81.53±0.65	81.41±1.84
SaC [5]	–	82.55±0.41	–
GSC [24]	73.4±1.20	83.2±0.4	–
LC-KSVD [35]	73.6	–	–
Ours	**74.24±0.96**	**83.27±0.83**	**85.29±1.49**

During our regularized AE network training, we fix the following parameters, i.e., learning rate = 1, batchsize = 100 or 200, momentum = 0.05, $\lambda_1 = 0.0001$, max iterative epochs ≤ 6. Now, we only have three free parameters: λ_2, μ_1, μ_2.

4.2 Classification Accuracy

Table 1 lists the average accuracies and standard deviations of different models. We can find that our model is better than other state-of-the-art models. Because we did not know the exact parameter settings and the implementation details of the compared models, the results of the compared models are borrowed from the cited references. It can be concluded that our proposed method is superior to other coding methods (reconstruction based coding, voting based coding, saliency coding, etc.) consistently. It is worthy to mention that our model is only based on single scale SIFT feature, while other methods are usually based on multi-scale SIFT features. Moreover, the maximal hidden node size (dictionary size) of our AE network is 3072, while some other methods use much larger dictionary than ours, e.g., GSC [24] uses a dictionary with 8192 codewords to obtain their results in Table 1.

We also explore accuracies under different hidden node size, i.e., the dimensionality of the coding vectors. We list the results on Table 2. It can be seen that different hidden node size has different performance. Best results are obtained with hidden node size 2048 for Caltech101 and 8-Sports datasets. While the best hidden node size is 3072 for scene15 dataset.

4.3 Impact of Hyper-Parameters

In this Subsection, we discuss the impact of the hyper-parameters, i.e., λ_2 in Eq. (7), μ_1, μ_2 in Algorithm 1. To save processing time, we only discuss these parameters on Caltech101 and Scene15 datasets. Figures 3 and 4 present the classification rate change tendency along different λ_2 and μ_1, μ_2.

Table 2. Classification rate (%) comparison on Caltech101, Scene15 and 8-Sports datasets under different size of hidden node.

Hidden node number	Caltech101(30train)	Scene15	8-Sports
1024	72.26±1.53	81.57±0.34	85.13±1.35
2048	**74.24±0.96**	82.61±0.18	**85.29±1.49**
3072	73.62±0.90	**83.27±0.83**	84.92±1.25

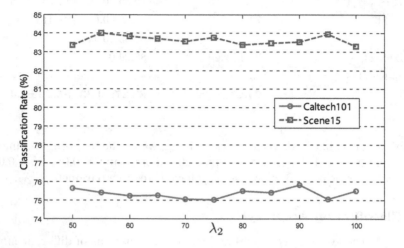

Fig. 3. Changing tendency of the classification rate along λ_2 on Caltech101 and Scene15 datasets (color figure online).

Classification results of one time experiment for Caltech101 and Scene15 datasets are drawn in Fig. 3 (red curve corresponding to Caltech101, blue curve corresponding to Scene15), with training-test set partition the same as the manner in Subsect. 4.1. Here, λ_2 takes $50, 55, \cdots, 100$, other relevant parameters of AE network are fixed. It can be seen that classification performance of our model w.r.t. λ_2 is stable, i.e., the fluctuation of accuracy is less than one percentage with the changing of λ_2.

To visualize the performance of the accuracy w.r.t. μ_1, μ_2, we show the $(\mu_1, \mu_2, \text{accuracy})$ maps of one time experiment both on Caltech101 and Scene15 datasets. The training-test partition manner is the same as the ones in Subsect. 4.1. The grids of μ_1, μ_2 used to draw the maps in Fig. 4 are in the range of $\mu_1 \in [0.001, 0.1]$ and $\mu_2 \in [0.001, 0.02]$, other parameters are fixed. It can be concluded from Fig. 4, our model is stable w.r.t. μ_1, and best μ_2 is located at interval: $[0.001, 0.006]$ for all datasets.

4.4 Comparison of Coding Speed

In this Subsection, we compare the coding (forward propagation) speed of our method with HAC [1], SAC [11], LSAC [4], SC [2], Approximate SC [2] (first

Table 3. Average single image processing time (second) on Caltech101 dataset under different dictionary size. The numbers in brackets are knn number of corresponding methods. SC(200) is the approximate SC [2] algorithm.

DictionarySize	HAC	SAC	LSAC(5)	SC	SC(200)	LLC(5)	SaC(5)	Ours
1024	0.196	0.047	0.191	1.355	2.007	0.343	0.179	**0.027**
2048	0.351	0.076	0.307	1.885	2.248	0.481	0.301	**0.045**
3072	0.502	0.112	0.449	3.382	2.437	0.721	0.437	**0.050**

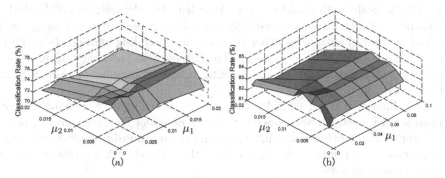

Fig. 4. Changing tendency of the classification rate along μ_1, μ_2 on (a) Caltech101 and (b) Scene15 datasets.

find the neighbor codewords, denoted as $\tilde{B}$, then coding the descriptors based on the sub-codebook $\tilde{B}$ instead of B), LLC [3] and SaC [5]. Average single image processing time is recorded for each method under different codebook (dictionary) size. Here, hidden layer size is the dictionary size for our AE network. We only reported the time on Caltech101 dataset. The average time on other datasets should be similar as Caltech101, because all three datasets have the same image magnitude, i.e., around 300-400 width and height. The experimental platform of comparing coding time is MATLAB8.1.0.604 (R2013a) in a server, with an Intel E5-2670 CPU (2.60 GHz and 16 cores) and 126.1 GB RAM.

To save dictionary learning time of other methods, K-means clustering is used to obtain the needed dictionaries of different size. Meanwhile, the weight $(W^{(1)}, b^{(1)})$ with different hidden node size (the same as dictionary size) should be learned. After that, we randomly select 10 images per class to test the coding speed of all these methods. The compared coding methods are implemented by us based on their public codes.

Results are listed in Table 3. It can be seen that our method is much faster than their counterparts. Moreover, weight learning time of our regularized AE network is also much faster than SC, LLC. In practical AE network learning process, less than six epoches are enough to gain good results, one epoch only takes several minutes. On the contrary, obtaining the dictionary by SC and LLC usually takes several hours or days. The fast inferring speed makes the proposed hybrid model more suitable for real application.

5   Conclusion and Future Work

In this paper, we propose a hybrid framework by combining traditional BoW+ SPM model with the regularized Auto-Encoder (AE) network. We use AE network to learn nonlinear transformation of local descriptors, which can be also seen as codebook learning in the viewpoint of BoW, by viewing the weights $W^{(1)}$ of AE network as the learned dictionary. During the AE network training, a random distortion based sparse and selective regularizer is also incorporated to guarantee the sparsity for each input descriptor and meanwhile the selectivity for each activate node in the hidden layer. After learning the weights $(W^{(1)}, b^{(1)})$ of the AE network, the inference speed (forward propagation) of local descriptors is very fast compared with some other state-of-the-art coding methods (e.g., HAC, SAC, LSAC, ScSPM, LLC and SaC). The classification accuracy of our model also consistently outperforms some recently proposed popular models (ScSPM, LLC, K-SVD, etc.).

In the future, we will consider incorporate discriminative information into regularized AE network and construct deep AE model for better coding of the descriptors. On the other hand, incorporating the relationship information (such as Laplacian constraint) of descriptors into the AE network learning process is also an interesting topic.

Acknowledgement. This work has been supported in part by the National Basic Research Program of China (973 Program) Grant 2012CB316302 and the Strategic Priority Research Program of the Chinese Academy of Sciences (Grant XDA06040102).

References

1. Csurka, G., Bray, C., Dance, C., Fan, L.: Visual categorization with bags of keypoints. In: ECCV, Workshop on Statistical Learning in Computer Vision, pp. 1–22 (2004)
2. Yang, J., Yu, K., Gong, Y., Huang, T.S.: Linear spatial pyramid matching using sparse coding for image classification. In: CVPR, pp. 1794–1801 (2009)
3. Wang, J., Yang, J., Yu, K., Lv, F., Huang, T.S., Gong, Y.: Locality-constrained linear coding for image classification. In: CVPR, pp. 3360–3367 (2010)
4. Liu, L., Lei, W., Liu, X.: In defense of soft-assignment coding. In: ICCV, pp. 2486–2493 (2011)
5. Huang, Y., Huang, K., Yu, Y., Tan, T.: Salient coding for image classification. In: CVPR, pp. 1753–1760 (2011)
6. Lowe, D.G.: Distinctive image features from scale-invariant keypoints. Int. J. Comput. Vis. **60**, 91–110 (2004)
7. Dalal, N., Triggs, B.: Histograms of oriented gradients for human detection. In: CVPR, vol. 1, pp. 886–893 (2005)
8. Bay, H., Tuytelaars, T., Van Gool, L.: SURF: speeded up robust features. In: Leonardis, A., Bischof, H., Pinz, A. (eds.) ECCV 2006, Part I. LNCS, vol. 3951, pp. 404–417. Springer, Heidelberg (2006)
9. Lazebnik, S., Schmid, C., Ponce, J.: Beyond bags of features: Spatial pyramid matching for recognizing natural scene categories. In: CVPR, pp. 2169–2178 (2006)

10. Huang, Y., Wu, Z., Wang, L., Tan, T.: Feature coding in image classification: A comprehensive study. IEEE Trans. Pattern Anal. Mach. Intell. **36**, 493–506 (2014)
11. van Gemert, J.C., Geusebroek, J.-M., Veenman, C.J., Smeulders, A.W.M.: Kernel codebooks for scene categorization. In: Forsyth, D., Torr, P., Zisserman, A. (eds.) ECCV 2008, Part III. LNCS, vol. 5304, pp. 696–709. Springer, Heidelberg (2008)
12. Gao, S., Tsang, I.W.H., Chia, L.T.: Laplacian sparse coding, hypergraph laplacian sparse coding, and applications. IEEE Trans. Pattern Anal. Mach. Intell. **35**, 92–104 (2013)
13. Galleguillos, C., Rabinovich, A., Belongie, S.: Object categorization using co-occurrence, location and appearance. In: IEEE Conference on Computer Vision and Pattern Recognition (2008)
14. Morioka, N., Satoh, S.: Compact correlation coding for visual object categorization. In: ICCV, pp. 1639–1646 (2011)
15. Su, Y., Jurie, F.: Visual word disambiguation by semantic contexts. In: ICCV, pp. 311–318 (2011)
16. Krizhevsky, A., Sutskever, I., Hinton, G.E.: Imagenet classification with deep convolutional neural networks. In: NIPS, pp. 1106–1114 (2012)
17. Hinton, G.E., Salakhutdinov, R.R.: Reducing the dimensionality of data with neural networks. Science **313**, 504–507 (2006)
18. Goh, H., Thome, N., Cord, M., Lim, J.-H.: Unsupervised and supervised visual codes with restricted boltzmann machines. In: Fitzgibbon, A., Lazebnik, S., Perona, P., Sato, Y., Schmid, C. (eds.) ECCV 2012, Part V. LNCS, vol. 7576, pp. 298–311. Springer, Heidelberg (2012)
19. Sohn, K., Jung, D.Y., Lee, H., Hero, A.O.: Efficient learning of sparse, distributed, convolutional feature representations for object recognition. In: ICCV, pp. 2643–2650 (2011)
20. Hinton, G.E.: Training products of experts by minimizing contrastive divergence. Neural Comput. **14**, 1771–1800 (2002)
21. Vincent, P., Larochelle, H., Lajoie, I., Bengio, Y., Manzagol, P.A.: Stacked denoising autoencoders: Learning useful representations in a deep network with a local denoising criterion. J. Mach. Learn. Res. **11**, 3371–3408 (2010)
22. Rumelhart, D., Hintont, G., Williams, R.: Learning representations by back-propagating errors. Nature **323**, 533–536 (1986)
23. Ngiam, J., Koh, P.W., Chen, Z., Bhaskar, S.A., Ng, A.Y.: Sparse filtering. In: NIPS, pp. 1125–1133 (2011)
24. Wu, Z., Huang, Y., Wang, L., Tan, T.: Group encoding of local features in image classification. In: ICPR, pp. 1505–1508 (2012)
25. Perronnin, F., Sánchez, J., Mensink, T.: Improving the fisher kernel for large-scale image classification. In: Daniilidis, K., Maragos, P., Paragios, N. (eds.) ECCV 2010, Part IV. LNCS, vol. 6314, pp. 143–156. Springer, Heidelberg (2010)
26. Perronnin, F., Dance, C.R.: Fisher kernels on visual vocabularies for image categorization. In: CVPR (2007)
27. Zhou, X., Yu, K., Zhang, T., Huang, T.S.: Image classification using super-vector coding of local image descriptors. In: Daniilidis, K., Maragos, P., Paragios, N. (eds.) ECCV 2010, Part V. LNCS, vol. 6315, pp. 141–154. Springer, Heidelberg (2010)
28. Yu, K., Zhang, T., Gong, Y.: Nonlinear learning using local coordinate coding. In: NIPS, pp. 2223–2231 (2009)
29. Lehky, S.R., Sejnowski, T.J., Desimone, R.: Selectivity and sparseness in the responses of striate complex cells. Vis. Res. **45**, 57–73 (2005)
30. Ng, A.: Sparse autoencoder. CS294 A Lecture notes (2011)

31. Vapnik, V.N.: The Nature of Statistical Learning Theory. Springer-Verlag New York Inc., New York (1995)
32. Fan, R.E., Chang, K.W., Hsieh, C.J., Wang, X.R., Lin, C.J.: Liblinear: A library for large linear classification. J. Mach. Learn. Res. **9**, 1871–1874 (2008)
33. Fei-Fei, L., Fergus, R., Perona, P.: Learning generative visual models from few training examples an incremental bayesian approach tested on 101 object categories. In: Proceedings of the Workshop on Generative-Model Based Vision (2004)
34. Li, L.J., Li, F.F.: What, where and who? classifying events by scene and object recognition. In: ICCV, pp. 1–8 (2007)
35. Jiang, Z., Lin, Z., Davis, L.S.: Label consistent k-svd: Learning a discriminative dictionary for recognition. IEEE Trans. Pattern Anal. Mach. Intell. **35**, 2651–2664 (2013)

Learning a Representative and Discriminative Part Model with Deep Convolutional Features for Scene Recognition

Bingyuan Liu$^{(\boxtimes)}$, Jing Liu, Jingqiao Wang, and Hanqing Lu

Institute of Automation, Chinese Academy of Sciences, Beijing, China
{byliu,jliu,jqwang,luhq}@nlpr.ia.ac.cn

Abstract. The discovery of key and distinctive parts is critical for scene parsing and understanding. However, it is a challenging problem due to the weakly supervised condition, *i.e.*, no annotation for parts is available. To address above issues, we propose a unified framework for learning a representative and discriminative part model with deep convolutional features. Firstly, we employ selective search method to generate regions that are more likely to be centered around the distinctive parts, which is used as parts training set. Then, the feature of each part region is extracted by forward propagating it into the Convolutional Neural Network (CNN). The CNN network is pre-trained by the large auxiliary ImageNet dataset and then fine-tuned on the particular scene images. To learn the parts model, we build a mid-level part dictionary based on sparse coding with a discriminative regularization. The two terms, *i.e.*, the sparse reconstruction error term and the label consistent term, indicate the representative and discriminative properties respectively. Finally, we apply the learned parts model to build image-level representation for the scene recognition task. Extensive experiments demonstrate that we achieve state-of-the-art performances on the standard scene benchmarks, *i.e.* Scene-15 and MIT Indoor-67.

1 Introduction

The task of scene recognition remains one of the most important but challenging problems in computer vision and machine intelligence. To solve this problem, how to build a suitable image representation is very critical. Conventional methods take advantage of the well engineered local features, such as SIFT [1] and HOG [2], to build Bag-of-Features (BoF) [3] image representation. However, this representation mostly captures local edges without enough mid-level and high-level information, which hinders the performance.

Recently, deep Convolutional Neural Network (CNN) has achieved great success in image classification by showing substantially higher accuracy on the ImageNet Large Scale Visual Recognition Challenge [4,5]. It is considered that the CNN may be used as a universal feature extractor for various vision tasks [6]. A number of recent works have also shown that CNN trained on sufficiently large and diverse datasets such as ImageNet can be successfully transferred to other

© Springer International Publishing Switzerland 2015
D. Cremers et al. (Eds.): ACCV 2014, Part I, LNCS 9003, pp. 643–658, 2015.
DOI: 10.1007/978-3-319-16865-4_42

visual recognition tasks, *e.g.*, human attribute classification [7] and object detection [8], with domain-specific fine-tuning by the limited amount of task-specific training data. In this paper, we generalize the CNN to the scene recognition domain and explore it for the distinctive part discovery and recognition.

To recognition scene categories, discovering distinctive parts to build image representation is very effective, such as screens in movie theater and tables in dining room. While the notion of part is widely used in object recognition, *e.g.* the Deformable Part Models (DPM) [9], it is still very difficult on the condition of scene classification, as there is only image-level label without further information on parts. For learning a good part model, two key requirements should be satisfied. One is the representative property, *i.e.*, the parts model should frequently occur within the dataset and typically indicate a particular category. The other one is the discriminative property. That is, the discovered mid-level part primitives are sufficiently different among diverse categories and help improve the final recognition task. In [10], they applied K-means to initialize the parts model and then train a linear SVM classifier for each cluster to select the most discriminative clusters. Juneja [10] proposed to initialize a set of parts by the selective search method [11] and then train part detectors to identify distinctive parts. Most previous methods adopted heuristic or iterative scheme, which firstly initial a representative model and then enhance its discrimination. However, we consider it is optimal to jointly encourage the two requirements and introduce a unified learning framework.

In this paper, we adapt the CNN features for parts discovery as analysis above, and introduce a unified learning framework jointly encouraging representative and discriminative properties. We firstly generate a particular parts training set that are more likely to be centered around distinctive parts by selective search [11], which is a method based on low-level image cues and over-segmentations. Then we employ affine warping to compute a fixed-size CNN input of each part proposal and obtain a fixed-length feature vector by the CNN forward operation, where the CNN network is pre-trained by the large auxiliary ImageNet dataset and fine-tuned on the particular scene image samples. Furtherly, we learn a mid-level part dictionary based on sparse coding, containing a sparse reconstruction error term and a label consistent regularization. The sparse reconstruction guarantees that the learned parts are significantly informative in the dataset, while the label consistent regularization encourages that different input from different categories have discriminative responses. Finally, we apply the learned parts model to build image-level representation for the scene recognition task. Extensive experiments on the benchmarks of Scene-15 and MIT Indoor-67 demonstrate the effectiveness of our method compared with related works. Combining with CNN features of the global image, we achieves state-of-the-art performances on both datasets.

2   Related Work

The introduction of some well engineered image descriptors (*e.g.* SIFT [1] and HOG [2]) have precipitated dramatic success and dominante most visual tasks in past decades. However, these kinds of features are unable to represent more complex mid and high level image structures. Over the recent years, a growing amount of researches focus on feature learning and selection [12,13], especially on building deep learning models for hierarchical image representations [14]. Deep Convolutional Neural Networks (CNN) is one of the most successful deep representation learning models, as it achieved great success in image classification by showing substantially higher accuracy on the ImageNet Challenge [4,5]. Some works still focus on further improving the CNN architectures and learning algorithm. Hinton et al. [15] proposed dropout by randomly omitting half of the feature detectors on each training case to prevent over-fitting, while Wan et al. [16] generalized this idea by setting a randomly selected subset of weights within the network to zero for regularizing large fully-connected layers. Some other works started to consider CNN as a universal image feature extractor for visual tasks [6]. Sun et al. [17] proposed to apply cascaded CNN for facial point detection, while Toshev et al. [18] adapted CNN for human pose estimation. In [8], CNN was explored as a region feature extractor and applied to solve object detection task. Most of these works use the highly effective "supervised pre-training/domain-specific fine-tuning" paradigm, which transfers CNN trained on sufficiently large and diverse datasets to other visual tasks. In this paper, we adapt the CNN features for the task of parts model learning in the scene recognition task.

Scene recognition and understanding is a fundamental task in computer vision. The key to solve this problem is how to obtain a suitable image representation. Many previous works are based on Bag of Features (BoF) model, which takes advantage of the traditional local features and the power of SVM classifier. Some efforts were made to improve the description power, such as quantizing local features with less information loss [19,20], building more effective codebook [21] and adopting kernel methods [22]. Other works attempted to incorporate some spatial information, such as the famous spatial pyramid match (SPM) [23]. Sharma et al. [24] defined a space of grids where each grid is obtained by a series of recursive axis aligned splits of cells and proposed to learn the spatial partition in a maximum margin formulation. An Orientational Pyramid Matching (OPM) model [25] was proposed to improve SPM, which uses the 3D orientations to form the pyramid and produce the pooling regions.

Since the distinctive parts are very important to recognize a typical scene, many researchers attempted to discovery and learn parts model for scene recognition. Zheng et al. [26] transfered the deformable part-based models [9] to build image representation. Singh et al. [10] used iterative procedure which alternates between clustering and training discriminative classifiers to discover discriminative patches, while Junejia et al. [27] apply exemplar SVM to train part detectors and iteratively identify distinctive parts from an initial set of parts. Lin et al. [28] proposed to jointly learn the part appearance and important spatial pooling regions. Different from the iterative scheme, we use a unified framework, jointly incorporating representative and discriminative properties.

3   The Proposed Model

In this section, we describe the details of our proposed model for learning distinctive parts for scene recognition. We will firstly present how to generate the particular training parts set prepared for parts learning and how to extract part features by CNN. Then our unified parts model learning algorithm is followed. At last, we will introduce how to employ the learned parts model to construct image-level representation.

3.1   Parts Training Set Generation

In our framework, an initial parts training set is needed to generate, prepared for part model learning. In the weakly supervised scene dataset (only image-level label without any label on parts), any sub-window in the training images is likely to contain a distinctive part. This simple way is to exhaustively include all the possible regions for parts learning. However, most of these regions don't contain valuable information, leading to high information redundancy and extra computation cost. We may also randomly sample a subset from all the possible regions to decrease the number, but this can not guarantee to cover all the useful regions.

To reduce the number of training samples as possible and contain most distinctive parts meanwhile, we turn to the selective search method [11]. Based on low-level image cues, the selective search method combines the strength of both an exhaustive search and segmentation to capture all possible object locations. Extending from objects to parts, we find the generated sub-windows of selective search on scene images tend to be centered around distinctive parts we want, as shown in Fig. 1. In particular, each training image is firstly resized into multiple

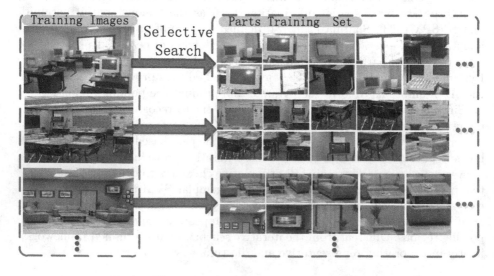

Fig. 1. The generation process of parts training set.

scales and then segmented into superpixels. A greedy algorithm is then employed which iteratively groups the two most similar regions together and calculates the similarities between this new region and its neighbors. The number of obtained region proposals ranges from 100 to 800 for each image. As evaluated in [11], this method is performed with very high recall, guaranteeing that almost every distinctive part is included. The overall generated part proposals for training are denoted as P in this paper.

3.2 Part Feature Extraction

Given a part proposal, we extract its feature by forward propagating it through the Convolutional Neural Network (CNN). We employ the Caffe [29] GPU implementation of the CNN architecture described in [4], which consists of five convolutional layers, two fully connected layers and uses the rectified linear unit (ReLu) as the activation function (please refer to [4] for more network details). Since the CNN requires inputs of a fixed $227 \times 227 \times 3$ pixel size, we resize each region to 227×227 RGB pixels, subtract the mean of the pixel values and then feed it into the network. The 4096-dimensional output of the seventh layer (the final fully connected layer) after the ReLU transformation is taken as the representation of the input part region (the performances of the previous layers are found worse in our experiments).

To train the CNN network, we apply the very effective "supervised pre-training/domain-specific fine-tuning" scheme. Firstly, we discriminatively pre-train the CNN on a large auxiliary dataset, $i.e.$ ImageNet 2012 benchmark, which includes roughly 1.2 million training samples from 1000 categories and $50,000$ images for evaluation. To generalize the pre-trained CNN to the new domain ($i.e.$ scene recognition), we fine-tune the network on the task dataset ($e.g.$ Scene-15 and MIT Indoor-67). The fine-tuning is performed by continuing the stochastic gradient descent learning process with new training samples, where all the CNN parameters is initialized by the pre-trained CNN except that the ImageNet-specific 1000-way softmax layer is replaced by a randomly initialized new softmax layer with the number of output units altered to the number of classes in the new dataset. As the domain dataset is small we further augment the training set by adding cropped, rotated and mirror samples. It is noted that the fine-tuning is started at a learning rate of 0.001 (1/10 of the initial pre-training rate), allowing the fine-tuning to make progress while not clobbering the initialization. Both the pre-training and fine-tuning in this paper is carried out using the Caffe GPU implementation.

3.3 Part Model Learning

Different from previous works, we hope to jointly encourage the representative and discriminative properties of the parts model. In another word, these two requirements mean that the learned parts frequently occur in each category and are able to distinguish different classes meanwhile. We denote the part training set as $P = \{p_1, p_2, \ldots, p_N\}$, where the number of training samples is denoted as N. The CNN feature of each part p_i is represented by a m-dimensional vector x_i. We directly impose the image label on the part proposals extracted within the image and denote the corresponding parts training label set as $Y = \{y_1, y_2, \ldots, y_N\}$.

With the parts training dataset prepared, we learn a mid-level parts dictionary based on sparse coding, while the discriminativity is motivated by a label consistent regularization. The unified part model learning objective with the two properties incorporated is defined as:

$$\min_{B,A,Z} \parallel X - BZ \parallel_2^2 + \alpha \parallel D - AZ \parallel_2^2$$
$$s.t. \forall i, |z_i|_1 \preceq T \tag{1}$$

This objective is comprised of two sections, $i.e.$, the reconstruction error term and label consistent regularization, where α controls the relative contribution. In Eq. 1, $B = [b_1, b_2, \ldots, b_k] \in R^{m \times K}$ represents the part dictionary and the size is denoted as K, while the latent code $Z = [z_1, z_2, \ldots, z_N] \in R^{K \times N}$ denotes the response vectors of the training part proposals. As the l_1 regularization constraint of z_i encourages it to be sparse (T denotes the sparse factor), the first term is a sparse coding term which is able to help learn a representative B. $D = [d_1, d_2, \ldots, d_N] \in R^{K \times N}$ in the second term are the discriminative sparse codes of training parts. We define that $d_i = [d_i^1, d_i^2, \ldots, d_i^K]^t = [0 \ldots 1, 1, \ldots 0]^t \in R^K$ is the discriminative code related to an training part x_i, if the non-zero values of d_i occur at those indices where the part and the model item b_k share the same label. For example, assuming there are 3 classes, 8 training samples and the dictionary size is 6, we denote $B = [b_1, b_2, \ldots, b_6]$ and $X = [x_1, x_2, \ldots, x_8]$. The x_1, x_2, b_1 and b_2 are from class 1, x_3, x_4, x_5, b_3 and b_4 are from class 2, and x_6, x_7, x_8, b_5 and b_6 are from class 3. Thus the D is set as:

$$D = \begin{pmatrix} 1 & 1 & 0 & 0 & 0 & 0 & 0 & 0 \\ 1 & 1 & 0 & 0 & 0 & 0 & 0 & 0 \\ 0 & 0 & 1 & 1 & 1 & 0 & 0 & 0 \\ 0 & 0 & 1 & 1 & 1 & 0 & 0 & 0 \\ 0 & 0 & 0 & 0 & 0 & 1 & 1 & 1 \\ 0 & 0 & 0 & 0 & 0 & 1 & 1 & 1 \end{pmatrix}_{6 \times 8} \tag{2}$$

In the second term, A is a linear transformation matrix, which transforms the latent sparse codes z to be most discriminative. As this term may measure the discriminative error of the latent sparse response and enforces that the sparse codes approximate the discriminative codes Q, it encourages the input from different classes to have different responses, thus enhancing the discriminative property.

For the optimization, we utilize the algorithm similar to [30]. We firstly rewrite Eq. 1 as:

$$\min_{B,A,Z} \parallel [X^T \sqrt{\alpha}D]^T - [B^t \sqrt{\alpha}A]^t Z \parallel_2^2$$
$$s.t. \forall i, |z_i|_1 \preceq T \tag{3}$$

Then the problem can be solved by the standard K-SVD [31] algorithm to find the optimal solution for all the parameters.

3.4 Image-Level Representation

With the learned part model, we regard it as a mid-level visual dictionary and build an image-level bag-of-part representation. As shown in Fig. 2, given a new image, we apply each part in the learned part dictionary as a template to slide over the input image in a densely sampled scheme and obtain the corresponding response map. The response value in each map is calculated by solving a sparse coding optimization:

$$\min_z \| x - Bz \|_2^2$$
$$s.t. |z|_1 \preceq T \tag{4}$$

where x is a sampled input patch, B is the learned parts dictionary and z is the obtained sparse codes where every dimension corresponds to a particular part template. In our implementation, the image is firstly sampled in multiple scales and response maps for each scale are obtained.

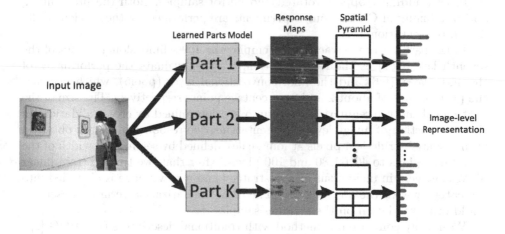

Fig. 2. The pipeline of building image-level representation.

After the mid-level parts score maps are obtained, we employ max-pooling to build global image representation. The max-pooling is carried out in a spatial pyramid fashion [23] ($1 \times 1, 2 \times 2$ grids). The output vector of each spatial region in every scale is finally concatenated into a long vector as the final image representation. This resulting representation may be further combined with the global CNN features of the image to enhance the performance.

4 Experiments

In the experiments, we evaluate our method on two public scene recognition benchmarks, *i.e.* Scene-15 and MIT-Indoor 67. In the following subsections, we firstly in-depth analyze our model by visualizing the parts model we learn and then evaluate the recognition performances.

In the CNN network training, the architecture we adopt is similar to that used by Krizhevsky *et al.* [4]. The only difference is that the sparse connections applied in the layers $3, 4, 5$ of the network [4] (due to the model being split across 2 GPUs) are replaced with dense connections in our model. The model is firstly pre-trained on a large auxiliary dataset (ImageNet ILSVRC 2012) with image-level supervision. In particular, our pre-trained CNN obtain an average accuracy of about 4 percentage points lower on the validation set than [4], which may be due to the little difference of the architecture and learning process. To adapt the CNN to the new domain, we perform domain-specific fine-tuning on the two datasets respectively. The only difference of architecture in fine-tuning is that the number of the final softmax layer is varied from 1000 to the number of classes in the specific datasets (15 for Scene-15 and 67 for MIT-Indoor 67). The initial learning rate of fine-tuning is set as 1/10th of the initial pre-training rate. Since the domain dataset is relatively small, we augment the training set by further adding cropped, rotated and mirror samples. Both the pre-training and fine-tuning of CNN in our experiments are performed by the efficient Caffe [29] implementation.

In the part feature extraction, we employ the 4096-dimensional output of the seventh layer (fc7) as the representation. We also evaluate the performance of the sixth layer (fc6) and the final convolutional layer (pool5), which decrease the performance of about 2 and 3 percentage points respectively. The size of the part model and the regularization term α are determined by cross validation. In the construction of image-level representations, the response maps are obtained with a spatial stride of 4 pixels at four scales, defined by setting the width of the sampling regions to $40, 60, 80$ and 100 pixels. After that, we turn to train linear SVM classifiers in one-versus-others strategy and a new image is classified into the category with the largest score. The SVM regularization term is chosen via 5-fold cross validation on the training samples.

We mainly compare our method with traditional descriptors (*i.e.* HOG [2]), the method without any discriminative motivation (*i.e.* K-means and sparse coding), and related works of mid-level parts mining [10,27] and scene recognition models [23,25,28].

4.1 Results on Scene-15 Dataset

We firstly experiment with a popular scene classification benchmark, *i.e.*, Scene-15 dataset, which is complied by several researchers [23,32]. This dataset is comprised of 15 classes of different indoor and outdoor scenes (*e.g.* kitchen, coast, highway), including totally $4,485$ gray-scale images with the number of each category ranging from 200 to 400. Following the standard experiment setup

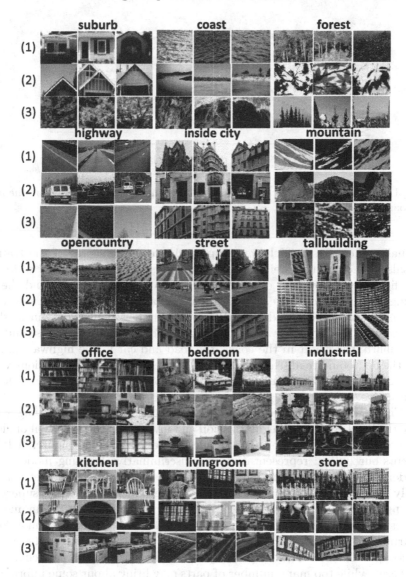

Fig. 3. The visualization of part model learned on Scene-15. We give 3 parts learned for each category, where each row in the figure corresponds to a particular part. Note how these capture key visual aspects of a typical scene.

of Lazebnik *et al.* [23], we take 100 images per class for training and the rest for testing. The regularization term α in Eq. 3 is set to 5 and the sparsity factor T is 10 according to our implementation. We repeat the procedure 5 times and report the mean and standard deviation of the mean accuracy.

In Fig. 3, we show some parts we have learned for each category. Most representative and distinctive parts we obtained are displayed for each class.

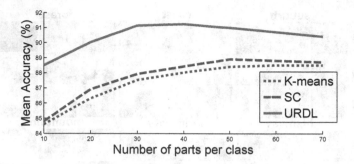

Fig. 4. The classification performance comparisons on Scene-15 with varying the number of parts per class.

To visualize the parts model, we compute the response scores of the training proposals on each part model and then sort these scores from highest to lowest. In this figure, each row of a class corresponds to a particular part and the top 3 scoring regions are displayed for each part. In another word, we visualize the part by evaluating which kinds of inputs it fires on. It is shown that our model is able to capture the key parts for each category. For example, the house and roof in the suburb, the water in the coast, the road and car in the highway and the bed in the bedroom are all captured. Also, different parts capture various visual aspects of a typical scene and different parts for different classes are visually discriminative.

In Fig. 4, we compare our model with K-means and sparse coding which neglect the label consistent regularization and investigate the variation of classification accuracy with number of parts selected per class. In this figure, "URDL" represents our unified representative and discriminative learning model, while "SC" denotes the method of sparse coding. It is shown that our method consistently outperform K-means and sparse coding which are both unsupervised clustering algorithms, demonstrating the label consistent term in our method improves the discriminative property. The mean accuracy increases as more parts are learned for the representation, but the peak is at around 40 parts per category for this dataset. This may relate to the diversity of the particular class and dataset, while too many number of parts may bring about some information redundancy or noise in the representation.

Table 1 shows the performance comparisons of our proposed method with related part learning models. It is shown that our efficient method outperform some very complex models, e.g. Hybrid-Parts [26] and ISPR [28]. "URDL(HOG feature)" denotes that we use traditional HOG feature to represent the parts instead of CNN features. This result shows that the CNN feature significantly improves the performance of more than 5 percentage points, as CNN feature is able to represent high-level image information. We compare our approach with more public reported performances on Scene-15 in Table 2. The "CNN-SVM" denotes the method of applying the CNN features of the whole images as

Table 1. Mean accuracy (%) comparison of parts representations on Scene-15.

Methods	Mean Accuracy
SPM [23]	81.4
Hybrid-Parts [26]	84.7
ISPR [28]	85.08 ± 0.01
CENTRIST [33]	83.88 ± 0.76
URDL(HOG feature)	85.92 ± 0.08
URDL	$\mathbf{91.15 \pm 0.02}$

Table 2. Mean accuracy (%) performance comparison on Scene-15.

Methods	Mean Accuracy
SPM [23]	81.40
Object Bank [34]	80.90
VC+VQ [35]	85.4
Hybrid-Parts+GIST-color+SP [26]	86.3
CENTRIST+LCC+Boosting [33]	87.8
LScSPM [20]	89.75 ± 0.50
IFV [36]	89.20 ± 0.09
ISPR+IFV [28]	91.06 ± 0.06
URDL	91.15 ± 0.02
CNN-SVM	92.20 ± 0.05
CNN+SPM-SVM	92.83 ± 0.04
URDL+CNN	$\mathbf{96.16 \pm 0.03}$

inputs to train SVM classifiers, while "CNN+SPM-SVM" indicates the method of extracting the CNN features of the spatial partitioned regions and then concatenating them to train SVM classifiers which is incorporated with some spatial layout information. Our best performance is reached when combining the part representation with the global CNN features. It is shown that the mean accuracy of our best result is about 96 %, which beats all the previous public performances and achieves stat-of-the-art in this dataset.

4.2   Results on MIT Indoor-67 Dataset

The MIT Indoor-67 dataset [37] is the currently largest indoor scene recognition dataset, including 15, 620 images in 67 categories. The categories are loosely divided into stores (*e.g.* bakery, toy store), home (*e.g.* bedroom, kitchen), public spaces (*e.g.* library, subway), leisure (*e.g.* restaurant, concert hall) and work (*e.g.* hospital, TV studio). The similarity of the objects present in different indoor scenes makes MIT-Indoor an especially difficult dataset compared to outdoor

Table 3. Mean accuracy (%) comparison of variant with number of parts per class on MIT Indoor-67.

Methods	Number of parts per class						
	10	20	30	40	50	60	70
URDL	57.5	58.0	58.9	60.5	61.0	61.2	60.8
URDL+CNN	67.9	68.4	69.1	70.8	71.5	71.9	71.3

Table 4. Mean accuracy (%) performance comparisons on MIT Indoor-67.

Methods	Mean Accuracy
ROI [37]	26.05
DPM [38]	30.40
CENTRIST [33]	36.90
Object Bank [34]	37.60
Patches [10]	38.10
Hybrid-Parts [26]	39.80
BoP [35]	46.10
ISPR [28]	50.10
Hybrid-Parts+GIST-color+SP [26]	47.20
BoP+IFV [35]	63.10
ISPR+IFV [28]	68.50
CNNaug-SVM [6]	69.00
URDL	61.20
CNN-SVM	68.50
CNN+SPM-SVM	69.09
URDL+CNN	**71.90**

scene datasets. Following the protocol of [37], we use the same training and test split where each category has about 80 training images and 20 test images. The regularization term α in Eq. 3 is set to 3 and the sparsity factor T is 20 according to our implementation. Performances are reported in terms of mean classification accuracy as in [37].

In the experiments on this dataset, we also evaluate the effect of the number of parts per class, as shown in Table 3. Similar to the results on Scene-15, the performances are improved as we increase the number of learned parts per class. The peak is reached at around 60 parts per category, which is more than that in Scene-15 due to the larger varieties and number of samples in MIT Indoor-67. Table 4 lists the performances comparison of our method with public results. It is noted that the performances of single-feature approaches are weak on this challenging dataset, such as ROI [37], DPM [38], CENTRIST [33], Object Bank [34], Patches [10], BoP [35] and ISPR [28]. Our performance of applying the

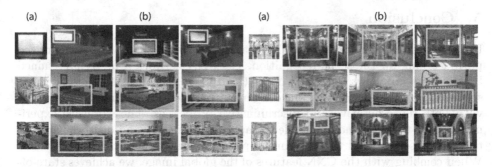

Fig. 5. Examples of the learned parts templates and detections on the test set images. (a) Learned parts templates. (b) Detections on the test set images.

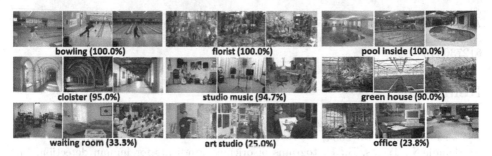

Fig. 6. Example images from classes with highest and lowest classification accuracy from MIT Indoor-67 dataset. The top 2 rows show example images from classes with highest accuracy, while the bottom row displays example images from classes with lowest accuracy.

single part representation (denoted as "URDL") beats all these methods and yields 61.20 %. When combining with the CNN feature of the global image, the performance outperforms all the public results and achieves 71.90 %.

Figure 5 shows examples of the learned parts and detections on some example images in the test set. It is displayed that the learned parts capture the key aspect of a particular scene, such as the screen in the movie theater and the bed in the bedroom. Compared to the results in [27], our model may endure more appearance variants, *i.e*, the diversity in the size, viewing angle, illumination and poses. This is mainly because CNN features capture very high-level image information. In Fig. 6, we display some example images from classes with highest and lowest classification accuracy from the MIT Indoor-67 dataset. Our method performs well on most classes with little clutter (like bowling and pool inside) or scenes with consistent key parts (like florist and cloister), and less successful on classes with extremely large intra-class variation (like art studio and office). Besides different scene categories may share similar key parts, such as the computer frequently appears in both office and computer room. Overall, our model improves the recognition performances for most categories.

5   Conclusion

In this paper, we generalize the CNN features for the task of weakly supervised parts learning for the scene recognition. The CNN network is firstly pre-trained by the large auxiliary ImageNet dataset and then fine-tuned on the particular scene datasets. Then we introduce a unified part learning framework together with both representative and discriminative properties. The extensive experiments show that our model is able to capture various key and distinct parts for the typical scenes, and the recognition performances outperform related works. When combing with the CNN features of the global image, we achieves state-of-the-art performances on the two standard scene benchmarks, *i.e.* Scene-15 and MIT Indoor-67.

Acknowledgement. This work was supported by 863 Program (2014AA015104) and National Natural Science Foundation of China (61332016, 61272329, 61472422, and 61273034).

References

1. Lowe, D.: Distinctive image features from scale-invariant keypoints. Int. J. Comput. Vision **60**, 91–110 (2004)
2. Dalal, N., Triggs, B.: Histograms of oriented gradients for human detection. In: CVPR (2005)
3. Csurka, G., Dance, C., Fan, L., Willamowski, J., Bray, C.: Visual categorization with bags of keypoints. In: ECCV 2004 Workshop on Statistical Learning in Computer Vision (2004)
4. Krizhevsky, A., Sutskever, I., Hinton, G.E.: Imagenet classification with deep convolutional neural networks. In: NIPS (2012)
5. Zeiler, M.D., Fergus, R.: Visualizing and understanding convolutional networks. CoRR abs/1311.2901 (2013)
6. Razavian, A.S., Azizpour, H., Sullivan, J., Carlsson, S.: CNN features off-the-shelf: an Astounding baseline for recognition. In: CVPR (2014)
7. Zhang, N., Paluri, M., Ranzato, M., Darrell, T., Bourdev, L.: PANDA: Pose aligned networks for deep attribute modeling. In: CVPR (2014)
8. Girshick, R., Donahue, J., Darrell, T., Malik, J.: Rich feature hierarchies for accurate object detection and semantic segmentation. In: CVPR (2014)
9. Felzenszwalb, P.F., Girshick, R.B., McAllester, D., Ramanan, D.: Object detection with discriminatively trained part-based models. IEEE Trans. Pattern Anal. Mach. Intell. **32**, 1627–1645 (2010)
10. Singh, S., Gupta, A., Efros, A.A.: Unsupervised discovery of mid-level discriminative patches. In: Fitzgibbon, A., Lazebnik, S., Perona, P., Sato, Y., Schmid, C. (eds.) ECCV 2012, Part II. LNCS, vol. 7573, pp. 73–86. Springer, Heidelberg (2012)
11. Uijlings, J., van de Sande, K., Gevers, T., Smeulders, A.: Selective search for object recognition. Int. J. Comput. Vision **104**, 154–171 (2013)
12. Li, Z., Liu, J., Yang, Y., Zhou, X., Lu, H.: Clustering-guided sparse structural learning for unsupervised feature selection. IEEE Trans. Knowl. Data Eng. **26**, 2138–2150 (2014)

13. Li, Z., Yang, Y., Liu, J., Zhou, X., Lu, H.: Unsupervised feature selection using nonnegative spectral analysis. In: AAAI (2012)
14. Bengio, Y., Courville, A.C., Vincent, P.: Representation learning: a review and new perspectives. IEEE Trans. Pattern Anal. Mach. Intell. **35**, 1798–1828 (2013)
15. Hinton, G.E., Srivastava, N., Krizhevsky, A., Sutskever, I., Salakhutdinov, R.: Improving neural networks by preventing co-adaptation of feature detectors. CoRR abs/1207.0580 (2012)
16. Wan, L., Zeiler, M., Zhang, S., LeCun, Y., Fergus, R.: Regularization of neural networks using dropconnect. In: ICML (2013)
17. Sun, Y., Wang, X., Tang, X.: Deep convolutional network cascade for facial point detection. In: CVPR (2013)
18. Toshev, A., Szegedy, C.: Deeppose: Human pose estimation via deep neural networks. In: CVPR (2014)
19. Yang, J., Yu, K., Gong, Y., Huang, T.: Linear spatial pyramid matching using sparse coding for image classification. In: CVPR (2009)
20. Gao, S., Tsang, I.W.H., Chia, L.T., Zhao, P.: Local features are not lonely - Laplacian sparse coding for image classification. In: CVPR (2010)
21. Wu, J., Rehg, J.M.: Beyond the Euclidean distance: creating effective visual codebooks using the histogram intersection Kernel. In: ICCV (2009)
22. Wang, P., Wang, J., Zeng, G., Xu, W., Zha, H., Li, S.: Supervised Kernel descriptors for visual recognition. In: CVPR (2013)
23. Lazebnik, S., Schmid, C., Ponce, J.: Beyond bags of features: spatial pyramid matching for recognizing natural scene categories. In: CVPR (2006)
24. Sharma, G., Jurie, F.: Learning discriminative spatial representation for image classification. In: BMVC (2011)
25. Xie, L., Wang, J., Guo, B., Zhang, B., Tian, Q.: Orientational pyramid matching for recognizing indoor scenes. In: CVPR (2014)
26. Zheng, Y., Jiang, Y.-G., Xue, X.: Learning hybrid part filters for scene recognition. In: Fitzgibbon, A., Lazebnik, S., Perona, P., Sato, Y., Schmid, C. (eds.) ECCV 2012, Part V. LNCS, vol. 7576, pp. 172–185. Springer, Heidelberg (2012)
27. Juneja, M., Vedaldi, A., Jawahar, C.V., Zisserman, A.: Blocks that shout: distinctive parts for scene classification. In: CVPR (2013)
28. Lin, D., Lu, C., Liao, R., Jia, J.: Learning important spatial pooling regions for scene classification. In: CVPR (2014)
29. Jia, Y.: Caffe: An open source convolutional architecture for fast feature embedding (2013). http://caffe.berkeleyvision.org/
30. Jiang, Z., Lin, Z., Davis, L.S.: Learning a discriminative dictionary for sparse coding via label consistent K-SVD. In: CVPR (2011)
31. Aharon, M., Elad, M., Bruckstein, A.: K-SVD: an algorithm for designing overcomplete dictionaries for sparse representation. IEEE Trans. Sig. Process. **54**, 4311–4322 (2006)
32. Fei-Fei, L., Perona, P.: A Bayesian hierarchical model for learning natural scene categories. In: CVPR (2005)
33. Yuan, J., Yang, M., Wu, Y.: Mining discriminative co-occurrence patterns for visual recognition. In: CVPR (2011)
34. Li, L.J., Su, H., Xing, E.P., Fei-Fei, L.: Object bank: a high-level image representation for scene classification and semantic feature sparsification. In: NIPS (2010)
35. Li, Q., Wu, J., Tu, Z.: Harvesting mid-level visual concepts from large-scale internet images. In: CVPR (2013)

36. Vedaldi, A., Fulkerson, B.: VLFeat: an open and portable library of computer vision algorithms (2008). http://www.vlfeat.org/
37. Quattoni, A., Torralba, A.: Recognizing indoor scenes. In: CVPR (2009)
38. Pandey, M., Lazebnik, S.: Scene recognition and weakly supervised object localization with deformable part-based models. In: ICCV (2011)

Image Representation Learning by Deep Appearance and Spatial Coding

Bingyuan Liu[1]([✉]), Jing Liu[1], Zechao Li[2], and Hanqing Lu[1]

[1] Institute of Automation, Chinese Academy of Sciences, Beijing, China
{byliu,jliu,luhq}@nlpr.ia.ac.cn
[2] School of Computer Science, Nanjing University of Science and Technology,
Nanjing, China
zechao.li@gmail.com

Abstract. The bag of feature model is one of the most successful model to represent an image for classification task. However, the discrimination loss in the local appearance coding and the lack of spatial information hinder its performance. To address these problems, we propose a deep appearance and spatial coding model to build more optimal image representation for the classification task. The proposed model is a hierarchical architecture consisting of three operations: appearance coding, max-pooling and spatial coding. Firstly, with an image as input, we extract a set of local descriptors and adopt the appearance coding to encode them into high-dimensional robust vectors. Then max-pooling is performed within the over spatial partitioned grids to incorporate spatial information. After that, spatial coding is carried out to increasingly integrate the region vectors to a global image signature. Finally, the resulting image representation are employed to train a one-versus-others SVM classifier. In the learning of the proposed model, we layerwisely pre-train the network and then perform supervised fine-tuning with image labels. The experiments on three image benchmark datasets (*i.e.* 15-Scenes, PASCAL VOC 2007 and Caltech-256) demonstrate the effectiveness of our proposed model.

1 Introduction

The task of recognizing semantic category of an image remains one of the most important but challenging problems in computer vision and machine intelligence. The crux of the problem is how to describe an image properly for the classification task. In recent years, Bag-of-Feature (BoF) [1] remains one of the most successful method. It extracts a set of local patch descriptors (*e.g.* SIFT [2] and HOG [3]), encode them into high dimensional vectors and pool to obtain an image-level signature. The standard BoF assigns each local descriptor to the closest entry in a visual codebook which is learned offline by clustering a large sampling set of descriptors with K-means. However, two major problems hinder the performance of this model, *i.e.*, the shortcomings brought by the appearance coding scheme and the lack of spatial information.

Given the simplicity, hard-assignment appearance coding scheme in BoF comes with the problem of quantization error. There have been several extensions

© Springer International Publishing Switzerland 2015
D. Cremers et al. (Eds.): ACCV 2014, Part I, LNCS 9003, pp. 659–672, 2015.
DOI: 10.1007/978-3-319-16865-4_43

to reduce this information loss by adopting better coding techniques as alternative. VanGemert *et al.* [4] proposed the concept of visual ambiguity and soft assign each descriptor into multiple visual words in the codebook. Yang *et al.* [5] adopt the sparse coding algorithm, which demonstrates effective in feature representation and discriminative task. Wang *et al.* [6] proposed to relax the restrictive constraint by locally-constrained linearity regularization. However, these methods are all performed in a purely unsupervised way without any high-level guidance, leading to the absence of discriminative information. Thus the resulting representation is not optimal for the classification, and a better coding model may explore both generative and discriminative properties.

Another inherent drawback is the lack of spatial layout information as the BoF model describes an image as an orderless collection of local features. To overcome this problem, one popular extension, known as Spatial Pyramid Matching (SPM) [7], has been shown effective by partitioning each image into a fixed sequence of increasingly finer grids and concatenating the BoF features in each grids to form a global image representation. It is obvious that the simple concatenation of the region features are not optimal to handle complex spatial distribution, and the spatial coding should also take advantage of both generative and discriminative characteristics, since different image classes usually have their own particular spatial distributions of local features.

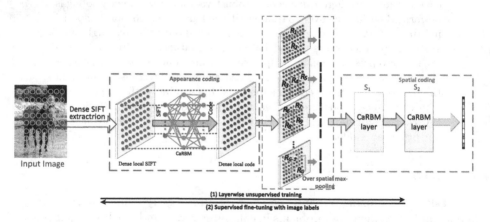

Fig. 1. The proposed deep appearance and spatial coding model. See Sect. 3 for details. (Better view in the color version) (Color figure online)

To address above issues, this paper proposes a deep appearance and spatial coding model to build representative and discriminative image representation. As shown in Fig. 1, the proposed model is a hierarchical architecture, consisting of three operations: appearance coding, over spatial max-pooling and spatial coding. The base module is Cardinality Restricted Boltzmann Machine [8], which is an extension to Restricted Boltzmann Machine with the attractive properties of sparse coding by introducing competition among its hidden units. With an image as input, our model firstly extracts local patch descriptors and employ the appearance coding to encode them into high-dimensional codes. To incorporate more optimal spatial layout information, we adopt the idea of over spatial max-pooling. We create various spatial partitions covering very flexible spatial distributions and perform max-pooling within each grid. The resulting features of each partitioned region are then concatenated as input to the next spatial coding module. At last, the layers of spatial coding are explored in a hierarchical structure to increasingly integrate the region vectors to a global image signature. To learn the deep model, we layerwisely pre-train it in an unsupervised way and then fine-tune the parameters with image labels to enhance the discrimination. In this way, our model better explores the generative and discriminative properties, making the obtained feature more optimal to represent the image and adapt to classification task. The output image representations are employed to train a one-versus-others SVM classifier to perform classification. We evaluate our model on three widely used benchmarks (*i.e.* 15-Scenes, PASCAL VOC 2007 and Caltech-256), and the extensive experiments demonstrate the effectiveness of our method in comparison with baselines and related works.

2   Related Work

The Bag-of-Feature(BoF) model [9] is directly borrowed from text retrieval community. In spite of the simplicity, it has been proven very effective to represent an image for large number of vision tasks. The standard BoF extracts a set of local descriptors, and assigns each to the closest entry in a visual codebook, which is learned offline by clustering a large sampling set of descriptors with K-means. Then all these resulting local codes are pooled into an image-level histogram representation. Over the past few years, many efforts have been done to improve the performance of the BoF model.

To overcome the information loss in the codebook learning and feature coding process, some researchers attempted to learn discriminative visual codebooks for image classification [10,11]. Co-occurrence information of visual words was also considered in a generative framework [12]. In [13], the idea of visual word ambiguity is introduced to soft assign each local descriptor to multiple visual words in the learned codebook. As sparse coding is proven effective in feature representation and discriminative tasks, Yang *et al.* [5] utilized it to encode the local features into high-dimensional sparse codes. This method can automatically learn the optimal codebook and search for the optimal coding weights for each local feature. Inspired by this, Wang *et al.* [6] proposed to use locality to constrain the sparse coding process which may be computed faster and yield better performance. Jiang *et al.* [14] proposed to improve the discriminatingly of dictionary via a label consistent regularization. Some other works [15,16] also tried to jointly learn the optimal codebooks and appearance codes. However, how to better explore the generative and discriminative properties of the data is still a difficult problem. In this paper, a combination of both unsupervised feature learning [17,18] and supervised learning is adopted.

As BoF represents an image as an orderless histograms of visual words, many subsequent researches have been done to incorporate spatial information. One direction is to incorporate the local spatial layout in image, *i.e.* the relative positions or pairwise positions of local features. Savarese *et al.* [19] explored the combination of correlograms and visual words to represent spatially neighboring image regions. Reference [20] proposed an efficient feature selection method based on boosting to mine high-order spatial features, while [21] proposed to jointly cluster feature space to build a compact local pairwise codebook capturing correlation between local descriptors and the spatial orders of local features were further considered in [22]. Since images often have spatial preferences, another direction is to incorporate global spatial layout property, *i.e.*, the absolute positions in image. Lazebnik *et al.* [7] pioneered this direction and proposed the Spatial Pyramid Matching (SPM) model. In SPM, the image is divided into uniform grids at different scales (*e.g.* $1 \times 1, 2 \times 2, 4 \times 4$), and the features are concatenated over all cells. This model is successful because it is demonstrated that the combinations of SPM with sparse coding [5], locality-constrained coding [6] and recently developed super vector [23] or fisher vector [24] models are very effective and achieved the state-of-the-art performance. However, the spatial partitions in SPM are too simple to adapt to complex nature situations and are chosen in an ad-hoc manner without any optimization [7]. To solve this problem, Harada *et al.* [25] proposed to form the image feature as a weighted sum of semi-local features over all pyramid levels and the weights are automatically selected to maximize a discriminative power. To design better spatial partition, Sharma *et al.* [26] defined a space of grids where each grid is obtained by a series of recursive axis aligned splits of cells and propose to learn the spatial partition in a maximus margin formulation. Reference [27] formulated the problem in a multi-class fashion with structured sparse regularizer for feature selection, while [28] proposed to learn category specific spatial partition in a one-versus-others classification scheme. In this paper, we explore the idea of over spatial partition and encode it into a deep representation. The most important difference of our model with the previous works is that we take advantage of both traditional BoF models and recently developed deep feature learning framework.

The feature learning models are usually build in a hierarchical framework by stacking shallow generative models with greedy layerwise scheme. One class of feature learning algorithms is based on the encoder-decoder architecture (*e.g.* Auto-encoder) [29]. The input is fed to the encoder which produces a feature vector and the decoder module then reconstructs the input from the feature vector with the reconstruction error measured. Deep Belief Networks(DBN) [30] build multiple layers of directed sigmoid belief nets with the top layer as a Restricted Boltzmann Machines. Lee *et al.* [31] extended DBN with convolution operation for the purpose of extracting latent features from raw image pixels. Yu *et al.* [32] proposed a hierarchical sparse coding model to learn image representations from local patches. Different from these models, we apply a stacked Cardinality Restricted Boltzmann Machine [8], which is an extension to Restricted Boltzmann Machine with the attractive properties of sparse coding by introducing competition among its hidden units. The most important difference of our model with the previous works is that we take advantage of both traditional BoF models and recently developed deep feature learning framework.

3 The Proposed Model

In this section, we describe the details of our proposed model for image representation and classification. As illustrated in Fig. 1, it is a hierarchial architecture, consisting of 3 operations: appearance coding, over spatial max-pooling and spatial coding. The base module of the deep model is Cardinality Restricted Boltzmann Machine(CaRBM).

3.1 Appearance Coding

Starting with an input image I, we densely extract a set of local patch descriptors (e.g. SIFT and HOG) and take each descriptor as input to the appearance coding layer. The appearance coding is a deep CaRBM module, encoding the input features into high-dimensional sparse and discriminative codes.

A Restricted Boltzmann Machine(RBM) [33] is a type of bi-partite undirected graphical model that is capable of learning a dictionary of patterns from unlabeled datas. It has a two-layer structure, defining a joint probability distribution over a hidden layer $h \in \{0,1\}^{N_h}$ and a visible layer $v \in \{0,1\}^{N_v}$:

$$P(v,h) = \frac{1}{Z}exp(v^\top Wh + v^\top b_v + h^\top b_h) \tag{1}$$

where Z is the partition function, $W \in R^{N_v \times N_h}$ represents the undirected weights and $b_v \in R^{N_v}, b_h \in R^{N_h}$ are the bias terms. As RBM is a popular density model for extracting features, a desirable property, i.e. sparsity, is neglected when applying it to discriminative task. CaRBM is an extension to RBM with the attractive properties of sparse coding by introducing competition among its hidden units. It combines RBM with cardinality potential, which is a class of highly structured global interactions by assigning preferences to counts over subsets of binary variables. The probability of the joint configuration in CaRBM is defined as follows:

$$P(v,h) = \frac{1}{Z}exp(v^\top Wh + v^\top b_v + h^\top b_h) \cdot \psi_k(\sum_{j=1}^{N_h} h_j) \tag{2}$$

where ψ_k is a potential given by $\psi_k(c) = 1$ if $c \leq k$ and 0 otherwise. This constrains that the conditional distribution $P(h|v)$ assigns a non-zero probability mass to a vector h only if $|h| \leq k$. In other words, a data vector v can be explained by at most k hidden units.

By letting the visible layer v correspond to dimensions of the input local descriptor, the CaRBM is able to encode it into a high-dimensional codes. Different from the standard visual coding, we directly map the descriptors into a high-dimensional space by the undirected weights matrix. Thus in the appearance layer, the dimension of the visible units is denoted as $N_v = X$(128 for SIFT) and the number of hidden units is denoted as $N_h = D$ which is usually much larger than X. In the appearance coding of our model, we build a two layer model by stacking the CaRBM, where the output of the first CaRBM is regarded as the input to the next layer. These deep coding scheme is more effective according to our implementation, and we finally concatenate the resulting codes of the two layer for further improvement.

To learn the appearance coding layer, we firstly train it in an unsupervised way and then perform fine-tuning to enhance discriminative property. In the unsupervised pre-training phase, the objective is to maximize the likelihood of training data. As the calculation of conditional distribution $P(h|v)$ is tractable by the sum-product algorithm [8], we may use algorithms like Persistent Contrastive Divergence(PCD) [34]. In the fine-tuning process, we associate each input descriptor with the image label. Different from RBM, the nonlinearity of CaRBM is not clear. Therefore an approximate Jacobian multiplication method is needed to compute gradients [8]. With the learned CaRBM, each local patch is encoded into a high dimensional code during inference process.

3.2 Over Spatial Max-pooling

In order to build a image-level signature, pooling operation is usually carried out to aggregate the local appearance codes. Traditional SPM partitions a given image into increasingly finer uniform grids (*i.e.* $1 \times 1, 2 \times 2, 4 \times 4$), and then pools within each region and concatenate all the region vectors as the final image representation. To overcome the limitation of the simple uniform partition, we propose to construct spatial partitions in a more flexible scheme incorporating as many geometric properties of the local features as possible.

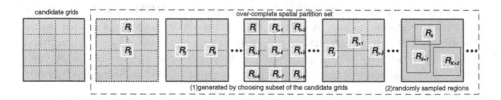

Fig. 2. The generation of over-complete spatial partition set.

As described in Fig. 2, we firstly apply uniform horizontal and vertical grids to divide the image into rectangular grids (the dotted grids). These grids are considered as the candidate grids to generate a certain kind of spatial partition. Then, a type of spatial partition is created by randomly choosing a subset of the candidate grids. By covering all the possible combinations of the grids, the spatial partition is able to present various spatial layout information. In addition, we generate some randomly sampled grids to provide more flexible spatial information. All these partitioned regions are collected as the over spatial partition set. Max-pooling is finally performed on the local appearance codes with each partitioned region and all the region vectors are concatenated as the input to the next spatial coding module. It is noted that the dimension of each region vector is D.

3.3   Spatial Coding

With the region vectors as input, spatial coding are then performed to integrate them into global image representations. If number of partitioned spatial region is k, then the input dimension of the spatial coding is kD. Since this input is highly redundant, we also turn to the sparse constrained CaRBM. As shown in Fig. 1, the spatial coding is comprised of two stacked CaRBM with the output of the first one taken as the input to the next. Instead of simply concatenating the regions vectors in SPM, our model explores the generative and discriminative properties of the spatial distribution to fuse the region vectors into a better representation. The pre-training is performed layer-by-layer by PCD algorithm to maximize the likelihood of the training dataset, while the fine-tuning is performed top down with the image label.

Finally, the obtained representations are employed to train a one-versus-others SVM to classify an image into the category with max score. The features of the two layers in spatial coding may be combined to further improve the performance.

4   Experiments

We start our experiments with an in-depth analysis of the proposed model on 15-Scenes dataset, after which we transpose the findings to experiments on PASCAL VOC 2007 and Caltech-256 dataset. Firstly, we evaluate the effectiveness of appearance coding compared with the hard-assignment [7], sparse coding [5], LLC [6] and RBM. Then, we demonstrate the effect of our spatial coding mainly compared with the popular SPM and some other works considering spatial information.

For fair comparison, the experiments are conducted closely following the standard settings [5,7,35]. We adopt a single local descriptor, the SIFT descriptor, by densely extracting local patches of 16×16 pixels over a grid with spacing of 4 pixels. The number of hidden units in appearance coding is fixed as $D = 1024$ for fair comparison, and the dimensions of hidden units for each CaRBM in spatial coding layers are equally set and denoted as S. The number of partitioned regions in the over spatial max-pooling is 60. The target sparsity is all set to 10 %. The SVM classifiers are trained with linear kernels in one-versus-others scheme and the trade-off parameters to the SVM regularization term are chosen via 5-fold cross validation on the training set.

4.1   Results on 15-Scenes

We start our experiments with a most popular scene classification benchmark, *i.e.* 15-Scenes. This dataset is complied by several researchers [7,36], including 15 scene categories (*e.g.* kitchen, coast, highway) with each class containing 200 to 400 images. Following the standard setup, 100 images per class are taken for training with the rest for testing. The performances are reported by repeating the experimental process 5 times with different randomly selected training and testing images.

Table 1. Classification rate (%) comparison of different coding methods on 15-Scenes.

Algorithms	Classification rate
Hard+SPM [7]	81.1 ± 0.3
Soft+SPM [37]	82.7 ± 0.4
SC+SPM [5]	80.8 ± 0.9
LLC+SPM	81.8 ± 0.60
SSRBM+SPM [16]	84.1 ± 0.8
Unsupervised RBM+SPM	82.5 ± 0.5
Unsupervised CaRBM+SPM	86.9 ± 0.2
Supervised CaRBM+SPM	$\mathbf{88.3 \pm 0.3}$

We firstly evaluate the effect of our appearance coding by comparing to the baselines and related works with only difference in the feature coding phase. The final image representations are all compiled by SPM after feature coding. The detailed performance comparison is shown in Table 1, where "Unsupervised RBM+SPM" and "Unsupervised CaRBM+SPM" denote the method of adopting RBM and CaRBM module to perform feature coding respectively, and "Supervised CaRBM+SPM" denotes the results after supervised fine-tuning. It is shown that our appearance coding method outperforms traditional method, such as hard assignment, soft assignment, sparse coding and LLC. Our method also beats SSRBM [16], which is a model of applying sparse regularized RBM. Compared with SSRBM, CaRBM accomplishes sparsity in a fundamentally different way and performs better according to our experiments. It is also shown that supervised fine-tuning brings a slight improvement, demonstrating that the discrimination are enhanced by fine-tuning process.

Secondly, with the coding scheme fixed as supervised CaRBM, we evaluate the effect of our spatial coding. Figure 3 shows the performance comparison by varying the dimension of the hidden units in the spatial layers. "S1" denotes the performance of the output feature in the 1st layer of spatial coding, while "S1+2" denotes the performance of combining the features of the 2 layers. The baselines are traditional SPM and the method of directly concatenating of all the region vectors (denoted as "CAT"). It is shown that the best performance

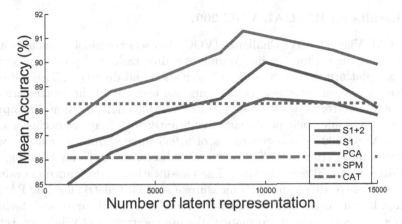

Fig. 3. Performance comparisons of the spatial layers with different dimensions of hidden units.

is achieved with the number of latent units set to about 9,000, which outperforms the *SPM* by nearly 3 percentage points. We also compare our approach to some dimension reduction technique, *e.g.* PCA. The classification accuracy is obviously improved by the CaRBM than PCA, due to the better exploration of generative and discriminative properties of the data. Table 2 shows the performance comparison between our best model with state-of-the-art results. Our best accuracy achieves 91.1%, which outperforms all the related results on this dataset. Compared with traditional BoF framework, our network needs more time to train, since both the appearance and spatial coding modules requires to be learned. However, in the test process, our model is efficient because only forward matrix multiplication operation is needed without any iteration. According to our evaluation, in "SC+SPM" [5], about 4 seconds are needed to obtain the pyramid representation for each image, while only 0.3 seconds are required in the proposed method.

Table 2. Classification rate (%) comparison on 15-Scenes.

Algorithms	Classification rate
Lazebnik et al. [7]	81.1 ± 0.3
Boureau et al. [38]	85.6 ± 0.3
Zhou et al. [39]	85.2
Goh et al. [16]	86.0 ± 0.5
Feng et al. [40]	83.2
Our (Unsupervised)	88.1 ± 0.3
Our (Supervised)	$\mathbf{91.1 \pm 0.2}$

4.2 Results on PASCAL VOC 2007

The PSCAL Visual Object Challenge (VOC) datasets are widely used as testbeds for evaluating algorithms for image understanding tasks and provide a common evaluation platform for both object classification and detection. This dataset is considered to be an extremely challenging one because all the images are daily photos obtained from Flicker where the size, viewing angle, illumination, appearances of objects and their poses vary significantly with frequent occlusions. The PASCAL VOC 2007 dataset consists of 9,963 images from 20 classes, which are divided into "train", "val" and "test" subsets, *i.e.* 25 % for training, 25 % for validation and 50 % for testing. The classification performance is evaluated using the Average Precision (AP) measure, a standard metric used by PASCAL challenge. It computes the area under the Precision/Recall curve, and the higher the score, the better the performance. We use the train and validation sets for training and report the mean average precision for the 20 classes on the test set as the performance evaluation. In the experiment setup, the size of the latent units in the appearance coding is 1024, while the size of each layer in spatial coding is set to 10,000.

Table 3. Recognition performance (AP in %) comparison on VOC 2007. (The table is divided into two parts due to the limitation of space).

Method	aero	bike	bird	boat	bottle	bus	car	cat	chair	cow	table
SPM[35]	68.7	57.0	39.9	64.6	22.0	58.8	73.9	53.8	52.4	38.6	49.2
LLC+SPM[35]	69.8	57.6	42.0	66.5	22.4	55.6	72.8	56.9	51.7	42.9	45.1
FK+SPM[35]	78.9	67.4	51.9	70.9	30.8	72.2	**79.9**	61.4	55.9	49.6	58.4
Object Bank[41]	68.7	53.4	34.6	61.8	19.8	49.9	75.0	42.1	48.7	28.7	50.2
Our(unsupervised)	77.3	67.3	51.2	72.1	31.8	70.5	76.0	59.3	55.8	48.4	57.9
Our(supervised)	**80.8**	**69.1**	**53.0**	**73.5**	**33.2**	**72.2**	78.3	**61.8**	**57.5**	**51.6**	**59.3**

Method	dog	horse	motor	person	plant	sheep	sofa	train	tv	Mean
SPM[35]	36.9	75.6	61.6	81.6	20.5	40.1	50.9	73.4	49.2	53.4
LLC+SPM[35]	39.5	74.1	62.0	80.9	24.5	38.8	49.4	71.2	51.0	53.8
FK+SPM[35]	44.8	78.8	**70.8**	84.9	31.7	**51.0**	56.4	80.2	57.5	61.7
Object Bank[41]	31.8	71.4	53.1	79.6	15.6	29.0	44.3	67.3	49.0	48.7
Our(unsupervised)	46.1	78.5	69.0	84.1	29.8	48.3	56.9	81.0	56.9	60.9
Our(supervised)	**48.6**	**80.6**	70.3	**86.4**	**32.3**	50.5	**59.5**	**83.2**	**58.5**	**63.1**

The performance comparisons of all the 20 classes are shown in Table 3. "SPM" denotes the method of applying hard assignment and SPM model, while "LLC+SPM" represents the method of using locality-constrained linear coding instead of hard assignment. "FK+SPM" denotes the method of using fisher kernel to encode the SIFT descriptors, which is the state-of-the-art feature coding method. In "Object Bank" [41], pre-trained object detectors are employed to extract image representations. As shown in the table, our method leads the performance for most categories. It is also demonstrated that the supervised fine-tuning is effective to improve the recognition performance. However, for some categories, such as car and sheep, our method decreases the accuracy. This is mainly on account of the highly diversity of the images in this challenging dataset.

4.3   Results on Caltech-256

The Caltech-256 [42] dataset totally holds 29, 780 images in 256 object categories, where the number of images in each category varies form 31 to 800. This dataset is very much challenging as it possesses highly intra-class variability and object location variability. Some example images are shown in Fig. 4. Following the standard experiment setup on this dataset, we train our model on 30 and 60 images per class and test on the rest. The other parameters setup is transposed from the former experiments on 15-Scenes.

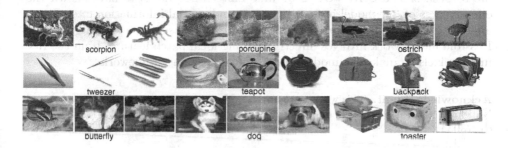

Fig. 4. Example images of Caltech-256 dataset.

Table 4. Classification rate (%) comparison on Caltech-256.

Algorithms	30 training	60 training
KSPM [7]	34.1	—
ScSPM [5]	34.0 ± 0.4	40.1 ± 0.9
LLCSPM [6]	41.2	47.7
GLP [40]	43.2	—
Our(Unsupervised)	46.5 ± 0.3	50.2 ± 0.4
Our(Supervised)	$\mathbf{48.7 \pm 0.2}$	$\mathbf{53.2 \pm 0.4}$

The performance comparison is shown in Table 4. In this challenging dataset, our method also consistently leads the performance on all the cases and outperforms the baseline ScSPM by more than 10 %. GLP [40] is a method of using discriminatively learned pooling operation to aggregate local features and our model also behaves better than it. The reason may be that our model explores more kinds of latent spatial layout and integrate the regions beyong the simple concatenation scheme. The results on this challenging object datasets demonstrate the effectiveness of the proposed deep image representation model.

5   Conclusion

In this paper, we address the issues of local feature coding and spatial information incorporation in the BoF model and propose a deep appearance and spatial coding model to build more representative and discriminative representation for image classification. We utilizes the Cardinality Restricted Boltzmann Machines, which is capable of combining generative and discriminative properties. With the CaRBM as the base module, our model includes appearance coding, over spatial max pooling and spatial coding operations, which is pre-trained in an unsupervised scheme and then fine-tuned with image labels. The extensive experiments on 15-Scenes, PASCAL VOC 2007 and Caltech-256 datasets have shown the effectiveness of our model in feature coding and spatial information integration, and the classification performances outperform the baselines and related works. Possible future work involves directly learning local patch features from the raw image pixels to make the model an end-to-end learning framework.

Acknowledgement. This work was supported by 863 Program (2014AA015104) and National Natural Science Foundation of China (61332016, 61272329, 61472422, and 61273034).

References

1. Csurka, G., Dance, C., Fan, L., Willamowski, J., Bray, C.: Visual categorization with bags of keypoints. In: ECCV 2004 Workshop on Statistical Learning in Computer Vision (2004)
2. Lowe, D.: Distinctive image features from scale-invariant keypoints. Int. J. Comput. Vision **60**, 91–110 (2004)
3. Dalal, N., Triggs, B.: Histograms of oriented gradients for human detection. In: CVPR (2005)
4. van Gemert, J.C., Geusebroek, J.-M., Veenman, C.J., Smeulders, A.W.M.: Kernel codebooks for scene categorization. In: Forsyth, D., Torr, P., Zisserman, A. (eds.) ECCV 2008, Part III. LNCS, vol. 5304, pp. 696–709. Springer, Heidelberg (2008)
5. Yang, J., Yu, K., Gong, Y., Huang, T.: Linear spatial pyramid matching using sparse coding for image classification. In: CVPR (2009)
6. Wang, J., Yang, J., Yu, K., Lv, F., Huang, T., Gong, Y.: Locality-constrained linear coding for image classification. In: CVPR (2010)
7. Lazebnik, S., Schmid, C., Ponce, J.: Beyond bags of features: Spatial pyramid matching for recognizing natural scene categories. In: CVPR (2006)
8. Swersky, K., Tarlow, D., Sutskever, I., Salakhutdinov, R., Zemel, R., Adams, R.: Cardinality restricted boltzmann machines. In: NIPS (2012)

9. Roth, P.M., Winter, M.: Survey of Appearance-Based methods for object recognition. Institute for Computer Graphics and Vision, Graz University of Technology, Technical report (2008)
10. Perronnin, F., Dance, C., Csurka, G., Bressan, M.: Adapted vocabularies for generic visual categorization. In: Leonardis, A., Bischof, H., Pinz, A. (eds.) ECCV 2006. LNCS, vol. 3954, pp. 464–475. Springer, Heidelberg (2006)
11. Jurie, F., Triggs, B.: Creating efficient codebooks for visual recognition. In: ICCV (2005)
12. Boiman, O., Shechtman, E., Irani, M.: In defense of nearest-neighbor based image classification. In: CVPR (2008)
13. van Gemert, J.C., Veenman, C.J., Smeulders, A.W.M., Geusebroek, J.M.: Visual word ambiguity. IEEE Trans. Pattern Anal. Mach. Intell. **32**, 1271–1283 (2010)
14. Jiang, Z., Lin, Z., Davis, L.S.: Learning a discriminative dictionary for sparse coding via label consistent k-svd. In: CVPR (2011)
15. Yang, J., Yu, K., Huang, T.S.: Supervised translation-invariant sparse coding. In: CVPR (2010)
16. Goh, H., Thome, N., Cord, M., Lim, J.-H.: Unsupervised and supervised visual codes with restricted boltzmann machines. In: Fitzgibbon, A., Lazebnik, S., Perona, P., Sato, Y., Schmid, C. (eds.) ECCV 2012, Part V. LNCS, vol. 7576, pp. 298–311. Springer, Heidelberg (2012)
17. Li, Z., Liu, J., Yang, Y., Zhou, X., Lu, H.: Clustering-guided sparse structural learning for unsupervised feature selection. IEEE Trans. Knowl. Data Eng. **26**, 2138–2150 (2014)
18. Li, Z., Yang, Y., Liu, J., Zhou, X., Lu, H.: Unsupervised feature selection using nonnegative spectral analysis. In: AAAI (2012)
19. Savarese, S., Winn, J., Criminisi, A.: Discriminative object class models of appearance and shape by correlatons. In: CVPR (2006)
20. Liu, D., Hua, G., Viola, P., Chen, T.: Integrated feature selection and higher-order spatial feature extraction for object categorization. In: CVPR (2008)
21. Morioka, N., Satoh, S.: Building compact local pairwise codebook with joint feature space clustering. In: Daniilidis, K., Maragos, P., Paragios, N. (eds.) ECCV 2010, Part I. LNCS, vol. 6311, pp. 692–705. Springer, Heidelberg (2010)
22. Morioka, N., Satoh, S.: Learning directional local pairwise bases with sparse coding. In: BMVC (2010)
23. Zhou, X., Yu, K., Zhang, T., Huang, T.S.: Image classification using super-vector coding of local image descriptors. In: Daniilidis, K., Maragos, P., Paragios, N. (eds.) ECCV 2010, Part V. LNCS, vol. 6315, pp. 141–154. Springer, Heidelberg (2010)
24. Perronnin, F., Dance, C.R.: Fisher kernels on visual vocabularies for image categorization. In: CVPR (2007)
25. Harada, T., Ushiku, Y., Yamashita, Y., Kuniyoshi, Y.: Discriminative spatial pyramid. In: CVPR (2011)
26. Sharma, G., Jurie, F.: Learning discriminative spatial representation for image classification. In: BMVC (2011)
27. Jia, Y., Huang, C., Darrell, T.: Beyond spatial pyramids: receptive field learning for pooled image features. In: CVPR (2012)
28. Liu, B., Liu, J., Lu, H.: Adaptive spatial partition learning for image classification. Neurocomputing **142**, 282–290 (2014)
29. Huang, F.J., lan Boureau, Y., Lecun, Y.: Unsupervised learning of invariant feature hierarchies with applications to object recognition. In: CVPR (2007)
30. Hinton, G.E., Osindero, S.: A fast learning algorithm for deep belief nets. Neural Comput. **18**, 1527–1554 (2006)

31. Lee, H., Grosse, R., Ranganath, R., Ng, A.Y.: Convolutional deep belief networks for scalable unsupervised learning of hierarchical representations. In: ICML (2009)
32. Yu, K., Lin, Y., Lafferty, J.: Learning image representations from the pixel level via hierarchical sparse coding. In: CVPR (2011)
33. Hinton, G., Salakhutdinov, R.: Reducing the dimensionality of data with neural networks. Science **313**, 504–507 (2006)
34. Tieleman, T.: Training restricted boltzmann machines using approximations to the likelihood gradient. In: ICML (2008)
35. Chatfield, K., Lempitsky, V., Vedaldi, A., Zisserman, A.: The devil is in the details: an evaluation of recent feature encoding methods. In: BMVC (2011)
36. Fei-Fei, L., Perona, P.: A bayesian hierarchical model for learning natural scene categories. In: CVPR (2005)
37. Liu, L., Wang, L., Liu, X.: In defense of soft-assignment coding. In: ICCV (2011)
38. Boureau, Y.L., Bach, F., LeCun, Y., Ponce, J.: Learning mid-level features for recognition. In: CVPR (2010)
39. Zhou, X., Cui, N., Li, Z., Liang, F., Huang, T.: Hierarchical gaussianization for image classification. In: ICCV (2009)
40. Feng, J., Ni, B., Tian, Q., Yan, S.: Geometric lp-norm feature pooling for image classification. In: CVPR (2011)
41. Li, L.J., Su, H., Xing, E.P., Fei-Fei, L.: Object bank: A high-level image representation for scene classification and semantic feature sparsification. In: NIPS (2010)
42. Griffin, G., Holub, A., Perona, P.: Caltech-256 object category dataset. Technical report 7694, California Institute of Technology (2007)

On the Exploration of Joint Attribute Learning for Person Re-identification

Joseph Roth and Xiaoming Liu[✉]

Department of Computer Science and Engineering, Michigan State University,
East Lansing, USA
{rothjos1,liuxm}@cse.msu.edu

Abstract. This paper presents an algorithm for *jointly* learning a set of mid-level attributes from an image ensemble by locating clusters of dependent attributes. Human describable attributes are an active research topic due to their ability to transfer between domains, human understanding, and improvement to identification performance. Joint learning may allow for enhanced attribute classification when there is inherent dependency among the attributes. We propose an agglomerative clustering scheme to determine *which* sets of attributes should be learned jointly in order to maximize the margin of performance improvement. We evaluate the joint learning algorithm on a set of attributes for the task of person re-identification. We find that the proposed algorithm can improve classifier accuracy over both independent or fully joint attribute classification. Furthermore, the enhanced classifiers also improve performance on the person re-identification task. Our algorithm can be widely applicable to a variety of attribute-based visual recognition problems.

1 Introduction

Person re-identification seeks to locate the same individual across multiple non-overlapping cameras within a short time frame [1]. As an enabling technique for video surveillance [2,3], it has many applications such as tracker linking, person retrieval, searching missing children in public spaces, etc. Depending on the applications, person re-identification can be posed in different scenarios. For example, classic *person re-identification* is image-to-image matching where one image is the occurrence of the person of interest in one of the cameras. *Zero-shot identification* is description-to-image matching where the only prior knowledge is a verbal description by an eyewitness.

While many prior work of person re-identification rely on low-level visual feature based image matching [4–8], recently human describable, mid-level attributes have become a promising approach for both re-identification [9] and zero-shot identification [10] scenarios. This is especially true for the latter where describable attributes are the *only* source of input information. These attributes have a number of advantages over low-level visual features. First, they enable the possibility of human-in-the-loop to assist decision making. Second, they can improve

© Springer International Publishing Switzerland 2015
D. Cremers et al. (Eds.): ACCV 2014, Part I, LNCS 9003, pp. 673–688, 2015.
DOI: 10.1007/978-3-319-16865-4_44

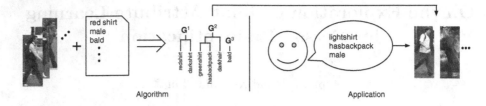

Fig. 1. Given an image ensemble with labels on a set of attributes, our *algorithm* automatically partitions the attribute set into various clusters and jointly learns a classifier for multiple attributes within each cluster. This leads to superior performance in both attribute classification and person re-identification *application* (e.g., zero-shot identification).

the system performance by fusion with low-level features. Third, human understanding of the attributes allows for their use as evidences in a courtroom.

In order to detect multiple attributes from an image, normally an array of classifiers are *independently* learned from training data - one classifier per attribute [9]. However, there are various potential *dependencies* among attributes that may enable a better approach to learning. Correlation in attribute occurrence may exist. For example, knowledge that a person is a male will impact the prior probability about the hair length. Another potential dependency is the subset of low-level features that define the attributes. Attributes about the same local area (e.g., wearing jeans or skirt) will likely share a common set of low-level features. Recent works recognize there exist dependencies [9,11], and few [12,13] seek to leverage them to *jointly* learn attribute classifiers from the features.

This paper aims to explore *whether* and *how* joint learning can improve attribute classification performance. As shown in Fig. 1, we propose an approach for jointly learning attributes by leveraging their dependencies. Given a set of images labeled with a set of attributes, we recognize that *not all* attributes have strong dependencies and therefore it is desirable to identify clusters of attributes for which joint learning will have greater impact. We propose a data-driven, agglomerative clustering scheme where each attribute begins in a separate cluster and we iteratively combine clusters based on the expected improvement from joint classification. This scheme efficiently partitions the attributes into K clusters, where K is estimated in a data-driven manner. We then train a set of classifiers, one for each cluster of related attributes. To predict the attributes for an unseen image, the image is given to the set of classifiers, which collectively assign all attribute labels. Using the person re-identification datasets, VIPeR [14] and PRID [15], we evaluate the joint learning on a challenging set of human labeled attributes [9] with little inter-attribute correlation. We demonstrate superior attribute classification performance of the proposed algorithm, and also improvement on zero-shot person identification using the predicted attributes.

In summary, this paper has two main contributions:

– We develop a joint attribute classification algorithm that leverages attribute dependencies to learn a set of attribute classifiers. Our algorithm can automatically determine the attribute combinations for joint learning.

– We demonstrate that joint learning improves classification accuracy of human labeled attributes for person re-identification and also improves zero-shot identification.

2 Related Work

Attribute-based visual analysis is a popular research topic. Computer vision has increasing interest in describing objects by a rich set of human describable attributes [16–18]. For example, [19] presented a system with 65 attributes for unconstrained face recognition, which performs well on the labeled faces in the wild dataset. Soft biometrics have been used to improve commercial face matchers [20]. For person re-identification, [9,10] explored the use of human describable attributes either computed directly from the low-level features or provided by a human operator. Most recently, [11] used human annotated soft biometrics as ancillary information to improve face recognition at a distance. In all of these works, the performances of the attribute classifiers are crucial to the overall performance of the problem at hand because attribute classification errors will propagate throughout the entire system.

All aforementioned applications have a separate, independently learned classifier for each attribute. Both [9,19] used an SVM to classify each attribute. Using independent classifiers is the naive approach for multi-attribute classification and may be inefficient since potentially different features need to be extracted for each classifier. With this insight, [21,22] proposed techniques to find optimal common sets of features in order to make multi-attribute classifications *computationally* efficient. These techniques find a subset of features, which jointly predict different classes where only one class will be present at a time. If $\mathbf{x}$ is the set of features used for classification and $\mathbf{y}$ is the output, these approaches seek to minimize $|\mathbf{x}|$, but do not place any criteria on the classification performance on $\mathbf{y}$. Also, in these works, $\mathbf{y}$ has only one attribute present in a given image whereas our work allows any number of attributes to be present.

A few multi-task learning works try to take advantage of dependencies in order to improve overall performance. These works have the same motivation for joint learning as us and try to maximize the classification performance on $\mathbf{y}$. Most notably [23] presented an approach for using support vector regression to jointly predict multidimensional output. They claimed this exploits the dependencies between variables and reduces the effects of noise in the input. In [24], image based regression (IBR) is proposed to use boosting to predict multiple outputs. One very recent work [25] automatically determines attribute dependency and learns a *single* classifier to jointly predict *all* attributes. These works differ from ours in that they assume *all* attributes should be learned jointly. In contrast, we recognize that *not all* attributes should be combined in order to improve performance, i.e., attributes without dependencies may hurt performance when learned jointly. Indeed, our experiment (Table 2) shows that *fully* joint learning does degrade performance.

A set of works [26–28] took advantage of the object labels along with the attribute labels in the joint learning framework to further improve performance for attribute learning. These object labels can act as latent variables or side information [29] for attribute classification since they are not directly in the feature set, but are known during training. For the task of person re-identification, we could use the identity information during training in the same manner if the database includes sufficient images of the same person. Unfortunately, the databases we use only have two images per person so we choose not to use the identity information while training.

There are a few recent works recognizing that fully joint learning may lead to overfit in attribute classification. The authors in [13] clustered attributes manually based on human understanding of relatedness. Features were encouraged to be shared among attributes within the same cluster, while attributes from different clusters were encouraged to use different features. In contrast, we use a data-driven approach to both clustering and feature selection. A data-driven approach was used in [12] to create attribute clusters and learn a separate classifier for each cluster. We use a data-driven approach to estimate the performance margin of clustering, whereas [12] used a regularization of the selected features to cluster attributes that reside in a low rank subspace of selected features.

3   Joint Attribute Learning

This section presents our approach for joint attribute learning. We start by formally defining the problem and objectives. Then we analyze one specific means of simultaneously predicting a set of multiple attributes. Finally, we present our hierarchical clustering scheme to efficiently identify the sets of attributes for joint learning, in order to best improve the attribute classification accuracy.

3.1   Problem Definition

Let us assume there are Q user-defined mid-level attributes to describe "person" in videos, and one example of such attributes is shown in Table 1. We denote the collection of attributes as $\mathbb{A} = \{1, 2, \cdots, Q\}$, where each integer corresponds to a particular attribute. The training data of the joint attribute learning includes the low-level visual features of N images $\mathbf{X} = \{\mathbf{x}_1, \mathbf{x}_2, \cdots, \mathbf{x}_N\}$, $\mathbf{x}_n \in \mathbb{R}_D$ and their corresponding attribute labels $\mathbf{Y} = \{\mathbf{y}_1, \mathbf{y}_2, \cdots, \mathbf{y}_N\}$, $\mathbf{y}_n \in \mathbb{R}_Q$. Here D is the feature dimension of the visual features. Each element of the Q-dim vector $\mathbf{y}_n$ can be either 0 or 1 for binary attributes such as gender and bald, or a real number scaled within $[0, 1]$ for ordinal attributes such as age and weight.

The first objective of joint attribute learning is to learn one classifier $\mathbf{G}(\mathbf{x})$: $\mathbb{R}_D \to \mathbb{R}_Q$ that minimizes attribute classification errors:

$$J(\mathbf{G}) = \sum_{n=1}^{N} \|\mathbf{y}_n - \mathbf{G}(\mathbf{x}_n)\|^2. \tag{1}$$

While this is a basic objective, it assumes that all attributes should be learned together, but in Sect. 3.3 we will show that K, rather than one, attribute classifier(s) should be learned to minimize $J()$. We will present an algorithm on how to estimate the optimal K value and partition Q attributes into K clusters. Note that when $K = Q$, this degenerates to the conventional approach where one classifier is trained for each individual attribute. For the clarity of presentation, in the next section we first present the fully joint attribute learning where $K = 1$.

3.2   Learning via Image Based Boosted Regression

Given a set of attributes, we seek to learn a classifier that predicts all attributes simultaneously. For this task, we use IBR, which has shown success in various vision applications [24] and its regressor formulation is also suitable for predicting both binary and ordinal attributes. We present a brief overview of the basic IBR algorithm. Given training data $\mathbf{X}$ and $\mathbf{Y}$, it learns a classifier in the form,

$$\mathbf{G}(\mathbf{x}) = \sum_{t=1}^{T} \alpha_i \mathbf{h}_t(\mathbf{x}), \tag{2}$$

where α_i is the weight, $\mathbf{h}_t(\mathbf{x})$ is the weak classifier that predicts all Q attributes simultaneously, and is comprised of Q 1-dim weak learners, i.e., $\mathbf{h}(\mathbf{x}) = [h_1(\mathbf{x}), h_2(\mathbf{x}), \cdots, h_Q(\mathbf{x})]^\mathsf{T}$.

We use the 1-dim decision stump weak learner $h(\mathbf{x})$, which has a low-level feature $g(\mathbf{x})$, a parity indicator $\tilde{p} \in \{-1, 1\}$, and a threshold θ. That is,

$$h(\mathbf{x}) = \begin{cases} +1 : \tilde{p}g(\mathbf{x}) \geq \tilde{p}\theta, \\ -1 : \text{otherwise.} \end{cases} \tag{3}$$

The low-level feature $g(\mathbf{x})$ may be from the color or texture of a localized region, or commonly used local descriptors.

During each boosting iteration, a weight α and weak classifier $\mathbf{h}(\mathbf{x})$ are chosen by minimizing the cost function,

$$J(\mathbf{G}) = \sum_{n=1}^{N} \|\mathbf{y}_n - \mathbf{G}(\mathbf{x}_n)\|_{\mathbf{B}_1}^2 + \lambda \sum_{n=1}^{N} \|\mu - \mathbf{G}(\mathbf{x}_n)\|_{\mathbf{B}_2}^2. \tag{4}$$

While the first term of this function is similar to Eq. 1, a regularization term with μ equal to the sample mean of $\mathbf{Y}$ is used to diminish overfitting. The matrices $\mathbf{B}_1$ and $\mathbf{B}_2$ are for normalization and are naturally related to the covariance matrix of the attribute set. For details on how to select α and $\mathbf{h}(\mathbf{x})$ from a pool of features and weak classifiers, we refer the readers to [24].

From this formulation, we see that joint learning occurs in part based on the choice of $\mathbf{B}_1$ and $\mathbf{B}_2$. If either is a non-diagonal matrix, it is computationally unfeasible to select the optimal weak classifier $\mathbf{h}(\mathbf{x})$. In contrast, if both $\mathbf{B}_1$ and $\mathbf{B}_2$ are identity matrices, each weak learner $h(\mathbf{x})$ can be optimally chosen independent of the other $Q - 1$ weak learners, and thus an incremental feature selection scheme can be employed. Based on this observation, [24] suggests a three-step approach to IBR, as shown in Fig. 2. In the first step, the multi-attribute labels $\mathbf{Y}$ are decorrelated via whitening. Specifically, let $\mathbf{D}$ and $\mathbf{V}$

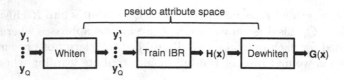

Fig. 2. Flow chart demonstrating a three-step approach to IBR. These steps correspond to Lines 24–26 in Algorithm 1.

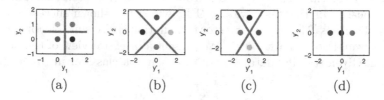

Fig. 3. Example demonstrating the effects of attribute correlation on their whitened attribute space. Red lines are decision boundaries. Figures are initial attribute space **Y** (a), and then transformed space **Y**$'$ with 0 (b), 0.5 (c), and 1 (d) correlation (Color figure online).

be the eigenvalue and eigenvector matrices of the covariance matrix of **Y**. We generate uncorrelated pseudo-attribute labels by

$$\mathbf{y}'_n = \mathbf{D}^{-1/2}\mathbf{V}^\mathsf{T}(\mathbf{y}_n - \mu). \tag{5}$$

The second step learns the regressor $\mathbf{H}(\mathbf{x}) = \sum \alpha_i \mathbf{h}_t(\mathbf{x})$ to predict the uncorrelated labels **Y**$'$, by setting $\mathbf{B}_1 = \mathbf{B}_2 = \mathbf{I}$. In the third step, the final attribute classifier $\mathbf{G}(\mathbf{x})$ can be obtained by dewhitening the estimated uncorrelated labels, $\mathbf{G}(\mathbf{x}) = \mu + (\mathbf{V}^\mathsf{T})^{-1}\mathbf{D}^{1/2}\mathbf{H}(\mathbf{x})$.

It is interesting to note that the joint learning is achieved in this implementation mainly because the whitening and dewhitening *share* the selected features across the attributes. Thus, we hypothesize that any standard regression technique can be applied to predict each one of Q attributes of **Y**$'$ independently. In Fig. 3 we demonstrate the effects of whitening on the **Y**$'$ attribute space ($Q = 2$) for different amounts of initial correlation.

While the learned regressor $\mathbf{G}(\mathbf{x})$ directly classifies ordinal attributes such as age and height, for binary attributes we must also find a threshold τ to perform classification. We select τ_q for attribute a_q that minimizes the error on the training data. Note that even in a case with all binary attributes, regression is still necessary because the **Y**$'$ space is ordinal.

3.3 Attribute Clustering

The aforementioned joint attribute learning assumes that on average the jointly learned classifier can achieve superior classification performance for Q attributes than Q independently learned attribute classifiers. However, it is important to note that this assumption may not always hold true. Let us consider two simple scenarios when $Q = 2$. First, the two attributes have dependencies and there is a difference between their independent classifier performances. Thus, the dependency between the attributes may be exploited by a joint classifier to improve the performance of the harder-to-classify attribute. Second, the two attributes have no dependency and they both have high independent classifier performance. If we apply joint learning in this scenario, the labeling noise in the training samples or bias in their sampling from the population may cause the joint classifier to assume there to be dependence when there is none. Hence, the joint learning may actually hurt the performance of attribute classification.

Therefore, our goal is to identify the contributing factors and predict *when* **joint learning will improve the attribute classification performance over independent learning, and to use this knowledge to** *partition* **the set of attributes into multiple clusters where the attributes within each cluster may be jointly learned to best improve performance.**

Mathematically we define this process as follows. Let a partitioning $\mathbb{C}$ split all Q attributes into K non-overlapping clusters, i.e., $\mathbb{C} = \{\mathbf{c}_1, \cdots, \mathbf{c}_K\}$, where $\mathbf{c}_k \subseteq \mathbb{A}$, $\cup_{k=1}^K \mathbf{c}_i = \mathbb{A}$, and $\mathbf{c}_{k_1} \cap \mathbf{c}_{k_2} = \emptyset$, $\forall 1 \leq k_1 \neq k_2 \leq K$. The objective of jointly learning K classifiers $\mathbb{G} = \{\mathbf{G}^1, \cdots, \mathbf{G}^K\}$ is to minimize the classification error,

$$J(\mathbb{G}, \mathbb{C}) = \sum_{k=1}^K \sum_{n=1}^N \|\mathbf{y}_n^k - \mathbf{G}^k(\mathbf{x}_n)\|^2, \tag{6}$$

where both $\mathbf{G}^k(\mathbf{x}_n)$ and $\mathbf{y}_n^k$ are the estimated and true labels of the attributes in the $\mathbf{c}_k$ cluster. As an extension of Eq. 1, this objective function is difficult to optimize since it depends on both $\mathbb{G}$ and $\mathbb{C}$. Therefore we propose a sub-optimal solution by estimating $\mathbb{C}$ and $\mathbb{G}$ sequentially. Most of the remaining section will present our approach to estimate $\mathbb{C}$ since learning $\mathbf{G}^k$ can be easily done by using the IBR approach in Sect. 3.2 or any other multi-attribute predictor.

The estimation of $\mathbb{C}$ is nontrivial due to the large solution space. The number of partitions for a Q-attribute set is equal to the Qth Bell number [30], which grows exponentially and is computationally unfeasible to enumerate as Q increases. Therefore, we propose a greedy approach similar to agglomerative hierarchical clustering. We start by placing each attribute in its own cluster and then iteratively merge the two clusters that are expected to benefit most from joint learning. The merging process stops when we arrive at a single cluster or more likely when the merging of any two clusters no longer has expected improvement.

Specifically, we denote a an attribute of the cluster $\mathbf{c}$, $p(a)$ the classification accuracy of a when learned independently, and $\widehat{p}(a, \mathbf{c})$ the accuracy when learned jointly as a part of $\mathbf{c}$. The performance margin of an attribute cluster is defined as the average margin of each attribute in the cluster,

$$m(\mathbf{c}) = \frac{1}{|\mathbf{c}|} \sum_{a_i \in \mathbf{c}} (\widehat{p}(a_i, \mathbf{c}) - p(a_i)). \tag{7}$$

Our objective is to find a partitioning $\mathbb{C}$ that maximizes the average performance margins across all clusters,

---

Algorithm 1. Joint attribute learning via attribute clustering.

Data: Attributes $\mathbb{A}$, training samples and labels $\mathbb{D} = \{\mathbf{X}, \mathbf{Y}\}$, validation samples and labels
$\quad\quad \mathbb{D}^v = \{\mathbf{X}^v, \mathbf{Y}^v\}$, a flag $useReg$.
Result: The partitioning $\mathbb{C}$, cluster classifiers $\mathbb{G}$, and thresholds $\mathbb{T}$.
/* Find partitioning   */
1 Initialize clusters $\mathbf{c}_1 = 1, \mathbf{c}_2 = 2, \cdots, \mathbf{c}_K = Q$ and $K = Q$;
2 Initialize margins $m(\mathbf{c}_1) = \cdots = m(\mathbf{c}_K) = 0$;
3 Train Q classifiers from $\mathbb{D}$ and compute $p(a)\ \forall a \in \mathbb{A}$ on $\mathbb{D}^v$;
4 **if** $useReg$ **then**
5 $\quad\lfloor$ Learn $R() : \mathbf{f} \to m(\mathbf{c})$ via $\mathbf{f}$ from $\mathbb{D}, \mathbb{D}^v$ and $m(\mathbf{c})$ from $\mathbb{D}^v$;

6 **repeat**
7 $\quad\mid\quad$ $bestGain = 0$;
8 $\quad\mid\quad$ **foreach** $k_1 = 1, \cdots, K - 1$ **do**
9 $\quad\mid\quad\quad$ **foreach** $k_2 = k_1 + 1, \cdots, K$ **do**
10 $\quad\mid\quad\quad\quad$ **if** $useReg$ **then**
11 $\quad\mid\quad\quad\quad\quad$ Compute $\mathbf{f}$ from $\mathbb{D}, \mathbb{D}^v$;
12 $\quad\mid\quad\quad\quad\quad$ Compute $m(\{\mathbf{c}_{k_1}, \mathbf{c}_{k_2}\})$ via $R(\mathbf{f})$;
13 $\quad\mid\quad\quad\quad$ **else**
14 $\quad\mid\quad\quad\quad\quad$ Train joint classifier on $\mathbb{D}$ via IBR;
15 $\quad\mid\quad\quad\quad\quad$ Evaluate $m(\{\mathbf{c}_{k_1}, \mathbf{c}_{k_2}\})$ on $\mathbb{D}^v$;
16 $\quad\mid\quad\quad\quad$ **if** $s(\mathbf{c}_{k_1}, \mathbf{c}_{k_2}) > bestGain$ **then**
17 $\quad\mid\quad\quad\quad\quad$ $bestGain = s(\mathbf{c}_{k_1}, \mathbf{c}_{k_2})$;
18 $\quad\mid\quad\quad\quad\quad$ $\mathbf{c}^t = \{\mathbf{c}_{k_1}, \mathbf{c}_{k_2}\}$;   ▷ Remember the best cluster

19 $\quad\mid\quad$ **if** $bestGain > 0$ **then**
20 $\quad\mid\quad\quad$ Merge two clusters into one, $\mathbf{c}_{k_1} = \mathbf{c}^t$, $\mathbf{c}_{k_2} = \emptyset$;
21 $\quad\mid\quad\quad$ $K = K - 1$;   ▷ One less total number of clusters

22 **until** $bestGain \leq 0$;
/* Train cluster-specific classifiers   */
23 **foreach** $k = 1, \cdots, K$ **do**
24 $\quad\mid\quad$ Whiten attribute labels from cluster $\mathbf{c}_k$ via Eq. 5;
25 $\quad\mid\quad$ Train regressor $\mathbf{H}^k(\mathbf{x})$ as Eq. 2 via IBR on $\mathbb{D}, \mathbb{D}^v$;
26 $\quad\mid\quad$ $\mathbf{G}^k(\mathbf{x}) = \mu + (\mathbf{V}^\mathsf{T})^{-1}\mathbf{D}^{1/2}\mathbf{H}^k(\mathbf{x})$;
27 $\quad\mid\quad$ Compute decision boundaries τ_q for binary attributes on $\mathbb{D}, \mathbb{D}^v$;
28 **return** $\mathbb{C} = \{\mathbf{c}_1, \cdots, \mathbf{c}_K\}$, $\mathbb{G} = \{\mathbf{G}^1(\mathbf{x}), \cdots, \mathbf{G}^K(\mathbf{x})\}$, $\mathbb{T} = \{\tau_1, \cdots, \tau_Q\}$.

$$\hat{\mathbb{C}} = \underset{\mathbb{C}}{\arg\min}\ J_1(\mathbb{C}) = \frac{1}{K}\sum_{k=1}^{K}(m(\mathbf{c}_k)|\mathbf{c}_k|), \tag{8}$$

where $|\mathbf{c}_k|$ is the cardinality of $\mathbf{c}_k$.

Our greedy approach starts with Q clusters, each with one distinct attribute. In each iteration, we search for a pair of clusters, which have the maximal expected improvement when combining them into one cluster compared to leaving them as two clusters. Hence, the expected improvement is computed by

$$s(\mathbf{c}_{k_1}, \mathbf{c}_{k_2}) = m(\{\mathbf{c}_{k_1}, \mathbf{c}_{k_2}\}) - \frac{|\mathbf{c}_{k_1}|m(\mathbf{c}_{k_1}) + |\mathbf{c}_{k_2}|m(\mathbf{c}_{k_2})}{|\mathbf{c}_{k_1}| + |\mathbf{c}_{k_2}|}. \tag{9}$$

The iteration continues until all $s(\mathbf{c}_{k_1}, \mathbf{c}_{k_2}) < 0$, which means that there is no expected performance improvement by combining any two existing clusters. Algorithm 1 summarizes our clustering and learning algorithm. In theory the complexity of each iteration is $O(K^2)$. However, with memoization of the $s(\mathbf{c}_{k_1}, \mathbf{c}_{k_2})$, each iteration after the first iteration has a complexity of $O(K)$, which becomes fairly efficient to compute.

The only thing remaining to implement Algorithm 1 is in Lines 11–15, i.e., how to estimate the performance margin of an attribute cluster, $m(\mathbf{c})$. We propose two methods for this estimation: a learned regressor based on the properties of the attribute set $\mathbf{c}$, and an empirical estimation based on its performance on a validation set, as detailed below.

Regression. To learn the regressor, we hypothesize that dependencies among attributes may impact the performance margin of joint learning, and these dependencies will be the features for regressor learning. First, the correlation among attributes may help since not all attributes are equally classifiable and the result of the "easier" attribute can benefit the prediction of the "harder" attribute. Thus we define f_0 to be the average of pair-wise correlation coefficients of any two attribute labels $\mathbf{Y}^k$ in the cluster $\mathbf{c}_k$, Second, this line of reasoning also suggests that the performance difference among the independently learned attributes could be indicative, which leads to $f_1 = \mathrm{var}(p(a)), \forall a \in \mathbf{c}$. Third, we note that the independent accuracy $p(a)$ can place restrictions on the joint performance. For example, if an attribute is 99 % accurate independently, it is less likely to be improved via joint learning. Hence we define $f_2 = \mathrm{mean}(p(a)), \forall a \in$ $\mathbf{c}$. Finally the correlation of the top selected features from the independently boosted classifiers also matters. If two attributes share many discriminative features, they will be less likely to help improve each other. But if their top features differ, they may potentially help create a more robust joint classifier. We define f_3 to be a 11-dim histogram of the pair-wise correlation coefficients of the top five selected features from each independently learned attribute's classifier. The collection of features $\mathbf{f} = [f_0, f_1, f_2, \mathbf{f}_3^{\intercal}]^{\intercal}$ becomes the input variable for the regressor $R(\mathbf{f})$, whose output variable is the expected performance margin $m(\mathbf{c}_k)$. Specifically we train a simple linear regressor by using $\mathbf{f}$ computed on $\mathbb{D}$, $\mathbb{D}^v$ and $m(\mathbf{c}_k)$ computed on $\mathbb{D}^v$, based on a small set of random clusters $\mathbf{c}$.

Validation. For the empirical estimation, we evaluate $p(a)$ and $\widehat{p}(a, \mathbf{c})$ on a separate validation set $\mathbb{D}^v$ for every attribute in the cluster, and then compute $m(\mathbf{c})$ directly. This scheme has a computational burden as it has to train a joint classifier each time it examines a potential cluster merge, but it will give us an accurate estimate of the performance margin. Using $R(\mathbf{f})$ to estimate the performance margin requires an upfront computational investment to train the regressor, but after it is trained, it efficiently examines potential merges. Ultimately, we seek to find an accurate prediction $R(\mathbf{f})$ of the margin through the regressor, which is one of the future research directions.

4   Experiments

Our experimental goal is to determine *whether* joint learning improves upon independent learning and *how* it works by exploring the aspects of the regressor that best predict the performance improvement for a set of attributes. We do present the results as reported by [9] solely for reference to show how our baseline

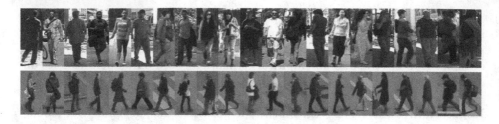

Fig. 4. Sample images from the VIPeR (top) and PRID (bottom) dataset of the 21 attributes used for person re-identification.

Table 1. 21 Mid-level attributes.

redshirt	blueshirt	lightshirt	darkshirt	greenshirt
nocoats	notlightdarkjeanscolour	darkbottoms	lightbottoms	
hassatchel	barelegs	shorts	jeans	male
skirt	patterned	midhair	darkhair	
bald	hashandbagcarrierbag	hasbackpack		

(independent learning) performance compares to the state of the art, but the most important question is if the joint learning technique can improve upon the independent formulation.

4.1 Experimental Setup

Datasets. We conduct experiments on the classic person re-identification datasets, VIPeR [14] and PRID [15], which contain 632 and 200 subjects respectively with a pair of images taken from different cameras (Cam A and Cam B) with arbitrary poses. The images are cropped and scaled to 128×48 pixels in size for VIPeR and 128×64 for PRID. Layne *et al.* [9] provided 21 manually labeled attributes for each image. Sample images from the databases are shown in Fig. 4 and the list of attributes is in Table 1.

Feature Representation. We extract the same low-level visual features as [5,9]. Images are split into 6 equal sized horizontal sections. For each section we compute 8 color channels and responses from 19 texture channels of Gabor and Schmid filters. Each channel is quantized by a 16-bin histogram. A total of 2592 low-level features **x** are extracted from each image, i.e., $D = 2592$.

Experimental Setup. Figure 5 displays the two different setups for our experiments. Setup 1 is intra-dataset and examines attribute classification within a single dataset. We elect to only examine VIPeR since it contains sufficient images to make decisions for the attributes, whereas PRID has multiple attributes with only a few positive examples. VIPeR also covers a wider range of camera viewpoints. This setup splits the subjects in five folds and we repeat the experiment

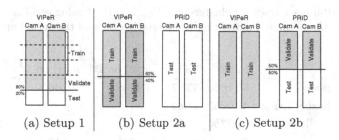

Fig. 5. Experimental setups. Shaded region is the data used to train final $\mathbb{G}$ used for classification. Vertical is across the subject space for each camera.

Table 2. Comparison of independent and joint learning techniques.

	Indep	Full	Reg	Valid
Setup 1: $Q = 16$	74.75 %	74.28 %	75.18 %	**75.31 %**
Setup 2a: $Q = 15$	65.63 %	64.98 %	67.83 %	**67.87 %**
Setup 2b: $Q = 15$	68.60 %	68.20 %	**70.43 %**	69.17 %

using one fold for testing each time. The validation set is used to learn the regressor and to predict the cluster margins for classification purposes. Setup 2 is inter-dataset and examines the ability to transfer attribute classifiers. This setup has two variations. Setup 2a uses completely different datasets for training and testing. Setup 2b uses half of PRID as the validation set to help training.

Evaluation Metrics. For attribute classification, we report *accuracy*, which is the number of correctly classified samples over the total number of samples. When evaluating person re-identification, we report the *expected rank*, which is the mean rank of genuine matches and provides an estimate of how many images a manual operator will have to examine to find the genuine match. We also report performance at rank n for re-identification, which is the probability that the genuine match appears within the top n matching results.

4.2 Attribute Classification

We evaluate joint attribute learning and report the accuracies for four different techniques in Table 2. (1) *Independent*, where each attribute is learned by a separate classifier, i.e., $K = Q$. (2) *Fully joint*, where all attributes are jointly learned in *one* cluster, i.e., $K = 1$. (3) *Regressor clustering*, where we use the regressor $R(\mathbf{f})$ to form the clustering. (4) *Validation clustering*, where the validation set is used for clustering.

Our hypothesis is that adaptively combining the attributes for joint learning will increase the performance of attribute classification. We evaluate using Setup 1 with the same 16 attributes as used by [9] where the remaining five attributes are not used due to extreme imbalanced samples. Our independent

Table 3. Attribute accuracy for clustering in Fig. 6 on the testing set. For each cluster, we also report the predicted margin on the validation set and the actual margin on the test set $\mathbb{D}^t$.

	Indep	Valid	$m(\mathbf{c})$ on $\mathbb{D}^v$	$m(\mathbf{c})$ on $\mathbb{D}^t$
male	55.16 %	53.97 %	4.41 %	−0.66 %
hasbackpack	48.02 %	47.62 %		
midhair	66.27 %	65.87 %		
lightshirt	76.98 %	80.95 %	2.17 %	2.18 %
greenshirt	83.73 %	84.13 %		
darkbottoms	76.98 %	75.00 %	1.88 %	0.79 %
lightbottoms	62.30 %	65.87 %		
redshirt	93.65 %	93.65 %	1.68 %	−1.38 %
blueshirt	86.51 %	83.73 %		
nocoats	67.86 %	73.41 %	1.04 %	2.68 %
darkhair	67.46 %	67.86 %		
notjeanscolor	80.16 %	82.54 %		
shorts	76.19 %	78.57 %		
darkshirt	85.71 %		—	
barelegs	75.00 %		—	
jeans	75.40 %		—	

result, 74.75 % is better than the 66.9 % as reported in [9]. For Setup 2, we can only use 15 attributes because the other six attributes of PRID have very few samples. We make a few comments based on the results reported in Table 2. First, fully joint learning has a negative impact on the classifier accuracy. Note that this observation is different to the very recent work [25] where fully joint learning has shown improvement. Part of the reason is that the chosen datasets have little overall correlation among attributes making joint learning difficult. We also note that conceptually [25] is a special case of our algorithm, because it is possible that all attributes are clustered into *one* cluster by our algorithm as long as the expected improvement s is positive. Second, both proposed clustering techniques improve over independent classifiers for all experiments. In Setup 1 we report the average accuracies from using each one of the five folds as the test set. Even though the relative improvement from the "Indep." to "Valid." is small, the p-value from one-tailed paired t-test is less than 0.05, which demonstrates this is a *statistically significant* performance increase.

We also examine a reduced subset of only five attributes in order to compare our greedy clustering with the global optimal clustering, which is obtained through brute force all possible attribute partitions. In this example, clustering with validation achieves 78.4 % accuracy barely below the global optimal clustering at 78.5 %.

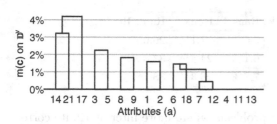
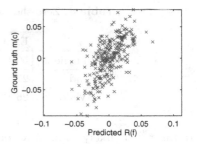

Fig. 6. Clustering of attributes as defined by the validation set and their expected margin for each cluster. Attributes 4, 11, and 13 are determined to be individual clusters by our algorithm.

Fig. 7. Predicted margin from clustering regressor versus ground truth margin. The Pearson correlation coefficient is 0.66.

4.3 Regression Versus Validation Based Clustering

We propose two means of estimating the performance margin of a cluster in the agglomerative clustering scheme, regression and validation. In Fig. 6 and Table 3, we show the chosen clusters as well as the per attribute accuracy improvement using the clustering with the validation set for one fold of the Setup 1 experiment. It can be observed that some of the clustering results are consistent with human intuition. For instance, darkbottoms and lightbottoms are negatively correlated and hence clustered together. Also, the inconsistency between the $m(c)$ on $\mathbb{D}^v$ and on $\mathbb{D}^l$ indicates the insufficient validation samples, and hence a more representative validation set will help us improve performances in the future.

Using a validation set to find the clusters can take several hours for $Q = 16$. We train $R(\mathbf{f})$ using less time than the validation approach, and once trained it takes a few minutes to cluster $\mathbb{A}$. In our experiments, we only train $R(\mathbf{f})$ on Setup 1 and use the same regressor for Setup 2a and 2b.

As discussed in Sect. 3.3, we define a regressor using dependencies between attributes to predict the performance margin of a cluster. We train the regressor with Setup 1, where we learn joint classifiers for all pairs of attributes and a random selection of sets of three attributes. The ground truth performance margins are computed on the validation set. Figure 7 displays the ability of the regressor to predict the actual margin. Of the four types of attribute dependencies modeled, the descending order of importance as defined by weights of the regressor $R(\mathbf{f})$ is feature correlation ($\mathbf{f}_3$), variance of independent classifier performance (f_1), mean independent classifier performance (f_2), and the attribute correlation (f_0). It might be counter-intuitive that attribute correlation would have the least impact on joint learning, but this is mainly an anomaly caused by the attributes having little correlation by design. There are too few attribute pairs with high correlation to impact the regressor. For example, the average inter-attribute correlation is only 0.07 in VIPeR. This low correlation makes joint attribute learning a very challenging problem, so if we can improve on this

Table 4. Zero-shot identification performance on VIPeR.

	ExpRank	Rank 1	Rank 5	Rank 10
Layne [9]	50.1	6.0%	17.1%	26.0%
Ind	27.11	6.1%	24.8%	37.8%
Valid	26.13	7.7%	26.3%	38.1%

dataset, it is likely to improve other problems where more inter-attribute correlation exists. Using a regressor to predict the performance margin demonstrates promise, but further exploration to improve the regressor prediction accuracy is still necessary.

4.4 Zero-Shot Identification

Improving attribute classification is good, but does joint learning also improve the applications of the attributes? We examine the zero-shot identification scenario [9], where only attribute descriptions of an eyewitness are available. Following the same experimental setup as [9], we use the provided human labels for the subjects $\mathbf{y}$ as the probe and use the raw regression output $\mathbf{G}(\mathbf{x})$ for VIPeR Cam B (Setup 1 test set) as the gallery. The distance metric is computed as the weighted sum of errors between $\mathbf{y}$ and $\mathbf{G}(\mathbf{x})$, i.e., $\tilde{s} = \sum_{k=1}^{K} e^{\widehat{p}(\cdot, \mathbf{c}_k)} \cdot |\mathbf{y}^k - \mathbf{G}^k(\mathbf{x})|$.

Table 4 reports the results averaged across all five folds for independent and the proposed clustering scheme with the validation set. Joint learning of the attributes improves both the expected rank (smaller is better) and the rank n accuracy (lager is better) at low ranks. To calibrate the zero-shot identification performance of our independently learned attributes, we show the performance of [9] as reported in the paper.

5   Conclusions

We have shown that joint learning of attributes can increase the average attribute classification performance. Our main contribution is the clustering scheme that identifies which sets of attributes should be jointly learned for maximum performance increase. For joint learning, we used IBR, but any multi-output classification algorithm can be substituted. We demonstrated the effectiveness of this joint attribute learning approach on the task of person re-identification and improved zero-shot identification performance.

A common characteristic of exploratory paper is to raise interesting questions and present opportunities for further work. This exploratory work is no exception. How will this translate to other multi-attribute problems such as the face attributes [19,31]? What other dependencies impact joint learning and can we leverage to improve the clustering prediction? Would accurate body alignment [32] have a positive impact on joint learning? Would we see a larger performance gain from joint learning if there is more inherent correlation among the user-defined attributes, especially on a larger dataset such as [33]? On the contrary, it is interesting to note that even a lack of correlation has the potential to improve joint classifier performance because that knowledge may lead to a selection of different low-level features to predict each attribute. Finally and most importantly, because our approach is independent to the definitions or types of attributes, we believe it is widely applicable to many attribute-based visual recognition problems, which warrants future research on this topic.

References

1. Cai, Q., Aggarwal, J.K.: Tracking human motion using multiple cameras. In: ICPR, pp. 68–72 (1996)
2. Liu, X., Tu, P., Rittscher, J., Perera, A., Krahnstoever, N.: Detecting and counting people in surveillance applications. In: AVSS (2005)
3. Tu, P.H., Doretto, G., Krahnstoever, N.O., Perera, A.G.A., Wheeler, F.W., Liu, X., Rittscher, J., Sebastian, T.B., Yu, T., Harding, K.G.: An intelligent video framework for homeland protection. In: Proceedings of SPIE Defense & Security Symposium, Conference on Unattended Ground, Sea, and Air Sensor Technologies and Applications IX, Orlando, Florida (2007)
4. Gheissari, N., Sebastian, T.B., Hartley, R.: Person reidentification using spatiotemporal appearance. In: CVPR, pp. 1528–1535 (2006)
5. Gray, D., Tao, H.: Viewpoint invariant pedestrian recognition with an ensemble of localized features. In: Forsyth, D., Torr, P., Zisserman, A. (eds.) ECCV 2008, Part I. LNCS, vol. 5302, pp. 262–275. Springer, Heidelberg (2008)
6. Madden, C., Cheng, E.D., Piccardi, M.: Tracking people across disjoint camera views by an illumination-tolerant appearance representation. Mach. Vis. Appl. 18, 233–247 (2007)
7. Prosser, B., Zheng, W.S., Gong, S., Xiang, T.: Person re-identification by support vector ranking. BMVC 21(1–21), 11 (2010)
8. Yang, Y., Yang, J., Yan, J., Liao, S., Yi, D., Li, S.Z.: Salient color names for person re-identification. In: Fleet, D., Pajdla, T., Schiele, B., Tuytelaars, T. (eds.) ECCV 2014, Part I. LNCS, vol. 8689, pp. 536–551. Springer, Heidelberg (2014)
9. Layne, R., Hospedales, T.M., Gong, S.: Attributes-based re-identification. In: Gong, S., Cristani, M., Yan, S., Loy, C.C. (eds.) Person Re-identification. Advances in Computer Vision and Pattern Recognition, pp. 93–117. Springer, Heidelberg (2014)
10. Thornton, J., Baran-Gale, J., Butler, D., Chan, M., Zwahlen, H.: Person attribute search for large-area video surveillance. In: HST, pp. 55–61 (2011)
11. Tome, P., Fierrez, J., Vera-Rodriguez, R., Nixon, M.S.: Soft biometrics and their application in person recognition at a distance. IEEE Trans. Inf. Forensics Secur. 9, 464–475 (2014)
12. Kang, Z., Grauman, K., Sha, F.: Learning with whom to share in multi-task feature learning. In: ICML, pp. 521–528 (2011)
13. Jayaraman, D., Sha, F., Grauman, K.: Decorrelating semantic visual attributes by resisting the urge to share. In: CVPR (2014)
14. Gray, D., Brennan, S., Tao, H.: Evaluating appearance models for recognition, reacquisition, and tracking. In: IEEE International Workshop on Performance Evaluation Tracking and Surveillance (2007)

15. Hirzer, M., Beleznai, C., Roth, P.M., Bischof, H.: Person re-identification by descriptive and discriminative classification. In: Heyden, A., Kahl, F. (eds.) SCIA 2011. LNCS, vol. 6688, pp. 91–102. Springer, Heidelberg (2011)
16. Farhadi, A., Endres, I., Hoiem, D., Forsyth, D.: Describing objects by their attributes. In: CVPR. (2009) 1778–1785
17. Dhar, S., Ordonez, V., Berg, T.L.: High level describable attributes for predicting aesthetics and interestingness. In: CVPR, pp. 1657–1664 (2011)
18. Parikh, D., Grauman, K.: Relative attributes. In: ICCV, pp. 503–510 (2011)
19. Kumar, N., Berg, A.C., Belhumeur, P.N., Nayar, S.K.: Attribute and simile classifiers for face verification. In: ICCV (2009)
20. Park, U., Jain, A.K.: Face matching and retrieval using soft biometrics. IEEE Trans. Inf. Forensics Secur. 5, 406–415 (2010)
21. Shalev-Shwartz, S., Wexler, Y., Shashua, A.: Shareboost: efficient multiclass learning with feature sharing. In: NIPS, pp. 1179–1187 (2011)
22. Torralba, A.B., Murphy, K.P., Freeman, W.T.: Sharing visual features for multiclass and multiview object detection. IEEE T-PAMI 29, 854–869 (2007)
23. Tuia, D., Verrelst, J., Alonso, L., Pérez-Cruz, F., Camps-Valls, G.: Multioutput support vector regression for remote sensing biophysical parameter estimation. IEEE J. Geosci. Remote Sens. Lett. 8, 804–808 (2011)
24. Zhou, S.K., Georgescu, B., Zhou, X.S., Comaniciu, D.: Image based regression using boosting method. ICCV 1, 541–548 (2005)
25. Liu, M., Zhang, D., Chen, S.: Attribute relation learning for zero-shot classification. Neurocomputing 139, 34–46 (2014)
26. Wang, Y., Mori, G.: A discriminative latent model of object classes and attributes. In: Daniilidis, K., Maragos, P., Paragios, N. (eds.) ECCV 2010, Part V. LNCS, vol. 6315, pp. 155–168. Springer, Heidelberg (2010)
27. Hwang, S.J., Sha, F., Grauman, K.: Sharing features between objects and their attributes. In: CVPR, pp. 1761–1768 (2011)
28. Wang, X., Ji, Q.: A unified probabilistic approach modeling relationships between attributes and objects. In: ICCV, pp. 2120–2127 (2013)
29. Chen, J., Liu, X., Lyu, S.: Boosting with side information. In: Lee, K.M., Matsushita, Y., Rehg, J.M., Hu, Z. (eds.) ACCV 2012, Part I. LNCS, vol. 7724, pp. 563–577. Springer, Heidelberg (2013)
30. Bell, E.T.: Exponential polynomials. Ann. Math. 35, 258–277 (1934)
31. Klare, B.F., Klum, S., Klontz, J., Taborsky, E., Akgul, T., Jain, A.K.: Suspect identification based on descriptive facial attributes. In: ICJB (2014)
32. Liu, X., Yu, T., Sebastian, T., Tu, P.: Boosted deformable model for human body alignment. In: CVPR, pp. 1–8 (2008)
33. Liao, S., Mo, Z., Hu, Y., Li, S.Z.: Open-set person re-identification (2014). arXiv:1408.0872v1 [cs.CV]

Complementary Geometric and Optical Information for Match-Propagation-Based 3D Reconstruction

Patricio A. Galindo[(✉)] and Rhaleb Zayer

INRIA Nancy, Villers-lès-Nancy, France
patricio.galindo@inria.fr

Abstract. In this work, we consider the problem of propagation-based matching for 3D reconstruction, which deals with expanding a limited set of correspondences towards a quasi-dense map across two views. In general, propagation based methods capture well the scene structure. However, the recovered geometry often presents an overall choppy nature which can be attributed to matching errors and abrupt variations in the estimated local affine transformations. We propose to control the reconstructed geometry by means of a local patch fitting which corrects both the matching locations and affine transformations throughout the propagation process. In this way, matchings that propagate from geometrically consolidated locations bring coherence to both positions and affine transformations. Results of our approach are not only more visually appealing but also more accurate and complete as substantiated by results on standard benchmarks.

1 Introduction

This paper revisits the problem of match propagation across a pair of views in the context of quasi-dense matching [1], and its extension to wide-baseline views which accounts for affine distortion [2]. We focus on these approaches due to their inherent simplicity and minimal requirements, however the proposed solutions can be applied to other propagation approaches. Alternative approaches such as [3,4] which require image rectification and further problem reformulations will not be addressed here.

Propagation-based matching is the workhorse of many surface reconstruction approaches e.g. [5–8]. In practice, it comes in different flavors, e.g. [1,9,10], but they all require corrective steps and/or postprocessing techniques to filter out mismatches. Furthermore, the resulting geometry exhibits a choppy nature which is often not addressed directly and is left to mesh reconstruction algorithms, e.g. [11]. Figures 1 and 2 show typical chaps and clefts observed when performing scene reconstruction using a state of the art propagation approach, in this case [2]. We are aware that the use of additional images can help reduce such effects relatively, e.g. [7,12], however, addressing the challenges of the fundamental problem on a pair of images remains necessary to take full advantage of the available data and can also be beneficial when additional views are accessible.

© Springer International Publishing Switzerland 2015
D. Cremers et al. (Eds.): ACCV 2014, Part I, LNCS 9003, pp. 689–703, 2015.
DOI: 10.1007/978-3-319-16865-4_45

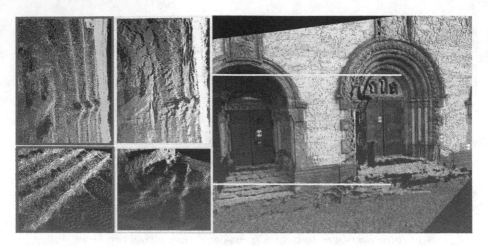

Fig. 1. Reconstruction from views 3–4 of the Herz-Jesu P8 dataset using [2] (right). Geometric artifacts are clearly visible in the closeups (middle). Whereas, the geometry of the scene is better captured with our approach (left).

In this paper, we argue that such problems can be resolved during the propagation process by including geometric cues which help consolidate the geometric reconstruction and the estimation of the local affine transformations, thus avoiding tedious post processing operations in the first place. The use of geometric information in propagation based methods is not new, for instance [13], proposes a splatting inspired approach based on local plane fitting. However, this approach is limited to narrow baselines and requires a relatively large number of images. Our approach, on the other hand, proceeds by fitting small surface patches on which initial 3D points are projected to adjust the matches and the local affine transformations. By operating in such way, the propagated information is confirmed by both optical and geometrical cues throughout the whole matching process.

In Sect. 2, we outline the propagation algorithm using only optical information and in Sect. 3, we proceed to outline and detail our approach. In Sect. 4, results are shown and discussed.

2   Background

To keep this exposition succinct and self contained, we briefly summarize the key ideas in quasi-dense propagation and we adopt the formalisms of [1,2]. The reader is referred to those papers and the references therein for a detailed description. Match propagation aims to obtain a larger number of matches between two views (I, I') starting from an initial set of matches (seeds) $S = \{s(\mathbf{x}, \mathbf{x}'), \mathbf{x} \in \mathbf{I}, \mathbf{x}' \in \mathbf{I}'\}$. When dealing with wide-baseline views, it is preferable to have the fundamental matrix between the views as well as the local affine transforms A associated with the individual seeds [2]. The affine transforms can

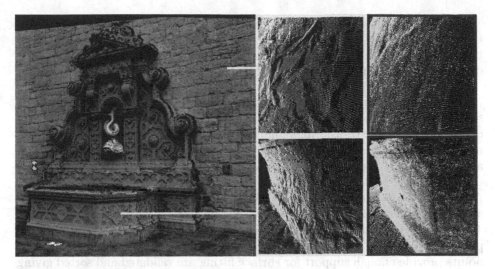

Fig. 2. Reconstruction from views 2–3 of the Fountain P11 dataset using [2] (left). Geometric artifacts are clearly visible in the closeups (middle). Whereas, the geometry of the scene is better captured with our approach (right).

be obtained using existing affine covariant region detectors [14]. In order to reduce geometric distortions, the reference view for each seed is defined so as the affine transformation across the image pair is always magnifying. Similarity is measured using the zero-mean normalized cross-correlation (ZNCC) of geometrically normalized image patches. Once the initialization data is set, the match propagation operates on a priority queue based on correlation scores of the seeds and proceeds by repeating the following steps:

- remove the seed s with best score from queue
- search new candidates in a neighborhood of s based on local affine transform
- compute correlation scores for all candidates
- append candidates to the matches and seeds if they have high correlation score, satisfy the epipolar constraint and are not yet filled
- update candidate's affine transform based on optical information
- mark the corresponding pixels as filled.

3   Geometry Based Image Match Propagation

3.1   Overview

The central idea of our approach is to couple geometric and optical information in a complementary fashion, in the sense that they correct and confirm each other. In this regard, when a sufficient number of data points are available in a localized region, a surface fitting can be performed and subsequently the matches and their affine transformation will be updated geometrically.

In practice, three main recurrent stages take place in our method: propagation, region search, and update by surface fitting. In the next paragraphs we briefly describe these stages and we later explain them in greater algorithmic detail in the next sub-sections.

(i) Propagation: In a propagation step the best seed (s) from the queue is selected and new candidates within a neighborhood of s are obtained using its corresponding affine transform. Candidates with correlation scores which pass a minimum threshold and comply with map occupancy and epipolar constraints are added to the queue (see Fig. 3) and are marked as unconfirmed matches.

(ii) Best candidate region querying: When new matches are found in the propagation step, the search for a suitable region for local surface fitting is initiated. This search is performed by sliding corresponding windows in the two image planes (depicted by the windows in Fig. 5). Candidate regions where the data points provide enough support for surface fitting are validated and sorted giving preference to the ones with the most confirmed points.

(iii) Local fitting and re-projection: When a suitable region is found in the previous step a local surface patch fitting is performed. A sub-set of the points representing the core of the region (see Fig. 5), are then projected onto the local surface patch. These new positions are re-projected to the image planes to update the correspondences.

Points that re-project too far in the image planes or yield a large change in their affine transformation remain marked as unconfirmed. Matches which improve their correlation scores are updated and marked as confirmed. This update serves the purpose of correcting point locations as well as steering subsequent propagation (see Fig. 4).

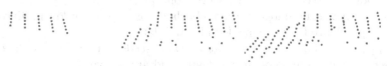

(a) Propagation step n   (b) Propagation step n+1   (c) Propagation step n+2

Fig. 3. Illustration of a few propagation steps before performing any geometric updates.

3.2   Propagation

In principle, the propagation stage proceeds similarly to the wide baseline matching proposed in [2] but presents three important differences. **First**, newly propagated matches are not defined as final matches; instead, they are stored as unconfirmed matches. **Second**, the seeds sorting operation gives preference to geometrically confirmed seeds and checks for correlation score in a secondary sorting step. **Third**, new matches stemming from a geometrically confirmed seed

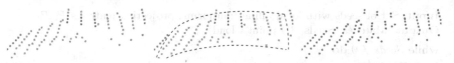

(a) Candidate region se- (b) Local surface fitting (c) New propagation re-
lected   places initial points

Fig. 4. Illustration of the geometric fitting steps. First, the candidate region is selected
(a), the support and the core are colored in green and blue respectively. Second,
local surface fitting is performed (b). Third, the core points are projected onto the
surface (c) (Color figure online).

can replace previous unconfirmed matches if their correlation score is higher.
Note that this second set of conditions do not come into play from the beginning since it takes several propagation steps to obtain a set of geometrically
confirmed matches. This categorization of points is depicted in Fig. 5 where blue
indicates confirmed points and red indicates unconfirmed (replaceable) ones. In
order to fix the ideas, we describe the steps of our propagation stage in Algorithms 1 and 2. Note that the 3D positions originating from each pair of matches
are obtained at this stage since they are needed for the later region search and
surface fitting.

3.3 Candidate Region Querying

The goal at this stage is to identify regions with adequate point distribution
and density to support a local patch fitting. The region querying is initiated
once a set of new unconfirmed points are obtained. In order to steer clear from
problematic regions during this search we avoid: (i) areas which present large
jumps, (ii) points which do not remain within their respective patch perimeter
when projected on the corresponding images planes. These requirements help
prevent fitting and consequentially smoothing sharp features, e.g. the stairs in
Fig. 9. On the other hand, we favor regions that present the most confirmed
points so that the large bodies of confirmed points expand first instead of creating
several isolated clusters of confirmed points. A typical scenario is shown in Fig. 5
where a set of confirmed matches (in blue) is surrounded by a set of unconfirmed
points (in red). The green windows represent the support region (outer square)
and the core window (inner square). Only unconfirmed points inside the core
window will be fit in the next stage. In the same figure, the points inside the
orange region represent newly matched points that enable a surface to be fit at
the depicted location.

The conditions that define wether surface fitting can be performed are:

- points inside the support and core regions defined on the first image should
  also lay inside the corresponding support and core regions defined on the
  second image

Input: Set of seeds with local affine transforms, projection matrices P_1, P_2
Output: Matches, Seeds, 3D point Cloud

while *Seeds* $\neq \emptyset$ **do**
    Sort(Seeds);
    foreach *seed* (x, x') **do**
        Local $= \emptyset$;
        `/* Local stores new candidates`   `*/`
        foreach (u, u') *in* $N(x, x')$ **do**
            if *SampsonDistance*$(u, u') < sd$ *and* $((map_1(u)$ *and* $map_2(u')$ *are*
            not filled) or (s is confirmed and correspondence occupying $map_1(u)$
            and $map_2(u')$ *is not))* **then**
                Compute $z = ZNCC(u, u')$ and standard deviations d, d';
                if $z > min\_correlation$ *and* $d > t$ *and* $d' > t$ **then**
                    store (u, u', z) in Local;
                end
            end
        end
        sort(Local);
        foreach $L(u, u')$ *in Local* **do**
            if $map_1(u)$ *and* $map_2(u')$ *are not taken* **then**
                $X \leftarrow Compute3D(u_1, u_2, P_1, P_2)$;
                $A_O \leftarrow$ UpdateAffineEstimationOptical(u, u');
                mark $map_1(u)$ and $map_2(u')$ as taken by an unconfirmed point;
                store (u, u', A_O) in Seeds;
                store (u, u', A_O) in Matches;
                store (X) in Cloud;
            end
        end
        while $R \leftarrow BestCandidateRegionQuerying(map_1, map_2, Cloud, Matches)$
        exists **do**
            FitSurfacePatch($R, Cloud, Seeds, Matches$);
        end
    end
end

Algorithm 1. Main match propagation. Parameter values used in all our experiments: $min\_correlation = 0.75$, $t = 2$, $sd = 1$. The FitSurfacePatch is summarized in Algorithm 2. The SampsonDistance is defined as in [15] and the Sort function follows the conditions set in Sect. 3.1

- there should be at least one point in the core that was not yet confirmed
- regions inside the support window but to the north, south, east and west of the core window should be sufficiently populated (at least 50 %)
- points inside the core window should be dense enough, any 2×2 window should contain at least one match (pixels).

The sizes of the windows in all of our experiments are 15×15 for the support and 5×5 for the core. These windows are defined in the view that presents the

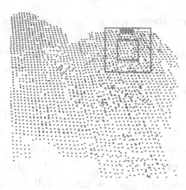

Fig. 5. Searching for best region to fit a surface patch. Confirmed points are depicted in blue, unconfirmed ones in red. Points in the orange region were obtained in the preceding propagation step. In green, support (outer) and core (inner) windows (Color figure online).

most fronto-parallel surface with respect to the image plane and are transformed to the other view using the affine transformation estimation of the point at the center of the window.

3.4 Fit Surface and Update

In this stage, we perform a surface fitting to the selected points inside a region obtained in the previous stage. For this purpose we use a least squares quadratic polynomial fitting of the form $ax^2 + by^2 + cxy + dx + ey + f$ [16]. Although it is possible to perform higher order fitting, we found in our experiments that quadratic fitting is fairly satisfactory for our purpose. The selected points used in this fitting stage are either part of the core region or of the support region. The core region encompasses a small set of points that are surrounded by a set of support points; this is because points should be fit and projected only when there is enough information to describe the local surface.

During the fitting process, the impact of each point in the least squares formulation can be controlled through a set of weights [16]. We formulate the weights as the product of three values: the correlation score of the corresponding matching points, the inverse 3D distance of the reconstructed point to the center of the region, and the nature of the point (confirmed or unconfirmed). More specifically, $w = z^3 \times (1 + is\_confirmed)/distance(X, X_c)$, where z is elevated to the third power in order to stretch the range. Once the surface is fit, each 3d point p is projected to a point p' that lies on the fitted surface.

Each newly obtained point p' can then be reprojected to the image planes I and I', obtaining the respective matching image positions u_r and u'_r. Furthermore, an estimation of the associated affine transformation is recovered. This affine transformation estimation (A_G) is obtained by sampling two additional points around p', projecting them to the image planes and computing the affine transformation that describes their local motion using the re-projection of p' as center of coordinates. Once these new estimations are obtained, we first require that the new 2D matching points induce only a small adjustment of the initial matching positions. Namely, $distance(u_r, u) < \gamma$ and $distance(u, u'_r) < \gamma$ (with $\gamma = 1.5$ pixels used in all our experiments). In this manner we ensure that points near surface edges do not drift away from their original location. Next, we verify if A_G does not represent a large change in transformation estimation with respect to the current estimation A. At the same time we need to verify that A_G does not yield a large shear. Specifically, we verify if $\theta \leq det(A)/det(A_G) \leq 1/\theta$, with $\theta = 0.5$ for all of our cases. We then define the eigen-values rations $eigratio_g = \frac{eig_1(A_G)}{eig_2(A_G)}$ and $eigratio = \frac{eig_1(A)}{eig_2(A)}$ and verify if $\theta \leq eigratio_g \leq 1/\theta$ and if $\theta \leq eigratio_g/eigratio1/ \leq \theta$. A point will remain as unconfirmed is it does not fulfill all of these requirements. Note that the common use of θ for all the previous tests is not required. Independent values can be used for the three verifications but in all of our experiments the same value was used.

The steps described above are summarized in Algorithm 2.

Input: region R, list of Matches, point Cloud, list of Seeds
Output: Updated: Cloud, Matches and Seeds
$w \leftarrow (z^3 \times 1/distance(X, X_c) \times (1 + is\_confirmed))$;
perform least squares surface fitting to obtain surface Q;
foreach *3D point p inside the core of region R* **do**
    obtain p' by projecting p to surface Q;
    if $distance(p', p) < \epsilon$ **then**
        $p'_1 \leftarrow$ re-project p' to I;
        $p'_2 \leftarrow$ re-project p' to I';
        $A_G \leftarrow$ compute affine transformation using Q and p';
        if A_G *does not represent a large change from A and does not represent too much distortion* **then**
            Obtain normalized windows using A_G;
            $z\_new \leftarrow ZNCC(p'_1, p'_2)$;
            if $z\_new > z\_old$ **then**
                $UpdateCloud(p')$;
                $UpdateMatches(p'_1, p'_2, A_G)$;
                $UpdateSeeds(p'_1, p'_2, A_G)$;
                mark $map_1(p'_1)$ and $map_2(p'_2)$ as taken by a confirmed point;
            end
        end
    end
end

Algorithm 2. *FitSurfacePatch* algorithm that performs matching correction by surface fitting and re-projection

4 Results

We tested our algorithm on various data sets comprising standard benchmarks as well as in-house acquired data. Typical results of our approach compared to those of Kannala and Brandt [2], Brox and Malik [17] and Tola et al. [18] are shown for the views 2–3 of the Fountain-P11 dataset (Figs. 6 and 7), and for the views 3–4 of the Herz-Jesu-P8 dataset (Figs. 8 and 9). Both datasets are provided in [19]. We benchmarked our results measuring depth estimation error with respect to the ground truth, in a similar way as in [12]. The benchmarked results are presented in Figs. 6 and 8 as error vs occupancy histogram graphs and as color coded depth estimation errors. We use the code provided by the authors of [2] to perform comparisons and we used similar values for the common parameters of the algorithms. We also use the code provided by the author of the variational matching method [17]. For the case of [18], we use the code provided by the author to compute the DAISY dense descriptor in combination with our own implementation of a descriptor matching method that searches for matches within rectified images. Since such approach does not accurately represents what is proposed in [18], we also compare our results to those presented in the later paper, following their own evaluation metrics (see Fig. 12). Notice that in both quantitative evaluations our method achieves better results.

In all cases our approach performs better than the state of the art pairwise propagation approach [2] and the other methods here tested. The depth error benchmarks presented in Figs. 6 and 8 clearly show that our method presents more accurate and more complete results.

In Fig. 6(top-right) it can be observed that our method attains 74.2 % of the viewed Fountain scene with an error of less than 0.1; while the method of Kannala and Brandt achieves only 68.3 %. In the same error vs occupancy graph we oppose our results to the combination of [2] with an MLS [16] in post-processing. This combination leads only to a small improvement for errors in the lower range but an overall decay in the quality of the results is observed.

In Fig. 8(top-right) our method's score for errors lower than 0.1 in the viewed Herz-Jesu scene is 63.6 %. The method of [2] as well as its combination with MLS post-processing yield only 58.4 % and 50.9 % of occupancy respectively.

The closeups to the fountain result presented in Fig. 7 illustrate the improvements gained by using our method. Our results do not exhibit the choppy characteristic of previous work and present a clearer and more accurate structure of the scene. The closeups to the Herz-Jesu result presented in Fig. 9 not only show that the quality is improved but also the total coverage. In this example the main stairs in the scene are accurately reconstructed thanks to the continuous interpretation and improvement of the matching results that lead to better propagations.

We also performed a comparison using two views of our own face dataset that comprises 1.3 mega-pixels images and two views (7 and 15) of the warrior dataset from [20]. Results are presented in Figs. 10 and 11 were uncolored closeups are presented next to the full views of the results. In both cases the results are significantly better when our approach is used.

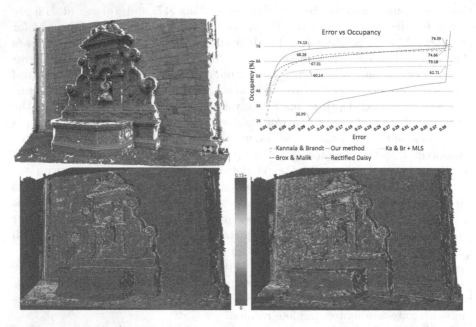

Fig. 6. Results of our approach on the Fountain P11 views 2–3 (top-left). On the top-right, a chart illustrating the depth error vs occupancy of our algorithm, [2,17,18] (rectified) and [2] with MLS as post-processing. On the bottom color coded depth error using our algorithm (left) and using [2] (right) (Color figure online).

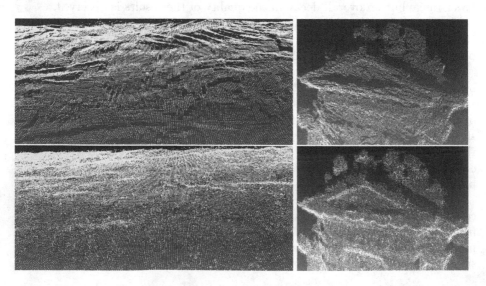

Fig. 7. Closeups on portions of the wall and fountain-top for the Fountain P11 views 2–3 using [2] (top) and using our method (bottom)

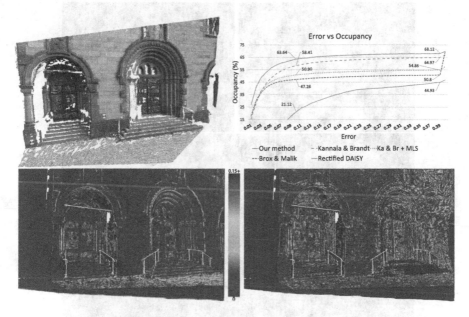

Fig. 8. Result of our approach on the Herz-Jesu P8 views 3–4 (top-left). On the top-right, a chart illustrating the depth error vs occupancy of our algorithm, [2,17,18] (rectified) and [2] with MLS as post-processing. On the bottom, color coded depth error using our algorithm (left) and using [2] (right) (Color figure online).

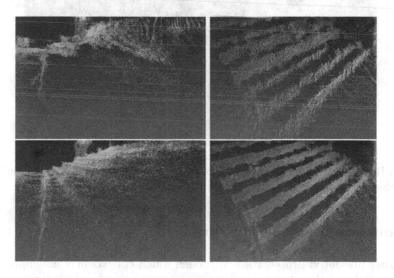

Fig. 9. Closeups on to results on Herz-Jesu P8 views 3–4 using [2] (top) and using our method (bottom). A closeup to a portion of the main stairs (left) and to the left-most stairs in the scene (right)

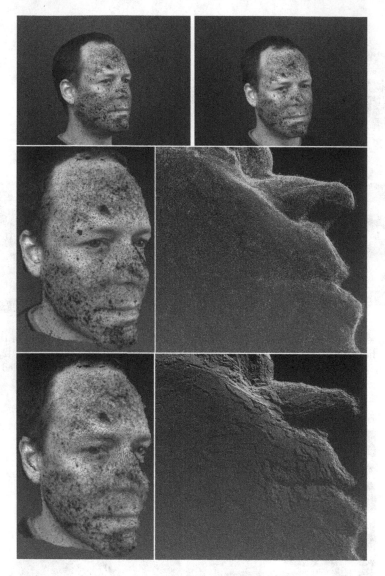

Fig. 10. Results on two views of our face dataset. The two views used (top), our result with a closeup to the cheek (middle), results using [2] (bottom)

5   Conclusion and Discussion

This paper presented propagation approach which congruently uses optical and geometric information to steer the propagation process. Although, many of underlying ideas are fairly simple, they lead to significant improvements both in the accuracy and completeness. Furthermore, as it could be argued that performing an equivalent MLS fitting as post processing would yield equivalent results,

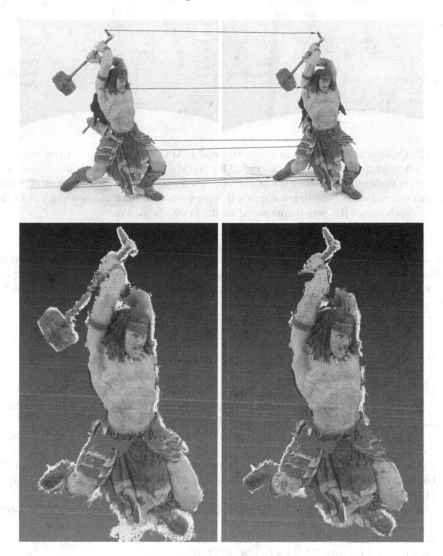

Fig. 11. Results on views 7 and 15 of the warrior dataset from [20]. The two views used are showed at the top row along with the 7 features matched. On the bottom row, our result (left) and results using [2] (right). Notice that our method returns less holes and it is able to reconstruct the warrior's hammer.

our comparisons to such a scenario, suggest that actually the results get worse. The reason being that in our case the subsequent matches depend on the fitting, whereas the use of fitting in post processing cannot alter how the matches are propagated.

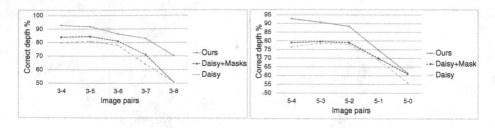

Fig. 12. Comparisons of our results to those of DAISY [18]. Results on the Fountain scene (left) and the Herz-Jesu scene (right) for pairs of images with increasing baselines. The charts present the percentage of correct depth estimations for each pair of views. A depth estimation is considered correct if it presents and error of less than 1 % of the scene's depth range [18] when compared to the laser scanned data.

Acknowledgments. The authors would like thank, the anonymous reviewers for their feedback on the paper, Juho Kannala for making his code publicly available, Christoph Strecha and Yasutaka Furukawa for their Multi-View datasets and Samuel Hornus for the face dataset. This work was funded by the ANR (Agence Nationale de la Recherche) under grant (PhysiGrafix ANR-09-CEXC-014-01).

References

1. Lhuillier, M., Quan, L.: Quasi-dense reconstruction from image sequence. In: Heyden, A., Sparr, G., Nielsen, M., Johansen, P. (eds.) ECCV 2002, Part II. LNCS, vol. 2351, pp. 125–139. Springer, Heidelberg (2002)
2. Kannala, J., Brandt, S.: Quasi-dense wide baseline matching using match propagation. In: CVPR, pp. 1–8 (2007)
3. Chen, Q., Medioni, G.: A volumetric stereo matching method: application to image-based modeling. In: CVPR, Fort Collins, United States, vol. 1, pp. 1029–1034 (1999)
4. Cech, J., Sara, R.: Efficient sampling of disparity space for fast and accurate matching. In: CVPR, pp. 1–8 (2007)
5. Lhuillier, M., Quan, L.: A quasi-dense approach to surface reconstruction from uncalibrated images. PAMI **27**, 418–433 (2005)
6. Yao, J., Cham, W.K.: 3D modeling and rendering from multiple wide-baseline images by match propagation. Sig. Process. Image Commun. **21**, 506–518 (2006)
7. Furukawa, Y., Ponce, J.: Accurate, dense, and robust multi-view stereopsis. In: CVPR, pp. 1–8 (2007)
8. Koskenkorva, P., Kannala, J., Brandt, S.: Quasi-dense wide baseline matching for three views. In: ICPR, ICPR 2010, Washington, DC, USA, pp. 806–809. IEEE Computer Society (2010)
9. Otto, G., Chau, T.: A 'region-growing' algorithm for matching of terrain images. Image Vis. Comput. **7**, 83–94 (1989)
10. Ferrari, V., Tuytelaars, T., Van Gool, L.: Simultaneous object recognition and segmentation by image exploration. In: Pajdla, T., Matas, J.G. (eds.) ECCV 2004. LNCS, vol. 3021, pp. 40–54. Springer, Heidelberg (2004)

11. Kazhdan, M., Bolitho, M., Hoppe, H.: Poisson surface reconstruction. In: Proceedings of the Fourth Eurographics Symposium on Geometry Processing, SGP 2006, Aire-la-Ville, Switzerland, Switzerland, pp. 61–70. Eurographics Association (2006)

12. Ylimaki, M., Kannala, J., Holappa, J., Heikkila, J., Brandt, S.: Robust and accurate multi-view reconstruction by prioritized matching. In: ICPR, pp. 2673–2676. IEEE (2012)

13. Habbecke, M., Kobbelt, L.: A surface-growing approach to multi-view stereo reconstruction. In: CVPR, pp. 1–8 (2007)

14. Mikolajczyk, K., Tuytelaars, T., Schmid, C., Zisserman, A., Matas, J., Schaffalitzky, F., Kadir, T., Gool, L.V.: A comparison of affine region detectors. IJCV **65**, 43–72 (2005)

15. Hartley, R.I., Zisserman, A.: Multiple View Geometry in Computer Vision, 2nd edn. Cambridge University Press, Cambridge (2004)

16. Barnhill, R., Farin, G., Jordan, M., Piper, B.: Surface/surface intersection. Comput. Aided Des. **4**, 3–16 (1987)

17. Brox, T., Malik, J.: Large displacement optical flow: descriptor matching in variational motion estimation. PAMI **33**, 500–513 (2011)

18. Tola, E., Lepetit, V., Fua, P.: Daisy: an efficient dense descriptor applied to wide-baseline stereo. PAMI **32**, 815–830 (2010)

19. Strecha, C., Von Hansen, W., Van Gool, L., Fua, P., Thoennessen, U.: On benchmarking camera calibration and multi-view stereo for high resolution imagery. In: CVPR, pp. 1–8 (2008)

20. Furukawa, Y., Ponce, J.: 3D photography dataset. http://www.cse.wustl.edu/furukawa/research/mview/index.html. Accessed 05 May 2014

Exploring Image Specific Structured Loss for Image Annotation with Incomplete Labelling

Xing Xu$^{(\boxtimes)}$, Atsushi Shimada, and Rin-ichiro Taniguch

Department of Advanced Information Technology, Kyushu University,
Fukuoka, Japan
xing@limu.ait.kyushu-u.ac.jp

Abstract. In this paper, we address the problem of image annotation with *incomplete labelling*, where the multiple objects in each training image are not fully labeled. The conventional one-versus-all SVM (OVA-SVM) that performs fairly well on full labelling decays drastically under the incomplete setting. Recently, structured learning method termed OVA-SSVM is proposed to boost the performance of OVA-SVM by modeling the structured associations of labels and show efficiency under incomplete setting. The OVA-SSVM assumes that each training sample includes a single label and adopts an loss measure of classification style that as long as one of the predicted label is correct, the overall prediction should be considered correct. However, this may not be appropriate for the multi-label annotation task. In this paper, we extend the OVA-SSVM method to the multi-label situation and design a novel image specific structured loss measure to account for the dependencies between predicted labels relying on the image-label associations. Then we develop an efficient optimization algorithm to learn the model parameters. Finally, we present extensive empirical results on two benchmark datasets with various degree of incompletion, and show that proposed method outperforms OVA-SSVM and achieves competitive performance compared with other state-of-the-art methods which are also designed for the issue of incomplete labelling.

1 Introduction

Automatic image annotation is an important research problem, where each image is associated with a set of labels and the target is to learn a model that assigns multiple labels to an unlabeled new image to describe its visual content. In particular, the human annotations play an significant role in training an annotation model as they provide empirical knowledge of the image-label associations. Although the quality of human annotations is quite crucial, one can not expect to accurately obtain all the labels for a given image, since human labelers usually tag only prominent labels and typically miss out on several objects present in the image. Here we pose a practical issue of *incomplete labelling* that the training images are not completely tagged with all relevant labels from vocabulary. As shown in Fig. 1, the images from two benchmark datasets have few human annotated labels and suffer from the problem of incomplete labelling.

© Springer International Publishing Switzerland 2015
D. Cremers et al. (Eds.): ACCV 2014, Part I, LNCS 9003, pp. 704–719, 2015.
DOI: 10.1007/978-3-319-16865-4_46

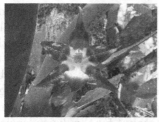 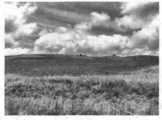

bloom, leave   clouds

Fig. 1. Example of incomplete labelling: two images are from benchmark datasets IAPRTC-12 [1] (left) and NUS-WIDE [2] (right). Potentially correct labels such as {*flower, plant, tree, trunk*}, {*sky, grass*} are missed from the ground truth of two images respectively.

The traditional annotation models such as generative models [3, 4] or nearest-neighbor based models [5–7] generally neglect the issue of incomplete labelling and treat the human annotated dataset as completely labeled. For these models, given a labeled training image, labels that are not presented in the groundtruth of that image make limited contribution to the annotation model. When applying these models on incompletely labeled dataset, the annotation performance can hardly achieve optimal because of the insufficient annotations of the dataset. Therefore, in our work, we intend to develop an annotation method that is more efficient for the incompletely labeled dataset. It should be noted that our problem setting is different from the researches of tag completion [8–10] or tag recommendation [11,12], where their goal is to complete partially tagged images offline or to recommend related tags to users online.

Regarding the methodology of annotation with incomplete labelling, one group of recent ongoing researches [13–16] directly modify conventional annotation prototypes such as multi-label ranking [13,16], binary SVM [14], and ridge regression [15], by incorporating additional consistency between visual and semantic cues in images to address the issue of incompletion. And the performance of these methods greatly depends on the assumption of consistency. Moreover, another group of works aim at boosting the conventional annotation models and adding new learning stage under the incomplete setting incrementally. The method utilized in the new learning stage could be multi-task learning [17], ensemble learning [18], and structured learning [19,20]. Here we would like to stress that structured learning method is an efficient scheme to handle the difficulties of incomplete labelling. Firstly, it captures the interdependencies of labels from the structure in the output space. Secondly, the weak learning manner allows it to explore the potential usages of missing labels, and those missing labels can be captured by latent variables [21].

Specifically, in the celebrated work termed OVA-SSVM of [20], structured learning method is adopted to boost the performance of pre-trained OVA-SVM classifiers under incomplete setting, and it designs a structured loss function of image classification style to benefit the prediction of missing labels. And promising prediction results are obtained on ImageNet [22] dataset where each training image has a single label. However, the OVA-SSVM method may not be well extended to more practical circumstances where each training image has multiple labels, due to limitation of its structured loss used. Therefore, in this paper, we put effort to improve OVA-SVM in three folds: (1) We extend the OVA-SSVM so that the number of labels per training image can be flexible, which is more practical to the multi-label annotation problem. (2) We design a novel image specific structured loss function which is more appropriate than previous flat structured loss used in OVA-SSVM to account for the dependencies between predicted labels relying on the specific image. (3) We develop efficient optimization algorithm with lower complexity by exploiting the properties of proposed structured loss. Empirical evaluations on two annotation datasets with various degree of incompletion demonstrate that proposed annotation method can boost conventional OVA-SVM classifiers, perform better than previous structured learning method OVA-SSVM, and achieve competitive performance compared with state-of-the-art methods designed for incompletely labeled dataset.

2   Problem Formulation

In this section, we will first introduce the conventional OVA-SVM used for image annotation task, then describe the OVA-SSVM method that uses structured learning to boost OVA-SVM classifiers under incomplete setting. Some notations used in the following sections are also defined in this section.

2.1   Conventional OVA-SVM

We are given an incompletely labeled dataset $\mathcal{T} = \{(x^1, Y^1), ..., (x^N, Y^N)\}$. Here $x^n \in \mathcal{X}$ represents the image feature vector, $Y^n \subseteq \mathcal{Y}$ is a set of labels, where $\mathcal{Y} = \{y_1, ..., y_C\}$ is the vocabulary of C labels. Note that Y^n is a subset of the ideally full set Ω^n of groundtruth labels for image x^n. Our goal is to learn an annotation model that, for an unseen image x, outputs an optimal set $\hat{Y}$ which includes K distinct labels.

A conventional annotation model consists of learning a series of binary OVA-SVM classifiers that distinguish a single label from all other. For a given label y_c, we denote the parameter vector of learnt OVA-SVM classifier as $w_{OVA}^{y_c}$, then to predict a set of K labels $\hat{Y}$ for an unseen image x, the annotation model simply returns the labels with the K highest scores performing on classifiers of all labels:

$$\hat{Y} = arg \max_{Y \in \mathcal{Y}} \sum_{y_c \in Y} x \cdot w_{OVA}^{y_c}, \tag{1}$$

where $Y \subseteq \mathcal{Y}$ represents any output set contain K labels. It is worth noting that the annotation model of OVA-SVM classifiers is suboptimal since that (1) the one-versus-all learning manner ignores the dependencies of labels, which implies that OVA-SVM optimizes the prediction of only a single output label, ignoring the "structure" altogether, (2) the performance of OVA-SVM classifiers drops drastically when incomplete labels for training image are provided.

2.2   OVA-SSVM

To overcome the disadvantages of conventional OVA-SVM and to exploit the structured associations in output label set Y, the structured learning method OVA-SSVM [20] considers that the training set consists of structured input-output pairs $T \in (\mathcal{X} \times \mathcal{Y})^N$. The prediction rule of optimal output labels $\hat{Y}$ for an unseen image x is

$$\hat{Y} = arg \max_{Y \in \mathcal{Y}} \Phi(x, Y) \cdot \boldsymbol{w} = arg \max_{Y \in \mathcal{Y}} \sum_{y \in Y} \phi(x, y) \cdot \boldsymbol{w}, \qquad (2)$$

where Φ is the joint feature vector that describes the relationship between input x and any structured output Y, ϕ is the joint feature vector for input x and single label y in Y, and $\boldsymbol{w}$ is the parameter vector to be learnt. In particular, given a set of pre-trained OVA-SVM classifiers $\{\boldsymbol{w}_{OVA}^{y_c}\}^{y_c \in \mathcal{Y}}$, the joint feature vector $\Phi(x, Y)$ in OVA-SSVM is defined as

$$\Phi(x, Y) = \sum_{y \in Y} x \circ \boldsymbol{w}_{OVA}^y, \qquad (3)$$

where $x \circ \boldsymbol{w}_{OVA}^y$ represents the Hadamard product of x and $\boldsymbol{w}_{OVA}^y$. Then the annotation model in Eq. 2 can be formulated as

$$\hat{Y} = arg \max_{Y \in \mathcal{Y}} \sum_{y \in Y} \langle x \circ \boldsymbol{w}_{OVA}^y, \boldsymbol{w} \rangle. \qquad (4)$$

We can learn from Eq. 4 that OVA-SSVM incrementally learns a single parameter vector $\boldsymbol{w}$ that re-weights the parameters of existing OVA-SVM classifiers $\{\boldsymbol{w}_{OVA}^{y_c}\}^{y_c \in \mathcal{Y}}$ and incorporates the structure nature of output Y through the joint feature vector $\Phi(x, Y)$.

Moreover, for the incomplete setting of T, the input-output relationship is not completely characterized by $(x, Y) \in \mathcal{X} \times \mathcal{Y}$. It is rational to introduce a set of unobserved latent variables, $Z = \{Z^1, ..., Z^N\}$, where Z^n represents the set of labels that appear in image x^n but were not annotated. The full set of labels for the image x^n is $\Omega^n = Y^n \cup Z^n$ (note that $Y^n \cap Z^n = \varnothing$). Now the joint feature vector $\Phi(x, \Omega)$ describes the relation among input x, output Y and latent variables Z, and it is defined as

$$\Phi(x, \Omega) = \sum_{y \in Y} x \circ \boldsymbol{w}_{OVA}^y + \sum_{z \in Z} x \circ \boldsymbol{w}_{OVA}^z \qquad (5)$$

To train OVA-SSVM, the parameter vector $\boldsymbol{w}$ is determined by minimizing the regularized risk on the training set T. Risk is measured through a user-provided structured loss function $\Delta(Y, Y^n)$ that quantifies how much the prediction Y differs from the given label set Y^n of image x^n. The resulting convex optimization problem is to minimize the objective function as

$$\min_{\boldsymbol{w}, \xi} \frac{\lambda}{2} \|\boldsymbol{w}\|^2 + \frac{1}{N} \sum_{n=1}^{N} \xi_n \qquad (6)$$

$$s.t \quad \boldsymbol{w} \cdot \Phi(x^n, \Omega^n) - \boldsymbol{w} \cdot \Phi(x^n, Y) \geq \Delta(Y, Y^n) - \xi_n, \quad \forall n, Y \in \mathcal{Y}.$$

The constraints of Eq. 6 identify the prediction Y with a score $\boldsymbol{w} \cdot \Phi(x^n, Y)$ that is smaller than the score $\boldsymbol{w} \cdot \Phi(x^n, \Omega^n)$ of the "full" groundtruth Ω^n by a soft margin equals to the loss $\Delta(Y, Y^n)$ with the slack variable ξ_n. The optimization problem can be solved efficiently using a constraint generation strategy: we can generate the constraint by identifying the most violated (incorrect) prediction $\bar{Y}$ from Y for the current parameter vector $\boldsymbol{w}$ on x^n. This amounts to solving

$$\bar{Y} = arg \max_{\hat{Y} \in \mathcal{Y}} \{\Delta(Y, Y^n) + \boldsymbol{w} \cdot \Phi(x^n, Y)\}. \tag{7}$$

Given the definition of user-provided structured loss Δ, we can use $\bar{Y}$ of all $x^n \in \mathcal{X}$ to approximate a lower bound of the objective in Eq. 6. Then we can compute the gradient of Eq. 6, and alternately optimize the latent variables Z and the parameter vector $\boldsymbol{w}$. In the next section, we will introduce proposed image specific loss term which is elaborately designed for incomplete labeled training data, and derive the corresponding optimization algorithm in the structured learning framework.

3   Proposed Structured Loss Under Incomplete Setting

3.1   Image Specific Structured Loss

Since the given label set Y^n may not describe all the object in image x^n, an annotation model should not be penalized for predicting "incorrect" labels that actually describe those objects in x^n. To address this issue, a structured loss function Δ is designed in OVA-SSVM. Given a set of predicted output labels Y for x^n, the OVA-SSVM method would not give penalty if one of the predicted labels $y \in Y$ is similar to any of the groundtruth labels $y^n \in Y^n$. The loss function is defined as

$$\Delta(Y, Y^n) = \min_{y \in Y} \min_{y^n \in Y^n} d(y, y^n), \tag{8}$$

where $d(y, y^n)$ is the error term measuring the difference between label y and y^n. In practice, $d(y, y^n)$ could be a flat error measure: $d(y, y^n) = 0$ if $y = y^n$, and 1 otherwise. And $d(y, y^n)$ could also be a hierarchical error measure: $d(y, y^n)$ is the shortest path distance between y^n and y in a taxonomic vocabulary tree.

Actually, there are several limitations of the structured loss of Eq. 8 for the incomplete setting. Firstly, to predict output labels Y, ensuring that only one of the predicted labels is similar to the groundtruth is not enough. In other words, it is expected that each of the predicted labels is similar to any (even all) of the groundtruth labels. Secondly, the error measure of $d(y, y^n)$ is either coarse to quantify the difference of labels (i.e. flat error measure), or rigorous to require the prior construction of taxonomic tree (i.e. hierarchical error measure). Thirdly, the error measure indicates that the variances of labels are based on the global statistics of training data, whereas for the incomplete setting, it is not sufficient to model the relatedness of missing labels and groundtruth labels.

In Fig. 2, we demonstrate two examples of label prediction using *flat* structured loss in OVA-SSVM. It can be observed that, although flat structured loss (in fifth column) is generated to be zero (since the predicted labels *bloom, man* match the incomplete groundtruth Y^n), the predicted result (in third column) is inferior which contains several incorrect labels, e.g. {*fruit, forest*}, {*woman, bottle, forest*}. Thus, it implies that numerically minimizing the structured loss of Eq. 8 could not guarantee all predicted labels to be similar to groundtruth labels.

| Image x^n | Incomplete labels Y^n | Predicted labels Y | | Structured loss Δ | |
		OVA-SSVM (Flat)	Proposed	Flat	Image specific
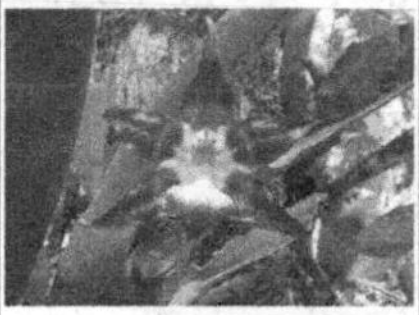	bloom, leave	bloom, flower, fruit, forest, branch	bloom (0), leave (0), trunk (0.531), flower (0.552), plant (0.765)	0	0.3696
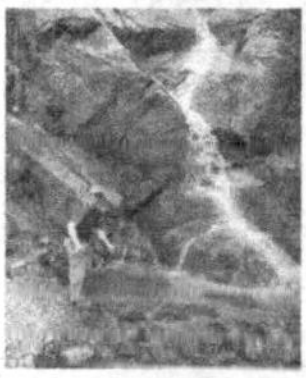	man, one, rock	man, woman, front, bottle, forest	man (0), rock (0), tee-shirt (0.647), hand (0.685), waterfall (0.689)	0	0.4042

Fig. 2. Examples of label prediction using flat loss (OVA-SSVM (Flat)) *vs.* image specific structured loss (proposed method). These two images are selected from IAPRTC-12 dataset. Note that in the fourth column, the image specific loss of each predicted label is also provided. And the loss values Δ in last two columns are calculated according to Eqs. 8 and 9 respectively.

To address the limitations of Eq. 8, we assume that each of the predicted labels is related to *all* of the groundtruth labels, and we desire the structured loss term to capture the variances of labels relying on the specific image content. Our proposed image specific loss function is formulated as

$$\Delta(Y, Y^n; x^n) = \frac{1}{|Y|} \frac{1}{|Y^n|} \sum_{y \in Y} \sum_{y^n \in Y^n} d(y, y^n; x^n). \tag{9}$$

Here the error measure $d(y, y^n; x^n)$ is image specific, representing the difference of label y and y^n particularly on image x^n. In addition, the structured loss $\Delta(Y, Y^n; x^n)$ ensures that each of the predicted labels in Y to be related to all the groundtruth labels in Y^n. Since the incomplete label set Y^n is small, here we restrict the structured loss of Eq. 9 to moderately consider the dependencies between each of the predicted labels and all labels in Y^n.

Inspired by the works [10,14], we cast measuring $d(y, y^n; x^n)$ to comparing the relatedness of image x^n to labels y and y^n. In particular, for a given label y_c, let $\mathcal{X}_c^+$ be the set of images that are annotated with label y_c, and the remaining images as $\mathcal{X}_c^- = \mathcal{X} \backslash \mathcal{X}_c^+$. For image x^n in $\mathcal{X}_c^+$, we define the relatedness of image x^n to label y_c as $R(x^n, y_c) = 1$ since x^n is annotated with y_c. And for image x^n belongs to $\mathcal{X}_c^-$ of y_c, we determine the relatedness score of $R(x^n, y_c)$ considering three factors: visual similarity, semantic similarity and image-label association in the visual neighborhood. Specifically, $R(x^n, y_c)$ consists of

- Visual similarity based relatedness score $R_V(x^n, y_c)$: We compute the visual distance $dist(\cdot)$ (scaled to range $[0, 1]$) of x^n with its nearest neighbor $x^* \in \mathcal{X}_c^+$, and define $R_V(x^n, y_c) = 1 - dist(x^n, x^*)$.
- Semantic similarity based relatedness score $R_S(x^n, y_c)$: We first compute the correlation score between pairwise labels y_i and y_j, $\forall y_i, y_j \in \mathcal{Y}$ as: co_occur $(y_i, y_j) = \frac{f_{i,j}}{f_i + f_j - f_{i,j}}$, where f_i and f_j are the count of occurrence of labels y_i and y_j, and $f_{i,j}$ is the count of co-occurrence of labels y_i and y_j. Let Y^n be the label set of image x^n, we define $R_S(x^n, y_c) = \max_{y^n \in Y^n} co\_occur(y_c, y^n)$.
- Reverse nearest neighbors based relatedness score $R_N(x^n, y_c)$: For a fixed value of $M(= 5)$, let p_m be the number of images in $\mathcal{X}_c^+$ that have x^n as their m^{th} nearest neighbor. Then we define $R_N(x^n, y_c) = \sum_{m=1}^{M} \frac{p_m}{m} / \sum_{m=1}^{M} p_m + \varepsilon$, where $\varepsilon > 0$ is a small number to avoid division by zero.

Finally, $R(x^n, y_c)$ is defined as the average of these three scores, similar as in [14]:

$$R(x^n, y_c) = average(R_V(x^n, y_c) + R_S(x^n, y_c) + R_N(x^n, y_c)). \qquad (10)$$

Now we can calculate the error measure $d(y, y^n; x^n)$ by comparing the relatedness scores of image x^n to labels y and y^n as

$$d(y, y^n; x^n) = R(x^n, y^n) - R(x^n, y) = 1 - R(x^n, y). \qquad (11)$$

Recalling that $y^n \in Y^n$ is the groundtruth label of x^n, thus it has highest relatedness score (equals to 1). It can be learnt that the calculation of Eq. 11 is directly determined by the relatedness score $R(x^n, y)$ of label y to image x^n. And if the predicted label y has larger relatedness score to x^n, it would have small difference with all the groundtruth labels. This is consistent with the proposed structured loss of Eq. 9, which now can be efficiently measured by the relatedness of predicted labels to the specific image.

Compared with the flat/hierarchical structured loss, our proposed structured loss of Eq. 9 has several advantages. Firstly, as shown in Fig. 2, although the loss values (in last column) are numerically larger than "zero" of flat structured loss (in fifth column), the predicted labels is more similar to the provided incomplete labels. This is because proposed structured loss moderately considers the predicting labels based on their relatedness to specific image content, and the relatedness measure is elaborately designed and more appropriate than the simple 0–1 measure. Secondly, the proposed structured loss is more flexible to the number of groundtruth labels as it accumulatively measures each of the predicted labels to all the groundtruth, while the flat structured loss focuses on the most dominant one in the predicted label to a single label of the groundtruth labels. Thirdly, the relatedness measure can be directly and precisely computed from labeled training images, while to construct the hierarchical measure, usually prior knowledge of taxonomy or large quantities of training data with full labelling is required.

3.2 Optimization Method

Given the proposed structured loss function of Eq. 9, we can generate the most violated constraint of prediction $\bar{Y}$ for image x^n according to Eq. 7 as the form

$$\bar{Y} = arg \max_{Y \in \mathcal{Y}} \{ \frac{1}{|Y|} \frac{1}{|Y^n|} \sum_{y \in Y} \sum_{y^n \in Y^n} d(y, y^n; x^n) + \sum_{y \in Y} \boldsymbol{w} \cdot \phi(x^n, y) \}$$

$$= arg \max_{Y \in \mathcal{Y}} \{ \frac{1}{|Y|} \sum_{y \in Y} (1 - R(x^n, y)) + \sum_{y \in Y} \boldsymbol{w} \cdot \phi(x^n, y) \}, \quad (12)$$

where the calculation of structured loss $\Delta(Y, Y^n; x^n)$ is converted to compute the relatedness scores of predicted label set Y to image x^n, as described in Sect. 3.1. We can obtain the solution of Y of Eq. 12 by simply sorting the term $\frac{1}{|Y|}(1 - R(x^n, y_c)) + \boldsymbol{w} \cdot \phi(x^n, y_c)$ for each label $y_c \in \mathcal{Y}$, and then choose the top K labels for $\bar{Y}$. Solving Eq. 12 greedily takes $\mathcal{O}(C \log C)$, thus it is faster than the constraints generation method in OVA-SSVM which takes $\mathcal{O}(C^2 \log C)$. After we have generated the most violated constraint $\bar{Y}$ for each image, the lower bound of the objective function in Eq. 6 can be derived as

$$J(\boldsymbol{w}) = \frac{\lambda}{2} \|\boldsymbol{w}\|^2 + \frac{1}{N} \sum_{n=1}^{N} \left[\Delta(\bar{Y} - Y^n) + \boldsymbol{w} \cdot \Phi(x^n, \bar{Y}) - \boldsymbol{w} \cdot \Phi(x^n, \Omega^n) \right], \quad (13)$$

and the gradient of $J(\boldsymbol{w})$ with respect to $\boldsymbol{w}$ is

$$\nabla_{\boldsymbol{w}} J(\boldsymbol{w}) = \lambda \boldsymbol{w} + \frac{1}{N} \sum_{n=1}^{N} \left[\boldsymbol{w} \cdot \Phi(x^n, \bar{Y}) - \boldsymbol{w} \cdot \Phi(x^n, \Omega^n) \right]. \quad (14)$$

It can be observed in Eqs. 13 and 14 that calculating $J(\boldsymbol{w})$ and its gradient involves in computing the joint feature vector $\Phi(x^n, \Omega^n)$ on "full" label set Ω^n of each image. And $\Phi(x^n, \Omega^n)$ can be efficiently computed according to Eq. 5 with latent variable Z^n. To learn the parameter vector $\boldsymbol{w}$ with latent variable Z^n, we follow the previous alternating optimization technique proposed in [19,20]. Specifically, we alternate between optimizing the parameter vector $\boldsymbol{w}^t$ by initializing the latent variable Z^n for each image in the tth iteration, and re-estimate the latent variable Z^n for the $(t+1)^{th}$ iteration given the learnt parameter vector $\boldsymbol{w}^t$. The pseudocode for solving the alternating optimization problem is depicted in Algorithm 1.

Algorithm 1. Alternating optimization of proposed method

Input: Incompletely labeled training data $\mathcal{T} = \{(x^n, Y^n)\}_{n=1}^N$, pre-trained binary classifiers $\{w_{OVA}^{y_c}\}_{c=1}^C$
Output: Parameter vector w
1: Initialize $w_0 = 1$ for iteration $t = 0$
2: **repeat**
3:    Set $t = t + 1$
4:    **for** $n = 1, ..., N$ **do**
5:       Assign latent variable $Z_t^n = \{arg\max_{Y \in \mathcal{Y}} w_{t-1} \cdot \Phi(x^n, Y)\} \backslash Y^n$ for x^n (preserving $K - |Y^n|$ missing labels)
6:    **end for**
7:    **for** $n = 1, ..., N$ **do**
8:       Generate the most violated constraint $\bar{Y}_t$ for x^n according to Eq. 12
9:    **end for**
10:    Compute objective $J_t(w)$ and gradient $\nabla_w J_t(w)$ according to Eqs. 13 and 14
11:    Minimize loss of Eq. 6 to calculate w_t
12: **until** Loss in Eq. 6 is converged

---

4   Experimental Evaluation

In this section, we evaluation the effectiveness of proposed method through comparing it with the previous OVA-SSVM and other state-of-the-art annotation methods under incomplete setting.

4.1   Experimental Setup

Datasets and Features. Our evaluation experiments are conducted on two publicly available benchmark datasets: IAPRTC-12 [1] and NUS-WIDE [2]. These two datasets are very challenging with significant diversity among the images that are obtained from the social web. Table 1 shows the general statistics of these two datasets, and it is worth noting that they cover both conditions of large vocabulary size and large number of images. In our experiments, for IAPRTC-12 dataset, we use the same multiple features as those in [5,6,14,15]. These multiple features consist of global and local features. The global features include histograms in RGB, HSV and LAB color space, and the GIST features; and the local features include the SIFT and hue descriptors obtained densely from multiscale grid, and from Harris-Laplacian interest points. For NUS-WIDE dataset, besides global GIST features, we also extract five types of SIFT based local features (C-SIFT, Opponent-SIFT, RGB-SIFT, RG-SIFT) using the public colorDescriptor tools [23]. The SIFT based features are computed without orientation invariance and the grid has a step size of three. The codebook for each SIFT based feature is generated from 7,000 randomly selected images, and quantized to 4,000 corresponding k-means clusters. For both datasets, we first separately perform L2 normalization for each type of feature, and then concatenate them to an fused feature vector (37,152-dimension for IAPRTC-12 and 20,512-dimension for NUS-WIDE) to represent each image.

Table 1. General statistics for the two datasets used for evaluation. The items in the second row are listed in the format "training/test", and items in the third and fourth rows are given in the format "mean/minimum/maximum"

	IAPRTC-12	NUS-WIDE
Total labels	291	81
No. of images	17,665/1,962	138,563/92,484
Labels per image	5.7/1/23	1.8/1/20
Images per label	34/153/4,999	2,512/333/16,425

Incomplete Setting. We consider the original IAPRTC-12 as fully labeled dataset since the average number of labels per image is more than 5 (5.7 in Table 1), which could be sufficient to describe multiple objects in an image. To simulate the incomplete setting, we randomly delete partial labels for each image, and the deletion process stands by the principle $\min(1, \lceil M \times (1 - ratio) \rceil)$ ensure that each image preserve at least one label. Here M denotes the number of original labels of an image, $\lceil \cdot \rceil$ denotes the ceiling function which gives the smallest integer not smaller than the given value, and $ratio$ represents the degree of incompletion. In our experiments, we set $ratio = \{10\,\%, 30\,\%, 50\,\%, 70\,\%, 90\,\%\}$, and it indicates that the larger the ratio is, the higher the degree of incompletion would be. For NUS-WIDE, as the average number of labels per image is less than 2 (1.8 in Table 1), which could be insufficient compared with the situation of IAPRTC-12, we treat the NUS-WIDE as incomplete labeled dataset, and directly utilize the original annotations for incomplete setting.

Binary Classifiers. As proposed method needs pre-trained binary classifier for each class as a starting point for structured learning, we follow previous works [14,20] and learn OVA-SVM classifiers for initialization. In particular, we train a linear OVA-SVM classifier for each label using Pegasos [24] algorithm and calibrate the raw confidence scores from the SVM classifiers to probabilities with Platt [25] algorithm. Finally, we obtain linear OVA-SVM classifiers with compatible probability scores and use them as initial input to proposed method.

Evaluation Metrics. Given an unlabeled test image, we first compute the score for each label using the learnt model, and then select five top-scoring ($K = 5$, $|Y| = 5$) labels according to Eq. 4. And we use two standard criteria to evaluate the performance: (1) average precision per label P, (2) average recall per label R. Note that the P and R scores are obtained by first computing precision and recall for each label and then averaging. In addition, as the number of labels in NUS-WIDE dataset is considerably small, we add another two criteria: *Hamming loss* and *Average AUC*, which take the performance of overall prediction and ranking into account. For all the adopted evaluation metrics except *Hamming loss*, larger numerical value indicates better performance.

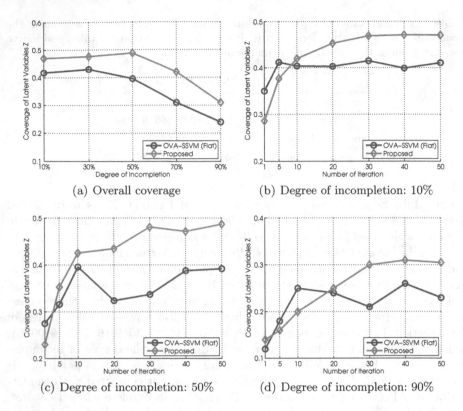

(a) Overall coverage   (b) Degree of incompletion: 10%

(c) Degree of incompletion: 50%   (d) Degree of incompletion: 90%

Fig. 3. Evaluation of coverage of latent variables with various degree of incompletion.

4.2 Evaluation on IAPRTC-12 Dataset

Assessment of Assigning Latent Variables. We first consider proposed method using image specific structured loss and OVA-SSVM (Flat) method using flat structured loss, to compare the efficiency of structured learning with latent variables. Specifically, we explore how closely the assigned latent variable Z^n matches those labels $\Omega^n \backslash Y^n$ deleted from the originally full annotations of image x^n when training as in Algorithm 1. We use a measure termed $Coverage = \frac{1}{N} \sum_{n=1}^{N} \frac{|Z^n \cap (\Omega^n \backslash Y^n)|}{|Z^n|}$ to represent the averaged intersection between Z^n and $\Omega^n \backslash Y^n$ for all training image $x^n \in \mathcal{X}$. Note that higher coverage indicates better assignments of latent variables.

Figure 3(a) shows the overall coverage of latent variable to the deleted labels in the full annotations with different degree of incompletion. It can be observed that (1) the coverage of latent variable of both methods increases when the degree of incompletion becomes lower, and this is reasonable because the more labels we have, the better we can predict the missing labels; (2) our proposed method consistently obtains higher coverage for missing labels than OVA-SSVM (Flat) which simply uses flat structured loss, as the image specific structured loss used in our method is more efficient to exploit various contextual information of labels and images under the incomplete setting. Furthermore, in Fig. 3(b)–(d), we explicitly demonstrate the changing of coverage of the latent variables through the iterations (as described in Algorithm 1) under different degree of incompletion: 10 %, 50 %, 90 %. We can learn that proposed image specific structured loss is appropriate to ensure our method to perform robustly, while OVA-SSVM (Flat) seems to be unstable through the iterations and results in inferior coverage. Especially, when the degree of incompletion is pretty high (e.g. 50 %, 90 %), the coverage of proposed method is significant better than OVA-SSVM (Flat), which solidly verifies the superiority of proposed method under the incomplete setting.

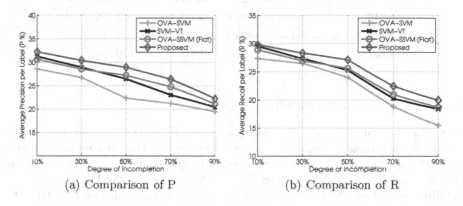

(a) Comparison of P   (b) Comparison of R

Fig. 4. Comparison of annotation performance with various degree of incompletion.

Overall Comparison with Various Degree of Incompletion. To make comprehensive comparison, we first explore the labeling results from binary classifiers: OVA-SVM and SVM-VT [14] (OVA-SVM combined with proposed image specific label relatedness as depicted in Sect. 3.1, without structured learning), then boost the binary classifiers by structured learning via flat structured loss (OVA-SSVM (Flat)) and image specific structured loss (proposed method).

Figure 4 shows the annotation results of four methods in terms of P and R with various degree of incompletion. Firstly, it can be seen that as the degree of incompletion decreases, the performance of all methods becomes better, since we have more labels for training. Secondly, our method can boost the performance of binary classifiers OVA-SVM and SVM-VT under incomplete setting, which verifies the efficiency of the incrementally structured learning. Thirdly, regarding the structured learning stage, proposed method performs remarkably better than OVA-SSVM (Flat) which uses the flat structured loss, especially when the degree of incompletion is considerably high (50 % ~ 90 %). The reason behind this is that we use more appropriate structured loss which efficiently accounts for the dependencies between the predicted labels under the incomplete setting.

Table 2. Annotation performance comparison among different methods on NUS-WIDE dataset. Previous and our best results are highlighted in bold.

Method	P (%)	R (%)	Average AUC	Hamming loss
JEC [5]	11.9	16.6	0.557	0.083
Tagprop [6]	13.2	23.8	0.707	0.074
OVA-SVM	12.3	22.8	0.782	0.079
M3L [26]	16.1	23.2	0.791	0.071
SVM-VT [14]	16.7	24.3	0.806	0.069
MLR-GL [13]	14.2	23.5	0.722	0.078
Fasttag [15]	**18.4**	21.3	**0.834**	0.067
LEML [16]	17.5	24.6	0.798	0.076
OVA-SSVM (Flat) [20]	16.9	24.1	0.772	0.070
Proposed	17.7	**25.6**	0.819	**0.064**

4.3 Evaluation on NUS-WIDE Dataset

Regarding experiments on incompletely labeled NUS-WIDE dataset, besides the four methods compared above, we also consider state-of-the-art annotation methods with assumptions of full labelling and incomplete labelling. Methods for full labelling include JEC [5], Tagprop [6], and M3L [26]. Methods for incomplete labelling consist of SVM-VT [14], MLR-GL [13], Fasttag [15] and LEML [16]. To make fair comparison, we use codes provided by the authors and follow the instructions in corresponding papers to tune model parameters.

Table 2 shows the annotation performance of different methods. And we can make the following observations: (1) The proposed method consistently boosts the binary SVM classifiers (OVA-SVM and SVM-VT) and also obtain better performance than OVA-SSVM (Flat). (2) The annotation methods including proposed method designed for incomplete labelling are generally superior to conventional annotation methods with full labelling, which again addresses the significance of tackling the issue of incompletion of practical annotation data. (3) The proposed method performs comparable or better than even the recently proposed methods with incomplete labelling, which corroborates the efficiency of structured learning on capturing the semantic correlations of labels when labels are incomplete.

Figure 5 gives qualitative samples of the annotation results of the proposed method on the two datasets. In particular, for IAPRTC-12 dataset, we preserve the original training images without the deletion process to evaluate the generalization of proposed method. From the samples we can see that, although the number of groundtruth labels are few, our method can still make correct prediction to them. In addition, our method can also reflect semantic connectedness among the predicted labels, e.g. {*field, landscape*}, {*gravel, road, stone*}, {*beach, sand, ocean*}, etc. This further demonstrates the effectiveness of proposed method using structured learning.

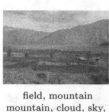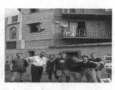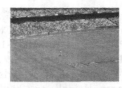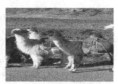

field, mountain	front, house, tourist	field, groundstand, spectator	road
mountain, cloud, sky,	house, building, street,	field, stadium, player,	llama, gravel, road
field, landscape	tourist, front	spectator, ground	stone, shrub

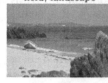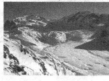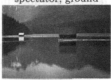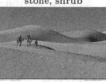

sand, sky	glacier, sky, snow	lake, water	sand
beach, sand, sky,	glacier, mountain, snow	lake, water, house,	sky, sand, animal,
rocks, ocean	rocks, sky	reflection, mountain	person, horse

Fig. 5. Samples of annotation results of the proposed method on IAPRTC-12 (the upper row) and NUS-WIDE (the lower row). The red labels are the groundtruth and black ones are top five labels predicted using proposed method.

5 Conclusion and Future Work

In this paper, to tackle the issue of incomplete labelling, we leverage the structured learning method to boost the performance of conventional OVA-SVM classifiers, and we formulate an image specific structured loss function which is more appropriate to explore the dependencies of predicted multiple labels. We further develop an efficient optimization algorithm with lower computational complexity to learn model parameters. Experimental evaluation verifies that the proposed annotation method is efficient to handle the issue of incomplete labeling and performs superior than several existing methods. In the future, we are planning to extend our method to the scenario where even some of the incomplete labels are incorrectly assigned to the training samples. This in turn would facilitate the annotation model to be robust against the defection of training data.

Acknowledgement. This work was partly supported by Grant-in-Aid for Scientific Research (B), Grant Number 24300074. We thank reviewers for the precious comments.

References

1. Grubinger, M.: Analysis and Evaluation of Visual Information Systems Performance. Ph.D. thesis, Victoria University (2007)
2. Chua, T.S., Tang, J., Hong, R., Li, H., Luo, Z., Zheng, Y.: Nus-wide: a real-world web image database from national university of singapore. In: Proceedings of the ACM International Conference on Image and Video Retrieval, p. 48 (2009)
3. Xiang, Y., Zhou, X., Chua, T.S., Ngo, C.W.: A revisit of generative model for automatic image annotation using markov random fields. In: IEEE Conference on Computer Vision and Pattern Recognition (CVPR), pp. 1153–1160 (2009)

4. Feng, S., Manmatha, R., Lavrenko, V.: Multiple bernoulli relevance models for image and video annotation. In: IEEE Conference on Computer Vision and Pattern Recognition (CVPR), vol. 2, pp. 1002–1009 (2004)
5. Makadia, A., Pavlovic, V., Kumar, S.: A new baseline for image annotation. In: Forsyth, D., Torr, P., Zisserman, A. (eds.) ECCV 2008, Part III. LNCS, vol. 5304, pp. 316–329. Springer, Heidelberg (2008)
6. Guillaumin, M., Mensink, T., Verbeek, J., Schmid, C.: Tagprop: discriminative metric learning in nearest neighbor models for image auto-annotation. In: IEEE 12th International Conference on Computer Vision (ICCV), pp. 309–316 (2009)
7. Verma, Y., Jawahar, C.V.: Image annotation using metric learning in semantic neighbourhoods. In: Fitzgibbon, A., Lazebnik, S., Perona, P., Sato, Y., Schmid, C. (eds.) ECCV 2012, Part III. LNCS, vol. 7574, pp. 836–849. Springer, Heidelberg (2012)
8. Wu, L., Jin, R., Jain, A.: Tag completion for image retrieval. IEEE Trans. Pattern Anal. Mach. Intell. (TPAMI) **35**, 716–727 (2013)
9. Lin, Z., Ding, G., Hu, M., Wang, J., Ye, X.: Image tag completion via image-specific and tag-specific linear sparse reconstructions. In: IEEE Conference on Computer Vision and Pattern Recognition (CVPR), pp. 1618–1625 (2013)
10. Xu, X., Shimada, A., Taniguchi, R.i.: Tag completion with defective tag assignments via image-tag re-weighting. In: IEEE International Conference on Multimedia and Expo (ICME), pp. 1–6 (2014)
11. Sigurbjörnsson, B., van Zwol, R.: Flickr tag recommendation based on collective knowledge. In: Proceedings of the 17th International Conference on World Wide Web (WWW), pp. 327–336 (2008)
12. Agrawal, R., Gupta, A., Prabhu, Y., Varma, M.: Multi-label learning with millions of labels: recommending advertiser bid phrases for web pages. In: Proceedings of the 22nd International Conference on World Wide Web (WWW), pp. 13–24 (2013)
13. Bucak, S.S., Jin, R., Jain, A.K.: Multi-label learning with incomplete class assignments. In: IEEE Conference on Computer Vision and Pattern Recognition (CVPR), pp. 2801–2808 (2011)
14. Verma, Y., Jawahar, C.V.: Exploring svm for image annotation in presence of confusing labels. In: British Machine Vision Conference (BMVC) (2013)
15. Chen, M., Zheng, A., Weinberger, K.: Fast image tagging. In: Proceedings of the 30th International Conference on Machine Learning (ICML), pp. 1274–1282 (2013)
16. Yu, H.F., Jain, P., Kar, P., Dhillon, I.S.: Large-scale multi-label learning with missing labels. In: Proceedings of the 30th International Conference on Machine Learning (ICML) (2013)
17. Binder, A., Samek, W., Müller, K.R., Kawanabe, M.: Enhanced representation and multi-task learning for image annotation. Comput. Vis. Image Underst. (CVIU) **117**, 466–478 (2013)
18. Dimitrovski, I., Kocev, D., Loskovska, S., Džeroski, S.: Detection of visual concepts and annotation of images using ensembles of trees for hierarchical multi-label classification. In: Ünay, D., Çataltepe, Z., Aksoy, S. (eds.) ICPR 2010. LNCS, vol. 6388, pp. 152–161. Springer, Heidelberg (2010)
19. Lou, X., Hamprecht, F.A.: Structured learning from partial annotations. In: Proceedings of the 29th International Conference on Machine Learning (ICML), pp. 1519–1526 (2012)
20. McAuley, J.J., Ramisa, A., Caetano, T.S.: Optimization of robust loss functions for weakly-labeled image taxonomies. Int. J. Comput. Vis. (IJCV) **104**, 343–361 (2013)

21. Yu, C.N.J., Joachims, T.: Learning structural svms with latent variables. In: Proceedings of the 26th International Conference on Machine Learning (ICML), pp. 1169–1176 (2009)
22. Deng, J., Dong, W., Socher, R., Li, L.J., Li, K., Fei-Fei, L.: Imagenet: a large-scale hierarchical image database. In: IEEE Conference on Computer Vision and Pattern Recognition (CVPR), pp. 248–255 (2009)
23. Van De Sande, K.E., Gevers, T., Snoek, C.G.: Evaluating color descriptors for object and scene recognition. IEEE Trans. Pattern Anal. Mach. Intell. (TPAMI) **32**, 1582–1596 (2010)
24. Shalev-Shwartz, S., Singer, Y., Srebro, N.: Primal estimated sub-gradient solver for SVM. In: Proceedings of the 24th International Conference on Machine Learning (ICML) (2007)
25. Platt, J.C.: Probabilistic outputs for support vector machines and comparisons to regularized likelihood methods. In: Advances in Large Margin Classifiers, pp. 61–74 (1999)
26. Hariharan, B., Zelnik-manor, L., Vishwanathan, S.V.N., Varma, M.: Large scale max-margin multi-label classification with priors. In: Proceedings of the 27th International Conference on Machine Learning (ICML) (2010)

Author Index

Printed in the United States
By Bookmasters

Printed in the United States
By Bookmasters